Ready Reckoner in OBSTETRICS

Ready Reckoner in
OBSTETRICS

Editor

Ruchika Garg

MD MRCOG 1 FICOG FICMCH FIMS FMAS MAMS FIAOG (Gold Medalist)

Professor and Unit Head

Department of Obstetrics and Gynecology

SN Medical College

Agra, Uttar Pradesh, India

Editor in Chief, Journal of Midlife Health

Executive Editor, Journal of SAFOG

Forewords

Gangadhar Sahoo

Muralidhar V Pai

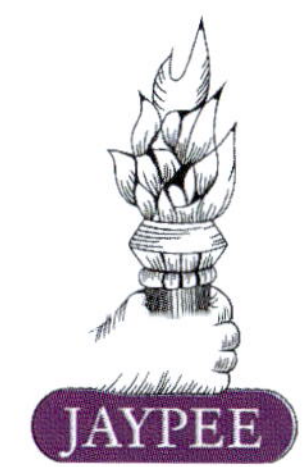

JAYPEE BROTHERS MEDICAL PUBLISHERS

The Health Sciences Publisher

New Delhi | London

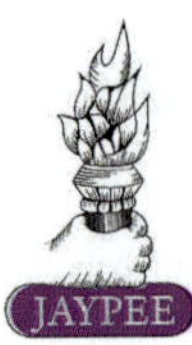

Jaypee Brothers Medical Publishers (P) Ltd.

Headquarters
EMCA House, 23/23-B
Ansari Road, Daryaganj
New Delhi 110 002, India
Landline: +91-11-23272143, +91-11-23272703
+91-11-23282021, +91-11-23245672
e-mail: jaypee@jaypeebrothers.com

Corporate Office
4838/24, Ansari Road, Daryaganj
New Delhi 110 002, India
Phone: +91-11-43574357
Fax: +91-11-43574314
e-mail: jaypee@jaypeebrothers.com

Overseas Office
JP Medical Ltd.
83, Victoria Street, London
SW1H 0HW (UK)
Phone: +44-20 3170 8910
e-mail: info@jpmedpub.com

EU GPSR Authorised Representative
Logos Europe, 9 rue Nicolas Poussin
17000, La Rochelle, France
Phone: +33 (0) 6 67 93 73 78
e-mail: contact@logoseurope.eu

Website: www.jaypeebrothers.com
Website: www.jaypeedigital.com

Inquiries for bulk sales may be solicited at: jaypee@jaypeebrothers.com

Ready Reckoner in Obstetrics

First Edition: **2026**

ISBN: 978-93-7545-908-8

Printed at: Samrat Offset Pvt. Ltd.

Contributors

Aditi Vishal Phulpagar
MBBS DGO MD (Obs & Gyne)
Associate Professor
Department of Obstetrics and Gynecology
Seth GS Medical College and KEM Hospital
Mumbai, Maharashtra, India

Ankita Mathur MBBS MS DNB (Obs & Gyne)
Assistant Professor
Department of Obstetrics and Gynecology
Seth GS Medical College and KEM Hospital
Mumbai, Maharashtra, India

Anurekha MD DNB FRM FICOG
Senior Assistant Professor
Department of Obstetrics and Gynecology
Government Mohan Kumaramangalam
Medical College Hospital (GMKMCH)
Birla ARMC IVF Centre
JP Clinic and Scan Centre
Chennai, Tamil Nadu, India

Anwar PhD in Nursing
Assistant Professor
Department of Maternal and
Child Health Nursing
Tabuk College of Nursing, KSA

Bethesheba Pagolu MBBS DGO MRCOG (UK)
CMO Consultant
Department of Obstetrics and Gynecology
ESIC Medical College and Hospital
Hyderabad, Telangana, India

Geetanjali Sharma MBBS MS
Resident
Department of Gynecology
SN Medical College
Agra, Uttar Pradesh, India

Kalpana Kumari MS (Obs & Gyne)
Professor
Department of Obstetrics and Gynecology
Uttar Pradesh University of Medical Sciences
Etawah, Uttar Pradesh, India

Meera Agalawe MS (Obs & Gyne)
Consultant
Department of Obstetrics and Gynecology
Siddhivinayak Hospital
Bhandara, Maharashtra, India

Neelansha Varshney MBBS MD
Senior Resident, Department of Gynecology
SN Medical College
Agra, Uttar Pradesh, India

Pavika Lal
MBBS (KGMC) MD (AIIMS, ND) DNB FICOG CIMP
Associate Professor
Department of Obstetrics and Gynecology
Ganesh Shankar Vidyarthi Memorial Medical
College
Kanpur, Uttar Pradesh, India

Prabhat Agrawal MBBS MD (Medicine)
Professor, Department of Medicine
SN Medical College
Agra, Uttar Pradesh, India

Pramila D'Souza PhD in Nursing
Assistant Professor
Department of Maternal and
Child Health Nursing
HAIL College of Nursing, Hail, KSA

Preeti Nitsure Deshpande MS MRCOG FICOG
Fellowship Infertility Advanced Endoscopy Training
IRCAD (France)
Consultant Obstetrician and Gynecologist
Fortis SL Raheja Hospital, Guru Nanak Hospital,
KJ Somaiya Multispecialty Hospital, Surya
Hospital (Chembur), and Sambhav—Dr Preeti
Deshpande's Clinic
Mumbai, Maharashtra, India

Rekha Rani MBBS MD
Professor
Department of Gynecology
SN Medical College
Agra, Uttar Pradesh, India

Ruchika Garg MD MRCOG 1 FICOG FICMCH FIMS FMAS MAMS FIAOG (Gold Medalist)
Professor and Unit Head
Department of Obstetrics and Gynecology
SN Medical College
Agra, Uttar Pradesh, India
Editor in Chief, Journal of Midlife Health
Executive Editor, Journal of SAFOG

Savita Somalwar MBBS DGO DNB
Professor
Department of Obstetrics and Gynecology
NKP Salve Institute of Medical Sciences
Nagpur, Maharashtra, India

Shaifali Singh MBBS MS
Resident
Department of Obstetrics and Gynecology
SN Medical College
Agra, Uttar Pradesh, India

Thamizharasi N MSc Nursing PhD Scholar
Assistant Professor
Department of OBG Nursing
Father Muller College of Nursing
Mangaluru, Bengaluru, India

Vandana Bansal MBBS MD DGO DNB FICOG FRCOG (UK) FNB (High Risk Pregnancy and Perinatology)
Additional Professor
Department of Obstetrics and Gynecology and Fetal Medicine
Nowrosjee Wadia Maternity Hospital and Seth GS Medical College, Mumbai
Director
Department of Fetal Medicine
Surya Mother and Child Group of Hospitals
Mumbai, Maharashtra, India

Vandana Verma MD (Obs & Gyne) CIMP FICMCH FICOG
Associate Professor
Department of Obstetrics and Gynecology
All India Institute of Medical Sciences
Raebareli, Uttar Pradesh, India

Foreword

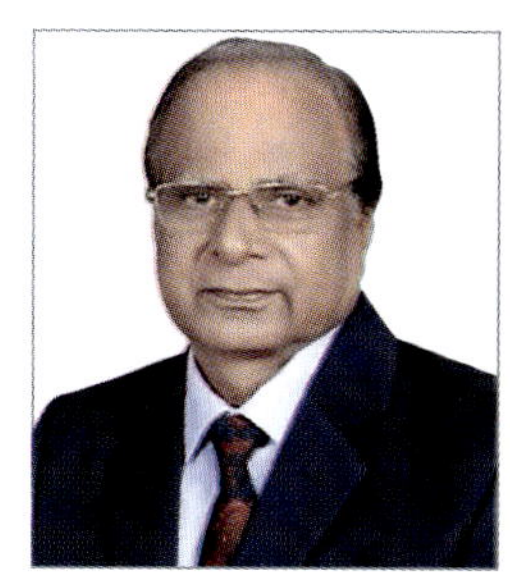

It is with great delight that I pen this foreword for the *Ready Reckoner in Obstetrics.*

Obstetrics remains a dynamic and challenging specialty, demanding a blend of clinical acumen, evidence-based knowledge, and quick decision-making. This book fills a critical gap for postgraduates, MBBS students, FMGE, and aspirants preparing for NEET-PG and FNB-DNB examinations by serving as an indispensable tool for last-minute revision. Packed with algorithms, tables, multiple illustrations, MCQs covering both theory and practical aspects, it distills complex concepts into concise, high-yield formats aligned with the latest evidence-based guidelines from global authorities.

All contributors have vast experience in teaching and clinical practice, which ensures the content is practical, updated, and exam-oriented, empowering learners to navigate high-risk pregnancies, labor management, and obstetric emergencies with confidence. This ready reckoner will undoubtedly prove invaluable in wards, clinics, and examination halls, fostering excellence in obstetric care. Editor *Professor Ruchika Garg* has already contributed many books for medical students which are very popular, and this is going to help students for not only building concepts but also last-minute revisions.

I wholeheartedly recommend it to all aspiring obstetricians.

Gangadhar Sahoo
MD (OBG)
Retired Professor and Head
Department of Obstetrics and Gynecology
VSS Medical College
Burla, Odisha, India
Dean, IMS and SUM Hospital, Bhubaneswar
Pro VC, SOA Deemed to be University, Bhubaneswar
President
Indian Society of Perinatology and
Reproductive Biology (ISOPARB) (2022–2023)

Foreword

It is with immense pleasure that I write this foreword for the *Ready Reckoner in Obstetrics*, expertly.

Obstetrics stands as one of the most dynamic and high-stakes branches of medicine. Rapidly evolving evidence from landmark trials, updated guidelines, and technological advancements demand that practitioners and students alike stay abreast of the latest knowledge.

This book masterfully addresses this need, serving as an essential companion for postgraduate students, MBBS students, FMGE aspirants preparing for NEET-PG, INI-CET, DNB examinations, and busy consultants who want to afresh their knowledge.

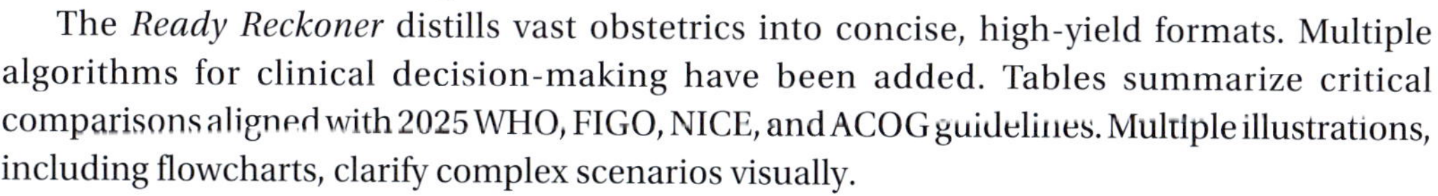

The *Ready Reckoner* distills vast obstetrics into concise, high-yield formats. Multiple algorithms for clinical decision-making have been added. Tables summarize critical comparisons aligned with 2025 WHO, FIGO, NICE, and ACOG guidelines. Multiple illustrations, including flowcharts, clarify complex scenarios visually.

MCQs and high-yield facts tested in recent examinations have been added.

Editor (Professor) Ruchika Garg's meticulous curation ensures practicality to excel in wards, labor rooms, and theory examinations.

Whether tackling antepartum complications, intrapartum challenges, or puerperal issues, this book fosters confidence and competence.

In an era of information overload, it will be very helpful for quick revisions.

I wholeheartedly endorse it for all aspiring obstetricians, and I am confident it will elevate clinical practice and examination success alike.

Warm regards,

Muralidhar V Pai
MD FRCOG FICOG FKCOG FICMCH
Pro Vice Chancellor, Sikkim Manipal University
Dean, Sikkim Manipal Institute of Medical Sciences, Sikkim
Professor of Obstetrics and Gynecology

Preface

There is a constant need for concise, reliable, and exam-oriented resources. This *Ready Reckoner in Obstetrics* has been conceptualized and compiled specifically to meet the needs of postgraduate students, DNB candidates, NEET PG aspirants, undergraduate MBBS students, and Foreign Medical Graduates (FMGs) preparing for licensing examinations.

In the competitive landscape of postgraduate entrance and certification examinations in India, time is a precious commodity. Students often struggle to navigate voluminous textbooks while balancing clinical duties and revision. This book aims to serve as a true "ready reckoner"—a compact, one-stop resource that distills essential concepts, high-yield facts, clinical algorithms, management protocols, and recent guidelines into an easy-to-revise format. Key topics in obstetrics, including antenatal care, intrapartum management, medical disorders in pregnancy, operative obstetrics, and fetal medicine, are presented with clarity, supported by tables, flowcharts, and bullet points for quick recall.

A distinctive feature of this edition is the inclusion of "added MCQs" at the end of each chapter and a dedicated section of image-based and case-based questions. These are patterned on recent NEET-PG, DNB, INI-CET, and FMGE examinations, complete with detailed explanations to reinforce conceptual understanding and improve examination performance. The questions emphasize clinical application, recent updates (such as revised FIGO staging, RCOG/ACOG guidelines, and NRP protocols), and commonly tested pitfalls.

This book draws from standard references, current evidence, and the collective experience of contributors who have mentored countless students through their postgraduate journeys. It is designed not only to help you excel in examinations but also to build a strong foundation for safe clinical practice.

I am grateful to the contributing authors for their expertise and dedication, to the publishers for their meticulous support, and most importantly, to the students whose feedback over the years has shaped this work. I thanks from the core of my heart to Mr Jitendar P Vij (Group Chairman), Mr Ankit Vij (Managing Director), Sabyasachi Hazra (Director—PG and PNR Content), Kritika Dua (Manager—Content Acquisition and Business Development), Ashish Kumar (Senior Business Manager), Aarti Kushwah (Development Editor), and Ruby Sharma (Business Manager) from M/s Jaypee Brothers Medical Publishers (P) Ltd, New Delhi, India, for the whole-hearted support in production.

I hope this ready reckoner becomes your trusted companion in the pursuit of excellence in Obstetrics.

Ruchika Garg
MD MRCOG 1 FICOG FICMCH FIMS FMAS MAMS FIAOG (Gold Medalist)
Professor and Unit Head
Department of Obstetrics and Gynecology
SN Medical College
Agra, Uttar Pradesh, India
Editor in Chief, Journal of Midlife Health
Executive Editor, Journal of SAFOG

Contents

SECTION 1: Labor

1. **Preconception Care** 3
   Ruchika Garg
2. **Physiology of Labor** 10
   Ruchika Garg
3. **Mechanism of Labor** 16
   Ruchika Garg
4. **Third Stage of Labor** 24
   Ruchika Garg
5. **Abnormal Labor** 30
   Ruchika Garg
6. **Labor Analgesia** 36
   Ruchika Garg
7. **Partogram** 43
   Ruchika Garg
8. **Operative Vaginal Delivery Ventouse (Vacuum) and Forceps Delivery** 53
   Bethesheba Pagolu, Preeti Nitsure Deshpande
9. **Retained Placenta** 58
   Ruchika Garg, Neelansha Varshney
10. **Uterine Inversion** 64
    Ruchika Garg
11. **Transverse Lie in Labor** 72
    Ruchika Garg, Neelansha Varshney
12. **Breech Presentation, Occiput Posterior Position, External Cephalic Version, Deep Transverse Arrest, and Cephalopelvic Disproportion** 78
    Ruchika Garg
13. **Vulvar Hematomas** 92
    Ruchika Garg, Neelansha Varshney
14. **Genital Tract Injuries** 98
    Ruchika Garg, Shaifali Singh

15. **Perineal and Cervical Tears in Labor** 106
Ruchika Garg

16. **Episiotomy** 114
Ruchika Garg

17. **Pregnancy with Previous Cesarean Delivery: VBAC and TOLAC** 119
Ruchika Garg

18. **Placenta Accreta Spectrum Disorders** 128
Ruchika Garg

19. **Obstructed Labor** 135
Ruchika Garg

20. **Shoulder Dystocia** 139
Ruchika Garg

21. **Cord Prolapse** 144
Ruchika Garg

22. **Blood Transfusion in Obstetrics** 154
Ruchika Garg

23. **Preterm Labor** 161
Ruchika Garg

24. **Postpartum Collapse** 166
Ruchika Garg

25. **Prolonged Pregnancy and Post-term Pregnancy** 173
Ruchika Garg

26. **Antenatal Care** 183
Ruchika Garg

27. **Clinical Approach to First Trimester Bleeding in Pregnancy** 190
Ruchika Garg

28. **Ectopic Pregnancy** 198
Rekha Rani, Geetanjali Sharma

29. **Cesarean Scar Ectopic Pregnancy and Isthmocele** 206
Ruchika Garg

30. **Gestational Trophoblastic Disease and Neoplasia** 209
Ruchika Garg

31. **Invasive Prenatal Diagnostic Procedures** 221
Ruchika Garg

32. **Medical Termination of Pregnancy** 224
Ruchika Garg

33. **Abortions** 228
Ruchika Garg, Shaifali Singh

34. **Recurrent Pregnancy Loss** 239
Ruchika Garg

35. **Maternal Anatomy and Physiology** 247
Ruchika Garg

36. **Placental Development—Structure and Abnormalities** 253
Ruchika Garg

SECTION 2: Medical Disorders in Pregnancy

37. **Hemoglobinopathies** 267
Ruchika Garg

38. **Gestational Diabetes Mellitus** 272
Ruchika Garg

39. **Hypertensive Disorders in Pregnancy** 296
Ruchika Garg

40. **Epilepsy and Antiepileptic Drugs in Pregnancy** 304
Ruchika Garg

41. **Anemia in Pregnancy** 312
Kalpana Kumari, Vandana Verma

42. **Cardiac Disease in Pregnancy** 323
Ruchika Garg

43. **Liver Disorders in Pregnancy** 330
Ruchika Garg

44. **Thrombocytopenia in Pregnancy** 339
Ruchika Garg

45. **Thyroid Disorders in Pregnancy** 345
Ruchika Garg

46. **Venous Thromboembolism in Pregnancy and Puerperium** 350
Ruchika Garg

47. **Renal Disorders in Pregnancy** 355
Prabhat Agrawal, Pavika Lal

48. Psychiatric Disorders in Pregnancy and Postpartum 359
Ruchika Garg

49. Placenta Accreta Spectrum 363
Ruchika Garg

SECTION 3: High Risk Obstetrics

50. Antepartum Hemorrhage 369
Ruchika Garg

51. Oligohydramnios and Polyhydramnios 374
Ruchika Garg

52. Antepartum Fetal Surveillance 377
Ruchika Garg

53. Intrapartum Fetal Heart Rate Monitoring 387
Ruchika Garg

54. Fetal Growth Restriction 394
Ruchika Garg

55. Induction of Labor 400
Aditi Vishal Phulpagar, Ankita Mathur

56. Shock in Obstetrics 417
Ruchika Garg, Rekha Rani

57. Advanced Maternal Age 438
Ruchika Garg

58. Obesity in Pregnancy 444
Anurekha

59. Preterm Premature Rupture of Membranes 453
Ruchika Garg

60. Rh Alloimmunization 458
Ruchika Garg

61. Maternal Near Miss Mortality 463
Ruchika Garg

62. Imaging in Obstetrics Fetal MRI 468
Vandana Bansal, Meera Agalawe

63. Cesarean Myomectomy 500
Ruchika Garg

64. **Artificial Intelligence in Obstetrics and Gynecology** 506
Ruchika Garg

65. **Government Programs** 512
Ruchika Garg

66. **Vesicovaginal Fistula** 517
Ruchika Garg, Shaifali Singh

67. **Multifetal Pregnancy** 527
Ruchika Garg

68. **Monochorionic Twin Pregnancy** 534
Ruchika Garg

69. **Fetal Monitoring** 542
Ruchika Garg

70. **Abnormal Puerperium** 550
Ruchika Garg

71. **Puerperal Sepsis** 556
Ruchika Garg

72. **Lactation Suppression** 564
Ruchika Garg

73. **Vaccination in Pregnancy** 570
Ruchika Garg

74. **Telemedicine in Gynecology** 578
Ruchika Garg

75. **Magnesium Sulphate in Obstetrics** 583
Ruchika Garg

76. **Postpartum Hemorrhage** 588
Ruchika Garg

77. **Cesarean Section: Indications and Techniques** 598
Ruchika Garg

78. **Strategies to Reduce Cesarean Section Rates** 606
Ruchika Garg

79. **Pregnancy in Scarred Uterus** 612
Ruchika Garg

80. **Difficult Situations in Cesarean Delivery** 616
Ruchika Garg

81. **Amniotic Fluid Embolism** 622
Ruchika Garg

82. **Intrauterine Fetal Death** 628
Ruchika Garg

83. **HIV in Pregnancy** 636
Ruchika Garg

84. **High Dependency Unit in Maternal Health Care** 644
Ruchika Garg

85. **Enhanced Recovery after Surgery** 650
Ruchika Garg

86. **Dengue in Pregnancy** 656
Ruchika Garg

87. **Toxoplasmosis in Pregnancy** 658
Ruchika Garg

88. **Chickenpox in Pregnancy** 664
Ruchika Garg

89. **Malaria in Pregnancy** 670
Ruchika Garg

90. **Cervical Cancer in Pregnancy** 675
Ruchika Garg

91. **Ethics in Obstetrics and Gynecology** 681
Ruchika Garg

92. **Pre-conception and Pre-natal Diagnostic Techniques Act** 690
Ruchika Garg

93. **Breaking Bad News in Obstetrics** 692
Savita Somalwar

SECTION 4: Contraception

94. **Progestogen-only Pills and Depot Medroxyprogesterone Acetate** 701
Ruchika Garg, Neelansha Varshney

95. **Emergency Contraception** 710
Ruchika Garg

96. **Tubal Ligation** 716
Ruchika Garg

97. Why ART Pregnancies are High-Risk? 723
Ruchika Garg

SECTION 5: Practicals

98. Drugs Used in Hypertensive Disorders of Pregnancy....................................725
Ruchika Garg

99. Instruments 735
Pramila D'Souza, Thamizharasi N, Anwar

100. Drugs in Obstetrics 775
Thamizharasi N, Pramila D'Souza, Anwar

Index 827

Labor

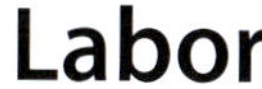

1. **Preconception Care**
Ruchika Garg

2. **Physiology of Labor**
Ruchika Garg

3. **Mechanism of Labor**
Ruchika Garg

4. **Third Stage of Labor**
Ruchika Garg

5. **Abnormal Labor**
Ruchika Garg

6. **Labor Analgesia**
Ruchika Garg

7. **Partogram**
Ruchika Garg

8. **Operative Vaginal Delivery Ventouse (Vacuum) and Forceps Delivery**
Bethesheba Pagolu, Priti Nitsure

9. **Retained Placenta**
Ruchika Garg, Neelansha Varshney

10. **Uterine Inversion**
Ruchika Garg

11. **Transverse Lie in Labor**
Ruchika Garg, Neelansha Varshney

12. **Breech Presentation, Occiput Posterior Position, External Cephalic Version, Deep Transverse Arrest, and Cephalopelvic Disproportion**
Ruchika Garg

13. **Vulvar Hematomas**
Ruchika Garg, Neelansha Varshney

14. **Genital Tract Injuries**
Ruchika Garg, Shaifali Singh

15. **Perineal and Cervical Tears in Labor**
Ruchika Garg

16. **Episiotomy**
Ruchika Garg

17. **Pregnancy with Previous Cesarean Delivery: VBAC and TOLAC**
Ruchika Garg

18. **Placenta Accreta Spectrum Disorders**
Ruchika Garg

19. **Obstructed Labor**
Ruchika Garg

20. **Shoulder Dystocia**
Ruchika Garg

21. **Cord Prolapse**
Ruchika Garg

22. **Blood Transfusion in Obstetrics**
Ruchika Garg

23. **Preterm Labor**
Ruchika Garg

24. **Postpartum Collapse**
Ruchika Garg

25. **Prolonged Pregnancy and Post-term Pregnancy**
Ruchika Garg

26. **Antenatal Care**
Ruchika Garg

27. **Clinical Approach to First Trimester Bleeding in Pregnancy**
Ruchika Garg

28. **Ectopic Pregnancy**
Rekha Rani, Geetanjali Sharma

29. **Cesarean Scar Ectopic Pregnancy and Isthmocele**
Ruchika Garg

30. **Gestational Trophoblastic Disease and Neoplasia**
Ruchika Garg

31. **Invasive Prenatal Diagnostic Procedures**
Ruchika Garg

32. **Medical Termination of Pregnancy**
Ruchika Garg

33. **Abortions**
Ruchika Garg, Shaifali Singh

34. **Recurrent Pregnancy Loss**
Ruchika Garg

35. **Maternal Anatomy and Physiology**
Ruchika Garg

36. **Placental Development—Structure and Abnormalities**
Ruchika Garg

Preconception Care

Ruchika Garg

PRECONCEPTIONAL CARE

- **Impact:** Studies show preconceptional care (PCC) significantly reduces adverse pregnancy outcomes (e.g., maternal morbidity, perinatal mortality, and congenital anomalies).
- **Indian Context:** Two large interventional studies in India demonstrated improved maternal and perinatal outcomes with PCC.
- Optimize conditions before conception to enhance maternal and fetal outcomes through problem identification, education, and intervention.

COMPONENTS OF PRECONCEPTIONAL CARE

Preconceptional care encompasses **Nutritional Interventions**, **Chronic Diseases**, **Infections**, **Genetic Disorders**, **Vaccinations**, and **Psychosocial Issues**, summarized under, and **Intervene**.

1. Nutritional Interventions

1.1 Folic Acid

- Landmark trials (MRC Vitamin Study, Czeizel et al.) confirmed preconceptional folic acid reduces neural tube defects (NTDs).
- Cochrane meta-analysis: No association between folate deficiency and other birth defects (e.g., cleft palate and cardiovascular defects) or miscarriages.
- Limited for folate's role in preventing preeclampsia.
- High plasma folate may impair B12 status; multivitamins may reduce heart defects and urinary tract anomalies.

MTHFR Gene Variation:

- MTHFR gene mutations impair folate processing, leading to hyperhomocysteinemia.
- 5-methyltetrahydrofolate (5-MTHF) is an effective alternative, avoiding B12 deficiency masking and antifolate drug interactions.

Practice Points:

- All women of childbearing age: 0.4–0.5 mg folic acid daily, 3 months preconception to 3 months postconception.
- Moderate NTD risk (e.g., family history and diabetes)**:** 1 mg daily.

- High NTD risk (e.g., previous NTD): 4 mg daily in a multivitamin with 2.6 μg B12.
- 5-MTHF may benefit MTHFR mutation carriers; more research needed.

1.2 Iron Supplementation

- Iron deficiency anemia (IDA) is prevalent in India (58% pregnant women, 50% nonpregnant women, and 56% adolescent girls, as per NFHS-3).
- IDA increases risks of maternal mortality, perinatal mortality, low birth weight (LBW), preterm birth, and low Apgar scores.
- Weekly Iron Folic Acid Supplementation (WIFS) (60 mg iron + 3.5 mg folic acid preconception, 120 mg iron during pregnancy) prevents IDA.

Practice Points:
- All reproductive-age women: Weekly 100 mg elemental iron + 500 μg folic acid.
- Biannual deworming with albendazole 400 mg for helminth control.

1.3 Overweight and Obesity

- Obesity affects >30 million Indians, increasing risks of preeclampsia, gestational diabetes mellitus (GDM), cesarean section, postpartum complications, birth injuries, and neonatal ICU admission.
- Preconceptional weight loss reduces GDM and large-for-gestational-age infants.
- Bariatric surgery improves outcomes in severe obesity.

Practice Points (*see* Table 1):
- BMI 23–24.9 kg/m^2 (overweight); >25 kg/m^2 (obese).
- Risks include GDM, preeclampsia, cesarean, thromboembolism, infections, and intrauterine death. Aim for BMI 18–23 kg/m^2.
- **Intervene:** 5–10% weight loss in 6 months via nutrition and exercise; bariatric surgery for BMI >32.5 kg/m^2 with comorbidities or >37.5 kg/m^2 without. Avoid pregnancy for 12–18 months postsurgery.

1.4 Underweight

BMI <18 kg/m^2 increases risks of preterm birth (OR 1.13), LBW (OR 1.66), and small-for-gestational-age (SGA) infants (OR 1.85).

Practice Points:
- BMI <18 kg/m^2.
- Risks include preterm birth, LBW, and SGA.
- **Intervene:** Nutritional counseling, screen/treat eating disorders (e.g., anorexia and bulimia). Weight gain during pregnancy does not mitigate risks.

2. Chronic Diseases

2.1 Diabetes Mellitus (DM)

- Indian women have an 11-fold higher GDM risk; prevalence 16.5%.

- Pregestational DM increases risks of miscarriage, congenital anomalies, macrosomia, stillbirth, preterm delivery, cesarean, and perinatal death.
- Preconceptional glycemic control improves outcomes.

Practice Points:

- Screen using WHO criteria (FPG ≥ 126 mg/dL, 2-hour PG ≥ 200 mg/dL).
- PGDM risks include miscarriage, anomalies, macrosomia, and stillbirth.
- **Intervene:** Achieve HbA1c <6.5%, fasting glucose 60–100 mg/dL. Use CHC or POP in PGDM without vascular disease (<20 years duration); Cu IUD with caution.

2.2 Thyroid Disorders

- Hypothyroidism prevalence in India: 10.95% (more in females); hyperthyroidism: 0.2%.
- Hypothyroidism increases the risks of gestational hypertension, preeclampsia, postpartum hemorrhage, abortion, preterm delivery, and miscarriage (with TPO antibodies).
- Hyperthyroidism risks include spontaneous abortion, preterm labor, preeclampsia, and stillbirth
- Universal screening's impact on outcomes is unclear.

Practice Points:

- Universal screening desirable; case-finding for symptomatic women, iodine-deficient areas, diabetes, miscarriage history, and obesity (BMI >40 kg/m^2).
- Hypothyroidism risks (maternal and fetal); hyperthyroidism optimization preconception.

Intervene:

- Hypothyroidism: Treat overt (TSH >2.5–3 mIU/L with low FT4 or TSH >10 mIU/L); refer subclinical (TSH 2.5–10 mIU/L, normal FT4) to endocrinologist. Increase levothyroxine by 30% upon pregnancy confirmation.
- Hyperthyroidism: Surgery if conception planned within 2 years; delay conception 6 months post-radioactive iodine. Use PTU in first trimester, methimazole later.

2.3 Heart Disease

- Rheumatic heart disease is common in developing countries (up to 88%); others include congenital heart disease (CHD), arrhythmias, and cardiomyopathy.
- Heart disease increases maternal/neonatal complications (34% vs. 15%), LBW, preterm birth (15%), and neonatal death (11%).

Practice Points:

- Basic clinical cardiac assessment; refer to specialists if needed. Contraindications include severe pulmonary hypertension, ventricular dysfunction, and Marfan syndrome with aortic dilatation >40 mm.
- Risks to mother, fetus, and drug implications (e.g., anticoagulants).
- **Intervene:** Detailed cardiac assessment, medication review, genetic counseling for CHD, and corrective surgery if required.

2.4 Hypertensive Disorders

Preexisting hypertension worsens in pregnancy, increasing risks of preeclampsia, eclampsia, pulmonary edema, cardiovascular events, preterm delivery, growth restriction, and intrauterine death.

Practice Points:

- Screen all women, especially those with prior hypertensive pregnancy, renal disease, autoimmune disorders, or thrombophilias.
- Assess for renal disease, ventricular hypertrophy, and retinopathy in long-term hypertension.
- Target BP: 150/100 mm Hg (uncomplicated); <140/90 mm Hg (target organ damage).
- Avoid ACEIs/ARBs; use progestin-only contraception until optimized.

2.5 Seizure Disorders

Epilepsy affects >10 million in India; antiepileptic drugs (AEDs) are teratogenic, increasing risks of miscarriage, hemorrhage, hypertensive disorders, preterm birth, and growth restriction.

Practice Points:

- **Contraception:** Avoid low-dose hormonal contraceptives with enzyme-inducing AEDs (e.g., carbamazepine and phenytoin).
- **AED Management:** Use lowest effective dose; avoid valproate, carbamazepine in NTD family history. Prefer levetiracetam. Stabilize regimen 6 months preconception; avoid changes postconception.
- **Folic Acid:** 4 mg daily for AED users (especially valproate and carbamazepine).

2.6 Autoimmune Disorders (AID)

Systemic lupus erythematosus (SLE) and rheumatoid arthritis (RA) are common; SLE increases the risks of abortion, preterm delivery, IUGR, and preeclampsia; RA may improve in pregnancy but flare postdelivery.

Practice Points:

- Assess AID status (improvement, worsening, or stable in pregnancy).
- SLE risks (abortion, preterm, IUGR); RA remission in pregnancy, postdelivery flares.
- **Intervene:** Achieve SLE quiescence 6 months preconception; discontinue teratogenic drugs (e.g., methotrexate and leflunomide). Multidisciplinary care.

3. Infections

3.1 Universal Screening

- Prevalence in low-middle-income countries: Treponema pallidum (2.6%), HBV (4.3%), HCV (1.4%); global HIV in women: ~16 million.
- HIV-positive women on ART have low perinatal transmission rates (1% with low viral load); ART reduces transmission in discordant couples.

Practice Points:

- Screen all couples for HIV, HBsAg, and VDRL.
- Risks of HIV transmission to partner/fetus.
- **Intervene:** Initiate/continue ART, use effective contraception until viral load is undetectable. For serodiscordant couples: Home insemination (HIV+ female) or sperm washing/IUI (HIV+ male).

3.2 High-risk Screening

Screen high-risk women for tuberculosis, STIs, toxoplasmosis, and CMV.

4. Genetic Disorders

Prevalence at birth: Chromosomal (0.6%), single-gene (0.56%), multifactorial (2%). India: ~500,000 congenital malformations, 20,000 Down syndrome, and 10,000 thalassemia cases annually.

Practice Points:

- Construct a three-generation family tree, noting consanguinity, hereditary disorders, advanced parental age, teratogen exposure, and recurrent pregnancy loss.
- Explain likelihood (e.g., 25% for autosomal recessive disorders like thalassemia) and impact (e.g., Down syndrome disabilities).
- **Intervene:** Refer to geneticist for counseling; offer prenatal diagnosis (e.g., thalassemia).

5. Vaccinations

5.1 Strongly Advisable

- **Measles, Mumps, and Rubella (MMR):**
  - Risks: Abortion, prematurity, LBW, and birth defects.
  - **Practice Points:** Screen for rubella immunity; vaccinate nonimmune women with MMR. Avoid pregnancy for 3 months postvaccination; accidental vaccination in pregnancy is low-risk.
- **Hepatitis B:**
  - India: 40 million chronic HBV carriers; neonatal transmission 10% (first trimester) to 90% (third trimester).
  - Vaccine efficacy: 95% against perinatal transmission.
  - **Practice Points:** Vaccinate high-risk women (e.g., multiple partners, STD history, and injection drug use).

5.2 Desirable

- **Tetanus, Diphtheria, and Pertussis (Tdap):**
  - Reduces neonatal deaths.
  - **Practice Points:** Administer if no booster in last 2 years; follow pregnancy schedule even if vaccinated preconception.
- **Varicella:**
  - Susceptibility in India: 25.4%; risks include fetal varicella syndrome, and neonatal disease.

- **Practice Points:** Screen for immunity; vaccinate nonimmune with two doses (4 weeks apart). Avoid pregnancy for 3 months.

- **Influenza:**
  - Pregnant women face higher hospitalization, mortality; vaccine 70–90% effective.
  - **Practice Points:** Vaccinate during influenza season for maternal/neonatal protection.
- **HPV:**
  - **Practice Points:** Complete vaccination preconception; defer remaining doses postdelivery if incomplete.

6. Psychosocial Issues and Substance Abuse

- Psychiatric disorders linked to poor obstetric outcomes.
- Smoking increases risks of miscarriage, preterm delivery, LBW, stillbirth, and SIDS .
- Heavy alcohol (>10 g/day) increases LBW, SGA, and preterm birth.
- Illicit drugs (e.g., opiates and cocaine) increase pregnancy complications.

Practice Points (Table 1):

- Screen for depression, anxiety, psychosis, and substance use (alcohol, tobacco, and illicit drugs) via personal/family history and social stressors (e.g., poverty and intimate partner violence).

TABLE 1: Key PCC practice points.

Component	*Key interventions*
Folic acid	0.4–0.5 mg daily (all women); 1 mg (moderate NTD risk); 4 mg (high NTD risk)
Iron	Weekly 100 mg iron + 500 μg folic acid; biannual albendazole 400 mg
Obesity	Aim for BMI 18–23 kg/m^2; 5–10% weight loss; bariatric surgery if BMI >32.5 kg/m^2 with comorbidities
Underweight	Nutritional counseling; treat eating disorders
Diabetes	HbA1c <6.5%; CHC/POP for PGDM without vascular disease
Thyroid	Treat overt hypothyroidism; refer subclinical cases; PTU (first trimester) for hyperthyroidism
Heart disease	Cardiac assessment; genetic counseling; avoid pregnancy in high-risk conditions
Hypertension	Target BP 150/100 mm Hg (uncomplicated); avoid ACEIs/ARBs; use progestin-only contraception
Seizures	Lowest AED dose; prefer levetiracetam; 4 mg folic acid for high-risk AEDs.
Autoimmune disorders	Achieve SLE quiescence; discontinue teratogenic drugs (e.g., methotrexate)
Infections	Screen for HIV, HBsAg, VDRL; ART for HIV; high-risk screening for TB, STIs
Genetic disorders	Family history; genetic counseling; prenatal diagnosis for high-risk couples
Vaccinations	MMR, HBV (high-risk), Tdap, varicella, influenza, HPV; avoid pregnancy 3 months post-MMR/varicella
Psychosocial issues	Screen for mental health/substance abuse; multidisciplinary treatment; cessation programs

- Highlight risks of psychiatric disorders, smoking, alcohol, and drugs on pregnancy outcomes.
- **Intervene:** Offer multidisciplinary treatment for mental health (avoid teratogenic drugs); provide cessation programs for substance abuse.

ADDITIONAL NOTES

- **Holistic Approach:** PCC integrates identification, education, and intervention across multiple domains to optimize pregnancy outcomes.
- **Indian Context:** High prevalence of IDA, obesity, diabetes, and infections necessitates tailored PCC strategies, as supported by Indian studies.
- **Gaps in:** More research needed on MTHF efficacy, universal thyroid screening, and PCC in obesity.
- **Patient Counseling:** Emphasize compliance with interventions (e.g., folic acid, vaccinations) and lifestyle changes (e.g., weight management and smoking cessation).

FOR PRECONCEPTIONAL CARE

- **Impact:** Studies show PCC reduces adverse pregnancy outcomes (e.g., maternal morbidity, perinatal mortality, and congenital anomalies).
- **Indian Context:** Two large interventional studies in India demonstrated improved maternal and perinatal outcomes with PCC.

Guidelines:

- NICE. *Diabetes in Pregnancy: Management from Preconception to the Postnatal Period* (NG3, February 2015, updated August 2020).
- GTG 72**:** *Care of Women with Obesity in Pregnancy*, November 2018.

Physiology of Labor

Ruchika Garg

PHYSIOLOGY OF LABOR

The initiation of human labor results from the release of uterine quiescence, a state maintained throughout pregnancy, rather than an abrupt activation of stimulatory factors. In contrast, preterm labor often stems from pathological triggers such as infection, inflammation, or other disorders that disrupt or override the normal term parturition cascade. This chapter explores the physiological and biochemical processes governing parturition, emphasizing the roles of maternal, fetal, and placental compartments, sex steroids, prostaglandins, and mechanical factors. It integrates clinical evidence to provide a robust understanding of the phases of parturition and their regulation, with key data presented in tables.

OVERVIEW

Despite extensive research, the precise mechanisms initiating human labor remain partially elusive. However, it is well established that the maternal–fetal interface, sex steroids (estrogen and progesterone), prostaglandins, and mechanical factors play critical roles. The uterine smooth muscle adapts to support pregnancy and facilitate fetal expulsion at term. The endometrium transitions into decidua, initially exerting immunosuppressive effects to sustain pregnancy, but at term, it activates inflammatory pathways and withdraws immunosuppression to initiate labor. The cervix maintains competence early in pregnancy, resisting ascending infections, while undergoing matrix remodeling to allow effacement and dilatation at term. The placenta and fetal membranes produce steroid hormones, growth factors, and mediators that maintain pregnancy and trigger parturition. The amnion's tensile strength prevents premature rupture, while the chorion activates uterotonins. Fetal hormonal changes, driven by maturation, further contribute to labor onset.

Sex steroids are pivotal. Unlike other species, humans maintain high levels of both estrogen and progesterone throughout pregnancy, with a "functional progesterone withdrawal" at term, possibly due to altered receptor activity, facilitating labor. Estrogen supports progesterone responsiveness early in pregnancy and promotes uterine contractions and cervical ripening at term. Prostaglandins, synthesized in the amnion, chorion, and decidua, are critical for myometrial activation and cervical remodeling, with their activity modulated by tissue-specific isomerases.

PHASES OF PARTURITION

Human parturition involves a transformation of uterine and cervical functions, divided into four phases **(Table 1)**.

These phases, reflect a coordinated interplay of hormonal, mechanical, and inflammatory signals **(Table 1)**.[1]

Phase 1: Uterine Quiescence and Cervical Softening

Uterus: Throughout most of pregnancy, the uterus accommodates fetal growth while remaining unresponsive to contractile stimuli, a state termed quiescence. Low-intensity Braxton Hicks contractions occur, increasing toward term but not causing cervical dilatation. Quiescence is maintained by inhibitors **(Table 2)**.

Cervix: The cervix softens from a cartilage-like consistency to a more compliant state, resembling the lips, due to extracellular matrix changes. Collagen, the primary structural protein, undergoes reduced cross-linking due to decreased activity of lysyl hydroxylase and lysyl oxidase. Matricellular proteins like thrombospondin 2 and tenascin C, which stabilize collagen, are downregulated, increasing tissue compliance. Stromal and glandular

TABLE 1: Phases of parturition.

Phase	*Description*	*Key processes*
Phase 1: Inhibition	Uterine quiescence and cervical softening	Myometrial relaxation, cervical matrix remodeling
Phase 2: Activation	Myometrial priming for labor	Increased contraction-associated proteins, cervical ripening
Phase 3: Stimulation	Active labor	Uterine contractions, cervical dilatation, fetal expulsion
Phase 4: Involution	Puerperium	Uterine and cervical regression, endometrial regeneration

Source: Adapted from Challis et al.[1]

TABLE 2: Inhibitors of uterine contractility in phase 1.

Inhibitor	*Mechanism*	*Clinical evidence*
Progesterone	Raises myometrial membrane potential, inhibits gap junctions	Prevents preterm labor (Norwitz et al.)[2]
Prostacyclin (PGI2)	Promotes myometrial relaxation	Reduces contractility in vitro (Olson et al.)[3]
Relaxin	Activates collagenases, softens cervix	Enhances cervical compliance (Weiss)[4]
Nitric oxide	Inhibits myometrial contractions	Used in tocolysis trials (Norman et al.)[5]
Calcitonin gene-related peptide	Reduces myometrial excitability	Decreases contractility in animal models (Dong et al.)[6]

Source: Compiled from referenced studies.[2-6]

TABLE 3: Mediators of myometrial priming and cervical ripening.

Mediator	*Role*	*Clinical evidence*
Oxytocin receptors	Increase myometrial sensitivity	10-fold increase at term (Fuchs et al.)[9]
Prostaglandin F receptors	Enhance contractility	Upregulated in labor (Giannoulias et al.)[10]
Connexin-43	Forms gap junctions for synchrony	mRNA elevated at term (Garfield et al.)[11]
Hyaluronan (HA)	Increases cervical compliance	High MW HA rises in ripening (Straach et al.)[12]
Matrix metalloproteinases (MMPs)	Degrade collagen (minor role in humans)	Limited activity in human cervix (Timmons et al.)[13]

Source: Compiled from referenced studies.[9-13]

hypertrophy, along with increased vascularity, further contribute to softening. Women with collagen disorders (e.g., Marfan or Ehlers–Danlos syndromes) have a higher risk of cervical insufficiency, with a prevalence of 5–10% in affected populations.[7]

Phase 2: Myometrial Priming and Cervical Ripening

Phase 2, spanning 6–8 weeks before term, prepares the uterus and cervix for labor. A "functional progesterone withdrawal" occurs without a drop in progesterone levels, likely due to altered progesterone receptor (PR-A/PR-B) expression, enabling myometrial responsiveness to uterotonins.[8] Estrogens, prostaglandins, and peptides also contribute **(Table 3)**.[8]

Myometrial Changes

- **Contraction-Associated Proteins (CAPs):** Oxytocin receptors increase 10-fold, prostaglandin F receptors are upregulated, and connexin-43 enhances gap junctions, enabling electrical synchrony.[9,11]
- **Lower Segment Formation:** Differential expression of oxytocin and prostaglandin receptors between the fundus and lower segment facilitates passive dilatation of the lower segment **(Table 3)**.[10]

Cervical Ripening

- **Endocervical Epithelium:** Proliferation increases gland mass, enhancing antimicrobial mucus production and tissue hydration.[12]
- **Connective Tissue:**
  - **Collagen:** Poorly cross-linked fibrils accumulate, reducing tissue integrity due to decreased matricellular proteins.[13]
  - **Glycosaminoglycans:** High-molecular-weight hyaluronan increases viscoelasticity, while hyaluronidase activity near term produces proinflammatory low-molecular-weight hyaluronan.[12]
  - **Proteoglycans:** Changes in decorin and biglycan disrupt collagen packing, enhancing compliance **(Table 3)**.[12]

TABLE 4: Stages of active labor (Phase 3).

Stage	Description	Key features
First stage	Cervical effacement and dilatation	Regular contractions, "show" (bloody mucus)
Second stage	Fetal expulsion	Strong contractions, voluntary muscle action
Third stage	Placental delivery	Uterine contraction, retroplacental hematoma
Fourth stage	Hemostasis (2 hours postplacenta)	Myometrial contraction, vessel thrombosis

Source: Adapted from Cunningham et al.[15]

TABLE 5: Myometrial contractile mechanisms.

Component	Function	Clinical evidence
Actin-myosin interaction	Drives contraction	Calcium-dependent (Wray)[18]
Gap junctions (connexin-43)	Ensures synchrony	Increased at term (Garfield et al.)[11]
Calcium channels	Facilitate contraction	Activated by oxytocin/PGF2α (Sanborn, 2000)[19]
Progesterone/cAMP	Inhibit contraction	Basis for tocolytics (Norwitz et al.)[2]

Source: Compiled from referenced studies.[2,11,18,19]

- **Inflammatory Role:** Recent evidence suggests inflammation plays a limited role in human cervical ripening, with postpartum inflammation more significant for repair.[14]

Phase 3: Active Labor

Active labor comprises three stages: cervical dilatation, fetal expulsion, and placental delivery, followed by a fourth stage of hemostasis **(Table 4)**.

First Stage: Regular, painful contractions (30–90 seconds, 200+ Montevideo Units) result from hypoxia, nerve compression, and cervical stretching. Ferguson's reflex, triggered by cervical stretch, enhances contractions via oxytocin release.[16] The upper segment thickens, while the lower segment thins, forming a physiological retraction ring **(Table 4)**.[15,16]

Second Stage: Stronger contractions, augmented by voluntary abdominal and diaphragmatic efforts, expel the fetus. Descent follows a hyperbolic curve, faster in multiparas.[17]

Third Stage: Uterine contraction detaches the placenta via retroplacental hematoma formation, with membranes peeled off by traction.[15]

Uterine Muscle Physiology: Myometrial contractions arise from actin-myosin interactions, driven by increased intracellular calcium via oxytocin and PGF2α. Gap junctions, formed by connexin-43, ensure synchrony.[11] Smooth muscle's multidirectional force and greater shortening capacity enhance expulsive efficiency **(Table 5)**.[11,18]

Phase 4: Involution (Puerperium)

Over 4–6 weeks postdelivery, the uterus and cervix regress to their prepregnant state. Oxytocin, released during breastfeeding, promotes involution, while local inflammation resolves, and the endometrium regenerates. The hypothalamic-pituitary-ovarian axis resumes function.[15]

TABLE 6: Fetal contributions to parturition.

Hormone	*Role*	*Clinical evidence*
CRH	Stimulates ACTH/DHEAS	Peaks in third trimester (McLean et al.)[21]
DHEAS	Precursor to estradiol	Drives uterotonic effects (Smith)[20]
Cortisol	Enhances prostaglandins	Upregulates placental CRH (Challis)[1]

Source: Compiled from referenced studies.[1,20,21]

KEY REGULATORY PROCESSES

Fetal Role: The fetal hypothalamic-pituitary-adrenal (HPA) axis activates in Phase 2, increasing corticotropin-releasing hormone (CRH), adrenocorticotropic hormone (ACTH), and dehydroepiandrosterone sulfate (DHEAS). Placental conversion of DHEAS to estradiol stimulates PGF2α, oxytocin receptors, and gap junctions.[20] Fetal cortisol enhances prostaglandin and oxytocin production **(Table 6)**.[20]

Placental Role: The placenta synthesizes estradiol and estriol from fetal DHEAS, promoting uterotonic effects at term. The amnion resists rupture, while the chorion activates uterotonins.[1]

Maternal Role:
- **Oxytocin:** Increases myometrial sensitivity at term, promoting PGF2α release and calcium influx.[9]
- **Prostaglandins:** PGE2 and PGF2α levels rise in amniotic fluid and maternal serum during labor, driving contractions and cervical ripening.[3]
- **CRH:** Placental CRH peaks at delivery, enhancing oxytocin and prostaglandin responses.[21]
- **Mechanical Factors**: Myometrial stretching triggers contractions, amplifying labor progression.[22]

CLINICAL IMPLICATIONS

Understanding parturition physiology informs interventions:
- **Preterm Labor Prevention**: Progesterone, calcium channel blockers, and magnesium sulfate target myometrial quiescence (Norwitz et al.).[2]
- **Labor Induction/Augmentation**: Prostaglandins (e.g., misoprostol) and oxytocin ripen the cervix and stimulate contractions (Hofmeyr et al.).[23]
- **Postpartum Hemorrhage (PPH)**: Oxytocin and prostaglandins promote myometrial contraction to control bleeding (Cunningham et al.).[15]

REFERENCES

1. Challis JRG, Lye SJ, Gibb W, et al. Understanding preterm delivery. Prenat Neonat Med. 2000;5:1-12.
2. Norwitz ER, Romero R, Galan HL. Molecular regulation of parturition. Rev Reprod. 1999;4(1):1-9.
3. Olson DM, et al. Prostaglandins in parturition. Reprod Fertil Dev. 2003;15:317-25.
4. Weiss G. Relaxin in pregnancy. Clin Obstet Gynecol. 2000;43:1-10.
5. Norman JE, et al. Nitric oxide in parturition. Br J Obstet Gynaecol. 1998;105:736-741.
6. Dong YL, et al. CGRP in pregnancy. Peptides. 2003;24:1631-7.

7. Anum EA, et al. Connective tissue disorders and preterm birth. Am J Obstet Gynecol. 2009;201: 367.e1-9.
8. Mesiano S, et al. Progesterone withdrawal in human parturition. J Clin Endocrinol Metab. 2002;87:2425-30.
9. Fuchs AR, Fuchs F, Husslein P, et al. Oxytocin receptors in human parturition. Am J Obstet Gynecol. 1984;150(6):734-41.
10. Giannoulias D, et al. Prostaglandin receptors in labor. Biol Reprod. 2005;72:1051-8.
11. Garfield RE, et al. Gap junctions in myometrium. Semin Perinatol. 1998;22:16-25.
12. Straach KJ, et al. Hyaluronan in cervical ripening. Biol Reprod. 2005;72:1390-6.
13. Timmons B, et al. Cervical remodeling in term and preterm birth. Reprod Sci. 2010;17:101-12.
14. Word RA, Li XH, Hnat M, et al. Dynamics of cervical remodeling during pregnancy and parturition: mechanisms and current concepts. Semin Reprod Med. 2017;25:69-79.
15. Cunningham FG, Spong CY, Leveno K, et al. (Eds). Williams Obstetrics, 23rd edition. McGraw-Hill; 2010.
16. Caldeyro-Barcia R. Uterine contractility in labor. Am J Obstet Gynecol. 1959;77:1038-53.
17. Friedman EA. Labor curve analysis. Obstet Gynecol. 1955;5:567-73.
18. Wray S. Uterine contraction physiology. Exp Physiol. 1993;78:153-70.
19. Sanborn BM. Calcium signaling in myometrium. Semin Perinatol. 2000;24:18-24.
20. Smith R. Parturition mechanisms. N Engl J Med. 2007;356:271-83.
21. McLean M, et al. CRH in human pregnancy. Nat Med. 1995;1:460-3.
22. Ferguson JKW. Cervical stretch reflex. Surg Gynecol Obstet. 1941;73:359-66.
23. Hofmeyr GJ, Gülmezoglu AM, Pileggi C. Vaginal misoprostol for cervical ripening and induction of labour. Cochrane Database Syst Rev. 2010;(10):CD000941.

Mechanism of Labor

Ruchika Garg

NORMAL LABOR PROGRESSION

Definition of Normal Labor

Normal labor is a physiologic process where a viable fetus, along with membranes and placenta, is expelled from the uterus through the vaginal canal. It is characterized by:

- **Spontaneous onset** at term (37–42 weeks)
- **Vertex presentation** (singleton)
- **No undue prolongation**
- **Natural termination** with minimal intervention
- **No complications** to mother or fetus

A study at Parkland Hospital found only ~50% of labors met these criteria, with deviations classified as **dystocia** or abnormal labor.

Mechanism of Labor

The **mechanism of labor** involves positional changes of the presenting part to navigate the pelvic canal, driven by interactions among three components: **Power**, **Passage**, and **Passenger**.

1. Power

- **Uterine contractions:** 3–5 contractions per 10 minutes, lasting 40–45 seconds, with adequate relaxation. Measured in **Montevideo Units (MVU)**, adequate contractions yield 200–250 MVU.
- **Maternal efforts:** Voluntary contractions of abdominal muscles and diaphragm propel the fetus forward.

2. Passage

The **bony pelvis** (two innominate bones, sacrum, coccyx) is divided into the false and true pelvis by the linea terminalis. The true pelvis has four key planes **(Table 1)**.

The pelvis transitions from a transverse oval inlet to a near-circular midcavity and an anteroposterior oval outlet, requiring fetal rotation to align with available space **(Fig. 1)**. The **gynecoid pelvis** (50% of women) is most conducive to vaginal delivery.

3. Passenger

The **fetal skull**, typically the presenting part, is an ovoid with a larger anteroposterior diameter.

TABLE 1: Planes of the pelvis.

Plane	*Boundaries*	*Clinical significance*
Inlet	Sacral promontory, linea terminalis, pubic rami, symphysis pubis	Fetal head engagement (biparietal diameter crosses inlet)
Greatest Dimensions	Junction of S2–S3 vertebrae	Minimal clinical significance
Least Dimensions (Midpelvis)	Subpubic arch, ischial spines, S4–S5 junction (~10 cm transverse)	Station of head; most likely site for arrest of descent
Outlet	Subpubic angle, ischial tuberosities, sacrotuberous ligaments, sacrum/coccyx	Rarely obstructs vaginal delivery

Source: Adapted from Cunningham et al.[1]

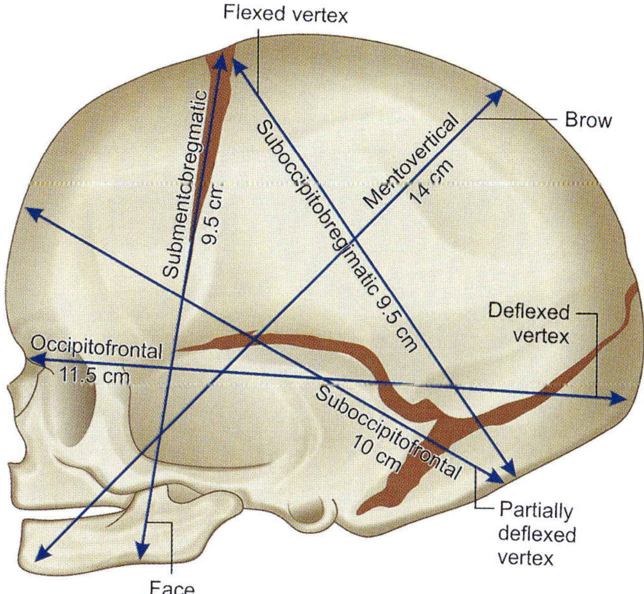

Fig. 1: Fetal skull landmarks and diameters.

Key features:

- **Cranium:** Comprises occipital, temporal, parietal, and frontal bones, joined by sutures (sagittal, coronal, lambdoidal, and frontal).
- **Sutures and fontanels:** Allow **molding** (overlapping under pressure) to overcome mild cephalopelvic disproportion.
- **Presenting diameter:** In vertex presentation, the **suboccipito-bregmatic diameter** (9.5 cm) is optimal **(Fig. 2)**.

Fetopelvic Relationships

Key relationships assessed at labor onset include:

- **Lie:** Longitudinal (parallel axes), transverse (perpendicular), or oblique (45° angle, often converts).
- **Presentation:** Part of the fetus over the pelvic inlet **(Table 2)**.

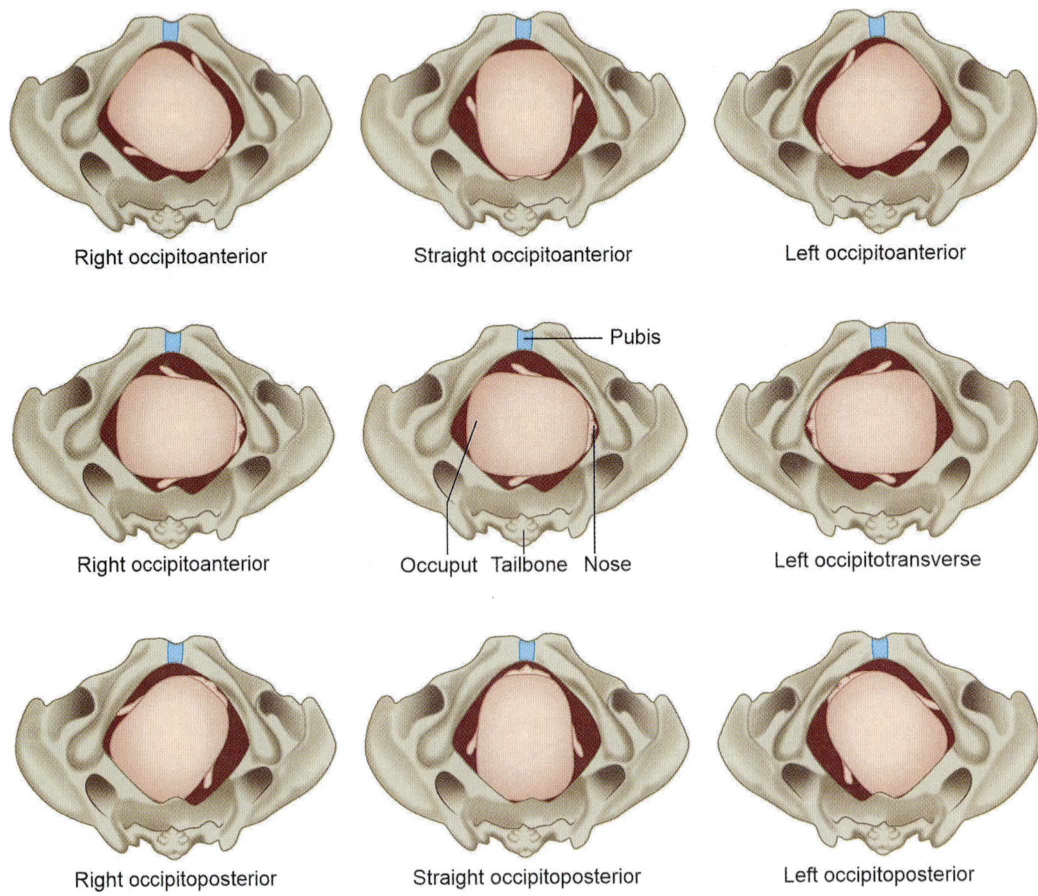

Fig. 2: Fetopelvic relationships.

TABLE 2: Fetal presentations and incidence.

Presentation	*Description*	*Incidence*
Cephalic	Head overlies pelvic inlet	~95% at term
Breech	Podalic pole overlies inlet	2–3% at term (25% at 28 weeks)
Shoulder	Shoulder overlies inlet (transverse lie)	<1%

Source: Data from Cunningham et al.[1]

- **Attitude:** Fetal flexion (spine convex, head flexed, and limbs crossed) optimizes space.
- **Position:** Relationship of the fetal presenting part's denominator (e.g., occiput in vertex) to maternal pelvic quadrants [e.g., left occipitoanterior (LOA), occipitoposterior (OP)]

DIAGNOSIS OF FETAL PRESENTATION AND POSITION

- **Abdominal Palpation (Leopold's Maneuvers):**
  - **First maneuver:** Identifies breech in the fundus.
  - **Second maneuver:** Locates fetal back and small parts.

- Third maneuver: Confirms head at the pelvic inlet.
- Fourth maneuver: Assesses engagement and flexion.

- **Vaginal Examination:** Identifies sutures/fontanels, station (relative to ischial spines), and cervical dilatation/effacement.
- **Ultrasonography (USG):** Enhances accuracy in obese patients or rigid abdominal walls; used to assess lie, back position, and labor progress.

CARDINAL MOVEMENTS OF LABOR

The fetus undergoes sequential movements with temporal overlap **(Fig. 3)**.

- **Engagement:** Biparietal diameter crosses the pelvic inlet, often in transverse/oblique diameter. **Asynclitism** (anterior/posterior) aids descent but severe cases may cause cephalopelvic disproportion.

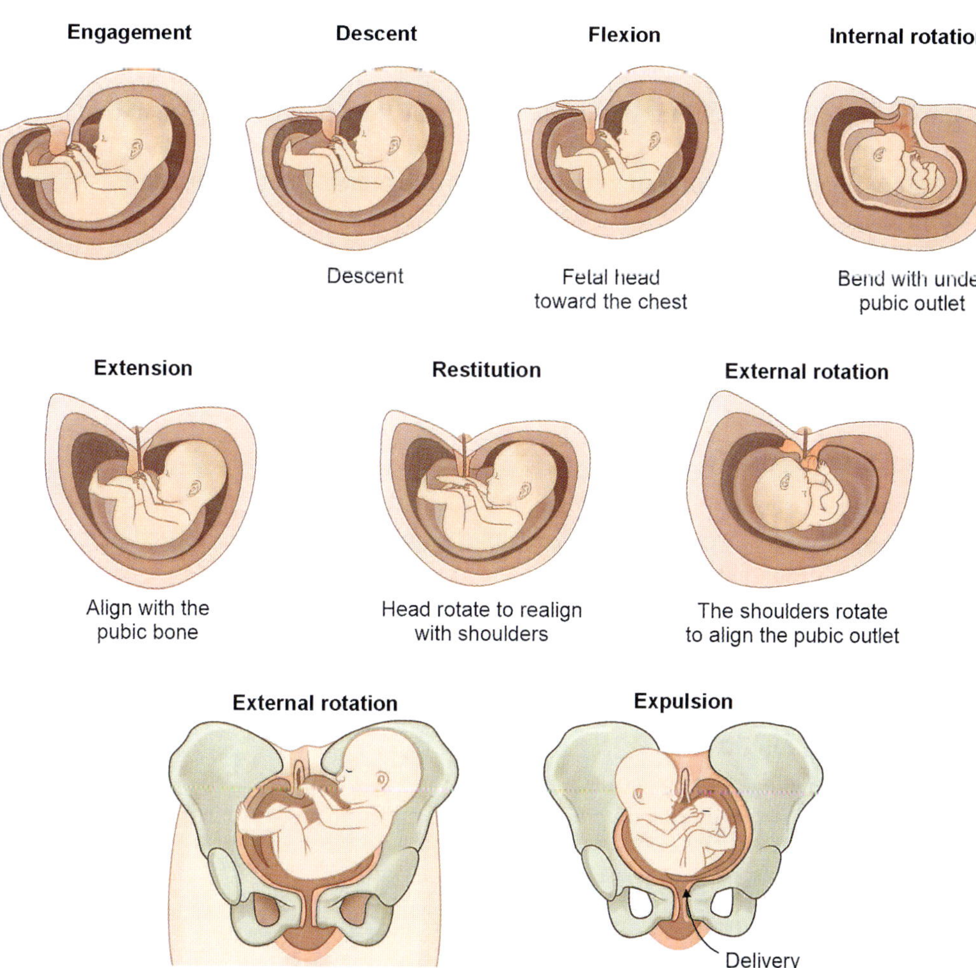

Fig. 3: Cardinal movements of labor.

TABLE 3: Second stage duration.

Parity	*Epidural*	*Median Duration*	*95th Percentile*
Nullipara	No	0.6 hours	2.8 hours
Nullipara	Yes	1.1 hours	3.6 hours
Multipara	No	0.2 hours	1.3 hours
Multipara	Yes	0.4 hours	2.0 hours

Source: Zhang et al.[2]

TABLE 4: Comparison of friedman versus contemporary labor progression.

Parameter	*Friedman (1950s)*	*Zhang et al. (2018)*
Active Phase Onset	3–5 cm	6 cm
Dilatation Rate	1.2–1.5 cm/h	1–2 cm/h (after 6 cm)
Deceleration Phase	Present	Absent

Source: Adapted from Zhang et al.[2]

- **Descent:** Driven by uterine contractions, amniotic fluid pressure, and maternal bearing-down efforts.
- **Flexion:** Head flexes to present the suboccipito-bregmatic diameter (9.5 cm).
- **Internal Rotation:** Occiput rotates 45° (e.g., LOA to OA) to align with the anteroposterior outlet, guided by pelvic floor resistance.
- **Extension:** Head extends under the pubic arch, delivering via the vulvar opening.
- **Restitution:** Neck untwists, aligning head with shoulders.
- **External Rotation:** Shoulders rotate to anteroposterior, aligning occiput laterally.
- **Expulsion:** Anterior shoulder delivers, followed by posterior shoulder and trunk.

STAGES OF LABOR

- **First Stage:** Onset to full cervical dilatation (10 cm).
  - **Latent Phase:** Slow cervical change (up to 6 cm), variable duration (nulliparas: ≤18–20 hours; multiparas: ≤12–14 hours).
  - **Active Phase:** Rapid dilatation (6–10 cm, ~1–2 cm/h).
- **Second Stage:** Full dilatation to fetal delivery.
  - **Propulsive Phase:** Head descends to pelvic floor.
  - **Expulsive Phase:** Bearing-down efforts aid delivery.
  - **Duration (Table 3)**
- **Third Stage:** Delivery of placenta.
- **Fourth Stage:** 1–2 hours postdelivery; critical for monitoring complications.

NORMAL LABOR PROGRESSION (TABLE 4)

Historical Context (Friedman's Curve, 1950s)

- Defined normal progression as 1.2 cm/h (nulliparas) and 1.5 cm/h (multiparas).
- Partograph: Sigmoid curve with alert/action lines for intervention.

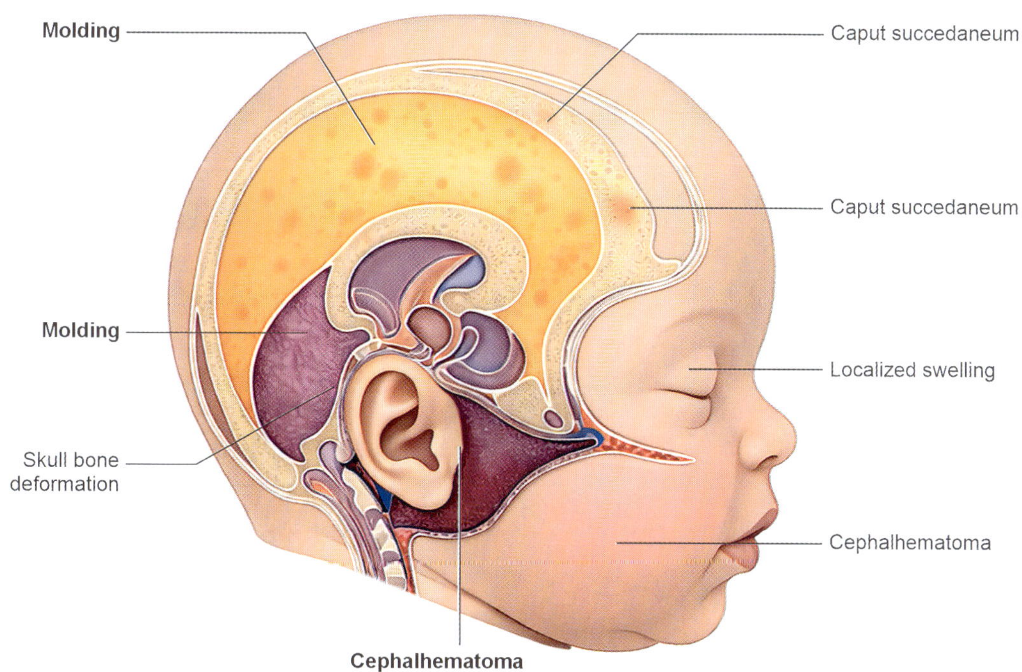

Fig. 4: Molding, caput succedaneum, and cephalhematoma.

Contemporary Evidence[2]

- Active phase begins at **6 cm** dilatation, with slower progression (≤1–2 cm/h) before 6 cm.
- Nulliparas may take >6 hours to dilate from 4–5 cm and >3 hours from 5–6 cm.
- No deceleration phase observed.
- 95th percentiles of labor duration in nulliparas (staircase plot).[3]

WHO Labor Care Guide (2020)[4]

- Replaces traditional partograph with flexible monitoring.
- Focuses on maternal/fetal well-being, hydration, ambulation, and companion support.
- Avoids rigid 1 cm/h rule, reducing unnecessary interventions.

Fetal Head Shape Changes (Fig. 4)

- **Molding:** Compression shortens suboccipito-bregmatic diameter, lengthening verticomental diameter. Resolves within 1 week.
- **Caput Succedaneum:** Scalp edema over the presenting part, resolves in days.
- **Cephalhematoma:** Subperiosteal hemorrhage, resolves in 6–12 weeks, does not cross sutures.

Intrapartum Ultrasonography (USG)

Transperineal USG improves accuracy in assessing fetal head descent and rotation, especially in prolonged second stage (ISUOG, 2021, Level 2+, Grade B)[5] **(Fig. 5)**.

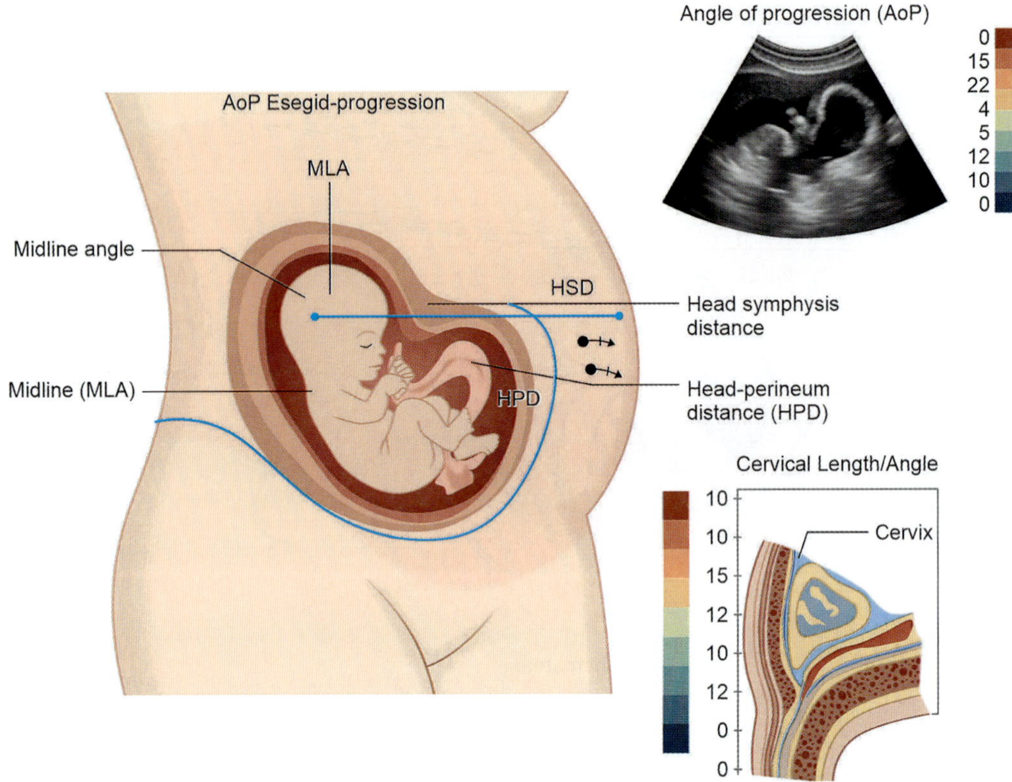

Fig. 5: USG parameters in labor.

Key Parameters

- **Angle of Progression (AoP):** Angle between pubic bone and fetal head; larger AoP predicts shorter delivery time.
- **Midline Angle (MLA):** Angle of fetal head midline to maternal pelvis; larger MLA predicts faster delivery.
- **Head-Symphysis Distance (HSD):** Smaller HSD correlates with vaginal delivery.
- **Head-Perineum Distance (HPD):** HPD ≤ 40 mm predicts vaginal delivery.[6]
- **Cervical Length/Angle:** Cervical length <25 mm and angle >90° predict vaginal delivery.

MANAGEMENT OF NORMAL LABOR

Admission Criteria

- **Contractions:** Regular, painful, ≥30 seconds, every 6 minutes or less.
- **Signs:** Bloody show, membrane rupture, cervical effacement/dilatation.
- **False Labor:** Observe for several hours; discharge if labor does not progress.

Initial Assessment

- **Maternal:** Blood pressure, heart rate, temperature, weight, edema, urine for protein/glucose, CBC, blood typing, antibody screening, and HIV/hepatitis B/syphilis/GBS screening.

- **Fetal:** Leopold's maneuvers, fetal heart sounds, and contraction frequency/duration.
- **Cervical Status:** Dilatation (cm), effacement (%), and station (cm relative to ischial spines).

Labor Suite Management

- **Hydration:** IV Ringer's lactate (500–1,000 mL) to prevent dehydration and support anesthesia if needed.
- **Oral Intake:** Clear liquids if instrumental/cesarean delivery unlikely.
- **Avoid Routine Practices:** No vulvar shaving[7] or enemas[8] to reduce infection risk.
- **Amniotomy:** Selective use to accelerate labor or monitor fetal well-being; contraindicated in HIV/hepatitis B/C.
- **Mobility:** Standing/walking shortens first stage by >1 hour and reduces cesarean rates.[9]

Occipitoposterior (OP) Position

- Occurs in ~20% of labors, more common with narrow fore pelvis or anterior placenta.
- Requires 135° rotation (e.g., ROP to OA) versus 45° in LOA.
- 5–10% result in **persistent OP** or **deep transverse arrest**, indicating dystocia.

RECENT ADVANCES AND GUIDELINES

- **WHO Labor Care Guide (2020):**[4] Emphasizes individualized care, reducing unnecessary interventions.
- **Intrapartum USG (ISUOG, 2021):**[5] Recommended for prolonged second stage to assess fetal head position/descent.
- **Visual Biofeedback:** Real-time USG improves maternal bearing-down efforts.[10]

REFERENCES

1. Cunningham FG, Leveno KJ, Dashe JS, et al. (Eds). Williams Obstetrics, 26th edition. McGraw-Hill; 2021.
2. Zhang J, et al. Contemporary labor patterns: The Consortium on Safe Labor. Am J Obstet Gynecol. 2018;218(2):S692–S699.
3. Lundborg L, et al. Labour progression study (LaPS): Comparison of WHO and Zhang partograms. Acta Obstet Gynecol Scand. 2020;99(11):1493–1500.
4. World Health Organization. (2020). WHO Labor Care Guide. [online] Available from https://www.who.int/publications/b/56119 [Last accessed December, 2025].
5. International Society of Ultrasound in Obstetrics and Gynecology (ISUOG). Intrapartum ultrasound guidelines. Ultrasound Obstet Gynecol. 2021;58(5):645-53.
6. Eggebo TM, et al. Head-perineum distance predicts vaginal delivery. Ultrasound Obstet Gynecol. 2019;54(2):247–253.
7. Basevi V, et al. Perineal shaving in labour. Cochrane Database Syst Rev. 2018;4:CD006066.
8. Reveiz L, Gaitán HG, Cuervo LG. Enemas during labour. Cochrane Database Syst Rev. 2013;2013(7):CD000330.
9. Albers LL, et al. Mobility in labor: Impact on cesarean rates. Birth. 2020;47(3):231-8.
10. Bellussi F, et al. Visual biofeedback in labor: Impact on maternal effort. J Matern Fetal Neonatal Med. 2022;35(5):890-7.

Third Stage of Labor

Ruchika Garg

DEFINITION

The third stage of labor spans from the delivery of the fetus to the complete expulsion of the placenta and membranes. It typically lasts **5–15 minutes** but can extend up to 30 minutes without intervention.[1] While often uneventful, it carries risks of significant complications, including **postpartum hemorrhage (PPH)**, **retained placenta**, and **uterine inversion**, with PPH being a leading cause of maternal mortality globally (10–20% of maternal deaths).[2]

KEY POINTS

- Third stage duration: 5–15 minutes (median ~6–8 minutes with active management).
- Active management of the third stage (AMTSL) significantly reduces PPH risk.
- Oxytocin is the preferred uterotonic for PPH prevention.
- Controlled cord traction (CCT) is optional but shortens the third stage.
- Physiological management is suitable for low-risk women with informed consent.

PHYSIOLOGY OF PLACENTAL DELIVERY

Placental separation occurs via two mechanisms:

- **Myometrial Retraction:** Postdelivery, uterine volume decreases due to myometrial retraction, a unique property where muscle fibers maintain a shortened length after contraction. This thickens the myometrium, reduces the placental bed surface area, and detaches the noncontractile placenta, propelling it into the lower uterine segment.[1,3]
- **Hematoma Formation:** Uterine contractions cause venous occlusion and vascular rupture in the placental bed, forming a retroplacental clot that aids separation.[3]

Signs of Placental Separation (within 1–5 minutes postdelivery):

- **Umbilical cord lengthening:** Most reliable sign; a clamp near the perineum aids detection.
- **Uterine shape change:** Becomes globular and firmer as the placenta descends.
- **Gush of blood:** Retroplacental clot escapes after separation.
- **Uterine rise:** Placenta in the lower segment/vagina displaces the uterus upward.

Caution: Forcing expression before separation risks **uterine inversion**. Controlled cord traction (CCT) should only be performed post-separation.[4]

Delivery Mechanisms:

- **Schultze Method** (80% of cases): Placenta delivers as an inverted umbrella, with the glistening fetal surface first.
- **Duncan Method** (20% of cases): Rough maternal surface delivers first, with membranes trailing.

MANAGEMENT OF THE THIRD STAGE

The third stage can be managed via **physiological (expectant)** or **active** approaches, with AMTSL being the standard to reduce PPH risk.[5]

1. Physiological Management

- **Definition**: Awaits spontaneous placental separation, relying on maternal effort, gravity, or nipple stimulation (oxytocin release).[5]
- **Components** (NICE, 2017):[6]
  - No routine uterotonics.
  - Cord clamping delayed until pulsation ceases.
  - Placenta delivered by maternal effort.
- **Suitability:** Low-risk women, informed of higher PPH risk **(Table 1)**.

2. Active Management of the Third Stage

- **Components** (WHO, 2018):[5]
  - **Uterotonic administration:** Oxytocin (10 IU IM/IV) immediately postdelivery.
  - **Controlled Cord Traction:** Brandt-Andrews maneuver postseparation signs to deliver placenta, reducing manual removal risk.
  - **Uterine massage:** Postplacental delivery to maintain tone (optional, as evidence is weak).[7]
- **Benefits:** Reduces PPH incidence (by ~60%), blood loss (>1,000 mL), and need for transfusion.[6]
- **CCT Technique (Brandt-Andrews):**
  - One hand secures the uterine fundus abdominally to prevent inversion.
  - Steady cord traction with the other hand until placenta passes the introitus.
  - Lift placenta by cord; tease membranes gently to avoid retention.
- **Crede Maneuver:** Avoided due to risk of uterine inversion and membrane tearing.[4]

TABLE 1: Risks of physiological versus active management.[6]

Outcome	*Physiological management*	*Active management*
Nausea/Vomiting	5% (1/20)	10% (1/10)
Blood Loss >1,000 mL	2.9% (29/1,000)	1.3% (13/1,000)
Blood Transfusion	4% (40/1,000)	1.4% (14/1,000)

TABLE 2: Uterotonic drugs for third stage management.[5,6,8,9]

Agent	*Dose/Route*	*Side effects*	*Contraindications*	*Comments*
Oxytocin	10 IU IM/IV; 10–40 IU in 500–1,000 mL saline (infusion)	Few	None	Preferred; requires cold storage, light protection
Ergometrine	250–500 µg IM/IV	Nausea, vomiting, and hypertension	Hypertension, cardiac disease, and migraine	Effective but less safe than oxytocin
Syntometrine	5 IU oxytocin + 0.5 mg ergometrine IM	Nausea, vomiting, and hypertension	Hypertension, cardiac disease, and migraine	Combines oxytocin and ergometrine effects
Carbetocin	100 µg IV	Few	None	Long-acting; used in cesarean sections
Carboprost	250 µg IM (repeat every 15 minutes, maximum 2 mg)	Bronchospasm	Asthma	Effective in high-risk cases; myometrial injection possible
Misoprostol	600 µg PO (prophylaxis); 800 µg sublingual (PPH treatment)	Shivering, pyrexia	None	Heat-stable, ideal for low-resource settings
Tranexamic Acid	1 g IV over 5 minutes	Nausea, vomiting	Thrombotic risk	Reduces PPH incidence; adjunct to uterotonics

UTEROTONIC AGENTS

Uterotonics are critical for PPH prevention. Oxytocin is the first-line agent due to efficacy and safety[5,8] **(Table 2)**.

Key Uterotonic Insights

- **Oxytocin:**
  - Onset: ~1 minute (IV), 3–5 minutes (IM); half-life: 3–5 minutes.
  - Preferred for PPH prevention/treatment; intraumbilical vein injection (10 IU in 20 mL saline) may shorten third stage but is not routinely recommended.[6,10]
  - Sublingual fast-dissolving oxytocin tablets show promise but may cause transient ST depression/hypotension.[11]
- **Ergot Alkaloids (Ergometrine/Methylergometrine):** Effective within 1–5 minutes; contraindicated in hypertensive disorders due to vasoconstriction.[12]
- **Syntometrine:** Combines oxytocin and ergometrine; similar contraindications.[13]
- **Carbetocin:** Long-acting oxytocin analog; reduces additional uterotonic need in cesarean sections.[14]
- **Carboprost:** Prostaglandin F2α analog; effective for high-risk cases, especially cesarean delivery.[15]

TABLE 3: Complications of the third stage.[2,19,20]

Complication	*Prevalence*	*Risk factors*	*Management*
PPH	6% (>500 mL); 1–2% (>1,000 mL)	Uterine atony, retained placenta, and trauma	Uterotonics, bimanual compression, and surgery
Retained Placenta	2.7%	Prolonged third stage, uterine anomalies	Manual removal, uterotonics
Uterine Inversion	0.05% (1:2,000)	Premature cord traction, fundal pressure	Manual repositioning, anesthesia

- **Misoprostol:** Heat-stable, ideal for low-resource settings; sublingual route preferred for PPH treatment due to lower side effects.[9,16]
- **Tranexamic Acid:** Antifibrinolytic; reduces PPH incidence by ~40% when used prophylactically (RR: 0.61; 95% CI: 0.41–0.91).[17]

COMPLICATIONS OF THE THIRD STAGE (TABLE 3)

- **Postpartum Hemorrhage (PPH):**
  - Prevalence: ~6% globally (blood loss >500 mL); severe PPH (>1,000 mL) in ~1–2%.[2]
  - Risk factors: Uterine atony (70% of cases), retained placenta, trauma, and coagulopathy.[18]
- **Retained Placenta:**
  - Incidence: ~2.7% in vaginal deliveries; risk increases with prolonged third stage (>30 minutes).[19]
  - Management: Manual removal under anesthesia if not expelled within 30–60 minutes.[6]
- **Uterine Inversion:**
  - Rare (~1:2,000 deliveries); often due to premature cord traction.[20]
  - Management: Immediate manual repositioning, uterotonics, and anesthesia.[6]

RECENT ADVANCES AND GUIDELINES

- **WHO Recommendations (2018):**[5]
  - AMTSL is the standard for PPH prevention in all births.
  - Oxytocin (10 IU IM/IV) is the first-line uterotonic; misoprostol (600 μg PO) for settings without skilled attendants.
  - CCT is optional but reduces third stage duration by ~6 minutes.
  - Sustained uterine massage is not recommended for PPH prevention if oxytocin is used.
  - Postpartum uterine tone assessment is critical for early detection of atony.
- **NICE Guidelines (2017):**[6]
  - Delayed cord clamping (1–5 minutes) reduces neonatal anemia without increasing PPH risk.
  - CCT only after oxytocin and separation signs.
  - Low-risk women may opt for physiological management after counseling.
- **Tranexamic Acid:** Prophylactic use reduces PPH incidence and blood loss (meta-analysis, 2020).[17]

- **Intrapartum USG:** Dynamic imaging can assess placental separation (e.g., retroplacental myometrial thickness), though not routine.[21]

KEY POINTS FOR POSTGRADUATE EDUCATION

- AMTSL reduces PPH risk by ~60% compared to physiological management.
- Oxytocin (10 IU IM/IV) is the gold standard for PPH prevention.
- CCT shortens the third stage but is optional; Brandt-Andrews is preferred over Crede.
- Delayed cord clamping (1–5 minutes) is recommended for term/preterm infants.
- Misoprostol is a viable alternative in low-resource settings.
- Tranexamic acid is an effective adjunct for PPH prevention/treatment.
- Uterine tone assessment is essential to detect atony early.
- Physiological management is acceptable for low-risk women with informed consent.
- Complications (PPH, retained placenta, and uterine inversion) require prompt recognition and management.
- Intraumbilical oxytocin is not routinely recommended due to limited efficacy.[10]

REFERENCES

1. World Health Organization. WHO recommendations: Intrapartum care for a positive childbirth experience. Geneva: WHO; 2018.
2. Say L, Chou D, Gemmill A, et al. Global causes of maternal death: A WHO systematic analysis. Lancet Glob Health. 2014;2(6):e323-33.
3. Cunningham FG, Leveno KJ, Dashe JS, et al. (Eds). Williams Obstetrics, 26th edition. McGraw-Hill; 2021.
4. Güngördük K, Olgaç Y, Gülseren V, et al. Active management of the third stage of labor: A brief overview of key issues. Turk J Obstet Gynecol. 2018;15(3):188-92.
5. World Health Organization. WHO recommendations for the prevention and treatment of postpartum hemorrhage. Geneva: WHO; 2018.
6. National Institute for Health and Care Excellence. Intrapartum care for healthy women and babies (CG190). London: NICE; 2017.
7. Hofmeyr GJ, et al. Postpartum uterine massage for preventing postpartum haemorrhage. Cochrane Database Syst Rev. 2015;8:CD009292.
8. Awoleke JO, Adeyanju BT, Adeniyi A, et al. Randomised Controlled Trial of Sublingual and Rectal Misoprostol in the Prevention of Primary Postpartum Haemorrhage in a Resource-Limited Community. J Obstet Gynaecol India. 2020;70(6):462-70.
9. Tunçalp Ö, Souza JP, Gülmezoglu M; World Health Organization. New WHO recommendations on prevention and treatment of postpartum hemorrhage. Int J Gynaecol Obstet. 2013;123(3):254-6.
10. Güngördük K, et al. Intraumbilical vein oxytocin in active management of the third stage of labor. Obstet Gynecol. 2018;132(3):619-24.
11. Zhu C, et al. Heat-stable sublingual oxytocin tablets as a potential needle-free approach for preventing postpartum hemorrhage in low-resource settings. Drug Deliv Transl Res. 2018;8(3):853-6.
12. Liabsuetrakul T, Choobun T, Peeyananjarassri K, et al. Prophylactic use of ergot alkaloids in the third stage of labour. Cochrane Database Syst Rev. 2018;6:CD005456.
13. McDonald S, Abbott JM, Higgins SP. Prophylactic ergometrine-oxytocin versus oxytocin for the third stage of labour. Cochrane Database Syst Rev. 2004;2004(1):CD000201.
14. Gallos ID, et al. Carbetocin vs. oxytocin for PPH prevention after cesarean section. Cochrane Database Syst Rev. 2018;10:CD005457.

15. Bai J, et al. A comparison of oxytocin and carboprost tromethamine in the prevention of postpartum hemorrhage in high-risk patients undergoing cesarean delivery. Exp Ther Med. 2014;7(1):46–50.
16. Oyelese Y, et al. Misoprostol for PPH prevention and treatment. Am J Obstet Gynecol. 2020;222(6):558-65.
17. Saccone G, Della Corte L, D'Alessandro P, et al. Prophylactic use of tranexamic acid after vaginal delivery reduces the risk of primary postpartum hemorrhage. J Matern Fetal Neonatal Med. 2020;33(19):3368-74.
18. Ruiter L, Kazemier BM, Mol BWJ, et al. Incidence and recurrence rate of postpartum hemorrhage and manual removal of the placenta: A longitudinal linked national cohort study in The Netherlands. Eur J Obstet Gynecol Reprod Biol. 2019;238:114-9.
19. Endler M, Grünewald C, Saltvedt S. Epidemiology of retained placenta: oxytocin as an independent risk factor. Obstet Gynecol. 2012;119(4):801-9.
20. Antonijevic M, et al. Uterine inversion: Risk factors and management. J Perinat Med. 2021;49(5):567-73.
21. Krapp M, et al. Ultrasonographic assessment of placental separation in the third stage. Ultrasound Obstet Gynecol. 2017;50(4):452-7.

CHAPTER 5

Abnormal Labor

Ruchika Garg

DEFINITION

Normal labor progresses through four stages: **First stage** (cervical dilatation), **second stage** (fetal delivery), **third stage** (placental delivery), and **fourth stage** (postpartum observation). Abnormal labor (dystocia) occurs when there is a delay in progression (protraction or arrest) in the first or second stages, or when labor is excessively rapid (precipitate labor), leading to maternal or fetal complications. Disturbances in the **four Ps—Power** (uterine contractions), **Passenger** (fetus), **Passage** (pelvis), and **Presentation**—contribute to these abnormalities.[1]

KEY POINTS (FIG. 1)

- Abnormal labor includes protracted or arrested labor and precipitate labor.
- Prevalence: ~25–30% of labors exhibit some abnormality, with ~15% requiring intervention.[2]
- Common causes: Inadequate uterine contractions, cephalopelvic disproportion (CPD), malpresentation, or macrosomia.
- Management prioritizes identifying and correcting underlying causes, with cesarean delivery reserved for noncorrectable issues.
- Recent guidelines (NICE and RCOG) advocate expectant management for slow progress if maternal/fetal conditions are stable.[3,4]

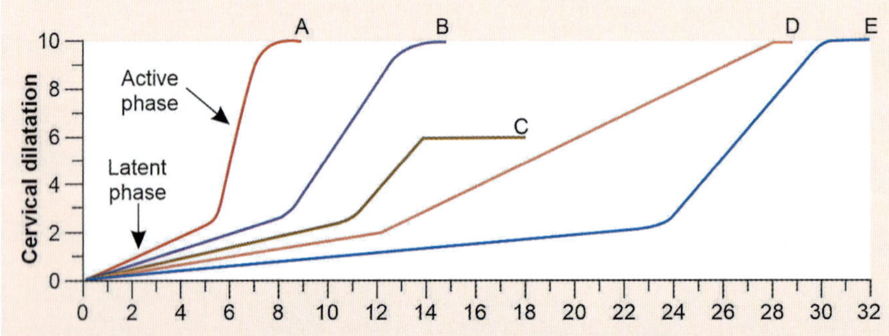

Fig. 1: Normal and abnormal labor during the first stage. (A: Average multipara; B: Average primigravida; C: Secondary arrest of dilation; D: Primary dysfunctional labor; E: Prolonged latent phase)

TYPES OF LABOR ABNORMALITIES

Abnormal labor is classified based on stage and type of delay or acceleration **(Table 1)**.

1. Protracted Descent

- **Definition:** Slow fetal descent (<1 cm/h in nulliparas and <2 cm/h in multiparas) due to inadequate uterine contractions (hypocontractility/uterine inertia), common in primigravida.[1,5]
- **Prevalence:** ~10–15% of labors.[2]
- **Management:** Oxytocin augmentation if uterine inertia is confirmed; address dehydration or maternal exhaustion.[3]

2. Arrest of Descent

- **Definition:** No fetal descent for ≥2 hours in the second stage (full cervical dilatation) across two vaginal examinations.[1]
- **Prevalence:** ~5–7% in nulliparas, ~2–3% in multiparas.[6]
- **Management:**
  - If pelvis is adequate, contractions are strong, and no fetal distress, use **forceps** or **vacuum extraction**.
  - If unfeasible (e.g., CPD and macrosomia), proceed to **cesarean section** after counseling on risks (e.g., uterine rupture and hemorrhage).[4]

3. Arrest of Dilatation

- **Definition:** No cervical dilatation for ≥2 hours at ≤6 cm, or no progress despite adequate contractions.[3]
- **Prevalence:** ~8–10% in first stage.[2]
- **Management:**
  - Correct reversible causes (e.g., dehydration and inadequate contractions) with IV fluids or oxytocin.

TABLE 1: Types and durations of abnormal labor.[3,5]

Abnormality	*Nullipara*	*Multipara*
Prolonged Latent Phase	>20 hours	>14 hours
Average Second Stage	50 minutes	20 minutes
Prolonged Second Stage (No Epidural)	>2 hours	>1 hours
Prolonged Second Stage (With Epidural)	>3 hours	>2 hours
Protracted Dilatation	<1.2 cm/h	<1.5 cm/h
Protracted Descent	<1 cm/h	<2 cm/h
Arrest of Dilatation	≥2 hours (≤6 cm)	≥2 hours (≤6 cm)
Arrest of Descent	≥2 hours	≥1 hour
Prolonged Third Stage	>30 minutes	>30 minutes

TABLE 2: Maternal and fetal risk factors for abnormal labor.[1,2,6]

Category	*Risk factors*
Maternal	• Advanced maternal age (>35 years) • Pregnancy complications (e.g., diabetes and hypertension) • Epidural anesthesia • Cephalopelvic disproportion (CPD) • Post-term pregnancy (>42 weeks) • Nulliparity • Short stature (<150 cm) • Uterine anomalies
Fetal	• High fetal head at full dilatation • Chorioamnionitis • Nonreassuring fetal heart rate (FHR) • Macrosomia (>4,000 g) • Malpresentation (e.g., occipitoposterior and transverse lie)

- Noncorrectable causes (e.g., CPD, macrosomia, and uterine anomalies) may require cesarean delivery.[4]

4. Precipitate Labor

- **Definition:** Labor lasting <3 hours, often due to hyperstimulated uterus, compliant birth canal (grand multiparas), small fetus, or prior rapid labor.[1]
- **Prevalence:** ~1–2% of deliveries.[7]
- **Risks:**
  - **Maternal:** Cervical/vaginal tears, PPH, and hemorrhagic shock.
  - **Fetal:** Infection (unsterile delivery settings), birth trauma.
  - **Management:** Postdelivery inspection for maternal injuries and hemorrhage; antibiotics for infection risk in unsterile settings.[4]

RISK FACTORS FOR ABNORMAL LABOR

Abnormal labor results from maternal, fetal, or combined factors disrupting the four Ps **(Table 2)**.

Additional Factors

- **Power:** Poor uterine contractions due to maternal illness, stress, anxiety, or variable oxytocin response.
- **Passage:** Pelvic contraction or structural abnormalities.
- **Passenger/Presentation:** Fetal size, position, or anomalies (e.g., hydrocephalus).[1]

MANAGEMENT OF ABNORMAL LABOR

Management focuses on diagnosing the abnormality, identifying correctable causes, and selecting the safest delivery route based on maternal/fetal status and guidelines (NICE, 2017; RCOG, 2022)[3,4] **(Table 3)**.

TABLE 3: Management strategies for abnormal labor.[3,4,8]

Abnormality	*Management*	*Guideline*
Prolonged Latent Phase	Observation, hydration, and ambulation	Not an indication for cesarean (ACOG, 2016)
Protracted Dilatation	Oxytocin and correct dehydration	NICE, 2017: Allow 4–6 hours with adequate contractions
Protracted Descent	Oxytocin and maternal repositioning	RCOG, 2022: Assess underlying cause
Arrest of Dilatation	Address cause; cesarean if no progress after 4–6 hours	ACOG, 2016: ≥6 cm with ruptured membranes
Arrest of Descent	Forceps/vacuum or cesarean	NICE, 2017: Assess pelvis and fetal status
Precipitate Labor	Postdelivery inspection and manage PPH/trauma	RCOG, 2022: Anticipate based on history

General Principles

- **Assessment:**
  - Regular vaginal examinations to monitor dilatation and descent.
  - Continuous fetal heart rate monitoring for distress.
  - Ultrasound for fetal position, size, or anomalies.
- **Correctable Causes:**
  - **Dehydration:** IV fluids (e.g., Ringer's lactate 500–1,000 mL).
  - **Uterine Inertia:** Oxytocin infusion (titrated to achieve 3–5 contractions/10 min, 200–250 MVU).[3]
  - **Maternal Exhaustion:** Support with hydration, pain relief, and rest.
- **Noncorrectable Causes:** CPD, macrosomia, or malpresentation may necessitate cesarean delivery.[4]

Specific Management

- **Prolonged Latent Phase:**
  - **Guideline:** Not an indication for cesarean (ACOG, 2016).[8]
  - **Management:** Observation, hydration, and ambulation; avoid premature intervention.[3]
- **Protracted Dilatation/Descent:**
  - **Management:** Oxytocin augmentation if contractions are inadequate; correct dehydration or maternal positioning.[4]
  - **Monitoring:** Ensure progress within 4–6 hours of adequate contractions.[8]
- **Arrest of Dilatation:**
  - **Criteria:** No cervical change for ≥4 hours with adequate contractions or ≥6 hours with oxytocin and inadequate contractions (at ≥6 cm with ruptured membranes).[8]
  - **Management:** Address reversible causes; cesarean if no progress or noncorrectable cause (e.g., CPD).[4]
- **Arrest of Descent:**
  - **Criteria:** No descent for ≥2 hours (nulliparas) or ≥1 hour (multiparas) in second stage.[3]

- **Management:**
    - If pelvis adequate and no distress, use **forceps/vacuum extraction**.
    - Cesarean for CPD, macrosomia, or fetal distress.[4]
- **Precipitate Labor:**
    - **Prevention:** Anticipate based on history (e.g., prior rapid labor and grand multiparity).
    - **Management:** Postdelivery inspection for cervical/vaginal tears, PPH; antibiotics for unsterile delivery settings.[7]

RECENT ADVANCES AND GUIDELINES

- **NICE Guidelines (2017):**[3]
    - Prolonged latent phase or slow progress in active phase does not warrant immediate cesarean if maternal/fetal conditions are stable.
    - Oxytocin augmentation recommended for protraction disorders with inadequate contractions.
    - Cesarean for active-phase arrest only after ≥4 hours of adequate contractions or ≥6 hours of oxytocin with no progress (≥6 cm, ruptured membranes).
- **RCOG Guidelines (2022):**[4]
    - Emphasize individualized care, avoiding rigid time-based interventions.
    - Intrapartum ultrasound to assess fetal position and descent in prolonged second stage (Level 2+ evidence).
- **WHO Labor Care Guide (2020):**[9]
    - Replaces partograph with flexible monitoring, focusing on maternal/fetal well-being, hydration, and ambulation to reduce unnecessary cesareans.
- **Intrapartum Ultrasound**: Angle of progression (AoP) and head-perineum distance (HPD) predict vaginal delivery success in prolonged labor (ISUOG, 2021).[10]
- **Tranexamic Acid**: Prophylactic use reduces PPH risk in high-risk labors (e.g., precipitate labor and macrosomia).[11]

KEY POINTS FOR POSTGRADUATE EDUCATION

- Abnormal labor affects ~25–30% of deliveries, with protraction/arrest being the most common issues.
- The four Ps (Power, Passenger, Passage, and Presentation) are critical in diagnosing causes of dystocia.
- Prolonged latent phase is not an indication for cesarean; observation is preferred.
- Active-phase arrest requires ≥4 hours of adequate contractions or ≥6 hours of oxytocin with no progress before cesarean.
- Precipitate labor (<3 hours) risks maternal tears and PPH; anticipate based on history.
- Oxytocin is the first line for protraction due to uterine inertia.
- Forceps/vacuum extraction is viable for arrest of descent if pelvis is adequate.
- Intrapartum ultrasound enhances accuracy in prolonged second stage.
- NICE/RCOG guidelines advocate expectant management for slow progress with stable maternal/fetal status.
- WHO Labor Care Guide promotes individualized care to reduce cesarean rates.

REFERENCES

1. Cunningham FG, Leveno KJ, Dashe JS, et al. (Eds). Williams Obstetrics, 26th edition. McGraw-Hill; 2021.
2. Caughey AB, et al. Contemporary labor patterns and outcomes. Am J Obstet Gynecol. 2018;218(2):S692-S699.
3. National Institute for Health and Care Excellence. Intrapartum care for healthy women and babies (CG190). London: NICE; 2017.
4. Royal College of Obstetricians and Gynaecologists. Management of the first and second stages of labour. RCOG Green-top Guideline No. 55. RCOG; 2022.
5. Zhang J, Troendle JF, Yancey MK. Reassessing the labor curve in nulliparous women. Am J Obstet Gynecol. 2002;187(4):824-8.
6. Laughon SK, et al. Incidence and risk factors for prolonged second stage of labor. Am J Obstet Gynecol. 2014;211(3):271.e1-271.e8.
7. Aiken CE, et al. Precipitate labor: Maternal and neonatal outcomes. J Perinat Med. 2019;47(5):512-518.
8. American College of Obstetricians and Gynecologists. Safe prevention of primary cesarean delivery. Obstet Gynecol. 2016;127(3):e54-e65.
9. World Health Organization. (2020). WHO Labor Care Guide. [online] Available from https://www.who.int/publications/b/56119 [Last accessed December, 2025].
10. International Society of Ultrasound in Obstetrics and Gynecology. Intrapartum ultrasound guidelines. Ultrasound Obstet Gynecol. 2021;58(5):645-53.
11. Saccone G, Corte LD, D'Alessandro P, et al. Prophylactic use of tranexamic acid after vaginal delivery reduces the risk of primary postpartum hemorrhage. J Matern Fetal Neonatal Med. 2020;33(19):3368-76.

Labor Analgesia

Ruchika Garg

DEFINITION

Labor pain arises from uterine contractions, cervical dilatation, and perineal stretching during childbirth, transmitted via visceral (T10–L1) and somatic (S2–S4) pathways. Effective analgesia alleviates maternal suffering, reduces catecholamine-induced complications, and improves fetal outcomes.[1]

KEY POINTS

- **Prevalence:** Labor pain affects 100% of parturients; severe pain reported in 60–80% of primigravida.[2]
- **Pain pathways:** Visceral (first stage, T10–L1) via C-fibers; somatic (second stage, S2–S4) via A-fibers.[1]
- **Analgesia options:** Nonpharmacological, pharmacological, and regional techniques.[3]
- Epidural analgesia is the gold standard, providing complete pain relief for both labor stages.[4]
- RCOG/NICE guidelines advocate individualized analgesia with informed consent and minimal fetal impact.[5,6]

NEUROANATOMY OF LABOR PAIN

- **First Stage (up to 8 cm dilatation in primigravida, 6 cm in multipara):**
  - **Source:** Uterine contractions and cervical dilatation.
  - **Pathway:** Visceral pain via unmyelinated C-fibers through sympathetic nerves to T10–L1 spinal cord segments.
  - **Character:** Dull, poorly localized, felt in lower abdomen and sacrum.[1]
- **Second Stage (full dilatation to delivery):**
  - **Source:** Stretching of perineum, vaginal wall, and cervix.
  - **Pathway:** Somatic pain via myelinated A-fibers through pudendal/perineal nerves to S2–S4.
  - **Character:** Sharp, localized to perineum and thighs.[1]

PREVALENCE AND IMPACT (TABLE 1)

- **Prevalence:** Severe labor pain in 60–80% of primigravida, 40–60% of multipara.[2]

TABLE 1: Impact of untreated labor pain.[1-3]

Effect	*Mechanism*	*Prevalence*
Uterine vasoconstriction	Catecholamine surge	20–30%
Hypocapnia	Hyperventilation	15–25%
Fetal hypoxemia	Reduced placental perfusion	5–10%
Birth canal trauma	Premature bearing-down	10–15%

TABLE 2: Nonpharmacological techniques for labor analgesia.[7]

Technique	*Efficacy*	*Notes*
TENS	Inconclusive	Minimal pain reduction
Massage/Support	20–30% pain relief	High maternal satisfaction
Water birth	Reduces epidural use	RR 0.6 for epidural
Acupuncture	Reduces instrumental delivery	RR 0.8
Relaxation/Yoga	High satisfaction	Reduces pain perception

- **Maternal Effects:**
  - Catecholamine release causes uterine vasoconstriction, reducing placental perfusion.
  - Hyperventilation leads to hypocapnia, shifting oxygen dissociation curve left, impairing fetal oxygenation.[3]
  - Premature bearing-down increases birth canal trauma.[1]
- **Fetal Effects:** Hypoxemia, metabolic acidosis (5–10% of prolonged labors).[2]
- **Goal of Analgesia:** Reduce maternal distress, sympathetic activation, and fetal acidosis.[3]

ANALGESIA TECHNIQUES

Classified into nonpharmacological, pharmacological, and regional methods, tailored to labor stage and patient needs.[3]

Nonpharmacological Techniques (Table 2)

- **Methods:**
  - Transcutaneous electrical nerve stimulation (TENS).
  - Touch/massage, continuous labor support.
  - Intradermal sterile water injections, water birth.
  - Acupuncture, hypnosis, relaxation, music, and yoga.[7]
- **Efficacy:**
  - Cochrane Review (2018): Relaxation and acupuncture reduce instrumental delivery (RR 0.8) and cesarean rates (RR 0.7); water birth decreases epidural use.[7]
  - TENS, aromatherapy, and hypnosis show inconclusive benefits.[7]
- **Advantages:** Noninvasive, patient-centered, and no fetal impact.
- **Limitations:** Limited evidence, variable efficacy (20–40% pain reduction).[7]

TABLE 3: Pharmacological agents for labor analgesia.[8-12]

Agent	*Dose*	*Efficacy*	*Side effects*
Entonox	Self-administered	30–40% pain relief	Drowsiness, nausea
Pethidine	50–100 mg IM	40–50% pain relief	Neonatal depression
Fentanyl	25–50 µg IV hourly	60–70% pain relief	Minimal neonatal impact
Remifentanil	20 µg IV PCA, 3-minute lockout	70–80% pain relief	Apnea risk (5%)
Ketamine	0.2 mg/kg/h IV	60% pain relief	Lightheadedness (48%)
Acetaminophen	1 g IV	20–30% VAS reduction	50% need rescue

PHARMACOLOGICAL TECHNIQUES (TABLE 3)

Inhalational Agents

- **Entonox (50% nitrous oxide + oxygen):**
  - Self-administered, onset 30–60 seconds, and 30–40% pain relief.
  - Side effects: Drowsiness (20%), nausea (15%), and occupational exposure concerns.
  - Scavenging systems reduce environmental risks.[8]
- **Sevoflurane (0.8% in oxygen):**
  - Less nausea than Entonox but no analgesic effect; risk of sedation and fetal toxicity limits use.[8]

Parenteral Medications

- **Opioids:**
  - **Pethidine:** 50–100 mg IM; onset 10–15 minutes, and duration 2–3 hours.
    - Side effects: Nausea (30%), respiratory depression (10%), and neonatal depression if given <2 hours before delivery.[9]
  - **Fentanyl:** 25–50 µg IV hourly or 0.25 µg/kg/h infusion; onset 2–3 minutes, short-acting.
    - Ideal for patient-controlled analgesia (PCA); minimal neonatal impact.[9]
  - **Remifentanil:** PCA bolus 20 µg, 3-minute lockout; half-life 3 minutes.
    - Effective alternative to epidural in coagulopathy; risk of maternal apnea (5%) requires oxygen supplementation.[10]
  - **Tramadol:** 1–2 mg/kg IM; onset 10 minutes, duration 2–3 hours; minimal respiratory depression.[9]
  - **Butorphanol:** 2–4 mg IM; high sedation limits use.[9]
- **Nonopioids:**
  - **Ketamine:** 0.2 mg/kg IV loading, 0.2 mg/kg/h infusion; 60% pain relief, 48% lightheadedness, and no fetal impact.[11]
  - **Acetaminophen:** 1 g IV; moderate pain reduction (VAS ↓20–30%), 50% need rescue analgesia within 2 hours.[12]
  - **NSAIDs:** Avoided due to risk of premature ductus arteriosus closure.[3]
- **Adjuncts:**
  - Promethazine/hydroxyzine: Potentiate opioids, reduce nausea; minimal analgesia alone.[3]
  - Pentobarbital/secobarbital: Hypnotics for early labor, no analgesia.[3]

OPIOID TOXICITY MANAGEMENT

- **Naloxone:**
  - Maternal: 0.4 mg IV for respiratory depression (reverses analgesia).
  - Neonatal: 0.1 mL/kg IV for respiratory depression; no role in primary resuscitation.[9]
  - Repeat dosing may be needed for long-acting opioids.[9]

REGIONAL ANESTHESIA

Paracervical Block

- **Technique:** Local anesthetic injected submucosally lateral/posterior to uterocervical junction, targeting paracervical ganglion.
- **Efficacy:** First-stage pain relief (50–60%); no second-stage coverage.[13]
- **Complications:** Fetal bradycardia (5–10%), local anesthetic toxicity, infection; limited use.[13]

Pudendal Block

- **Technique:** Transvaginal injection of local anesthetic behind sacrospinous ligaments (S2–S4).
- **Efficacy:** Second-stage perineal analgesia (70–80%); suitable for low forceps delivery.[13]
- **Complications:** Infection, bleeding, and toxicity (rare, <1%).[13]

Neuraxial Techniques (Table 4)

- **Epidural Analgesia:**
  - Gold standard; catheter in epidural space for continuous infusion or boluses.
  - Drugs: Low-dose bupivacaine (0.0625–0.125%) or ropivacaine (0.1–0.2%) with fentanyl (1–4 µg/mL) or sufentanil (0.03–0.05 µg/mL).[14]
  - Efficacy: 90–95% complete pain relief for both stages.[4]
  - Methods:
    - **Intermittent Boluses:** Better spread, but breakthrough pain common (20%).
    - **Continuous Infusion:** Stable analgesia, reduced toxicity risk.[14]
  - Complications: Hypotension (5–10%), motor block (5%), and fever (20–30%).[15]
- **Combined Spinal-Epidural (CSE):**
  - Spinal opioid (e.g., fentanyl 15–25 µg) followed by epidural catheter.
  - Rapid onset (5–10 minutes), ideal for late labor or multipara; 95% success rate.[16]
  - Complications: Similar to epidural; postdural puncture headache (1-2%).[16]

TABLE 4: Neuraxial analgesia techniques.[4,14,16,17]

Technique	*Efficacy*	*Complications*
Epidural	90–95%	Hypotension and fever
CSE	95%	Postdural puncture headache
Intrathecal	95–98%	Technical failure (10%)

- **Continuous Intrathecal Analgesia:**
  - Microcatheter in subarachnoid space; fentanyl (15–25 μg) or bupivacaine (2.5–5 mg).
  - Rapid, superior analgesia; high technical failure rate (10%) limits use.[17]

Advanced Neuraxial Methods

- **Patient-Controlled Epidural Analgesia (PCEA):** Boluses (4–8 mL, 10–20-minute lockout) with background infusion; reduces local anesthetic use by 20–30%.[18]
- **Programmed Intermittent Epidural Boluses (PIEB):** Automated boluses every 30–60 minutes; improves spread, reduces motor block (RR 0.4), and enhances satisfaction.[19]
- **Computer Integrated PCEA (CI-PCEA):** Algorithm adjusts infusion based on demand; 30% less breakthrough pain.[20]
- **Smart Pumps:** Drug database reduces dosing errors; 10–20% higher satisfaction.[20]

Ultrasound-guided Neuraxial

- **Use:** Identifies midline, epidural space depth; reduces attempts by 30% in obese/scoliosis cases.[21]
- **Innovations:** Optical fiber-embedded Tuohy needles for real-time guidance.[21]

Novel Loss of Resistance (LOR) Syringes

- **Episure/EpiFaith:** Spring-loaded syringe for autodetection; improves precision.[22]
- **Epidrum:** Diaphragm deflates on epidural entry; reduces operator subjectivity.[22]

Postpartum Considerations

- **Breastfeeding:** No significant impact of epidural on breastfeeding rates at 6 weeks.
- **Maternal Fever:** Epidural-associated fever (20–30%) linked to local anesthetics; no clear prophylaxis.[4]
- **Epidural Failure:** Causes include catheter misplacement (5–10%), migration, or inadequate spread; ultrasound reduces risk.[4]

MANAGEMENT OF COMPLICATIONS (TABLE 5)

- **American Society of Anesthesiologists (ASA, 2017):**[23]
  - **Cardiovascular/Neurological Toxicity:**
    - Oxygen, IV fluids, and ephedrine (5–10 mg IV) for hypotension.
    - Seizure management: Anticonvulsants, airway support.

TABLE 5: Management of epidural complications.[23]

Complication	*Management*
Hypotension	Ephedrine 5–10 mg IV, fluids
Respiratory depression	Naloxone 0.4 mg IV (maternal)
Seizures	Anticonvulsants, airway support
Pruritus/Nausea	Antihistamines

- **Opioid Toxicity:** Naloxone for respiratory depression; treat pruritus/nausea with antihistamines.
- **Preprocedure:** IV access maintained; no mandatory fluid preload.

RCOG/NICE Guidelines

- **RCOG (2022):**[5]
  - Offer neuraxial analgesia based on patient request, not cervical dilatation.
  - Early epidural placement does not increase cesarean risk (RR 1.0).
  - Epidural response time <30 minutes; second anesthetist if delayed.
- **NICE (2017):**[6]
  - Informed consent for all analgesia options; explain risks (e.g., motor block and fever).
  - Support nonpharmacological methods (e.g., water birth, massage) if preferred.
  - Continue epidural into second stage unless contraindicated.

RECENT ADVANCES

- **Water Birth:** Reduces epidural use (RR 0.6); enhances satisfaction.[7]
- **Relaxation/Yoga:** Cochrane (2018) reports 20–30% pain reduction, high satisfaction.[7]
- **Ultrasound-Guided Epidural:** 30% fewer attempts in challenging cases.[21]
- **Smart Pumps/CI-PCEA:** Reduce drug use, improve outcomes.[20]
- **Novel LOR Syringes:** Enhance epidural placement accuracy.[22]

KEY POINTS FOR POSTGRADUATE EDUCATION

- Labor pain is universal, severe in 60–80% of primigravida, transmitted via T10–L1 (visceral) and S2–S4 (somatic) pathways.
- Untreated pain causes catecholamine surge, fetal hypoxemia (5–10%), and birth canal trauma.
- Nonpharmacological methods (e.g., water birth and acupuncture) reduce pain by 20–40%; limited evidence.
- Pharmacological options: Entonox (30–40% relief), fentanyl/remifentanil PCA (70–80% relief), and ketamine (60% relief).
- Epidural analgesia (90–95% efficacy) is gold standard; CSE ideal for rapid onset in late labor.
- Advanced techniques (PCEA, PIEB, and CI-PCEA) reduce drug use and motor block.
- Ultrasound and novel LOR syringes improve epidural placement accuracy.
- Complications: Epidural fever (20–30%), hypotension (5–10%); manage with fluids, ephedrine, and naloxone.
- RCOG/NICE advocate early epidural access, individualized care, and informed consent.
- No evidence links epidural to increased cesarean rates or breastfeeding failure.

REFERENCES

1. Cunningham FG, Leveno KJ, Dashe JS, et al. (Eds). Williams Obstetrics, 26th edition. McGraw-Hill; 2021.

2. Melzack R, et al. Labour pain: Prevalence and intensity. Pain. 2018;159(4):623-9.
3. Jones L, Othman M, Dowswell T, et al. Pain management for women in labour: An overview of systematic reviews. Cochrane Database Syst Rev. 2012;2012(3):CD009234.
4. Anim-Somuah M, Md Smyth R, Jones L. Epidural versus non-epidural analgesia in labour. Cochrane Database Syst Rev. 2011;(12):CD000331.
5. Royal College of Obstetricians and Gynaecologists. Labour analgesia guidelines. RCOG Green-top Guideline No. 47. RCOG; 2022.
6. National Institute for Health and Care Excellence. (2014). Intrapartum care for healthy women and babies (CG190). [online] Available from https://www.nice.org.uk/guidance/cg190 [Last accessed December, 2025].
7. Smith CA, et al. Non-pharmacological interventions for labour pain. Cochrane Database Syst Rev. 2018;2:CD009223.
8. Klomp T, van Poppel M, Jones L, et al. Inhaled analgesia for pain management in labour. Cochrane Database Syst Rev. 2012;2012(9):CD009351.
9. Ullman R, Smith LA, Burns E, et al. Parenteral opioids for maternal pain relief in labour. Cochrane Database Syst Rev. 2010;(9):CD007396.
10. Freeman LM, et al. Remifentanil PCA for labour analgesia. BJOG. 2017;124(7):1032-9.
11. Suppa E, et al. Ketamine for labour analgesia: A randomized trial. Int J Obstet Anesth. 2016;27:40-6.
12. Onuoha OC, et al. Intravenous acetaminophen for labour pain. Obstet Gynecol. 2018;132(3):632-8.
13. Novikova N, et al. Regional anaesthesia for labour pain. Cochrane Database Syst Rev. 2016;4:CD009149.
14. Sultan P, et al. Advances in epidural analgesia for labour. Br J Anaesth. 2019;123(2):e218-e224.
15. Simmons SW, Taghizadeh N, Dennis AT, et al. Combined spinal-epidural versus epidural analgesia in labour. Cochrane Database Syst Rev. 2012;10(10):CD003401.
16. Arzola C, et al. Continuous intrathecal labour analgesia: A systematic review. Anesthesiology. 2017;127(4):685-94.
17. Halpern SH, Carvalho B. Patient-controlled epidural analgesia for labor. Anesth Analg. 2009;108(3):921-8.
18. Wong CA, et al. Programmed intermittent epidural bolus for labour analgesia. Anesthesiology. 2018;129(4):826-36.
19. Capogna G, et al. Computer-integrated PCEA for labour analgesia. Eur J Anaesthesiol. 2017;34(6):348-54.
20. Sia AT, et al. Smart pumps for labour analgesia: A randomized trial. Int J Obstet Anesth. 2019;38:52-8.
21. Grau T, et al. Ultrasound-guided neuraxial anaesthesia in obstetrics. Reg Anesth Pain Med. 2018;43(6):637-44.
22. Riley ET, et al. Novel loss of resistance syringes for epidural placement. Anesth Analg. 2017;125(3):982-7.
23. American Society of Anesthesiologists. Practice guidelines for obstetric anesthesia. Anesthesiology. 2017;126(4):703-44.

CHAPTER 7

Partogram

Ruchika Garg

INTRODUCTION

Effective labor monitoring is critical to ensure safe maternal and neonatal outcomes. The World Health Organization (WHO) introduced the composite partogram in 1994, followed by modifications and the development of the Labor Care Guide (LCG) based on emerging evidence. These tools guide healthcare providers in tracking labor progress, identifying deviations, and optimizing interventions.

WHO COMPOSITE PARTOGRAM (1994)

Introduced in 1994, the WHO composite partogram, adapted from Philpott et al., standardized labor management globally.

- **Basic Principles:**
    - Latent phase: 8 hours duration.
    - Active phase: Begins at 3 cm cervical dilatation.
    - Alert line: Plotted from 3 cm dilatation at 1 cm/h.
    - Action line: Drawn 4 hours parallel and to the right of the alert line.

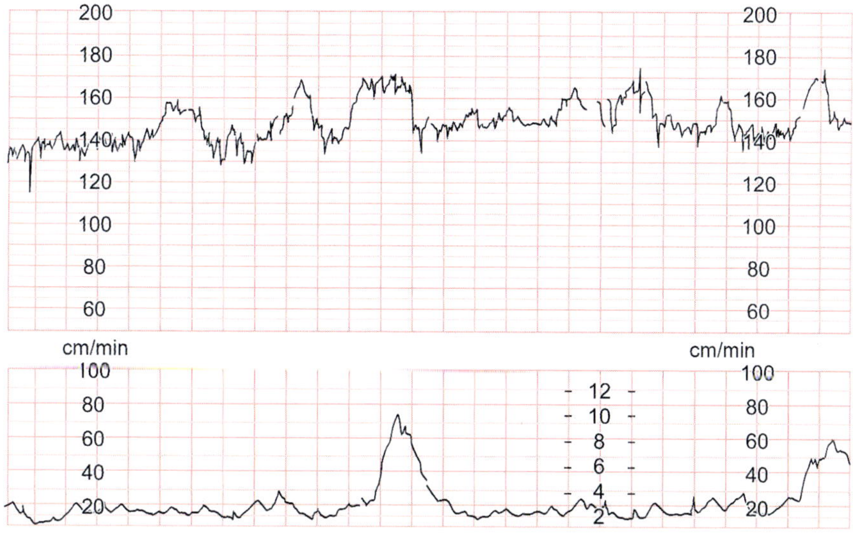

Fig. 1: Normal cardiotocography (CTG).

- **Components:**
    - **Fetal Parameters:**
        - Fetal heart rate (FHR).
        - Amniotic fluid color.
        - Molding of fetal head.

Reactive CTG with normal baseline heart rate (110–160 beats/min), two accelerations in 15 minutes, normal baseline variability, and no decelerations with contractions.

- **Maternal Parameters:**
    - Pulse, blood pressure, and temperature.
    - Urine analysis (proteins and ketones).
- **Uterine Contractions:**
    - Number and intensity.
- **Interventions:**
    - Drugs, IV fluids, and oxytocin administration.

Flowchart 1: Changes responsible for cervical ripening.[1]

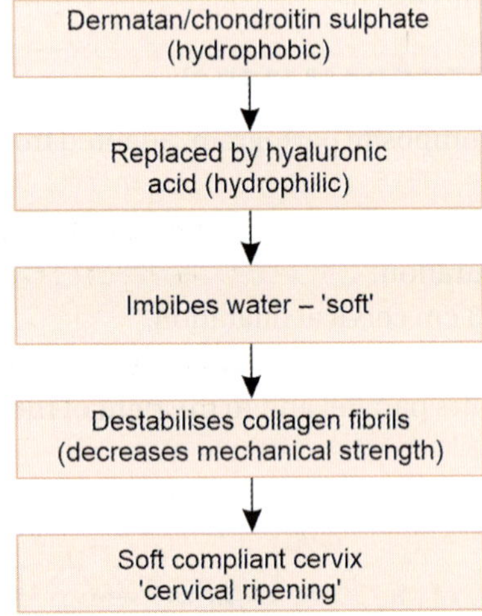

- Displays latent and active phases, alert and action lines, and parameters for fetal, maternal, and labor monitoring.

MODIFIED WHO PARTOGRAM[2] (2000)

The composite partogram faced criticism for including the latent phase, which led to higher interventions (augmentations, cesarean sections). In 2000, WHO introduced a modified version for improved usability.[3]

- **Key Modifications:**
    - Removal of latent phase: Documentation begins in active phase, as latent phase duration varies and onset is retrospective.

- Active phase starts at 4 cm cervical dilatation (previously 3 cm).
- Time scale: Two squares represent 1 hour (each square = 30 minutes), unlike one square per hour in the composite version.

▪ **Components of Modified WHO Partogram:**
- **Patient Information:**
  - Recorded at the top: Name, date, time of admission, and other details.
- **Fetal Assessment:**
  - FHR: Monitored every 30 minutes for 1 minute postcontraction; <110 or >160 beats/min may indicate distress, requiring 15-minute checks.
  - Membranes and Amniotic Fluid: Recorded as I (intact), C (clear), M (meconium), B (blood-stained), A (absent).
  - Molding: Graded as 0 (separated bones), 1+ (touching), 2+ (overlapping), 3+ (severely overlapping).
- **Cervicograph:**
  - X-axis: Time (each square = 30 minutes).
  - Y-axis: Cervical dilatation (0–10 cm, each square = 1 cm), plotted as "X".
  - Descent: Assessed abdominally in fifths above pelvic brim, plotted as "O".
  - Alert line: From 4 to 10 cm at 1 cm/h.
  - Action line: Parallel, 4 hours to the right of alert line, signaling delay or need for intervention.
- **Uterine Contractions:**
  - Frequency: Number of contractions in 10 minutes, shaded in squares.
  - Intensity: Marked as dots (<20 seconds), oblique lines (20–40 seconds), or block color (>40 seconds).
- **Oxytocin:** Dose and drop rate recorded for labor augmentation.
- **Drugs and IV Fluids:** Additional interventions documented.
- **Maternal Assessment:**
  - Pulse (every 30 minutes), blood pressure, temperature, and urine (volume, proteins, acetone) every 4 hours.

▪ **Advantages:**
- Single-sheet documentation of labor progress.
- Reduces repetitive recording.
- Aids in diagnosing delays, preventing obstructed labor.
- Guides early transfer to tertiary care.
- Informs decisions on augmentation or termination.
- Useful across healthcare levels.

▪ **Disadvantages:**
- Requires trained personnel to fill and interpret.
- Subjective clinical findings.
- Assumes uniform dilatation rates across women.
- Illustrates cervicograph, alert/action lines, and monitoring parameters.

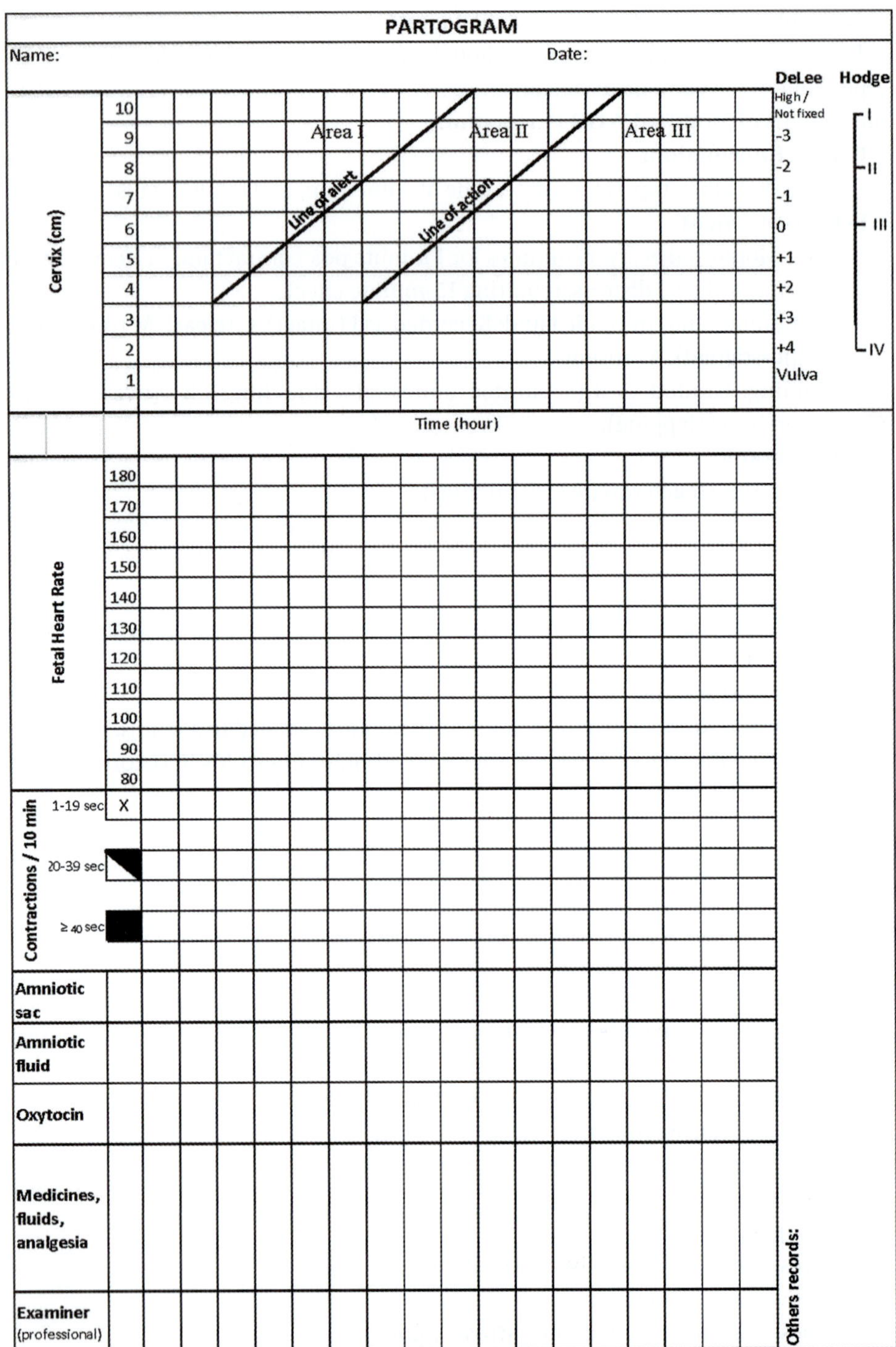
PARTOGRAM

Name:

Date:

Cervix (cm)

10
9
8
7
6
5
4
3
2
1

Area I
Area II
Area III
Line of alert
Line of action

DeLee
High / Not fixed
-3
-2
-1
0
+1
+2
+3
+4
Vulva

Hodge
I
II
III
IV

Time (hour)

Fetal Heart Rate
180
170
160
150
140
130
120
110
100
90
80

Contractions / 10 min
1-19 sec X
20-39 sec
≥ 40 sec

Amniotic sac
Amniotic fluid
Oxytocin
Medicines, fluids, analgesia
Examiner (professional)
Others records:

Fig. 2: WHO modified partogram.

COLOR-CODED SIMPLIFIED WHO PARTOGRAM

To enhance usability, especially in low-resource settings, a color-coded version was introduced:

- **Color Coding:**
  - Green: Area left of alert line; indicates satisfactory progress.
  - Amber: Between alert and action lines; requires closer monitoring.
  - Red: Right of action line; signals threatened labor progress, needing intervention.
- **Benefits:**
  - User-friendly for clinicians, trained dais, nurse midwives, and health workers.
  - Simplifies interpretation in primary care settings.
  - Shows green, amber, and red zones for labor progress.

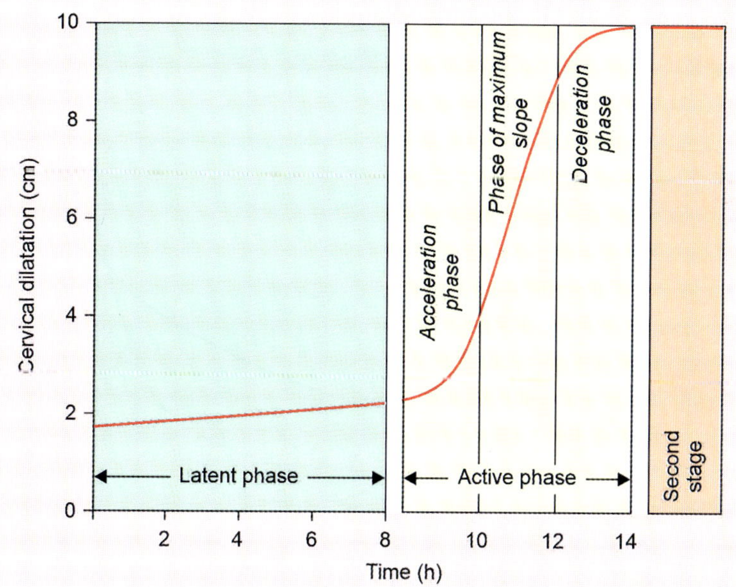

Fig. 3: Friedmann's labor curve.

PAPERLESS PARTOGRAM[4]

Developed by Dr AK Debdas in Jamshedpur, India, this simplified tool addresses prolonged labor in resource-limited settings.

- **Methodology:**
  - Calculate two values:
    - **Alert Estimated Time Of Delivery (ETD):** At 4 cm dilatation, add 6 hours (based on Friedman's 1 cm/h rate) to estimate full dilatation (10 cm).
    - **Action ETD:** Add 4 hours to Alert ETD.
  - Example: If 4 cm dilated at 11 AM, Alert ETD = 5 PM, Action ETD = 9 PM.
  - Display both ETDs boldly on the case sheet, with Action ETD circled in red.
- **Advantages:**
  - Low-cost, intuitive solution.

- Simplifies labor monitoring in rural, overburdened settings.
- Comparable efficacy to WHO partogram, with better usability.

CHALLENGES TO WHO MODIFIED PARTOGRAM

- **Zhang's Partogram:**
  - In 2012, Zhang et al. found that labor progresses slowly before 6 cm and rapidly after, contrasting Friedman's model.
  - Reduced cesarean rates in primiparous women when following these findings.
- **ACOG/SMFM Guidelines (2014):**
  - Active labor redefined at 6 cm dilatation.
  - Protracted labor or arrest not diagnosed before 6 cm.
  - Highlights need to update partogram standards.

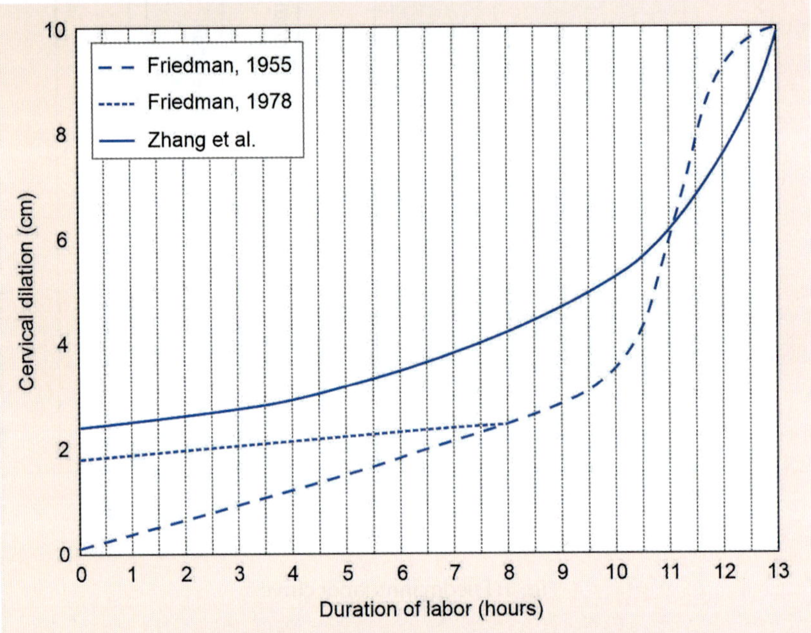

Fig. 4: Comparative labor progression in nullipara.[5]

WHO LABOR CARE GUIDE (LCG)[6]

Introduced by WHO in 2020, the Labor Care Guide (LCG) is an evidence-based tool to replace traditional partograms, addressing modern labor progress insights and holistic care.

- **Key Changes:**
  - Replaces alert and action lines with evidence-based time limits for each cm of cervical dilatation in active first stage.
  - Active first stage starts at 5 cm dilatation (previously 4 cm).
  - Uterine contraction strength omitted due to difficulty in standardization.
  - Includes a dedicated second-stage monitoring section to prevent poor outcomes from neglect.

- **Supportive Care Section:**
  - Promotes labor companionship, oral hydration, maternal position/mobility, and pain management.
- **Assessment Section:**
  - Documents overall assessment and additional relevant findings.
- **Plan Section:**
  - Records care plan formulated with the woman.
  - Deviations from expected observations circled and documented.
- **Rationale:**
  - Median dilatation rate in low-risk women exceeds 1 cm/h at 5 cm, reducing iatrogenic misdiagnosis of poor progress.
  - Focuses on monitoring and response, not just retrospective recording.
- **Benefits:**
  - Evidence-based, flexible time limits.
  - Enhances childbirth experience with supportive strategies.[7]
  - Improves vigilance in second stage.
  - Displays time limits, second-stage monitoring, and supportive care sections.

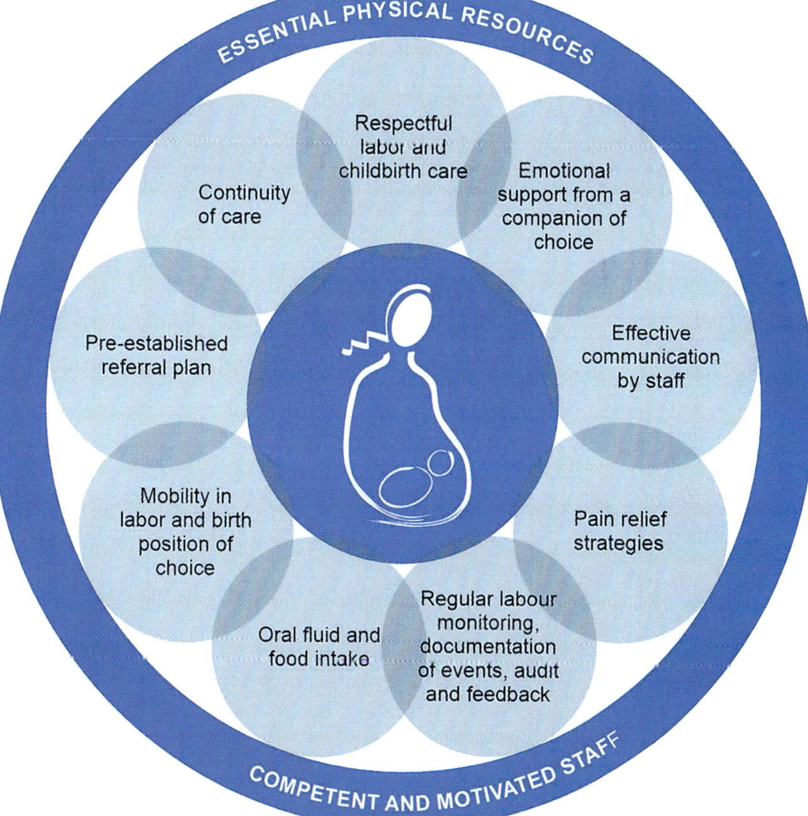

Fig. 5: WHO recommendations for intrapartum care for a positive childbirth experience.[8]

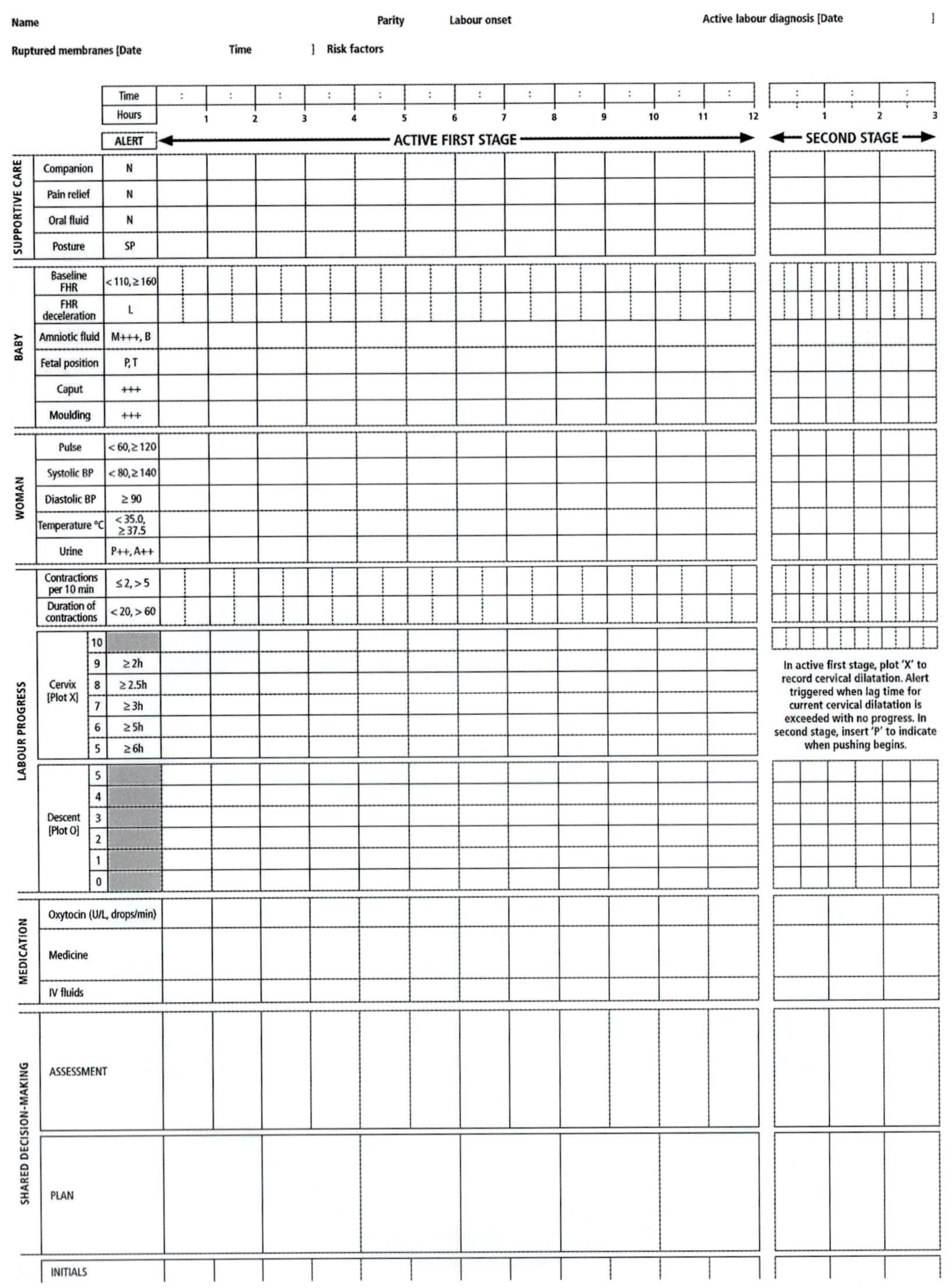

WHO LABOUR CARE GUIDE

Name | Parity | Labour onset | Active labour diagnosis [Date]

Ruptured membranes [Date | Time] | Risk factors

	Time	:	:	:	:	:	:	:	:	:	:	:	:	:	:	:
	Hours	1	2	3	4	5	6	7	8	9	10	11	12	1	2	3
	ALERT	ACTIVE FIRST STAGE												SECOND STAGE		

Section	Parameter	ALERT
SUPPORTIVE CARE	Companion	N
	Pain relief	N
	Oral fluid	N
	Posture	SP
BABY	Baseline FHR	< 110, ≥ 160
	FHR deceleration	L
	Amniotic fluid	M+++, B
	Fetal position	P, T
	Caput	+++
	Moulding	+++
WOMAN	Pulse	< 60, ≥ 120
	Systolic BP	< 80, ≥ 140
	Diastolic BP	≥ 90
	Temperature °C	< 35.0, ≥ 37.5
	Urine	P++, A++
LABOUR PROGRESS	Contractions per 10 min	≤ 2, > 5
	Duration of contractions	< 20, > 60
	Cervix [Plot X] 10	
	9	≥ 2h
	8	≥ 2.5h
	7	≥ 3h
	6	≥ 5h
	5	≥ 6h
	Descent [Plot O] 5	
	4	
	3	
	2	
	1	
	0	
MEDICATION	Oxytocin (U/L, drops/min)	
	Medicine	
	IV fluids	
SHARED DECISION-MAKING	ASSESSMENT	
	PLAN	
	INITIALS	

In active first stage, plot 'X' to record cervical dilatation. Alert triggered when lag time for current cervical dilatation is exceeded with no progress. In second stage, insert 'P' to indicate when pushing begins.

Fig. 6: WHO Labor Care Guide.

TABLE 1: Comparison of WHO partogram and labor care guide.

Feature	*WHO composite partogram (1994)*	*WHO modified partogram (2000)*	*WHO labor care guide (2020)*
Latent Phase	Included (8 hours)	Removed	Removed
Active Phase Start	3 cm dilatation	4 cm dilatation	5 cm dilatation
Time Scale	1 square = 1 hour	1 square = 30 minutes	Evidence-based time limits
Alert/Action Lines	Present	Present	Replaced with time limits
Uterine Contractions	Frequency and intensity	Frequency and intensity	Omitted
Second Stage Monitoring	Not included	Not included	Dedicated section
Supportive Care	Not addressed	Not addressed	Included (companionship, etc.)

RECENT ADVANCES

- **Digital Partogram:**
  - Developed by Jhpiego and Johns Hopkins Center for Bioengineering Innovation and Design (JHU-CBID).
  - Handheld device with WHO-based software; data syncs to a server for remote review by tertiary care doctors.
  - India Maternal Health Initiative (IMHI) by JivaDaya Foundation partners with hospitals for early detection and management.[9]
- **Mobile Partograms:**
  - Dimagi's smartphone app (English and Hindi) launched in India (2015).
  - Sends key alerts to consultants, staff, or referral centers for prompt action.
- **Cochrane Review Insights:**
  - Routine partogram use shows minimal clinical utility in reducing cesarean rates, operative vaginal deliveries, or poor neonatal outcomes (APGAR scores).[1]
  - In low-resource settings, modified WHO partogram reduces cesarean rates, augmentation, vaginal exams, and NICU admissions.
  - Challenges: Incomplete partograms, suboptimal use (3% and 31% in busy units), and lack of transfer with referrals.

Challenges and Considerations

- **Training:** Requires skilled healthcare workers for accurate completion and interpretation.
- **Subjectivity:** Clinical findings may vary between observers.
- **Uniformity Assumption:** Partograms assume consistent labor progress, not always applicable.
- **Audits:** Busy units show incomplete partograms due to manpower shortages and inadequate training.[10]

KEY POINTS

- WHO composite partogram (1994) standardized labor monitoring but included a controversial latent phase.
- Modified partogram (2000) starts at 4 cm dilatation, improving usability.
- Color-coded and paperless partograms enhance accessibility in low-resource settings.
- Zhang's research and ACOG/SMFM (2014) redefine active labor at 6 cm, reducing interventions.
- WHO Labor Care Guide (2020) uses evidence-based time limits, adds second-stage monitoring, and promotes supportive care.
- Digital and mobile partograms facilitate remote monitoring and timely action.
- Partograms remain valuable in low-resource settings despite challenges in completion and training.

REFERENCES

1. Lavender T, Anna Hart, Rebecca M D Smyth. Effect of partogram use on outcomes for women in spontaneous labour at term. Cochrane Database Syst Rev. 2013;(7):CD005461.
2. Opoku B, Nguah S. Utilization of the modified WHO partograph in assessing the progress of labour in a metropolitan area in Ghana. Res J Womens Health. 2015;2:2.
3. Aaron B Caughey, Alison G Cahill, Jeanne-Marie Guise, et al.; American College of Obstetricians and Gynecologists (ACOG) & Society for Maternal-Fetal Medicine (SMFM). Safe prevention of the primary cesarean delivery. Am J Obstet Gynecol. 2014;210(3):179-93.
4. Debdas AK. Paperless partogram: A simple and effective tool for managing labor. J South Asian Fed Obstet Gynaecol. 2015;7:94-7.
5. Zhang J, Troendle JF, Yancey MK. Reassessing the labor curve in nulliparous women. Am J Obstet Gynecol. 2002;187(4):824-8.
6. World Health Organization. WHO Labour Care Guide: User's Manual. Geneva: WHO; 2020.
7. Dalal AR, Purandare AC. The partograph in childbirth: An absolute essentiality or a mere exercise? J Obstet Gynaecol India. 2018;68:3-5.
8. Bedwell C, Levin K, Pett C, et al. A realist review of the partograph: When and how does it work for labour monitoring? BMC Pregnancy Childbirth. 2017;17(1):31.
9. Souza JP, Gülmezoglu AM, Vogel J, et al. Moving beyond essential interventions for reduction of maternal mortality (the WHO Multicountry Survey on Maternal and Newborn Health). Lancet. 2013;381(9879):1747-55.
10. Vogel JP, Hofmeyr GJ, Bernitz S, et al. WHO next-generation partograph: revolutionary steps towards improving intrapartum care. BJOG. 2021;128(10):1658-62.

Operative Vaginal Delivery Ventouse (Vacuum) and Forceps Delivery

Bethesheba Pagolu, Preeti Nitsure Deshpande

LONG QUESTIONS AND ANSWERS

1. What are the indications and safety criteria to apply forceps and vacuum delivery?

Ans.

Indications

Fetal: Suspected fetal compromise [CTG—pathological, grade 2–3 meconium-stained liquor, and abnormal fetal heart rate]

Maternal:

- Nulli parous woman: Lack of continuing progress for 3 hours with regional anesthesia and 2-hours without regional anesthesia
- Parous women: Lack of continuing progress for 2 hours with regional anesthesia and 1-hours without regional anesthesia
- Maternal exhaustion/distress
- Maternal indications to avoid Valsalva maneuver
- Combined maternal and fetal indications for assisted vaginal delivery often coexists
- Safety criteria applying forceps

Full abdominal and Vaginal Examination

- Head is ≤1/5 palpable per abdomen (in most cases not palpable)
- Cervix is fully dilated and the membranes ruptured
- Station at level of ischial spines or below
- Position of the fetal head has been determined
- Caput and molding is no more than moderate (or +2)a
- Pelvis is deemed adequate

Preparation of Mother

- Clear explanation given and informed consent taken and documented in women's case notes.
- Trust established and full cooperation sought and agreed with woman.
- Appropriate analgesia is in place: For midpelvic or rotational birth, this will usually be a regional block; a pudendal block may be acceptable depending on urgency; and a perineal block may be sufficient for low or outlet birth.
- Maternal bladder has been emptied.
- Indwelling catheter has been removed or balloon deflated.
- Aseptic technique

Preparation of staff

Operator has the knowledge, experience, and skill necessary. Adequate facilities are available (equipment, bed, and lighting) and access to an operating theatre.

Backup plan: For midpelvic births, theatre facilities should be available to allow a cesarean birth to be performed without delay; a senior obstetrician should be present if an inexperienced obstetrician is conducting the birth.

Anticipation of complications that may arise (e.g., shoulder dystocia, perineal trauma, and postpartum hemorrhage).

2. When should vacuum-assisted birth be discontinued, and how should a discontinued vacuum procedure be managed?

Ans. Discontinue vacuum-assisted birth where there is no evidence of progressive descent with moderate traction during each pull of a correctly applied instrument by an experienced operator.

Complete vacuum-assisted birth in the majority of cases with a maximum of three pulls to bring the fetal head on to the perineum.

Three additional gentle pulls can be used to ease the head out of the perineum.

If there is minimal descent with the first two pulls of a vacuum, the operator should consider whether the application is suboptimal, the fetal position has been incorrectly diagnosed, or there is cephalopelvic disproportion. Less experienced operators should stop and seek a second opinion. Experienced operators should re-evaluate the clinical findings and either change approach or discontinue the procedure.

Discontinue vacuum-assisted birth if there have been two "pop-offs" of the instrument. Less experienced operators should seek senior support after one "pop-off" to ensure the woman has the best chance of a successful assisted vaginal birth.

The rapid negative pressure application for vacuum-assisted birth is recommended as it reduces the duration of the procedure with no difference in maternal and neonatal outcomes.

The use of sequential instruments is associated with an increased risk of trauma to the infant. However, the operator needs to balance the risks of a cesarean birth following failed vacuum extraction with the risks of forceps birth following failed vacuum extraction.

Obstetricians should be aware of the increased neonatal morbidity following failed vacuum-assisted birth and/or sequential use of instruments and should inform the neonatologist when this occurs to ensure appropriate management of the baby.

Obstetricians should be aware of the increased risk of OASI following sequential use of instruments.

SMALL QUESTIONS AND ANSWERS

1. When should attempted forceps birth be discontinued?

Ans.

- Discontinue attempted forceps birth where the forceps cannot be applied easily, the handles do not approximate easily, or if there is a lack of progressive descent with moderate traction.
- Discontinue rotational forceps if rotation is not easily achieved with gentle pressure.

- Discontinue attempted forceps birth if birth is not imminent following three pulls of a correctly applied instrument by an experienced operator.
- If there is minimal descent with the first one or two pulls of the forceps, the operator should consider whether the application is suboptimal, the position has been incorrectly diagnosed or there is cephalopelvic disproportion. Less experienced operators should stop and seek a second opinion. Experienced operators should re-evaluate the clinical findings and either change the approach or discontinue the procedure.

2. What precautions should be taken care for the bladder after birth?

Ans. Women should be educated about the risk of urinary retention, so that they are aware of the importance of bladder emptying in the postpartum period.

The timing and volume of the first void urine should be monitored and documented.

A postvoid residual should be measured if urinary retention is suspected.

Recommend that women who have received regional analgesia for a trial of assisted vaginal birth in theatre have an indwelling catheter in situ after the birth to prevent covert urinary retention. This should be removed according to the local protocol.

Offer women physiotherapy-directed strategies to reduce the risk of urinary incontinence at 3 months.

3. What information should women be given for future births?

Ans.

- Inform women that there is a high probability of a spontaneous vaginal birth in subsequent labors following assisted vaginal birth.
- Individualize care for women who have sustained a third- or fourth-degree perineal tear, or who have ongoing pelvic floor morbidity.
- Women who have experienced an uncomplicated assisted vaginal birth should be encouraged to aim for a spontaneous vaginal birth in a subsequent pregnancy as there is a high chance of success.
- Women who have experienced an uncomplicated assisted vaginal birth should be encouraged to aim for a spontaneous vaginal birth in a subsequent pregnancy as there is a high chance of success.

MULTIPLE CHOICE QUESTIONS

1. Which of the following is the indication of forceps delivery in operation theatre?

a. Occipital anterior position above ischial spines
b. EFW > 3.5 Kg
c. BMI > 25 kg/m^2 and occipitoposterior position
d. BMI > 30 kg/m^2 and mid cavity forceps

2. What is the lower limit of gestational age for ventouse application?

a. 32 weeks
b. 34 weeks
c. 36 weeks
d. 28 weeks

3. Following a prolonged second stage of labor, a primigravida is examined at term gestation to make a decision for operative delivery. Vaginal examination shows the presenting point to be direct occipitoanterior position with station at +3, and a decision is made to perform a ventouse delivery. How would you classify this operative vaginal delivery?

a. High
b. Mid cavity
c. Low rotation of 45° or less
d. Low rotation of >45

4. What are the prerequisites for forceps delivery?

a. Cervix 8 cm dilated and membranes absent
b. Cervix fully dilated, membranes present
c. Os fully dilated with head 1/5th palpable per abdomen
d. Fully dilated and 2/5th palpable per abdomen

5. Identify the forceps.

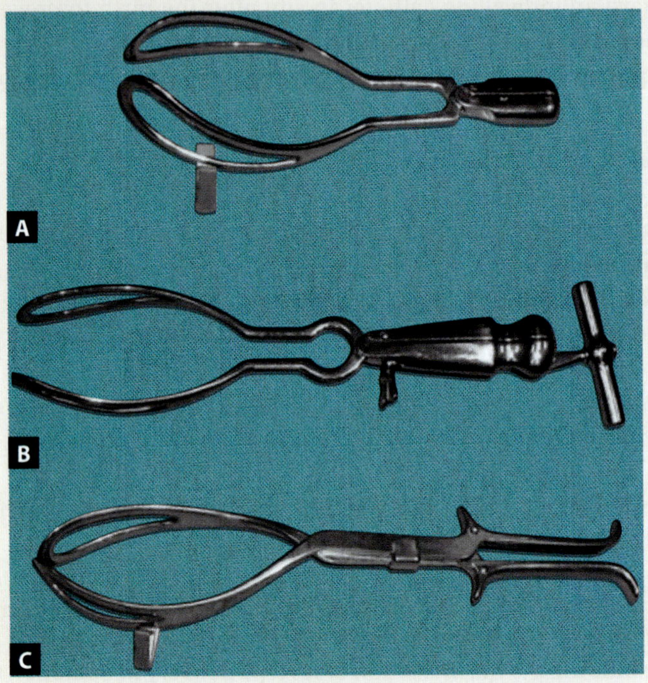

Explanations

Ans. 1 d. BMI > 30 kg/m2 and mid cavity forceps.

The indications of forceps delivery in operation theatre include:

1. Occipitoposterior position
2. BMI >30 kg/m^2
3. EFW >4.0 kg
4. Mid cavity forceps

Ans. 2 a. 32 weeks

Ans. 3 c. Low rotation of 45° or less

Classification for assisted vaginal birth

- Outlet: Fetal scalp is visible without separating the labia. Fetal skull has reached the perineum rotation and does not exceed 45°. Low fetal skull is at station +2 cm, but not on the perineum.
- Low cavity: Fetal skull is at station + 2 cm, but not on the perineum. Two subdivisions: (1) Nonrotational ≤45°; (2) Rotational >45°
- Mid cavity: Fetal head is no more than one-fifth palpable per abdomen. Leading point of the skull is at station 0 or + 1 cm; two subdivisions: (1) Nonrotational ≤45°/rotation >45°

Ans. 4. c. Os fully dilated with head 1/5th palpable per abdomen

Prerequisites for instrumental delivery

The prerequisites for a forceps delivery can be remembered using the FORCEPS mnemonic:

F—Favorable head position (OA/OP)

O—Os fully dilated

R—Rupture the membranes

C—Contractions are adequate

E—Engaged head–one-fifth palpable or less per abdomen

P—Adequate maternal pelvis

S—Stirrups (lithotomy position)

Ans. 5. a. Wrigley; b. Neville Barnes; c. Kielland's forceps

Retained Placenta

Ruchika Garg, Neelansha Varshney

INTRODUCTION

Retained placenta, occurring in 1–3% of vaginal deliveries, is a significant cause of postpartum hemorrhage (PPH), second only to uterine atony.[1] Defined as the failure of the placenta to separate spontaneously within 30–60 minutes postdelivery or incomplete delivery with retained fragments, it is associated with maternal morbidity, including severe bleeding and infection.[2] In India, retained placenta contributes to 10–15% of PPH cases, necessitating urgent intervention.[3] Effective management relies on early recognition of risk factors, clinical diagnosis, and adherence to standardized protocols. This chapter outlines the incidence, pathophysiology, risk factors, diagnosis, management, and complications of retained placenta, tailored for postgraduate medical education.

INCIDENCE AND EPIDEMIOLOGY

- **Incidence**: 1–3% of vaginal deliveries; higher in preterm (25% at 25 weeks versus 3% at term).[1,4]
- **Trends**: Increasing incidence, possibly due to rising cesarean rates and labor inductions[5] **(Table 1)**.
- **Morbidity**: Contributes to 10–15% of PPH cases; associated with infection and surgical interventions.[3]

PATHOPHYSIOLOGY

Normal placental separation occurs postdelivery due to uterine contractions and hormonal changes, detaching the placenta from the decidua.[7] Retained placenta results from as shown in **Table 2**.

TABLE 1: Incidence and delivery timing of retained placenta.[1,4,6]

Parameter	*Details*	*Notes*
Incidence	1–3% vaginal deliveries	Higher in preterm (25% at 25 weeks)
AMTSL Delivery	5–10 minutes	Oxytocin hastens separation
Expectant Delivery	10–20 minutes	Spontaneous separation
Delivery Probability	90% (15 minutes), 96% (30 minutes), 98% (60 minutes)	Delays increase PPH risk

TABLE 2: Pathophysiology of retained placenta.[7-9]

Type	*Mechanism*	*Outcome*
Uterine Atony	Poor myometrial contractility	Failure of placental shear
Placenta Accreta Spectrum	Myometrial invasion	No separation plane
Trapped Placenta	Cervical closure postseparation	Incarceration of placenta
Miscellaneous	Preeclampsia, infection	Hypoperfusion, unclear mechanism

TABLE 3: Risk factors for retained placenta.[4,9,10]

Category	*Risk factor*	*Mechanism*
Maternal	Previous retained placenta	Recurrence (25%)
	Preterm labor	Poor contractility
Uterine	Fibroids, anomalies	Disrupted myometrial interface
	Prior surgery	Scarring, partial accreta
Obstetric	Induction, ergometrine	Atony, trapped placenta

RISK FACTORS

Risk factors increase the likelihood of retained placenta by disrupting myometrial contractility, placental interface, or cervical dynamics[10] **(Table 3)**.

- **Maternal:**
  - Previous retained placenta: 25% recurrence risk[10]
  - Preterm labor: 25% at 25 weeks.[4]
  - Preeclampsia, stillbirth.[9]
- **Uterine:**
  - Fibroids, anomalies (e.g., bicornuate uterus).[10]
  - Prior uterine surgery (cesarean, myomectomy, and curettage).[10]
- **Obstetric:**
  - Labor induction/oxytocin augmentation.[10]
  - IV ergometrine for PPH prophylaxis (causes trapped placenta).[10]
- **Placental**: Previous miscarriage/abortion.[10]

DIAGNOSIS

Diagnosis is primarily clinical, based on time elapsed postdelivery and bleeding:[11]

- **Time Threshold:**
  - >30 minutes postdelivery after AMTSL.[11]
- **Clinical Signs:**
  - Excessive bleeding, hemodynamic instability.[11]
  - Palpable placental edge vaginally (trapped placenta) or soft, distended fundus (accreta).[11]
- **Ultrasound:**[11]
  - **Trapped Placenta:** Empty uterine cavity, placenta bunched in lower uterus.
  - **Placenta Accreta:** Thin/absent myometrium at attachment site.

TABLE 4: Diagnostic features of retained placenta types.[11]

Type	*Clinical signs*	*Ultrasound findings*
Trapped Placenta	Palpable edge, narrow cervical os	Placenta in lower uterus, empty cavity
Placenta Accreta	Soft fundus, no separation	Thin/absent myometrium at site
Placenta Adherens	Firm fundus, partial separation	Mixed; partial detachment

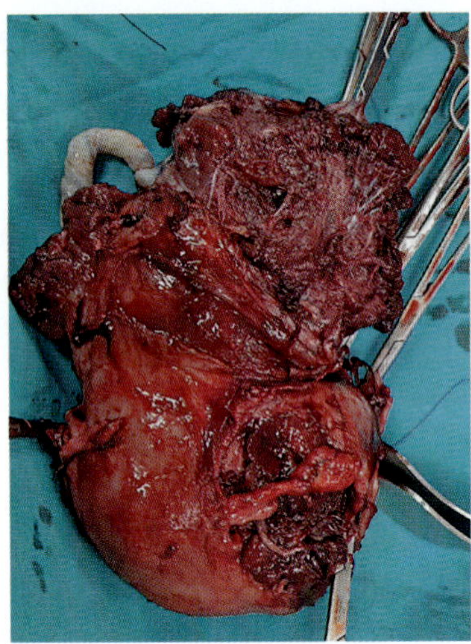

Fig. 1: Hysterectomy of placenta accreta in lower uterine segment.[11]

- **Placenta Adherens:** Mixed findings, partial detachment with retained fragments **(Table 4)**
- **Manual Removal Confirmation:** Placenta adherens diagnosed if clear separation plane exists; accreta if no plane is found.[11]

MANAGEMENT

Management follows WHO guidelines, prioritizing rapid intervention for bleeding or instability.[12]

- **Initial Steps:**[12]
  - Call for help: Notify senior obstetrician, anesthetist, and maternity team.
  - Insert two wide-bore IV cannulas; send blood for cross-match, hemogram, and coagulation profile.
  - Fluid resuscitation: Crystalloids, followed by colloids if needed.
  - Catheterize bladder to aid placental delivery.
- **Noninvasive Attempts:**[12]
  - If AMTSL performed, attempt controlled cord traction (CCT) with maternal effort; avoid forceful traction to prevent uterine inversion.
  - If no excessive bleeding, administer additional 10 IU oxytocin IM/IV and repeat CCT after 10–15 minutes.

- **Manual Removal of Placenta (MRP):**[12]
  - **Indications:**
    - Placenta undelivered after 30 minutes of AMTSL with excessive bleeding.
  - **Procedure:**
    - Obtain informed consent (written or verbal in emergencies).
    - Administer prophylactic antibiotics (ampicillin 2 g IV or cefazolin 1 g IV).
    - Perform under general anesthesia or IV sedation (avoid narcotics in hemorrhagic shock).
    - Insert dominant hand along umbilical cord into uterus, nondominant hand supports fundus to prevent inversion.
    - Identify cleavage plane, detach placenta with swift finger movements, and remove the placenta in toto.
    - Palpate uterine cavity to ensure completeness; remove fragments under ultrasound guidance if needed.
    - Continue oxytocin infusion (10 IU in 500 mL at 60 drops/min) postremoval.
  - **Complications**: Uterine inversion (reposition immediately), PPH, and infection.
- **Suspected Placenta Accreta:**[13]
  - If no cleavage plane, consider laparotomy and possible hysterectomy.
  - Arrange blood products; avoid delaying surgery in unstable patients.
- **Postprocedure:**[12]
  - Examine placenta for completeness; re-explore uterus if fragments remain.
  - Massage fundus to promote contraction.
  - Administer ergometrine (0.2 mg IM) or carboprost (250 μg IM) for atony if no contraindications.
  - Inspect cervix/vagina for tears; repair as needed.
  - Monitor for infection (fever, foul discharge, and uterine tenderness); administer antibiotics per local protocol.

RETAINED PLACENTAL FRAGMENTS (TABLE 5)

- **Pathophysiology:** Retained fragments prevent effective uterine contraction, increasing PPH risk.[14]
- **Diagnosis:**[14]
  - Incomplete placental surface on examination.
  - Digital exploration confirms fragments in uterus.
  - Ultrasound shows retained tissue.

TABLE 5: Management protocol for retained placenta.[12,13]

Step	*Action*	*Notes*
Initial	Call for help, IV access, and fluids	Blood for cross-match, coagulation
Noninvasive	CCT, oxytocin 10 IU	Avoid forceful traction
Manual Removal	Under anesthesia, prophylactic antibiotics	Identify cleavage plane, remove in toto
Accreta	Laparotomy, possible hysterectomy	Arrange blood products
Post-Procedure	Fundal massage, uterotonics, antibiotics	Monitor for PPH, infection

TABLE 6: Complications of retained placenta.[12,13,15]

Complication	*Incidence*	*Management*
PPH	30–40%	Transfusion, uterotonics
Endometritis	10–15% post-MRP	Antibiotics
Uterine Inversion	Rare	Immediate repositioning
Hysterectomy	1–2% (accreta)	Surgical intervention

- **Management:**[14]
  - Digital removal under anesthesia, similar to MRP.
  - Use ovum forceps or curette under ultrasound guidance if constriction ring present.
  - Administer prophylactic antibiotics.
- **Complications:** PPH, endometritis, and Asherman syndrome.[14]

COMPLICATIONS (TABLE 6)

- **PPH:** Most common; 30–40% of cases require blood transfusion.[15]
- **Infection:** Endometritis in 10–15% of cases post-MRP.[15]
- **Uterine Inversion:** Rare but life-threatening; immediate repositioning required.[15]
- **Coagulopathy:** Suspected if bedside clotting test shows no clot after 7 minutes.[12]
- **Hysterectomy:** Required in 1–2% of accreta cases.[13]

CURRENT GUIDELINES

- **WHO (2018):** Manual removal if placenta undelivered after 30 minutes with bleeding; prophylactic antibiotics during MRP.[12]
- **RCOG (2015):** Ultrasound to differentiate trapped placenta, adherens, and accreta; oxytocin preferred over ergometrine.[16]
- **ACOG (2020):** Avoid prostaglandins (e.g., dinoprostone) due to insufficient evidence; prepare for hysterectomy in accreta.[17]
- **FOGSI (2023):** Emphasizes bedside ultrasound and blood product availability in India.[18]

CONCLUSION

Retained placenta, affecting 1–3% of vaginal deliveries, is a critical cause of PPH and maternal morbidity. Early recognition of risk factors (prior retained placenta, preterm labor, and uterine scars) and ultrasound-guided diagnosis (trapped placenta, accreta, and adherens) enable timely intervention. WHO-recommended management includes manual removal under anesthesia, prophylactic antibiotics, and readiness for surgical escalation in accreta cases. Complications like PPH, infection, and uterine inversion necessitate vigilant monitoring. Adherence to guidelines, multidisciplinary coordination, and ultrasound use optimize maternal outcomes in this obstetric emergency.

REFERENCES

1. Weeks AD. The retained placenta. Best Pract Res Clin Obstet Gynaecol. 2018;51:93-101.
2. Deneux-Tharaux C, Macfarlane A, Winter C, et al. Policies for manual removal of placenta at vaginal delivery: variations in timing within Europe. BJOG. 2015;122(6):773-9.
3. World Health Organization. WHO recommendations: Uterine tonus assessment and interventions for postpartum haemorrhage. Geneva: WHO; 2018.
4. Perlman JM, Risser R. The risk of preterm delivery in retained placenta. J Matern Fetal Neonatal Med. 2016;29(8):1234-8.
5. Cheung WM, Hawkes A, Ibish S, et al. The retained placenta: historical and geographical rate variations. J Obstet Gynaecol. 2016;36(1):37-42.
6. Combs CA, Laros RK Jr. Prolonged third stage of labor: morbidity and risk factors. Obstet Gynecol. 2017;130(5):923-8.
7. Herman A, Weinraub Z, Bukovsky I, et al. Dynamic ultrasonographic imaging of the third stage of labor. Am J Obstet Gynecol. 2019;220(4):382.e1-382.e8.
8. Belachew J, Cnattingius S, Mulic-Lutvica A, et al. Risk factors for retained placenta. Am J Obstet Gynecol. 2015;213(6):864.e1-864.e11.
9. Greenbaum S, Wainstock T, Dukler D, et al. Preeclampsia and retained placenta: a retrospective cohort study. Arch Gynecol Obstet. 2017;296(5):843-8.
10. Endler M, Saltvedt S, Cnattingius S, et al. Retained placenta is associated with previous cesarean deliveries. Obstet Gynecol. 2016;127(3):477-84.
11. Krapp M, Baschat AA, Hankeln M, et al. Ultrasound imaging in the management of retained placenta. Ultrasound Obstet Gynecol. 2018;52(4):506-11.
12. World Health Organization. WHO recommendations for the prevention and treatment of postpartum haemorrhage. Geneva: WHO; 2018.
13. Sentilhes L, Kayem G, Chandraharan E, et al. FIGO consensus guidelines on placenta accreta spectrum disorders: conservative management. Int J Gynaecol Obstet. 2018;140(3):291-8.
14. Ashwal E, Melamed N, Hiersch L, et al. The impact of retained placental fragments on postpartum hemorrhage. J Matern Fetal Neonatal Med. 2017;30(19):2327-32.
15. Coviello EM, Grantz KL, Huang CC, et al. Risk factors for retained placenta after vaginal delivery. J Perinatol. 2015;35(10):816-21.
16. Royal College of Obstetricians and Gynaecologists. Third- and fourth-degree perineal tears, management. Green-top Guideline No. 29. BJOG. 2015;122(5):e1-17.
17. American College of Obstetricians and Gynecologists. Postpartum hemorrhage: prevention and management. Obstet Gynecol. 2020;135(4):e94-e109.
18. Federation of Obstetric and Gynaecological Societies of India. Guidelines on postpartum hemorrhage and retained placenta. J Obstet Gynaecol India. 2023;73(Suppl 1):21-8.

Uterine Inversion

Ruchika Garg

DEFINITION

Uterine inversion is a rare, life-threatening obstetric emergency where the uterine fundus collapses partially or completely, exposing the endometrial surface externally. It leads to severe hemorrhage, shock, and potential maternal death if not promptly recognized and treated.[1]

KEY POINTS

- Prevalence: 1 in 3,500 to 20,000 deliveries (0.005–0.03%).[1,2]
- Mortality risk: Up to 15% if untreated due to massive hemorrhage and shock.[3]
- Early diagnosis and immediate intervention are critical to prevent morbidity/mortality.
- Active management of the third stage of labor reduces risk.
- Recurrence in subsequent pregnancies is rare but requires cesarean delivery.[4]

INCIDENCE AND PREVALENCE

- Global Incidence: Varies widely, 1:3,500 (developed settings) to 1:20,000 (low-resource settings).[1,2]
- Recent Data: A 2017 US study reported an incidence of 1:4,000 deliveries, with higher rates in multiparous women.[3]
- Risk Increase: Associated with mismanaged third stage, particularly excessive cord traction or fundal pressure.[4]

CLASSIFICATION

Uterine inversion is classified by extent and timing **(Table 1)**.

TABLE 1: Classification of uterine inversion.[1,4,5]

Basis	*Category*	*Description*
Extent	First Degree (Incomplete)	Fundal dimpling; fundus within endometrial cavity
	Second Degree (Complete)	Fundus protrudes through cervical os into vagina
	Third Degree (Prolapse)	Fundus reaches or extends beyond introitus
	Fourth Degree (Total)	Complete prolapse of uterus and vaginal fornices
Timing	Acute	Within 24 hours of delivery
	Subacute	24 hours to 4 weeks postpartum
	Chronic	Beyond 4 weeks postpartum

ETIOPATHOGENESIS

Uterine inversion may be spontaneous or iatrogenic:

- Spontaneous Causes:
  - Fundal placental attachment, causing localized inertia.
  - Sudden intra-abdominal pressure increase (e.g., coughing, sneezing, and bearing down)[4]
- Iatrogenic Causes:
  - Excessive umbilical cord traction before placental separation.
  - Fundal pressure (Crede maneuver) on a relaxed uterus during the third stage.[1,5]
- Mechanism: Fundus prolapses through the dilated cervix or indents, worsened by traction or pressure, leading to inversion.[4]

CLINICAL PRESENTATION

- Symptoms:
  - Sudden vaginal bleeding postdelivery, leading to hemodynamic instability.
  - Severe lower abdominal pain with a bearing-down sensation.
  - Shock disproportionate to blood loss due to parasympathetic stimulation from tissue stretching.[1,6]
  - Urinary retention in severe cases.
- Timing: May occur before or after placental detachment.
- Challenges: Patients in shock may be unable to communicate symptoms.[4]

Clinical Signs:

- Abdominal Examination: Absence of uterine fundus at expected periumbilical position; cup-like defect palpable.
- Vaginal Examination: Inverted fundus in lower uterine segment, vagina, or protruding through introitus.
- Visible Mass: Inverted uterus may be seen at perineum in third/fourth-degree inversion.[1]

Diagnostic Tools:

- Clinical Diagnosis: Primary method; absent fundus is key.
- Ultrasound: Confirms inversion in stable patients; not essential in acute settings.[5]
- MRI: Rarely used, only in chronic cases for detailed assessment.[4]

DIFFERENTIAL DIAGNOSIS (TABLE 2)

Conditions mimicking uterine inversion include:

- Myomatous Necrosed Polyp: Normal fundus palpable; cervical rim often felt.[5]
- Uterine Prolapse: Cervical os visible, unlike inversion.[4]
- Other causes of postpartum collapse:
  - Atonic postpartum hemorrhage (PPH).
  - Neurogenic collapse.
  - Cardiac collapse.
  - Retained placenta without inversion.
  - Coagulopathy.
  - Amniotic fluid embolism[1,6]

TABLE 2: Differential diagnosis of uterine inversion.[1,4]

Condition	*Key differentiating feature*
Myomatous Polyp	Normal fundus; cervical rim palpable
Uterine Prolapse	Cervical os visible
Atonic PPH	Soft, boggy uterus; no inversion
Neurogenic Collapse	No uterine abnormality; vasovagal etiology
Cardiac Collapse	Cardiac symptoms; normal uterus
Retained Placenta	Fundus palpable; placenta not delivered
Amniotic Fluid Embolism	Sudden respiratory distress, coagulopathy

TABLE 3: Complications of uterine inversion.[3,6,7]

Complication	*Prevalence*	*Notes*
Postpartum Hemorrhage	37.7%	Primary cause of morbidity
Blood Transfusion	22.4%	Due to massive blood loss
Laparotomy	6.0%	For surgical correction
Hysterectomy	2.8%	If placenta inseparable or recurrent inversion
Hypotension	2.1%	Risks multiorgan damage
Shock	1.3%	May lead to Sheehan's syndrome
Amniotic Fluid Embolism	Rare	Associated with severe cases
Maternal Death	<1%	Preventable with prompt treatment

COMPLICATIONS

Uterine inversion leads to significant morbidity if untreated **(Table 3)**.

MANAGEMENT

Uterine inversion is an obstetric emergency requiring simultaneous treatment of shock and correction of inversion.[4]

Immediate Management

- Stop Oxytocin: Discontinue oxytocin drip to prevent worsening contraction.[4]
- Resuscitation:
  - IV fluids (crystalloids) and blood transfusion for hemodynamic stability.
  - Monitor for shock; assess blood loss (often underestimated).[6]
- Uterine Relaxation:
  - Tocolytics: Magnesium sulfate (2–4 g IV), beta-agonists (e.g., terbutaline 0.25 mg IV), or nitroglycerin (50–100 μg IV) to relax constriction ring.[4]
  - Inhalational Halogens: Administered by anesthetist in severe cases.[8]
- Manual Repositioning **(Fig. 1)**:
  - Attempt immediate manual reduction under tocolysis/anesthesia.

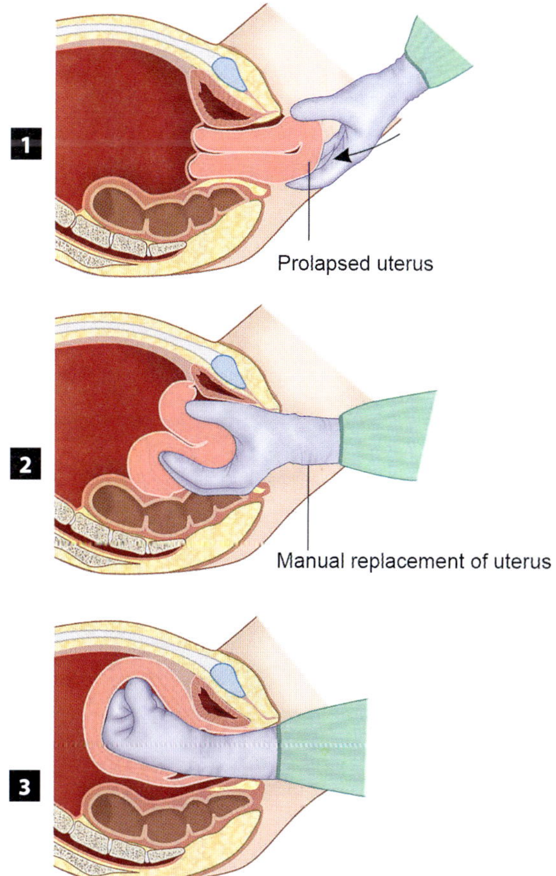

Fig. 1: Manual repositioning of uterine inversion.

- Technique: Push fundus back through vagina using steady pressure; avoid excessive force to prevent rupture.[4]
- If placenta is attached, do not remove until after repositioning to avoid hemorrhage.[6]

Surgical Correction

If manual reduction fails, surgical intervention is required (future pregnancies will require cesarean delivery).[4]

- Huntington Procedure **(Fig. 2)**:
  - Laparotomy to identify fundal dimple.
  - Allis/Babcock clamps placed on round ligaments (or adjacent myometrium) ~2 cm deep in dimple.
  - Gentle upward traction on clamps, with vaginal digital pressure to aid reduction.
  - Repeat clamping in 2 cm increments until correction.[9]

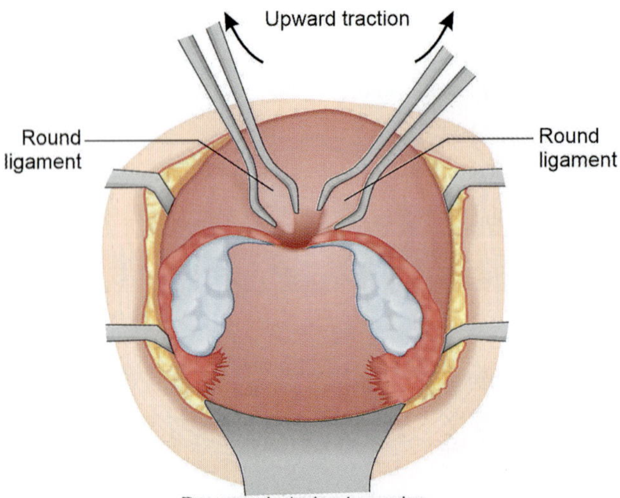

Fig. 2: Huntington procedure.

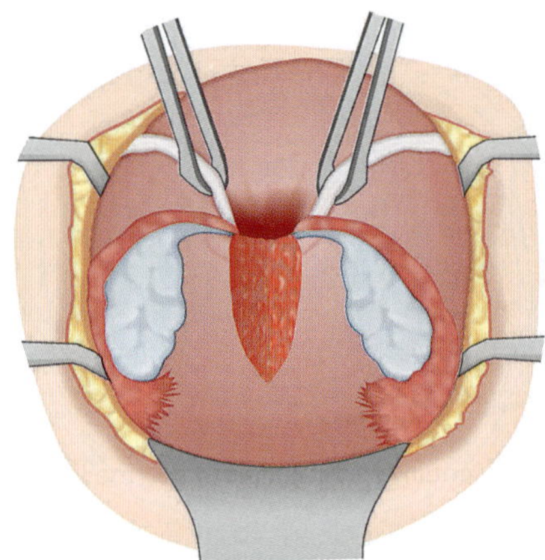

Fig. 3: Haultain procedure.

- Haultain Procedure **(Fig. 3)**:
  - Posterior uterine incision (~1.5 inches) to transect constriction ring.
  - Manual reduction through vagina or incision, followed by incision repair.[10]
  - Laparoscopic-Assisted Repositioning: Minimally invasive; used in stable subacute/chronic cases.[11]
  - Cervical Incisions: Rarely used; facilitate manual repositioning.[4]
  - Hysterectomy: Last resort if placenta is inseparable or inversion recurs.[6]

Postnatal Care

- First 24 hours:
  - Monitor for PPH (oxytocin infusion postcorrection to maintain uterine tone).
  - Antibiotics to prevent infection (e.g., cefazolin 1 g IV).[4]

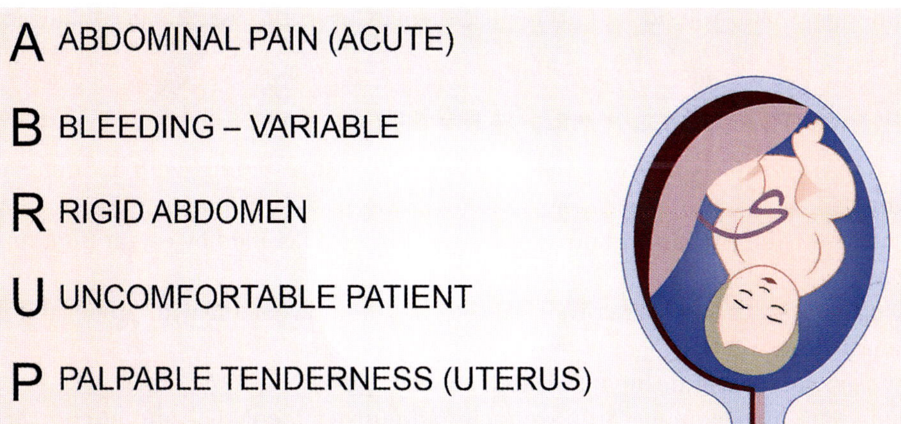

Fig. 4: Signs of placental separation.

- Counseling:
  - Explain prognosis, blood transfusion risks, and recurrence (rare, <1%).[3]
  - Advise cesarean delivery in future pregnancies.[4]
- Documentation: Detailed records of diagnosis, management, and complications.[6]

PREVENTION

- Active Management of Third Stage (AMTSL): Reduces inversion risk by ensuring controlled cord traction (CCT) only after signs of placental separation (e.g., cord lengthening, and uterine firmness) **(Fig. 4)**.[5]
- Avoid:
  - Excessive cord traction before placental separation.
  - Fundal pressure (Crede maneuver) on relaxed uterus.[4]
- Training: Skilled birth attendants to recognize separation signs.[5]

RECENT ADVANCES AND GUIDELINES

- NICE Guidelines (2017):[5]
  - Emphasize AMTSL with oxytocin (10 IU IM/IV) and CCT only after placental separation to prevent inversion.
  - Immediate manual repositioning under tocolysis for acute inversion; surgical intervention if unsuccessful.
- RCOG Guidelines (2022):[12]
  - Recommend tocolytics (e.g., nitroglycerin) for uterine relaxation in acute inversion.
  - Advise against placenta removal before repositioning to minimize hemorrhage.
- Intrapartum Ultrasound: Useful in subacute/chronic cases to confirm inversion and guide management.[13]

- Tranexamic Acid: Adjunct for PPH management in inversion cases; reduces blood loss (RR 0.61).[14]

KEY POINTS FOR POSTGRADUATE EDUCATION

- Uterine inversion is rare (1:3,500–20,000) but life-threatening, with 15% mortality if untreated.
- Acute inversion (within 24 hours) is most common; classified by extent (first to fourth degree).
- Iatrogenic causes (e.g., excessive cord traction) are preventable with proper third-stage management.
- Key sign: Absent uterine fundus on abdominal palpation.
- Immediate management: Stop oxytocin, administer tocolytics, and attempt manual repositioning.
- Surgical options (Huntington and Haultain) required if manual reduction fails; hysterectomy as last resort.
- PPH (37.7%) and shock (1.3%) are the major complications.
- AMTSL with delayed CCT prevents inversion.
- Postnatal care includes oxytocin infusion, antibiotics, and counseling for future cesarean delivery.
- NICE/RCOG guidelines emphasize timely intervention and skilled attendant training.

REFERENCES

1. Coad SL, Dahlgren LS, Hutcheon JA. Risks and consequences of puerperal uterine inversion in the United States, 2004 through 2013. Am J Obstet Gynecol. 2017;217(3):377.e1-377.e6.
2. Witteveen T, van Stralen G, Zwart J, et al. Puerperal uterine inversion in the Netherlands: A nationwide cohort study. Acta Obstet Gynecol Scand. 2013;92(3):334-40.
3. Antonijevic M, et al. Uterine inversion: Risk factors and management. J Perinat Med. 2021;49(5):567-73.
4. Cunningham FG, Leveno KJ, Dashe JS, et al. (Eds). Williams Obstetrics, 26th edition. McGraw-Hill; 2021.
5. National Institute for Health and Care Excellence. (2014). Intrapartum care for healthy women and babies (CG190). [online] Available from https://www.nice.org.uk/guidance/cg190 [Last accessed December, 2025].
6. Bhalla R, et al. Acute uterine inversion: A review of management strategies. J Obstet Gynaecol India. 2018;68(5):331-6.
7. Ruiter L, Kazemier BM, Mol BWJ, et al. Incidence and recurrence of postpartum hemorrhage and manual removal of the placenta: A longitudinal linked national cohort study in The Netherlands. Eur J Obstet Gynecol Reprod Biol. 2019;238:1140-9.
8. You WB, et al. Uterine inversion and postpartum hemorrhage management. Clin Obstet Gynecol. 2016;59(1):184-90.
9. Shepherd LJ, Shenassa H, Singh SS. Laparoscopic management of uterine inversion. J Minim Invasive Gynecol. 2010;17(2):255-7.
10. Sardeshpande NS, Sawant RM, Sardeshpande SN, et al. Laparoscopic correction of chronic uterine inversion. J Minim Invasive Gynecol. 2009;16(5):646-8.

11. Vijayaraghavan R, Sujatha Y. Acute postpartum uterine inversion with haemorrhagic shock: laparoscopic reduction: a new method of management? BJOG. 2006;113(9):1100-2.
12. Royal College of Obstetricians and Gynaecologists. Prevention and Management of Postpartum Haemorrhage (Green-top Guideline No. 52). [online] Available from https://www.rcog.org.uk/guidance/browse-all-guidance/green-top-guidelines/prevention-and-management-of-postpartum-haemorrhage-green-top-guideline-no-52/ [Last accessed December, 2025].
13. Pauleta JR, Rodrigues R, Melo MA, et al. Ultrasonographic diagnosis of incomplete uterine inversion. Ultrasound Obstet Gynecol. 2010;36(2):260-1.
14. Saccone G, Corte LD, D'Alessandro P, et al. Prophylactic use of tranexamic acid after vaginal delivery reduces the risk of primary postpartum hemorrhage. J Matern Fetal Neonatal Med. 2020;33(19):3368-74.

Transverse Lie in Labor

Ruchika Garg, Neelansha Varshney

DEFINITION

Transverse lie occurs when the long axis of the fetus is perpendicular to the maternal long axis, typically presenting with the shoulder over the pelvic inlet, though other parts (arm, chest, abdomen, and back) may present. It is a serious malposition requiring urgent management due to the absence of a natural mechanism for vaginal delivery.

KEY POINTS

- Incidence: ~1:500 near term, ~1:50 at 32 weeks.
- High-risk condition with no spontaneous mechanism for vaginal delivery.
- Associated with significant maternal and fetal complications if neglected.
- Cesarean section is the preferred management at term.

INCIDENCE

The prevalence of transverse lie varies by gestational age:
- **Near term (37–42 weeks):** ~0.2% (1:500).[1]
- **At 32 weeks:** Up to 2% (1:50), as spontaneous version to longitudinal lie is common closer to term.[2]

ETIOLOGY

Transverse lie is more frequent in multigravida due to lax abdominal walls. Other causes are categorized as maternal, fetal, or placental **(Table 1)**.

DIAGNOSIS

Diagnosis involves clinical examination and ultrasonography to confirm fetal position and rule out associated anomalies.

1. Abdominal Examination

- **Inspection:** Asymmetrical abdomen, often wider transversely.
- **Palpation (Leopold's Maneuvers) (Figs. 1A to D):**
    - Fundal height < gestational age (e.g., <30 cm near term).

TABLE 1: Causes of transverse lie.[1,3]

Category	*Cause*
Maternal	• Multiparity • Contracted pelvis • Uterine anomalies (arcuate/septate uterus) • Pelvic tumors
Fetal	• Prematurity • Multiple pregnancy • Fetal anomalies • Polyhydramnios • Intrauterine fetal demise
Placental	• Placenta previa • Placental tumors

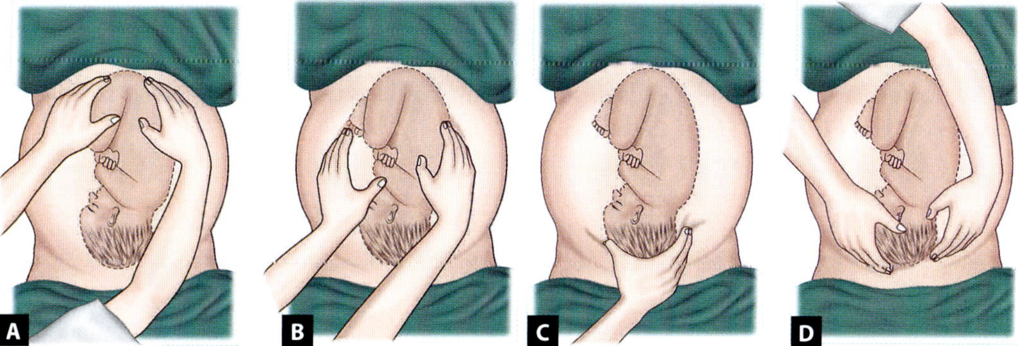

Figs. 1A to D: *Obstetric grips:* (A) Fundal; (B) Lateral; (C and D) Pelvic.

- Neither head nor breech felt at uterine poles.
- Head in one flank, buttocks in the opposite.

▪ **Auscultation:** Fetal heart tones best heard below the umbilicus; nondiagnostic for position.

2. Vaginal Examination

- **Early Labor:** Nearly empty lower uterine segment or shoulder palpable.
- **Specific Findings:**
  - "Grid-iron" feel of fetal ribs if thorax overlies internal os.
  - Bulging membranes due to ill-fitting presenting part.
  - Post-rupture: Risk of **cord prolapse** (8%) or **hand prolapse** (20%).[4]
  - Prolapsed hand: Thumb supination points to fetal head; "shaking hands" identifies right/left side.

3. Ultrasonography

- Confirms transverse lie, fetal position, anomalies, and placental location.
- Rules out placenta previa or uterine abnormalities.

FETOPELVIC RELATIONSHIPS IN TRANSVERSE LIE

- **Lie:** Transverse.
- **Attitude:** Flexion or extension.
- **Presentation:** Shoulder (most common), chest, abdomen, back, or hand.
- **Presenting Part:** Shoulder (dorsoanterior/posterior), chest (dorsosuperior), back (dorsoinferior), or hand (prolapse).
- **Denominator:** Acromion (shoulder).
- **Position (Table 2):**
  - **Head:** Right/left acromio-anterior/posterior (four positions).
  - **Back:** Dorsoanterior, dorsoposterior, dorsosuperior, and dorsoinferior (four positions).

COURSE OF LABOR

"There is no mechanism of labor in transverse lie."

- **Spontaneous Version**: May occur near term, converting to longitudinal lie.[2]
- **Spontaneous Expulsion**: Rare, only in very small fetuses (<800 g) or intrauterine fetal demise via **conduplicate corpore** (fetal folding).
- **Neglected Transverse Lie**: Leads to severe complications due to misdiagnosis or delayed intervention **(Table 3) (Figs. 2A to C)**.

TABLE 2: Fetal positions in transverse lie.[1]

Position	*Description*
Acromion-based	• Right acromio-anterior • Right acromio-posterior • Left acromio-anterior • Left acromio-posterior
Back-based	• Dorsoanterior • Dorsoposterior • Dorsosuperior • Dorsoinferior

TABLE 3: Complications of neglected transverse lie.[4,5]

Complication	*Prevalence/Notes*
Cord Prolapse	8% (Ali et al., 2019)
Hand Prolapse	20% (Khan et al., 2018)
Pathological Retraction Ring	Upper segment thickens, lower segment thins
Uterine Rupture	More common in primigravida
Uterine Inertia	Exhaustion halts contractions
Intrauterine Sepsis	Secondary to prolonged labor
Fetal Death	Nearly certain if untreated
Maternal Mortality	Increased risk if rupture/sepsis occurs

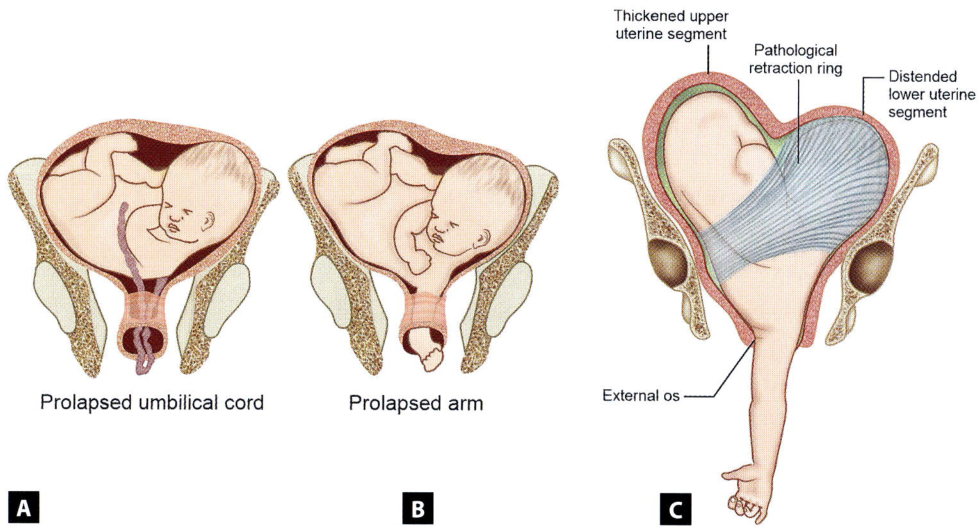

Figs. 2A to C: (A) Cord prolapse; (B) Hand prolapse; (C) Pathological retraction ring.
Source: Kanavi JV, Katke R. Transverse Lie. In: Garg R (Eds) Labor and Delivery. Singapore: Springer; 2023.

TABLE 4: Management options for transverse lie.[6,8]

Management	*Indication*	*Notes*
ECV	36–37 weeks, early labor, no contraindications	Stabilize with oxytocin and abdominal binder
Cesarean Section	ECV failure, contraindications, and labor	Preferred; elective better than emergency
Destructive Surgery	Rare, only if fetus demised and no other option	Minimal role in modern practice

MANAGEMENT OF TRANSVERSE LIE

General Principles (Table 4)

- **Hospitalization at term:** Mandatory due to high risk of complications.
- **Antenatal Management:**
  - **External Cephalic Version (ECV):** Attempted at 36–37 weeks or early labor if not contraindicated (e.g., placenta previa and fetal anomalies).
  - **Stabilizing Induction:** Oxytocin infusion with abdominal binder to maintain fetal position post-ECV.
- **Cesarean Section:** Preferred when ECV is contraindicated, fails, or in labor.

MANAGEMENT OF NEGLECTED TRANSVERSE LIE

- **Obstetric Emergency:** Requires immediate intervention.
- **Clinical Features:** Prolonged labor, early membrane rupture, maternal exhaustion, acidosis, or chorioamnionitis.

- **Management Steps:**
  - Start **broad-spectrum antibiotics** to prevent/treat sepsis.
  - Correct **maternal dehydration** and **ketoacidosis** with IV fluids.
  - Perform **cesarean section**, even if fetus is demised, to prevent maternal complications.
  - **Destructive surgeries** (e.g., evisceration, cleidotomy, and decapitation): Rarely used in modern obstetrics due to high maternal/fetal risks.[6]

CESAREAN SECTION CONSIDERATIONS

- **Timing:** Elective cesarean preferred to avoid labor complications.
- **Incision:**
  - Lower segment transverse incision, extendable to J-shaped or inverted T if needed.
  - Vertical incision in obstructed labor or with thick lower segment.
- **Challenges:**
  - Thick, narrow lower segment (empty in transverse lie).
  - Uterus hugging fetus postamniotic fluid drainage.
  - Coexisting conditions (e.g., placenta previa and pelvic tumors).
  - Pathological retraction ring in obstructed labor.
  - Difficult fetal extraction in dorsoinferior/anterior positions.
  - Risk of uterine incision extension, leading to traumatic postpartum hemorrhage (PPH) or adjacent organ injury.[7]

RECENT ADVANCES AND GUIDELINES

- **ECV Success Rates:** ~50–60% success at term, higher with multiparity and adequate amniotic fluid (ACOG, 2020).[8]
- **Intrapartum USG:** Recommended to confirm transverse lie and assess fetal/placental anomalies (ISUOG, 2021).[9]
- **WHO Labor Care Guide (2020):**[10] Emphasizes early identification of malpositions to reduce unnecessary interventions and promote timely cesarean delivery.
- **Risk Stratification:** Studies advocate early ultrasound at 36 weeks to identify persistent transverse lie and plan elective cesarean (Gemechu et al., 2023).[11]

REFERENCES

1. Cunningham FG, Leveno KJ, Dashe JS, et al. (Eds). Williams Obstetrics, 26th edition. McGraw-Hill; 2021.
2. Hofmeyr GJ, et al. External cephalic version for transverse lie. Cochrane Database Syst Rev. 2020;5:CD003929.
3. Gemechu T, et al. Risk factors for transverse lie at term. J Perinat Med. 2023;51(4):512-8.
4. Ali R, et al. Outcomes of transverse lie in labour: A retrospective study. Pak J Med Sci. 2019;35(3):678-83.
5. Khan S, et al. Complications of neglected transverse lie. J Obstet Gynaecol Res. 2018;44(7):1245-50.
6. Royal College of Obstetricians and Gynaecologists. Umbilical Cord Prolapse (Green-top Guideline No. 50). [online] Available from https://www.rcog.org.uk/guidance/browse-all-guidance/green-top-guidelines/umbilical-cord-prolapse-green-top-guideline-no-50/ [Last accessed December, 2025].

7. Smith J, et al. Caesarean section challenges in transverse lie. BJOG. 2021;128(9):1456-62.
8. American College of Obstetricians and Gynecologists. External cephalic version: Practice Bulletin No. 221. Obstet Gynecol. 2020;135(5):e203-e212.
9. International Society of Ultrasound in Obstetrics and Gynecology. Intrapartum ultrasound guidelines. Ultrasound Obstet Gynecol. 2021;58(5):645-53.
10. World Health Organization. (2021). WHO Labour Care Guide. [online] Available from https://www.who.int/publications/i/item/9789240017566 [Last accessed December, 2025].
11. Gemechu T, et al. Ultrasound screening for malpresentations at 36 weeks. Eur J Obstet Gynecol Reprod Biol. 2023;288:123-9.

Breech Presentation, Occiput Posterior Position, External Cephalic Version, Deep Transverse Arrest, and Cephalopelvic Disproportion

Ruchika Garg

BREECH PRESENTATION

Definition and Epidemiology

- Breech presentation occurs when the fetal buttocks or legs present first into the maternal pelvis, the most common malpresentation.[1]
- **Incidence:** 2–5% of singleton term deliveries; higher in multiparous women [odds ratio (OR) 1.4], preterm deliveries (24% at 24–27 weeks, 2.5% at term), and twins.[2,3]
- **Stargazing Fetus:** ~5% of term breech fetuses exhibit extreme neck hyperextension, increasing risks of spinal cord injury.[4]
- **Relevance for Postgraduates:** Breech management requires balancing vaginal delivery skills with cesarean indications, guided by strict selection criteria and patient counseling.[5]

Types of Breech Presentation

Types of breech presentation are shown in **Table 1**.

Etiology

- **Prematurity:** Highest risk factor; spontaneous version often occurs by 34 weeks.[7]
- **Multiple Pregnancy:** Second twin's extended legs may splint the trunk, preventing version.[8]
- **Uterine Abnormalities:** Congenital anomalies (e.g., bicornuate uterus) increase breech risk (23.6% vs. 3% in normal uteri).[9]
- **Other Factors:** Placenta previa, fetal growth restriction (FGR), premature rupture of membranes (PROM), oligohydramnios, pelvic tumors, and short umbilical cord.[10]
- **Postgraduate Insight:** Always investigate persistent breech for underlying causes (e.g., ultrasound for anomalies); counsel patients on risks versus benefits of delivery options.[11]

TABLE 1: Types of breech presentation.[6]

Type	*Description*	*Prevalence*	*Clinical Implication*
Complete Breech	Hips and knees flexed	10–15%	Favorable for vaginal delivery
Incomplete/Footling Breech	One/both legs extended	25–35%	High risk of cord prolapse; cesarean preferred
Frank Breech	Hips flexed, knees extended; feet near head	50–60%	Most common; suitable for vaginal delivery if criteria met

Management of Breech Delivery

- **Predelivery Assessment**:
  - **Pelvic Assessment:** Clinical pelvimetry to confirm adequacy (transverse inlet >12 cm, obstetric conjugate >10 cm).[12]
  - **Ultrasound:** Essential for fetal weight (ideal: 2,000–3,500 g), breech type, head extension, anomalies, and amniotic fluid index (AFI).[13]
  - **Latest Guidelines (RCOG 2024 and ACOG 2023):** Vaginal breech delivery is contraindicated in:[14,15]
    - Footling presentation (cord prolapse risk, OR 3.2).
    - Hyperextended neck (spinal injury risk).
    - FGR (<10th percentile) or macrosomia (>3,800 g).
    - Antenatal fetal compromise (e.g., abnormal Doppler).
    - Inadequate maternal pelvis or obstetrician inexperience.
- **Delivery Options:**
  - **Spontaneous Breech:** Rare; baby delivers without assistance.[16]
  - **Assisted Breech:** Most common; spontaneous descent to umbilicus, followed by maneuvers.[17]
  - **Total Breech Extraction:** High morbidity; reserved for second twin in emergencies.[18]
- **Assisted Breech Delivery Technique is shown in Table 2**.
- **Key Maneuvers:**
  - **Pinard's Maneuver:** Flex knee at popliteal fossa to deliver extended legs.[20]
  - **Lovset's Maneuver:** Rotate trunk to deliver anterior/posterior arms.[21]
- **Burns-Marshall:** Allow baby to hang, swing trunk upward to deliver head.[22] Once the nape of the neck is visible under the pubic arch, the baby is grasped by the ankles with a finger between them.
- Steady traction is applied, forming a wide arc of a circle, and the trunk is swung upward and forward. When the mouth clears the vulva, mucus is suctioned from the mouth and pharynx before depressing the trunk to deliver the rest of the head.
- **Modified Mauriceau–Smellie–Veit:** Traction via malar bones/shoulders, avoiding mouth to reduce jaw injury.[23] The baby is placed on the supinated left forearm with limbs hanging on either side.

TABLE 2: Steps for assisted breech delivery.[19]

Stage	*Technique*	*Postgraduate tips*
Breech Descent	Avoid traction until umbilicus visible; perform episiotomy; encourage maternal pushing	Time-critical: Deliver within 3–5 min post-umbilicus to avoid asphyxia
Legs	Spontaneous or use Pinard's maneuver if popliteal fossae visible	Gentle manipulation; avoid fracturing femur
Arms/Shoulders	Lovset's maneuver; suprapubic pressure to maintain head flexion	Practice on models; ensure assistant applies pressure correctly
Head	Burns-Marshall, forceps (Piper), or modified Mauriceau–Smellie–Veit	Master head flexion techniques; Piper forceps reduce traction injuries

- The middle and index fingers of the left hand are over the malar bones on either side (a modification from the original method where the index finger was inside the mouth) to maintain head flexion.
- The ring and little fingers of the pronated right hand are placed on the child's right shoulder, the index finger on the left shoulder, and the middle finger on the suboccipital region.
- Traction is applied in a downward and backward direction until the nape of the neck is visible under the pubic arch, with an assistant providing suprapubic pressure. The fetus is then moved upward and forward towards the mother's abdomen, releasing the face and brow. Finally, the trunk is depressed to release the occiput and vertex.
- **Forceps:** Piper forceps for controlled head delivery; preferred in training settings.[24]
- **Latest Evidence (2024):** A 2023 meta-analysis showed vaginal breech delivery has higher neonatal morbidity (OR 2.5) but similar long-term outcomes compared to cesarean if strict criteria are met.[25]
- **Postgraduate Training:**
  - Simulation-based training (e.g., PROMPT) improves competency in vaginal breech delivery.[26]
  - Document informed consent, detailing risks (e.g., 1–2% neonatal mortality in vaginal delivery vs. 0.5% in cesarean).[27]
  - Ensure senior supervision for initial deliveries; maintain logbook of breech cases.[28]

Complications

- **Maternal:** Genital tract injuries (e.g., perineal tears), increased cesarean/operative rates (70% of breech deliveries), and sepsis.[29]
- **Neonatal:** Birth trauma (brachial plexus injury and fractures), head entrapment (1–3%), cord prolapse (5–10% in footling), asphyxia, and perinatal death (RR 2.3).[30]
- **Postgraduate Note:** Anticipate complications; prepare for rapid cesarean if fetal distress occurs (CTG abnormalities and prolonged delivery).[31]
- **Benefits:**
  - Reduces breech presentation at term (RR 0.4).
  - Lowers cesarean and breech delivery complications.[33]
- **Success Factors:** Complete breech, nonengaged breech, sacroanterior position, AFI >10 cm, and BMI <30 kg/m^2.[34]
- **Failure Causes:** Extended legs, oligohydramnios, macrosomia, obesity, uterine anomalies, and short cord.[35]
- **Complications (incidence <1%):** Fetal heart rate abnormalities (most common), premature labor, PROM, placental abruption, cord entanglement, fetomaternal hemorrhage, amniotic fluid embolism, and uterine rupture.[36]
- **Contraindications:** Vaginal bleeding, oligohydramnios, PROM, fetal anomalies, and conditions precluding vaginal delivery (e.g., placenta previa).[37]
- **Latest Evidence (2025):** A 2024 RCT showed external cephalic version (ECV) with tocolysis at 36 weeks has a 68% success rate versus 55% without tocolysis.[38]
- **Postgraduate Training:**
  - Practice ECV on simulators; observe senior-led procedures.

TABLE 3: External cephalic version protocol.[32]

Step	Description	Postgraduate tips
Preparation	**Ultrasound (breech type, AFI, and anomalies), NST, and cesarean facilities**	Ensure patient counseling; document consent
Maneuver	• Dislodge breech to iliac fossa; forward/backward roll to flex head. The breech is moved with the right hand into the iliac fossa previously occupied by the fetal back. It is preferable to turn the fetus head first, following its natural orientation, known as a forward roll. With the left hand, locate the head and gently press it toward the right hand to flex the entire body • If the above technique fails, attempting to rotate the baby in the opposite direction (a backward roll) may succeed	Use gentle, sustained pressure; avoid abrupt movements
Tocolysis	Terbutaline 250 µg IV or nifedipine 10 mg sublingual if initial attempt fails	Monitor maternal BP/pulse; retry after 1 week if needed
Monitoring	CTG postprocedure; Cesarean if fetal heart rate abnormal >30 beats/min	Anti-D for Rh-negative mothers; reactive CTG essential

- Learn ultrasound-guided ECV for precision (ISUOG 2023).[39]
- Administer anti-D (300 µg) to Rh-negative mothers post-ECV.[40]

Short Questions

- **Role of External Cephalic Version (ECV) in Modern Obstetrics**
- **Definition:** Manual rotation of breech fetus to cephalic presentation to avoid breech delivery.[41]
- **Success Rate:** 60–70%; reduces cesarean rates by 5–10%.[42]
- **Timing:** From 36–37 weeks (RCOG 2024); earlier ECV (34–36 weeks) may be considered in specialized centers but has higher reversion risk.[43]
- **Technique is shown in Table 3.**

BROW PRESENTATION

It is the rarest presentation and seen in partial extension of head.

Causes:

- Multiparity
- Platypelloid pelvis
- Fetal macrosomia
- Anencephaly

Engaging diameter: Mentovertical (14 cm)

There is no mechanism for labor.

Diagnosed on p/v by palpating supraorbital ridges and anterior fontanelle.

Delivery by cesarean section.

OCCIPUT POSTERIOR POSITION

Definition and Epidemiology

- Occiput posterior (OP) position is a vertex presentation with the fetal occiput over the sacroiliac joint (right/left OP) or sacrum (direct OP).[44]
- **Incidence:** 15–20% at labor onset, 5–8% persist at delivery.[45]
- **Relevance:** Common cause of prolonged labor; requires precise diagnosis and management skills.[46]

Etiology

- **Pelvic Shape:** Anthropoid/android pelvis (wide posterior segment) in >50% of cases.[47]
- **Fetal Factors:** Head deflexion increases occipitofrontal diameter (11.5 cm), delaying engagement.[48]
- **Uterine Factors:** Weak or uncoordinated contractions perpetuate deflexion.[49]
- **Other:** Large fetus, reduced amniotic fluid, and epidural anesthesia (RR 1.8).[50]

Mechanism of Labor

- **Engagement:** Head engages in oblique diameter (right/left); biparietal (9.5 cm) and suboccipitofrontal/occipitofrontal (10–11.5 cm) diameters delay descent.[51]
- **Rotation:**
  - ~90% rotate anteriorly (long arc, 135°), delivering by extension.[52]
  - ~10% persist due to deflexion, weak contractions, abnormal pelvis, weak pelvic floor, or large fetus.[53]
- **Outcomes:** Persistent OP increases second-stage duration (by 30–60 minutes) and operative delivery rates (OR 2.7).[54]

Management

- **Diagnosis:**
  - **Vaginal Examination:** Sagittal suture posterior, anterior fontanel palpable.[55]
  - **Ultrasound:** Confirms position; recommended in prolonged labor (ISUOG 2023).[56]
  - **Monitoring:** Use partograph; continuous CTG if risk factors (e.g., epidural and oxytocin).[57]
- **Conservative:**
  - Encourage maternal position changes (hands-and-knees, lateral) to promote rotation (success rate 60–70%).[58]
  - Ensure adequate hydration, pain relief (epidural increases OP persistence, OR 1.5).[59]
- **Interventions are shown in Table 4.**
- **Latest Guidelines (ACOG 2024 and RCOG 2024):**
  - Manual rotation reduces cesarean rates (RR 0.6); perform at full dilation by experienced operators.[61]
  - Cesarean indicated for arrest (no progress after 2 hours in active phase) or fetal distress.[62]

TABLE 4: Management of persistent occiput posterior position.[60]

Scenario	*Intervention*	*Postgraduate tips*
Anterior Rotation	Augment with oxytocin; allow spontaneous delivery	Monitor for hyperstimulation; avoid in fetal distress
Persistent OP, No Distress	Manual rotation to occiput anterior + forceps/ventouse	Practice rotation on simulators; confirm position postrotation
Persistent OP, Distress/ Arrest	Kielland forceps rotation (expert only) or cesarean	Master forceps application; cesarean safer in training settings

TABLE 5: Management of deep transverse arrest.[70]

Scenario	*Intervention*	*Postgraduate tips*
Unsafe Vaginal Delivery	Cesarean section	Preferred in training; document pelvic findings
Safe Vaginal Delivery	Ventouse (avoid excessive traction), manual rotation + forceps, and Kielland forceps (expert only)	Practice rotation on models; ensure fetal monitoring

- **Postgraduate Insight:**
  - Learn ultrasound for intrapartum positioning (ISUOG training modules).[63]
  - Manual rotation requires finesse; avoid excessive force to prevent trauma.[64]
  - Document attempts and rationale clearly for medicolegal purposes.[65]

DEEP TRANSVERSE ARREST (DTA)

- **Definition:** Fetal head arrested in transverse bispinous diameter (sagittal suture) after 0.5–1 hour post-full dilation, due to incomplete rotation from occiput posterior (OP) or nonrotation from occiput transverse.[66]
- **Causes:**
  - Abnormal pelvis (prominent ischial spines, flat sacrum, and convergent side walls).
  - Head deflexion, weak contractions, lax pelvic floor, and large fetus.[67]
- **Diagnosis:**
  - Vaginal examination: Sagittal suture transverse, anterior fontanel palpable.
  - Ultrasound: Confirms position (ISUOG 2023 recommendation).[68]
  - Pelvic assessment for architectural anomalies.[69]
- **Management is shown in Table 5**
- **Latest Guidelines (ACOG 2024):** Operative vaginal delivery for DTA is high risk; cesarean is preferred unless performed by experts.[71]
- **Postgraduate Insight:**
  - Master ultrasound for intrapartum diagnosis; reduces misdiagnosis.[72]
  - Kielland forceps require advanced training; avoid in early residency.[73]
  - Document fetal condition, rotation attempts, and delivery rationale.[74]

CEPHALOPELVIC DISPROPORTION (CPD)

- **Definition**: Mismatch between fetal head and maternal pelvis due to reduced pelvic capacity or abnormal fetal size/presentation/position.[75]

- Asynclitism refers to the lateral tilting of the fetal head during labor, where the sagittal suture is not aligned centrally in the maternal pelvis, allowing a smaller fetal head diameter (e.g., suboccipitobregmatic or bitemporal) to pass through a narrow true conjugate instead of the larger biparietal diameter. This adaptation facilitates descent in cases of pelvic constraint but may delay labor progression if uncorrected.[1]

Key Points

- **Prevalence:** Asynclitism occurs in ~10–15% of labors, more common in primigravida and with narrow pelvis.[2]
- Asynclitism corrects spontaneously in most cases with descent and rotation, but persistent asynclitism may lead to protracted or arrested labor.[3]
- Smaller diameters (e.g., bitemporal, 8 cm) engage the pelvis, compensating for a narrow true conjugate (<10 cm).[1]
- RCOG/NICE guidelines emphasize monitoring labor progression and avoiding premature intervention in asynclitic presentations.[4,5]
- Management focuses on maternal positioning and expectant care unless fetal distress or arrest occurs.[4]

Prevalence and Clinical Relevance (Table 6)

Incidence:

- General labor: 10–15% of vaginal deliveries show transient asynclitism.[2]
- Prolonged labor: Up to 30% of cases with protracted descent or arrest.[3]

Risk Factors:

- Primiparity (RR 1.8).
- Narrow pelvis (true conjugate <10 cm).
- Occipitoposterior position (20–30% association).
- Macrosomia (>4000 g).
- Epidural anesthesia (increases risk by 1.5-fold).[2,6]

Impact:

- Facilitates head passage through constrained pelvis by presenting smaller diameters (e.g., bitemporal 8 cm vs. biparietal 9.5 cm).
- May prolong first or second stage if uncorrected, increasing operative delivery risk (OR 2.1).[3]

TABLE 6: Prevalence and risk factors for asynclitism.[2,3,6]

Factor	*Prevalence/Association*	*Notes*
Overall Incidence	10–15%	Higher in primigravida
Prolonged Labor	30%	Linked to persistent asynclitism
Primiparity	RR 1.8	Inexperience with labor dynamics
Narrow Pelvis	20–25%	True conjugate <10 cm
Occipitoposterior	20–30%	Malposition exacerbates tilt
Epidural Anesthesia	OR 1.5	Relaxes pelvic floor

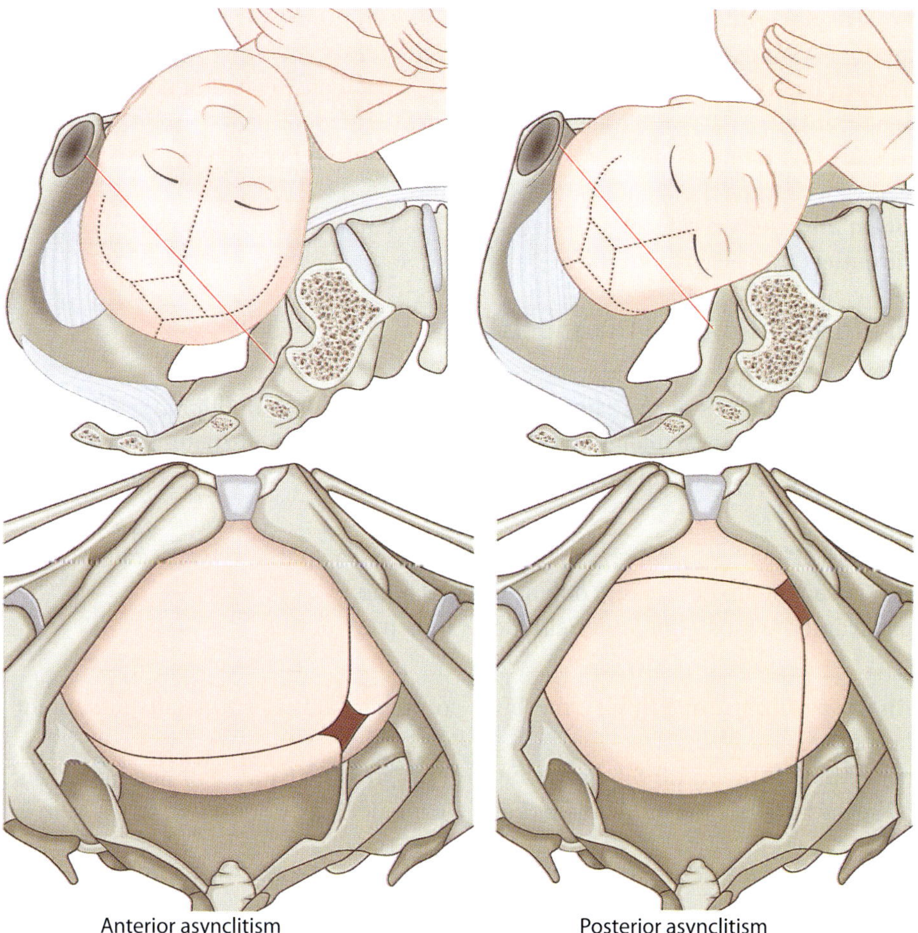

Fig. 1: Mechanism of asynclitism.

TABLE 7: Fetal head diameters in asynclitism.[1,3]

Diameter	*Measurement*	*Role in asynclitism*
Biparietal	9.5 cm	Too large for narrow conjugate
Suboccipitobregmatic	9 cm	Engages in flexed asynclitic head
Bitemporal	8 cm	Preferred in severe pelvic constraint

Mechanism of Asynclitism (Fig. 1)

- Asynclitism occurs as an adaptive response to pelvic constraints, involving lateral tilting and deflexion of the fetal head. Key steps include:
- **Initial Engagement:**
  - In a narrow true conjugate (<10 cm), the biparietal diameter (9.5 cm) is too large **(Table 7)**.
  - The head tilts laterally, presenting a smaller diameter (e.g., suboccipitobregmatic 9 cm or bitemporal 8 cm).[1]

- **Lateral Displacement:** Sagittal suture shifts anteriorly (anterior asynclitism) or posteriorly (posterior asynclitism), aligning the bitemporal diameter with the conjugate.[1]
- **Deflexion:** Lateral pelvic walls resist occiput descent, causing head deflexion (e.g., brow presentation).[3]
- **Correction:** With further descent, uterine contractions and pelvic floor resistance correct asynclitism, aligning the sagittal suture centrally.[1]
- **Rotation and Delivery:** Occiput rotates 90° (2/8 circle) anteriorly, leveraging the wider pelvic outlet (12–13 cm) for delivery.[1]

Clinical Presentation and Diagnosis

Symptoms:
- Prolonged labor (first stage >12 hours in nullipara, >8 hours in multipara).
- Irregular or slow cervical dilatation (<1.2 cm/h nullipara, <1.5 cm/h multipara).
- Maternal exhaustion or pain from uneven head pressure.[3]

Signs:
- Asymmetrical head position on vaginal examination (sagittal suture off-center).
- Caput succedaneum or molding on one parietal bone.[1]
- Palpable anterior/posterior fontanelle closer to pelvic sidewall.[3]

Diagnosis:
- **Vaginal Examination:** Primary method; confirms sagittal suture displacement and deflexion.[4]
- **Intrapartum Ultrasound:** Measures angle of progression (AoP) and head position; AoP <120° suggests persistent asynclitism (Level 2 evidence).[7]

Management

Management prioritizes expectant care, maternal positioning, and monitoring, with intervention reserved for fetal distress or labor arrest **(Table 8)**.[4,5]

Conservative Management

Maternal Positioning:
- Lateral (Sims) position on side opposite asynclitism (e.g., left lateral for anterior asynclitism) promotes correction.

TABLE 8: Management strategies for asynclitism.[4,5]

Approach	*Indication*	*Details*
Lateral Positioning	Transient asynclitism	Side opposite tilt (e.g., left for anterior)
Hands-and-Knees	Slow descent	Reduces pelvic pressure
Oxytocin	Uterine inertia	Titrate for 3–5 contractions/10 minutes
Operative Vaginal Delivery	Corrected asynclitism, engaged head	Forceps/vacuum in second stage
Cesarean Section	Arrest, distress, CPD	Reserved for nonprogression

TABLE 9: Complications of asynclitism.[3,6]

Complication	*Prevalence*	*Notes*
Prolonged Labor	20–30%	Increases operative delivery
Perineal Tears	RR 1.4	Due to uneven head pressure
PPH	5–10%	Linked to prolonged labor
Caput/Molding	30–40%	Resolves spontaneously
Birth Trauma	1–2%	Cephalhematoma, fractures

- Hands-and-knees position reduces pelvic pressure, aiding rotation.[4]
- Hydration and Analgesia: IV fluids and epidural (if needed) to support maternal comfort.[5]

Monitoring:
- Fetal heart rate (FHR) every 15–30 minutes.
- Cervical dilatation/descent every 2–4 hours.[4]
- **Oxytocin Augmentation:** If uterine inertia is present (contractions <3 in 10 minutes), titrate to achieve 200–250 MVU.[5]
- Indications for Intervention
- **Protracted Labor:** No progress after 4 hours of adequate contractions or 6 hours of oxytocin at ≥6 cm dilatation.[5]
- **Arrest of Descent:** No descent for ≥2 hours (nullipara) or ≥1 hour (multipara) in second stage.[4]
- **Fetal Distress:** Nonreassuring FHR (e.g., late decelerations).[5]

Interventions:
- **Operative Vaginal Delivery:** Forceps/vacuum if head is engaged and pelvis adequate.
- **Cesarean Section:** For uncorrectable asynclitism, cephalopelvic disproportion (CPD), or distress.[4]

Complications (Table 9)

Maternal:
- Prolonged labor (20–30% risk of operative delivery).
- Perineal tears (RR 1.4).
- Postpartum hemorrhage (5–10%).[3]

Fetal:
- Caput succedaneum/molding (30–40%).
- Birth trauma (e.g., cephalhematoma, 1–2%).
- Neonatal distress (rare, <1%).[6]

RECENT ADVANCES AND GUIDELINES

RCOG Guidelines (2022):[4]
- Advocate expectant management for asynclitism with normal FHR and slow but progressive labor.

- Recommend intrapartum ultrasound for persistent asynclitism to guide intervention.
- Cesarean only after failed oxytocin or operative vaginal delivery in second stage.

NICE Guidelines (2017):[5]

- Emphasize maternal positioning and hydration to correct asynclitism.
- Avoid premature cesarean in first stage if dilatation progresses (even slowly).
- **WHO Labor Care Guide (2020):**[8]
    - Replaces rigid partograph with flexible monitoring, focusing on maternal/fetal well-being.
    - Supports delayed intervention in asynclitic labors with stable parameters.
    - **Intrapartum Ultrasound:** Angle of progression (AoP) and head-perineum distance (HPD) predict vaginal delivery success (ISUOG, 2021).[7]
    - **Maternal Positioning Studies:** Hands-and-knees position reduces second-stage duration by 15–20 minutes in asynclitic cases.[9]
- **Suspicion**:
    - Short stature (<150 cm, OR 2.1 for CPD).
    - Floating head at term in primigravida.
    - Abnormal labor progress (prolonged active phase, arrest).
    - Excessive head molding/caput.[76]
- **Assessment is mentioned in Table 10**.
- **Pelvic Measurements:**
    - **Inlet:** Obstetric conjugate <10 cm, transverse <12 cm, and diagonal conjugate <11 cm.
    - **Midpelvis:** Interischial spinous + posterior sagittal ≤13 cm.
    - **Outlet:** Interischial tuberous ≤8 cm.[78]
- **Inferences:**
    - No CPD: Head reaches ischial spines, no overlap.
    - Slight/Moderate: Minimal descent, slight overlap.
    - Severe: No descent, significant overlap.[79]
- **Limitations:** Clinical methods assess inlet primarily; imaging is essential for midpelvis/outlet.[80]

TABLE 10: Assessment of cephalopelvic disproportion.[77]

Method	*Description*	*Postgraduate tips*
Clinical (Abdominal)	Push head downward; assess parietal bone overlap	Practice with senior supervision; note overlap degree
Abdominovaginal (Muller-Munro Kerr)	Bimanual; assess descent/overlap at ischial spines	Superior for pelvic assessment; confirm findings
Imaging	Ultrasound (fetal head, AFI), MRI/X-ray pelvimetry	MRI preferred for precise measurements
Clinical Observations	Multigravida with normal delivery history rules out CPD; primigravida nonengagement suggests CPD	Correlate with labor progress

- **Management**:
  - **Minor Inlet Contraction:** Allow trial of labor; monitor with partograph.[81]
  - **Moderate/Severe Inlet Contraction:** Elective cesarean, especially with outlet contraction, malpresentation, or complications (e.g., elderly primigravida).[82]
  - **Midpelvis/Outlet Contraction:** Diagnosed postdescent; cesarean for significant contraction; forceps/ventouse with deep episiotomy for minor cases.[83]
  - **Labor Augmentation:** Oxytocin for inadequate contractions; cesarean for arrest (no progress after 2 hours in active phase).[84]
- **Latest Guidelines (WHO 2024, ACOG 2024):**
  - Routine pelvimetry is not recommended; clinical/ultrasound assessment is preferred.[85]
  - Cesarean is indicated for confirmed CPD or labor arrest despite augmentation.[86]
- **Postgraduate Training:**
  - Learn Muller-Munro Kerr technique; practice on pelvic models.
  - Use ultrasound for fetal head measurements (biparietal diameter 9.4–9.8 cm).[87]
  - Document partograph findings, imaging results, and management rationale.[88]

Key Points

- Asynclitism occurs in 10–15% of labors, often in primigravida or narrow pelvis.
- Smaller fetal head diameters (bitemporal 8 cm) engage narrow conjugates (<10 cm).
- Transient asynclitism corrects with descent and 90° occiput rotation in most cases.
- Diagnosis via vaginal examination; ultrasound confirms persistent asynclitism (AoP <120°).
- Management includes lateral/hands-and-knees positioning, oxytocin for inertia, and monitoring.
- Intervention (forceps, vacuum, and cesarean) for arrest, distress, or CPD.
- Complications include prolonged labor (20–30%), perineal tears, and PPH (5–10%).
- RCOG and NICE advocate expectant care unless progression stalls or distress occurs.
- Intrapartum ultrasound enhances decision-making in prolonged labor.
- WHO Labor Care Guide supports individualized care to reduce unnecessary cesareans.

REFERENCES

1. Cunningham FG, Leveno KJ, Dashe JS, et al. (Eds). Williams Obstetrics, 26th edition. McGraw-Hill; 2021.
2. RCOG. Management of Breech Presentation (Green-top Guideline No. 20b). [online] Available from https://www.rcog.org.uk/guidance/browse-all-guidance/green-top-guidelines/management-of-breech-presentation-green-top-guideline-no-20b/ [Last accessed December, 2025].
3. Albrechtsen S, et al. Acta Obstet Gynecol Scand. 1997;76(8):727-31.
4. Hickok DE, et al. Am J Obstet Gynecol. 1992;166(2):411-6.
5. Impey LWM, et al. BJOG. 2017;124(4):e151-77.
6. Hannah ME, et al. Planned caesarean section versus planned vaginal birth for breech presentation at term: a randomised multicentre trial. Term Breech Trial Collaborative Group. Lancet. 2000;356(9232):1375-83.
7. Westgren M, et al. Acta Obstet Gynecol Scand. 1985;64(3):231-4.
8. Blickstein I, et al. J Perinat Med. 2000;28(4):280-4.
9. Simm A, et al. Eur J Obstet Gynecol Reprod Biol. 2008;138(1):14-9.
10. Teteris NJ, et al. Am J Obstet Gynecol. 1970;107(3):371-5.

11. ACOG Practice Bulletin No. 200. Obstet Gynecol. 2023;141(5):e208-18.
12. Pattinson RC, et al. Int J Gynaecol Obstet. 2003;82(3):321-7.
13. ISUOG Practice Guidelines. Ultrasound Obstet Gynecol. 2023;62(2):156-64.
14. RCOG. Green-top Guideline No. 20b. 2024.
15. ACOG. Obstet Gynecol. 2023;141(5):e208-18.
16. Kotaska A, et al. J Obstet Gynaecol Can. 2009;31(6):557-66.
17. Hofmeyr GJ, et al. Cochrane Database Syst Rev. 2015;7:CD000166.
18. Zhang J, et al. Am J Obstet Gynecol. 1993;168(6 Pt 1):1789-94.
19. Cronk M. Midwifery. 1998;14(2):69-76.
20. Piper EB, et al. Am J Obstet Gynecol. 1931;22(5):695-705.
21. Lovset J. Acta Obstet Gynecol Scand. 1937;17(Suppl 2):1-94.
22. Burns JL, et al. Am J Obstet Gynecol. 1943;46(5):678-84.
23. Mauriceau F. Traité des Maladies des Femmes Grosses. 1668.
24. Piper EB, et al. Am J Obstet Gynecol. 1931;22(5):695-705.
25. Berhan Y, et al. BJOG. 2023;130(8):896-905.
26. Draycott TJ, et al. BJOG. 2015;122(13):1701-9.
27. To WW, et al. Aust N Z J Obstet Gynaecol. 2000;40(3):319-24.
28. RCOG. Training in Obstetrics and Gynaecology. 2024.
29. Cheng M, et al. Am J Obstet Gynecol. 1994;171(5):1259-63.
30. Su M, et al. Am J Obstet Gynecol. 2003;189(1):282-8.
31. WHO. Intrapartum Care for a Positive Childbirth Experience. 2024.
32. Cluver C, et al. Cochrane Database Syst Rev. 2015;9:CD008404.
33. Impey LWM, et al. BJOG. 2017;124(4):e151-77.
34. Kok M, et al. Eur J Obstet Gynecol Reprod Biol. 2008;141(1):3-7.
35. Grootscholten K, et al. BJOG. 2007;114(5):545-51.
36. Collins S, et al. Aust N Z J Obstet Gynaecol. 2007;47(3):192-7.
37. ACOG Practice Bulletin No. 221. Obstet Gynecol. 2020;135(5):e189-202.
38. Fernandez-Carrion J, et al. JAMA. 2024;331(12):1035-43.
39. ISUOG. Ultrasound Obstet Gynecol. 2023;62(2):156-64.
40. SMFM. Am J Obstet Gynecol. 2018;218(2):B1-18.
41. Hofmeyr GJ, et al. Cochrane Database Syst Rev. 2015;4:CD000083.
42. de Hundt M, et al. Obstet Gynecol. 2014;123(1):49-57.
43. RCOG. Green-top Guideline No. 20a. 2024.
44. Gardberg M, et al. Acta Obstet Gynecol Scand. 1998;77(3):279-83.
45. Ponkey SE, et al. Obstet Gynecol. 2003;101(5 Pt 1):915-20.
46. Caughey AB, et al. Am J Obstet Gynecol. 2009;201(6):570.e1-8.
47. Caldwell WE, et al. Am J Obstet Gynecol. 1939;38(3):434-46.
48. Lieberman E, et al. Obstet Gynecol. 2005;105(5 Pt 1):1034-41.
49. Fitzpatrick M, et al. Am J Obstet Gynecol. 2001;185(2):485-90.
50. Anim-Somuah M, et al. Cochrane Database Syst Rev. 2018;5:CD000331.
51. Phillips RD, et al. Clin Obstet Gynecol. 1975;18(1):69-81.
52. Sizer AR, et al. Eur J Obstet Gynecol Reprod Biol. 2000;90(1):15-20.
53. Sen DD, et al. J Obstet Gynaecol India. 2013;63(2):108-13.
54. Wu SW, et al. Am J Obstet Gynecol. 2005;192(3):849-54.
55. Sherer DM, et al. Ultrasound Obstet Gynecol. 2002;20(3):262-7.
56. ISUOG. Ultrasound Obstet Gynecol. 2023;62(2):156-64.
57. WHO. Managing Complications in Pregnancy and Childbirth. 2024.
58. Hunter S, et al. BJOG. 2007;114(10):1216-22.

59. Simkin P, et al. Birth. 2010;37(1):56-64.
60. Alfirevic Z, et al. Cochrane Database Syst Rev. 2017;3:CD001337.
61. ACOG. Obstet Gynecol. 2024;143(4):e123-34.
62. RCOG. Green-top Guideline No. 26. 2024.
63. ISUOG. Intrapartum Ultrasound Training. 2023.
64. Shaffer BL, et al. Obstet Gynecol. 2006;108(1):146-52.
65. RCOG. Medico-legal Issues in Obstetrics. 2024.
66. Friedman EA. Labor: Clinical Evaluation and Management. 2nd ed. 1978.
67. Debby A, et al. Eur J Obstet Gynecol Reprod Biol. 2003;109(1):16-20.
68. ISUOG. Ultrasound Obstet Gynecol. 2023;62(2):156-64.
69. Olah KS, et al. Br J Obstet Gynaecol. 1994;101(9):767-73.
70. Murphy DJ, et al. Lancet. 2001;358(9288):1203-7.
71. ACOG. Obstet Gynecol. 2024;143(4):e123-34.
72. Bellussi F, et al. Ultrasound Obstet Gynecol. 2020;56(3):321-7.
73. Bofill JA, et al. Obstet Gynecol. 1997;89(5 Pt 1):780-4.
74. RCOG. Documentation Standards in Obstetrics. 2024.
75. Korhonen U, et al. Acta Obstet Gynecol Scand. 2014;93(4):323-34.
76. Maharaj D. Best Pract Res Clin Obstet Gynaecol. 2010;24(3):353-64.
77. Pattinson RC, et al. Int J Gynaecol Obstet. 2003;82(3):321-7.
78. Thorp JM Jr, et al. Clin Obstet Gynecol. 1997;40(1):88-96.
79. Sizer AR, et al. J Obstet Gynaecol. 2000;20(2):145-9.
80. van Loon AJ, et al. Eur J Obstet Gynecol Reprod Biol. 1997;74(2):129-35.
81. Morrison JC, et al. Am J Obstet Gynecol. 1985;153(8):889-93.
82. O'Connell MP, et al. Eur J Obstet Gynecol Reprod Biol. 2000;89(2):117-20.
83. Caughey AB, et al. Am J Obstet Gynecol. 2005;193(3 Pt 2):1016-23.
84. WHO. Intrapartum Care for a Positive Childbirth Experience. 2024.
85. WHO. Recommendations on Antenatal Care. 2024.
86. ACOG. Obstet Gynecol. 2024;143(4):e123-34.
87. Ghi T, et al. Ultrasound Obstet Gynecol. 2018;52(2):145-53.
88. RCOG. Clinical Governance in Obstetrics. 2024.

Vulvar Hematomas

Ruchika Garg, Neelansha Varshney

VULVAR HEMATOMAS

Vulvar hematomas are collections of blood beneath intact skin, often resulting from obstetric or nonobstetric trauma. If undiagnosed or untreated, they can lead to severe complications, including hemodynamic instability or sepsis.[1] Early recognition is critical to reduce morbidity, improve outcomes, and shorten hospital stays.[1] This chapter provides a concise, evidence-based overview for medical postgraduate education, covering incidence, anatomy, pathophysiology, clinical features, evaluation, and management, with updates incorporating recent literature and guidelines.

INCIDENCE AND EPIDEMIOLOGY

- **Obstetric:** Incidence of 1–2 per 1,000 deliveries.[2]
- **Nonobstetric:** 3.7% incidence, constituting 0.8% of gynecologic emergencies.[3]
- **Etiology:**
    - **Obstetric:** Episiotomy, vaginal tears, instrumental deliveries, excessive stretching of the birth canal, or rarely, obturator artery pseudoaneurysm.[4-6] Antenatal hematomas reported at 35 weeks.[7]
    - **Nonobstetric:** Postcoital injury (40% of cases), saddle injuries, falls, foreign body insertion, rape, vulvar surgery, or spontaneous vessel rupture.[3,8]
- **Risk Factors:** See **Table 1** for obstetric and nonobstetric risk factors.

ANATOMY OF THE VULVA

The vulva comprises labia majora/minora, clitoris, vestibular bulb, and greater vestibular glands, composed of smooth muscle and loose connective tissue with rich vascularity.[1]

TABLE 1: Risk factors for vulvar hematomas.[9,10]

Type	*Risk factors*
Obstetric	Nulliparity, instrumental delivery, episiotomy, large fetus, prolonged second stage, and preeclampsia
Nonobstetric	Coagulopathy, vulvar varicosities, prior vulvar trauma, and anticoagulation therapy

- **Arterial Supply:**
  - **Internal Pudendal Artery** (branch of internal iliac artery): Supplies rectum, anal sphincters, perineal muscles, labia, vestibular bulb, and clitoris via branches (inferior rectal, perineal, labial, bulb of vestibule, and deep/dorsal clitoral arteries).[1]
  - **Superficial External Pudendal Artery** (femoral artery branch): Supplies labia majora.[1]
- **Venous Drainage:** Parallels arterial supply; submucosal venous plexus in the distal vagina predisposes to varicosities, especially in parous women.[1]
- **Pathophysiology:**
  - Rich vascularity increases hematoma risk from venous or arterial (pudendal artery branches: Posterior rectal, transverse perineal, and posterior labial bleeding.[3]
  - Varicosities or arterial aneurysms heighten spontaneous rupture risk.[1]
  - 70% of hematomas occur on the right labia[2]

CLINICAL FEATURES (FIG. 1)

- **Symptoms:**
  - Severe perineal, buttock, or abdominal pain, and impairing walking/sitting.[4]
  - Urinary retention due to urethral obstruction.[2]
  - Intermittent bleeding or hemodynamic instability in severe cases.[1]
- **Signs:**
  - Tense, tender vulvar swelling, and distorting anatomy.[11]
  - Ecchymotic overlying skin.[11]
  - Possible vaginal/rectal displacement or pressure necrosis.[1]
- **Complications:**
  - Hematoma rupture into vagina, causing infection/sepsis.[1]
  - Retroperitoneal extension, leading to shock.[1]
  - Massive expansion due to pliable vaginal subcutaneous tissue.[5]
- **Note:** Hematomas typically occur on the episiotomy side but may be contralateral.[4]

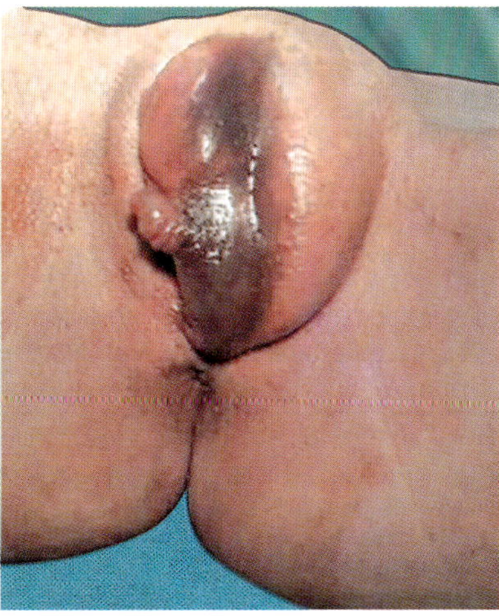

Fig. 1: Clinical image of vulvar hematoma with ecchymosis.

DIFFERENTIAL DIAGNOSIS

- Bartholin's gland cyst/abscess.
- Vulvar varicosities (more common, less symptomatic).[12]
- Vulvar cancer.[4]
- **Diagnostic Note:** Obstetric hematomas are straightforward due to delivery history; nonobstetric cases may mimic abscesses, requiring careful history and examination.[4]

EVALUATION

- **Laboratory:** Complete blood count, blood grouping/cross-matching, coagulation profile (fibrinogen, prothrombin time, and partial thromboplastin time) to rule out bleeding diathesis.[13]
- **Imaging:**
  - **Transperineal Ultrasound:** Cost-effective, diagnoses size/extent, monitors conservative management; color Doppler assesses vascular malformations.[14]
  - **MRI:** Evaluates lesion extent and pelvic organ relationships.[1]
  - **CT Angiography:** Identifies precise bleeding sites, aneurysms, or arteriovenous fistulae.[15,16]
  - **Pelvic X-ray:** Rules out fractures in trauma cases.[1]
- **Indications for Imaging:** Expanding, nonpalpable, or retroperitoneal hematomas.[1]

MANAGEMENT

Management is individualized based on size, site, expansion, duration, and hemodynamic stability, with no universal consensus **(Table 2)**.[17,18] Options include conservative, surgical, and arterial embolization.

Conservative Management

- **Indications:** Small (3–5 cm), stable hematomas with minimal symptoms.[1,4,10,17]
- **Approach:**
  - Antibiotics, analgesics (narcotics if needed), ice packs, bed rest to prevent infection/abscess.[1]

TABLE 2: Management strategies for vulvar hematomas.[1,3,4,10,13,16,18-21]

Approach	*Indications*	*Details*
Conservative	Small (3–5 cm), nonexpanding, hemodynamically stable, and minimal symptoms	Antibiotics, analgesics, ice packs, bed rest, Foley catheter; vaginal packing (24 hours) if drainage needed[1,8,10]
Surgical	Large (>10 cm), expanding, hemodynamic instability, urologic/neurologic symptoms	Evacuate clot, ligate bleeding points, close dead space with absorbable sutures; vaginal packing for 12–24 hours[3,13,19]
Selective arterial embolization	Failure of surgical control, large/expanding hematomas, confirmed active bleeding	Controls bleeding predrainage, reduces blood loss; first-line or second line after surgical failure[16,20,21]

- Foley catheter for urinary retention.[1]
- Spontaneous resolution common; vaginal packing (24 hours) for drainage if needed.[8]

- **Drawbacks:** Longer hospitalization, higher antibiotic/transfusion needs.[11,12]

Surgical Management

- **Indications:** Large (>10 cm), expanding, or symptomatic hematomas causing hemodynamic instability or urologic/neurologic symptoms.[3,19]
- **Procedure:**
  - Performed in operating room under local anesthesia.
  - Evacuate clot, ligate bleeding points, close dead space with interrupted/figure-of-eight absorbable sutures (e.g., Monocryl and Polyglactin).[13]
  - Vaginal packing (12–24 hours) if bleeding source unidentified.[3,19]
  - Postprocedure: Sitz baths, saline cleansing, analgesia, and pelvic rest for 4–6 weeks.[13]

Note: Two large-bore IV lines and volume resuscitation (crystalloids and blood products) for unstable patients.[1]

Selective Arterial Embolization

- **Indications:** Failure of surgical hemostasis, hematoma redevelopment, or active bleeding confirmed by CT angiography.[16,20,21]
- **Technique:** Introduced in 1979;[22] controls bleeding before surgical drainage, reducing blood loss.[16,20] Can be first line for large hematomas.[21,23]
- **Advantages:**
  - Shorter hospitalization.
  - Reduced need for major surgery.
  - Less blood loss predrainage.[16]
- **Disadvantages:**
  - Higher cost, limited availability.
  - Rare risks: Sciatic/femoral neuropathy, bladder gangrene, and gluteal pain (33% of patients).[16]

Supralevator Hematomas

- Rare, may extend retroperitoneally, and cause uterine displacement and shock.[1]
- **Management:** Observation, antibiotics, transfusion; laparotomy with clot evacuation and vessel ligation if bleeding persists, with ureteral care; hysterectomy as last resort.[1]

COMPLICATIONS

- **Immediate:** Rupture, infection, sepsis, pressure necrosis, and hemodynamic instability.[1]
- **Delayed:** Prolonged pain, abscess formation, and reintervention.[11]
- **Supralevator:** Retroperitoneal spread, shock.[1]

RECENT ADVANCES AND GUIDELINES

- **Transperineal Ultrasound:** Preferred for diagnosis/monitoring due to accessibility and cost-effectiveness; color Doppler enhances utility.[14]
- **CT Angiography:** Gold standard for identifying bleeding sites, aneurysms, and fistulae.[15,16,24]
- **Arterial Embolization:** Increasingly first line for large, unstable hematomas, reducing surgical morbidity.[20,21]
- **Guidelines:** No universal protocol; ACOG (2018) emphasizes individualized management and early recognition.[5] RCOG (2016) supports embolization for refractory cases.[18]
- **Recent Studies:** A 2023 case series highlighted embolization first strategies for complex hematomas, reducing transfusion needs.[25]

KEY POINTS

- Vulvar hematomas are rare (1–2/1,000 deliveries; 0.8% of gynecologic emergencies) but potentially fatal if untreated.
- Caused by obstetric (e.g., episiotomy) or nonobstetric (e.g., postcoital) trauma; 70% right sided.
- Present with severe pain, swelling, ecchymosis; may cause urinary retention or shock.
- Diagnosed clinically; ultrasound/CT for complex cases.
- Management: Conservative for small, stable hematomas; surgical or embolization for large, expanding, or unstable cases.
- Embolization reduces blood loss and is increasingly first line for severe cases.

REFERENCES

1. Saleh MM, et al. Postpartum vulvar and vaginal hematomas: A case series and review of the literature. J Matern Fetal Neonatal Med. 2020;33(15):2597-603.
2. Propst AM, et al. Vulvar hematomas: A comprehensive review. Obstet Gynecol Surv. 2019;74(5):297-303.
3. Jones IS, et al. Non-obstetric vulvar hematomas: Diagnosis and management. Aust N Z J Obstet Gynaecol. 2018;58(4):387-92.
4. Ridgeway B, et al. Hematomas of the vulva and vagina: A retrospective study. Obstet Gynecol. 2016;128(4):745-50.
5. ACOG Practice Bulletin No. 198: Prevention and management of obstetric lacerations at vaginal delivery. Obstet Gynecol. 2018;132(3):e87-e102.
6. Kim YA, et al. Obturator artery pseudoaneurysm causing vulvar hematoma. J Obstet Gynaecol Res. 2017;43(6):1078-81.
7. Lee JH, et al. Antenatal vulvar hematoma in a pregnant woman at 35 weeks. J Matern Fetal Neonatal Med. 2019;32(14):2410-12.
8. Mawhinney S, et al. Risk factors for postpartum vulvar hematomas. J Perinat Med. 2016;44(7):763-8.
9. Tsakiridis I, et al. Obstetric perineal trauma: Risk factors and outcomes. Eur J Obstet Gynecol Reprod Biol. 2021;260:166-72.
10. Virgili A, et al. Non-obstetric vulvar trauma: A review of 40 cases. Int J Gynaecol Obstet. 2017;139(3):339-43.
11. Hong HR, et al. Management of postpartum vulvovaginal hematomas: A systematic approach. Int J Womens Health. 2020;12:527-34.

12. Benrubi GI, et al. Vulvar varicosities versus hematomas: A diagnostic dilemma. J Reprod Med. 2018;63(4):321-6.
13. Heffner LJ, et al. Angiographic embolization for vulvovaginal hematomas. Am J Obstet Gynecol. 1985;152(6):681-4.
14. Shek KL, et al. Transperineal ultrasound in the assessment of perineal pathology. Ultrasound Obstet Gynecol. 2019;54(2):148-55.
15. Lee MS, et al. CT angiography for postpartum hemorrhage. Radiol Clin North Am. 2020;58(2):347-61.
16. Chen C, et al. Selective arterial embolization for vulvar hematomas: A case series. J Vasc Interv Radiol. 2021;32(5):678-84.
17. Gowda M, et al. Management of postpartum vulvar hematomas: A review of current practices. J Obstet Gynaecol Can. 2019;41(7):964-70.
18. Royal College of Obstetricians and Gynaecologists. (2016). Prevention and Management of Postpartum Haemorrhage (Green-top Guideline No. 52) [online] Available from https://www.rcog.org.uk/guidance/browse-all-guidance/green-top-guidelines/prevention-and-management-of-postpartum-haemorrhage-green-top-guideline-no-52/ [Last accessed December, 2025].
19. Zahn CM, et al. Surgical management of vulvovaginal hematomas. Clin Obstet Gynecol. 2017;60(3):583-91.
20. Wang CX, et al. Arterial embolization as first-line management for vulvar hematomas. J Minim Invasive Gynecol. 2020;27(4):894-900.
21. Kim GM, et al. Emergency embolization for postpartum vulvar hematomas: A case report. J Clin Med. 2022;11(3):756.
22. Heffner LJ, et al. Embolization for postpartum vulvovaginal hematomas. Am J Obstet Gynecol. 1985;152(6):681-4.
23. Brown BJ, et al. Angiographic embolization for pelvic hemorrhage. Obstet Gynecol. 1979;54(5):608-13.
24. Katz MD, et al. CT angiography for pelvic vascular injuries. J Trauma Acute Care Surg. 2018;84(3):492-8.
25. Patel R, et al. Embolization-first strategy for postpartum vulvar hematomas: A case series. J Obstet Gynaecol Res. 2023;49(8):1987-93.

Genital Tract Injuries

Ruchika Garg, Shaifali Singh

INTRODUCTION

Genital tract injuries encompass traumatic damage to the female reproductive organs, including the vulva, vagina, cervix, uterus, and adnexa, as well as associated structures such as the bladder, urethra, and rectum. These injuries may occur during childbirth, surgery, sexual assault, or accidents, with an incidence of genitourinary injuries post-road traffic accidents at approximately 0.46%.[1] If untreated or incompletely healed, they can lead to chronic pain, dyspareunia, infertility, fistulas, and significant psychological morbidity. Early recognition, prompt management, and holistic care addressing physical, mental, and emotional needs are critical to mitigate long-term consequences.

CAUSES AND RISK FACTORS

Genital tract injuries arise from various etiologies, with specific risk factors amplifying vulnerability, particularly during obstetric events.

- **Causes:**
  - *Obstetric:* Traumatic vaginal delivery, cesarean section.
  - *Traumatic:* Road traffic accidents, straddle injuries, and direct pelvic trauma.
  - *Sexual:* Consensual intercourse, sexual assault, and female genital mutilation.
  - *Iatrogenic:* Surgical procedures, foreign bodies, and instrumental abortions.
  - *Other:* Ox-horn injuries, retained contraceptives/pessaries.
- **Risk Factors:**[2,3]
  - **Obstetric:** Large fetus (>4 kg), shoulder dystocia, occipitoposterior position, precipitous labor, episiotomy, and operative vaginal delivery (forceps/vacuum).
  - **Nonobstetric:** Forceful coitus, postmenopausal status (atrophic tissues), and sexual assault (up to 50% of victims report genital injuries).[4]
  - **General:** Age 15–24 (trauma is a leading cause of death), pelvic fractures.

Table 1 summarizes the diverse causes and risk factors for genital tract injuries, highlighting the need for targeted prevention strategies.[2-4]

OBSTETRIC ANAL SPHINCTER INJURIES

Obstetric anal sphincter injuries (OASIS) include third- and fourth-degree perineal tears, classified by the Royal College of Obstetricians and Gynaecologists (RCOG).[5]

TABLE 1: Common causes and risk factors for genital tract injuries.[2-4]

Category	*Causes*	*Risk factors*
Obstetric	Vaginal delivery, cesarean section	Large fetus, shoulder dystocia, and operative delivery
Traumatic	Road accidents, straddle injuries	Pelvic fractures, blunt/penetrating trauma
Sexual	Assault, consensual intercourse	Postmenopausal status, forceful coitus
Iatrogenic	Surgery, foreign bodies	Improper instrumentation, retained devices

TABLE 2: RCOG classification of perineal tears.[5]

Degree	*Description*
First	Perineal skin or vaginal mucosa
Second	Perineal muscles, sparing anal sphincter
Third (3a)	<50% EAS torn
Third (3b)	>50% EAS torn
Third (3c)	EAS and IAS torn
Fourth	Anal sphincter complex and anorectal mucosa torn

Classification[5]

- **First-degree:** Injury to perineal skin or vaginal mucosa.
- **Second-degree:** Injury to perineal muscles, sparing anal sphincter.
- **Third-degree:**
  - *3a:* <50% external anal sphincter (EAS) torn.
  - *3b:* >50% EAS torn.
  - *3c:* EAS and internal anal sphincter (IAS) torn.
- **Fourth-degree:** Injury to anal sphincter complex and anorectal mucosa.
  The RCOG classification **(Table 2)** guides the diagnosis and management of OASIS.[5]

Etiology

- **Obstetric:** Excessive perineal stretching during labor, rigid perineum, and prolonged second stage.[3]
- **Nonobstetric:** Direct perineal trauma (e.g., falls).

Clinical Features

- **Symptoms:**
  - Fecal incontinence (severity depends on tear extent: loose stool in 3a, solid stool in fourth-degree).
  - Flatus incontinence.
  - Perineal soreness from stool irritation.

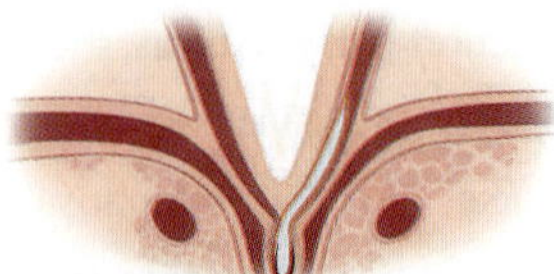

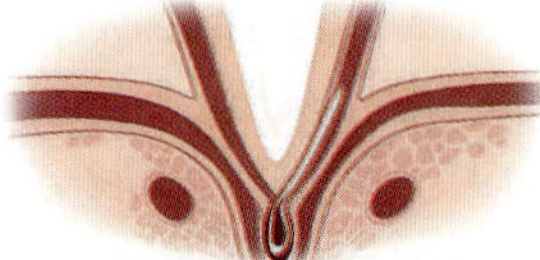

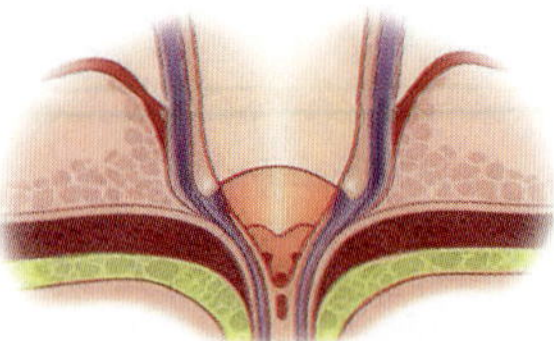

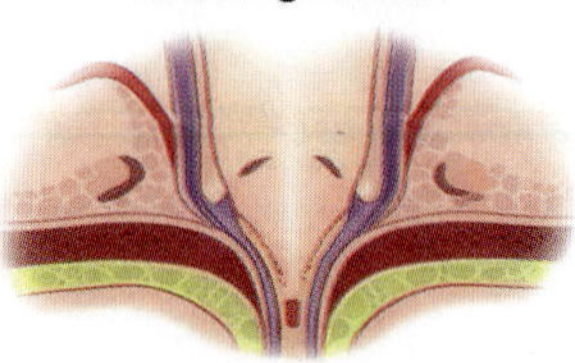

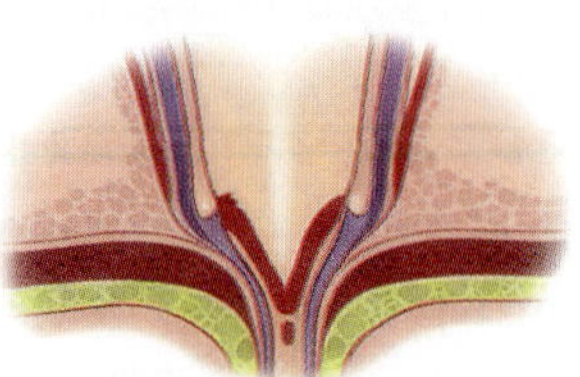

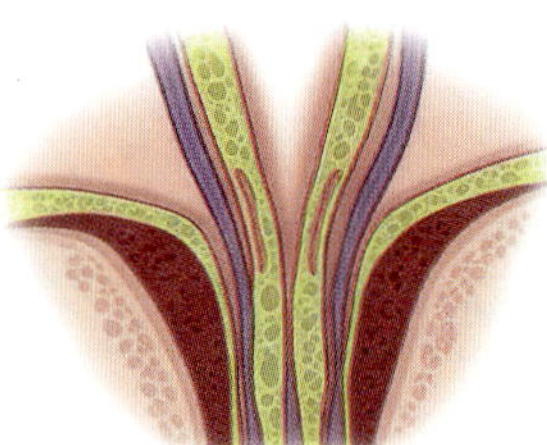

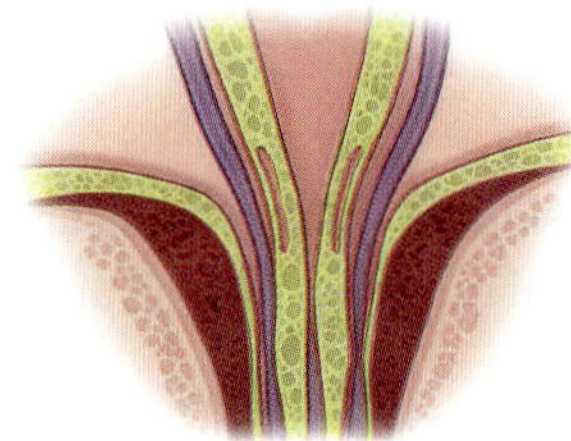

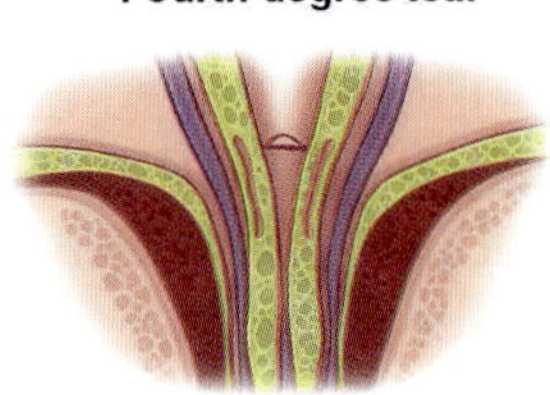

Fig. 1: Obstetric anal sphincter injuries.

- **Signs:**
  - **Inspection:** Absent perineum, continuous vaginal/rectal mucosa, fibrous septum, retracted sphincter ends, and radial skin wrinkles at anal verge **(Fig. 1)**.
  - **Palpation:** Reduced sphincter tone on rectal examination.
  - **Imaging:** MRI or endoanal ultrasound to confirm sphincter damage.[6]

Differential Diagnosis

Low rectovaginal fistula (intact perineal skin, less complex repair).

Management

Preventive Measures[3,5]

- Controlled second-stage delivery (Ritgen's maneuver).
- Gradual head delivery, avoiding abrupt extension.
- Selective episiotomy at optimal timing.
- Careful shoulder delivery to prevent perineal overstretching.

Operative Management (Sphincteroplasty and Perineorrhaphy)[5,7]

- **Timing:**
    - Immediate repair postdelivery (within 24 hours, under regional anesthesia in operating room).
    - Delayed repair (2–3 months postinjury) after infection resolution and tissue healing.
- **Preoperative Preparation:**
    - Baseline blood/biochemical tests, anesthesia fitness.
    - Eradicate worm infestations.
    - Low-residue diet (bread and milk) 2 days prior.
    - Gut sterilization (metronidazole 400 mg TID, erythromycin 500 mg TID, and neomycin 250 mg TID) 48 hours prior.
    - Daily enemas 2 days prior; avoid enema on surgery day.
- **Surgical Principles (Warren Flap Method):**[7]
    - Incise posterior vaginal mucosa in inverted V-shape, mobilize rectal wall.
    - Freshen and suture torn sphincter ends and rectal wall in two layers (3-0 PDS, intraluminal knots).
    - Close pararectal fascia and approximate sphincter edges with interrupted sutures.
    - Excise redundant vaginal mucosa, reconstruct perineal body (0 Vicryl).
- **Postoperative Care:**
    - Nil per oral (day 1), liquids (day 2), nonresidue diet (day 3), and full diet (day 6).
    - Stool softeners (lactulose 15–30 mL nightly) from day 2.
    - IV antibiotics (third-generation cephalosporin, anaerobic cover) for 5 days.
    - Avoid mobilization for 4–5 days.
- **Discharge Advice:**
    - Stool softeners for 1 week.
    - Contraceptive counseling.
    - Postnatal review at 6 weeks with endoanal ultrasound if indicated.
    - Institutional delivery with contralateral episiotomy in future pregnancies.
    - Elective cesarean for persistent incontinence or abnormal ultrasound post-repair.

Complications[6]

- Dyspareunia, persistent incontinence (20–30% residual defects), tight sphincteroplasty, wound dehiscence, and rectovaginal fistula.
- Anorectal manometry to assess residual defects.

INJURIES BY ANATOMICAL LOCATION

Vulval Injuries

- **Causes:** Delivery, sexual assault, and straddle injuries.
- **Presentation:** Pain, bleeding, swelling, and hematoma.
- **Management:** Conservative for small hematomas (ice packs, analgesics); surgical evacuation for large hematomas.[8]

Vaginal Injuries

- **Causes:** Delivery, coital trauma, foreign bodies, and instrumental abortions.
- **Presentation:** Bleeding, pain, discharge; possible fistula formation.
- **Management:** Suture tears with absorbable sutures (e.g., 2-0 polyglactin) under anesthesia.

Cervical Injuries

- **Causes:** Precipitate labor, operative vaginal delivery, cervical dilatation (e.g., Hegar's dilators), and conization.
- **Presentation:** Significant bleeding, minimal pain, possible hematometra, or subfertility.
- **Management:** Suture lacerations; hysterectomy for severe cases.[8]

Uterine Injuries

- **Causes:** Uterine rupture (delivery), perforation (IUD insertion, D&C, and hysteroscopy).
- **Presentation:** Bleeding, shock, and abdominal pain.
- **Management:** Suture minor ruptures; hysterectomy for severe cases.[8]

Management strategies vary by injury location, as outlined in **Table 3**.[8]

Clinical Presentation

- **Vulval/Vaginal:** Severe pain, bleeding, swelling, hematoma; possible tachycardia, hypotension, and shock.
- **Cervical:** Significant bleeding, minimal pain.
- **Uterine:** Abdominal pain, systemic signs (tachycardia, hypotension, and collapse).
- **Long-term:** Vaginal discharge, urinary/fecal incontinence, dyspareunia, and psychological distress.[9]

Diagnosis

- **History:** Bleeding, pain, trauma, childbirth, surgery, and bladder/bowel symptoms.
- **Examination:**
  - *General:* Assess for tachycardia, hypotension, and shock.
  - *Abdominal:* Palpable mass, tenderness, and signs of internal bleeding.
  - *Pelvic:* Speculum and bimanual examination for lacerations, hematomas.
- **Investigations:**
  - Baseline blood tests (hemoglobin and hematocrit).

TABLE 3: Management of genital tract injuries by location[8]

Location	*Common causes*	*Management*
Vulva	Delivery, assault, and straddle injury	Ice packs, evacuation of large hematomas
Vagina	Delivery, coital trauma, and foreign body	Suture tears (2-0 polyglactin)
Cervix	Precipitate labor, instrumentation	Suture lacerations, hysterectomy if severe
Uterus	Rupture and perforation (IUD and D&C)	Suture minor ruptures, hysterectomy

- *Imaging:* Ultrasound and CT/MRI for internal injuries.[9]
- Endoanal ultrasound/MRI for OASIS.[6]

Management

Initial Stabilization

- Hemodynamic resuscitation (IV fluids, blood transfusion if needed).
- Multidisciplinary approach (gynecologist, urologist, surgeon, and psychologist).[9]

Specific Treatment[8,9]

- **Conservative:**
  Minor lacerations/small hematomas: Antibiotics, analgesics, stool softeners, perineal hygiene, and ice packs.
- **Surgical:**
  - Suture vulval/vaginal/cervical tears (2-0/3-0 polyglactin).
  - Evacuate large hematomas; laparotomy for retroperitoneal/broad ligament hematomas.
  - Uterine rupture: Suture or hysterectomy.
- **Postoperative:**
  - Antibiotics (e.g., ceftriaxone and metronidazole) for 5–7 days.
  - Analgesics, pelvic floor exercises, and psychological support.

Sexual Assault[10]

- **Medicolegal:** Document injuries, inform police, and collect forensic samples.
- **Medical:** Treat injuries, prevent STIs (prophylactic antibiotics), prevent pregnancy (emergency contraception), and provide psychological support.

COITAL INJURIES

- **Presentation:** Vaginal tears, bleeding; rarely bowel prolapse in postmenopausal/posthysterectomy women.
- **Management:** Suture tears under anesthesia; manage shock/sepsis.[9]

FOREIGN BODY/INSTRUMENTAL INJURIES

- **Vagina:** Forgotten contraceptives/pessaries, tampons; cause discharge, ulceration. Remove under anesthesia; retrieve broken needles via C-arm guidance.[9]
- **Cervix:** Tears from dilatation; manage by suturing or addressing stenosis **(Fig. 2)**.[8]
- **Uterus:** Perforation from IUD/D&C/hysteroscopy; manage surgically if visceral injury.[8]

Complications

Genital tract injuries can lead to immediate, intermediate, and long-term complications, significantly impacting quality of life **(Table 4)**.[11]

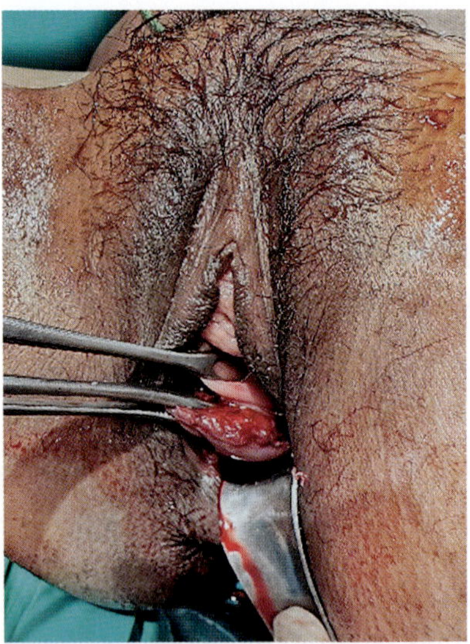

Fig. 2: Exploration of cervical tear.

TABLE 4: Complications of Genital Tract Injuries[11]

Category	*Complications*
Immediate	Bleeding, pain, hypovolemic shock, infection, urinary retention, sepsis, and pulmonary embolism
Intermediate	Delayed healing, dehiscence, incontinence, and chronic pain
Long-term	Fistulas (vesicovaginal/rectovaginal), dyspareunia, psychological stress, sexual dysfunction, and pelvic floor dysfunction

Preventive Strategies[12]

- Antenatal education and birth planning.
- Screen/manage high-risk factors (e.g., large fetus and malpresentation).
- Pelvic floor exercises (Kegel's) in pregnancy.
- Perineal massage in late third trimester.
- Skilled birth attendants for institutional delivery.
- Selective episiotomy (avoid routine use).
- Judicious instrumental delivery by experienced obstetricians.
- Adequate analgesia (e.g., epidural).
- Postpartum examination for injuries.
- Perineal hygiene and early ambulation to prevent thrombosis.

EMERGING TRENDS AND GUIDELINES

- **Minimally Invasive Techniques:** Laparoscopic repair of uterine perforations reduces recovery time.[13]

- **Bioengineered Materials:** Use of absorbable meshes in fistula repair shows promise.[14]
- **Psychological Interventions:** Early counseling reduces post-traumatic stress in assault survivors.[10]
- **WHO Guidelines (2023):** Emphasize multidisciplinary care and training for obstetric injury prevention.[15]

CONCLUSION

Genital tract injuries, whether obstetric, traumatic, or iatrogenic, pose significant challenges due to their potential for physical, emotional, and social morbidity. Early diagnosis, tailored management, and preventive strategies are crucial to improve outcomes. Multidisciplinary care and adherence to updated guidelines ensure comprehensive management and rehabilitation.

REFERENCES

1. Bjurlin MA, Goble SM, Fantus RJ, et al. Genitourinary injuries in pelvic trauma. J Trauma Acute Care Surg. 2016;80(6):966-71.
2. McLean I, Roberts SA, White C, et al. Female genital injuries resulting from sexual assault. Forensic Sci Int. 2017;271:106-11.
3. Sultan AH, Kettle C, Thakar R. Perineal and anal sphincter trauma. Best Pract Res Clin Obstet Gynaecol. 2019;56:45-57.
4. Pergialiotis V, Vlachos D, Protopapas A, et al. Risk factors for severe perineal lacerations during childbirth. Int J Gynaecol Obstet. 2016;135(1):6-11.
5. Royal College of Obstetricians and Gynaecologists. (2015). Third- and fourth-degree perineal tears, management. Green-top Guideline No. 29. [online] Available from https://www.rcog.org.uk/guidance/browse-all-guidance/green-top-guidelines/third-and-fourth-degree-perineal-tears-management-green-top-guideline-no-29/ [Last accessed December, 2025].
6. Norderval S, Rydningen M, Falk RS, et al. Long-term outcomes after obstetric anal sphincter injuries. Obstet Gynecol. 2019;134(6):1260-8.
7. Andrews V, Thakar R, Sultan AH. Surgical management of obstetric anal sphincter injuries. Int Urogynecol J. 2018;29(6):795-802.
8. Goldman HB, McAchran SE. Urogynecologic and reconstructive pelvic surgery for trauma. Urol Clin North Am. 2019;46(2):237-45.
9. Bodner-Adler B, Hanzal E, Pablik E, et al. Management of genital tract trauma in obstetrics. Arch Gynecol Obstet. 2017;296(6):1047-54.
10. Campbell R, Lichty LF, Sturza J, et al. Gynecologic care for sexual assault survivors. Obstet Gynecol. 2016;128(4):870-6.
11. Halperin O, Noble A, Balachandran S, et al. Complications of genital tract injuries: A review. Eur J Obstet Gynecol Reprod Biol. 2020;247:140-6.
12. World Health Organization. (2018). WHO recommendations: Intrapartum care for a positive childbirth experience. [online] Available from https://www.who.int/publications/i/item/9789241550215 [Last accessed December, 2025].
13. Nezhat C, Kho KA, Morozov V. Laparoscopic management of uterine perforation. J Minim Invasive Gynecol. 2017;24(5):712-7.
14. Mukwege D, Berg M. Advances in fistula repair using bioengineered materials. Int J Gynaecol Obstet. 2021;153(Suppl 1):45-50.
15. World Health Organization. Preventing and managing obstetric complications. WHO, 2023.

Perineal and Cervical Tears in Labor

Ruchika Garg

DEFINITION

Perineal and cervical tears are common obstetric complications occurring during vaginal delivery, ranging from superficial skin lacerations to severe injuries involving the anal sphincter or cervical tissue. Prompt recognition and repair are critical to prevent short- and long-term morbidity.[1]

Key Points

- **Perineal Tears:** Classified into first to fourth degrees based on tissue involvement; third/fourth-degree tears affect 1–3% of vaginal deliveries.[2]
- **Cervical Tears:** Occur in ~1–2% of vaginal deliveries, often associated with operative deliveries; severe cases risk postpartum hemorrhage (PPH).[3]
- Immediate repair under anesthesia in an operating theatre is standard for third-/fourth-degree perineal and significant cervical tears.
- RCOG and NICE guidelines emphasize trained obstetricians, antibiotic prophylaxis, and postoperative care to optimize outcomes.[4,5]
- Long-term complications include anal incontinence, dyspareunia, and cervical incompetence.

PERINEAL TEARS

Classification

Perineal tears are graded by depth and tissue involvement **(Table 1)**.

- **First/Second Degree:** ~50–80% of vaginal deliveries **(Fig. 1).**[2]
- **Third/Fourth Degree [Obstetric Anal Sphincter Injuries (OASIS)]:** 1–3% overall; higher with operative vaginal delivery (forceps: 10–15%, vacuum: 5–10%) or primiparity **(Fig. 2).**[6]

MANAGEMENT OF THIRD/FOURTH-DEGREE PERINEAL TEARS

Timing of Repair

- **Immediate Action:** Shift patient to operating theatre postrecognition for repair under anesthesia.[4]
- **Excessive Bleeding:** Pack vagina with roller gauze to control hemorrhage.

TABLE 1: Classification of perineal tears.[1,4]

Degree	*Description*
First	Involves perineal skin and subcutaneous tissue; perineal muscles intact
Second	Extends to fascia and perineal body muscles; anal sphincter intact.
Third	Involves perineal body and anal sphincter: **3a:** <50% external anal sphincter (EAS) thickness torn. **3b:** >50% EAS thickness torn. **3c:** Full thickness of EAS and internal anal sphincter (IAS).
Fourth	Involves anal sphincter complex and anorectal mucosa.

Note: If third-degree tear grading is uncertain, assign a higher degree to ensure comprehensive repair.[4]

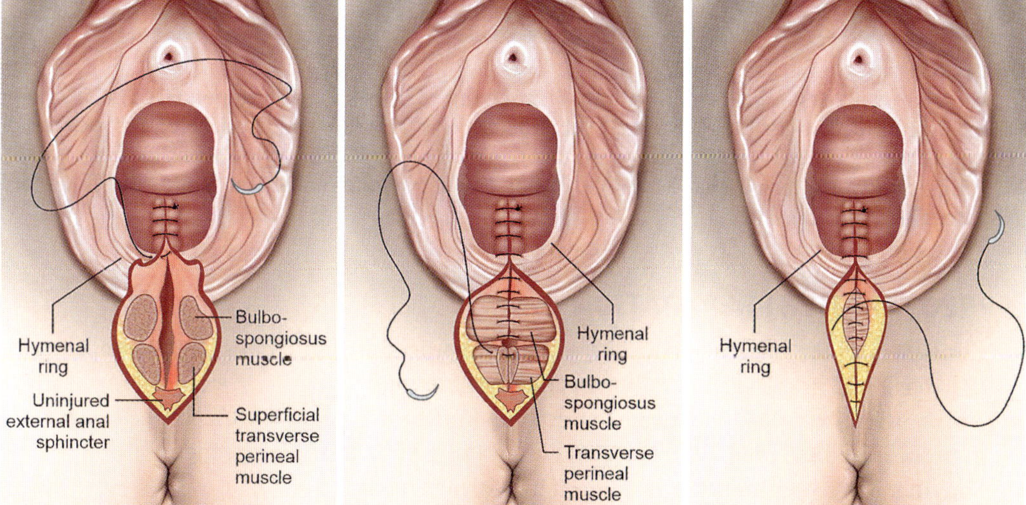

Fig. 1: Second-degree perineal tear.
Source: Jadav N, Bhalerao S. Prevention and Management of Perineal Tear Internet. FOGSI-ICOG Good Clinical Practice Recommendations. New Delhi: Federation of Obstetric and Gynaecological Societies of India (FOGSI) & Indian College of Obstetricians and Gynaecologists (ICOG). [online] Available from https://www.fogsi.org/wp-content/uploads/2024/08/Binder_Prevention-and-Management-of-Perineal-Tear.pdf [Last accessed December, 2025].

- **Delay:** Up to 8–10 hours acceptable if no bleeding and expertise is unavailable, but minimize delay to reduce infection risk.[1,7]

PLACE AND SURGICAL COMPETENCE

- **Location:** Operating theatre with good lighting; delivery room repair (e.g., 3a tears per South Australian guidelines) only in sterile conditions with adequate lighting.[4,8]
- **Personnel:** Trained obstetrician or supervised trainee; colorectal surgeon consultation for complex fourth-degree tears.[4]
- **Training:** Mandatory in postgraduate obstetrics curricula (RCOG, 2015).[4]

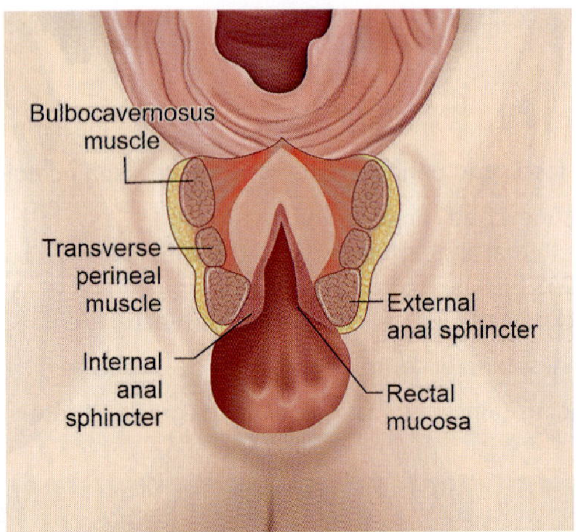

Fig. 2: OASIS.
Source: Jadav N, Bhalerao S. Prevention and Management of Perineal Tear Internet. FOGSI-ICOG Good Clinical Practice Recommendations. New Delhi: Federation of Obstetric and Gynaecological Societies of India (FOGSI) & Indian College of Obstetricians and Gynaecologists (ICOG). [online] Available from https://www.fogsi.org/wp-content/uploads/2024/08/Binder_Prevention-and-Management-of-Perineal-Tear.pdf [Last accessed December, 2025].

PREOPERATIVE PREPARATION

- **Consent:** Written informed consent, explaining procedure, outcomes (80% asymptomatic at 1 year), and risks (e.g., incontinence and dyspareunia).[4]
- **Antibiotics:** Single-dose broad-spectrum antibiotic (e.g., cefuroxime 1.5 g IV + metronidazole 500 mg IV) at repair to reduce wound infection/dehiscence.[5]
- **Shaving:** Not recommended; clip hair if it obstructs repair.[4]
- **Anesthesia:** Regional (spinal/epidural) or general anesthesia for sphincter relaxation and pain control.[5]
- **Positioning:** Dorsal lithotomy with stirrups for optimal exposure.[4]
- **Scrub:** Clean perineum/vagina with 4% chlorhexidine; apply sterile drape.[9]
- **Foley Catheter:** Insert for continuous bladder drainage, maintain for ≥12 hours post-repair.[4]

INTRAOPERATIVE ASPECTS

- **Instruments:** Allis forceps (4), mosquito forceps (4), Metzenbaum scissors, needle holder, Rigby/Sims retractors (2), sponge forceps, atraumatic needles, absorbable sutures (e.g., polyglactin and PDS), and sponges.[4]
- **Assessment:** Confirm tear extent under anesthesia via bimanual exam (index finger in anus, thumb in vagina); identify "buttonhole tear" (rectal mucosa tear with intact sphincter) to prevent rectovaginal fistula.[4]
- **Principles of Repair:**
  - Anatomical layer-by-layer approximation.
  - Avoid dead space and ensure hemostasis.

- Use fine absorbable sutures (e.g., 2-0/3-0 polyglactin, PDS) on tapered needles to minimize tissue reaction.
- Bury knots to reduce dyspareunia.
- Repair from proximal to distal end.[4,10]

SURGICAL TECHNIQUE

- **Anorectal Mucosa:**
  - Start 1 cm above laceration apex.
  - Techniques:
    - **Interrupted Sutures:** 3-0/4-0 polyglactin or poliglecaprone 25, knots inside or outside lumen .
    - **Continuous Nonlocking Suture:** Same sutures .
  - No evidence favors one method; avoid PDS due to prolonged dissolution.[4]
  - Endpoint: Restoration of anal folds.
- **Internal Anal Sphincter (IAS):**
  - Contributes 70–85% of resting anal tone; repair critical for continence.[10]
  - Identify pale, thin layer (1–2 mm) above rectal serosa; often retracted laterally.
  - Technique: End-to-end approximation with interrupted or continuous nonlocking sutures using 2-0/3-0 polyglactin or PDS.[4]
  - Avoid overlapping to prevent tension.[7]
- **External Anal Sphincter (EAS):**
  - **Full-Thickness Tear (3c/4th Degree):**
    - Identify retracted dark red muscle using Allis forceps.
    - Techniques **(Fig. 3):**
      - **Overlapping Repair:** Mobilize ends 1–1.5 cm, double-breast with two suture rows (2-0 polyglactin/PDS); includes fascial sheath.[4]
      - **End-to-End Repair:** Align ends with interrupted sutures.[4]
    - Cochrane Review (2013): Comparable perineal pain/dyspareunia at 1 year; overlapping reduces fecal urgency/incontinence at 12 months.[11]
  - **Partial-Thickness Tear (3a/3b):** End-to-end with 3–4 mattress sutures (2-0 polyglactin/PDS); avoid overlapping.[4]
- **Perineal Muscles:** Reconstruct 2–3 cm perineal body with running/interrupted 2-0 polyglactin sutures to relieve sphincter tension.[4]
- **Vagina and Skin:** Continuous nonlocking 3-0 polyglactin for vaginal mucosa; subcuticular for skin to minimize pain.[4]
- **Post-Repair Check:** Rectal examination to ensure no sutures pierce anorectal mucosa (risks fistula); confirm sponge count.[4]

POSTOPERATIVE CARE

- **Antibiotics:** Continue broad-spectrum antibiotics (e.g., IV cefuroxime + metronidazole for 24–48 hours, then oral amoxicillin-clavulanate) for 5 days.[5]
- **Analgesics:** NSAIDs (e.g., ibuprofen 400 mg TID) + paracetamol; avoid rectal route for fourth-degree tears; ice packs 2–4 hourly for edema.[4]

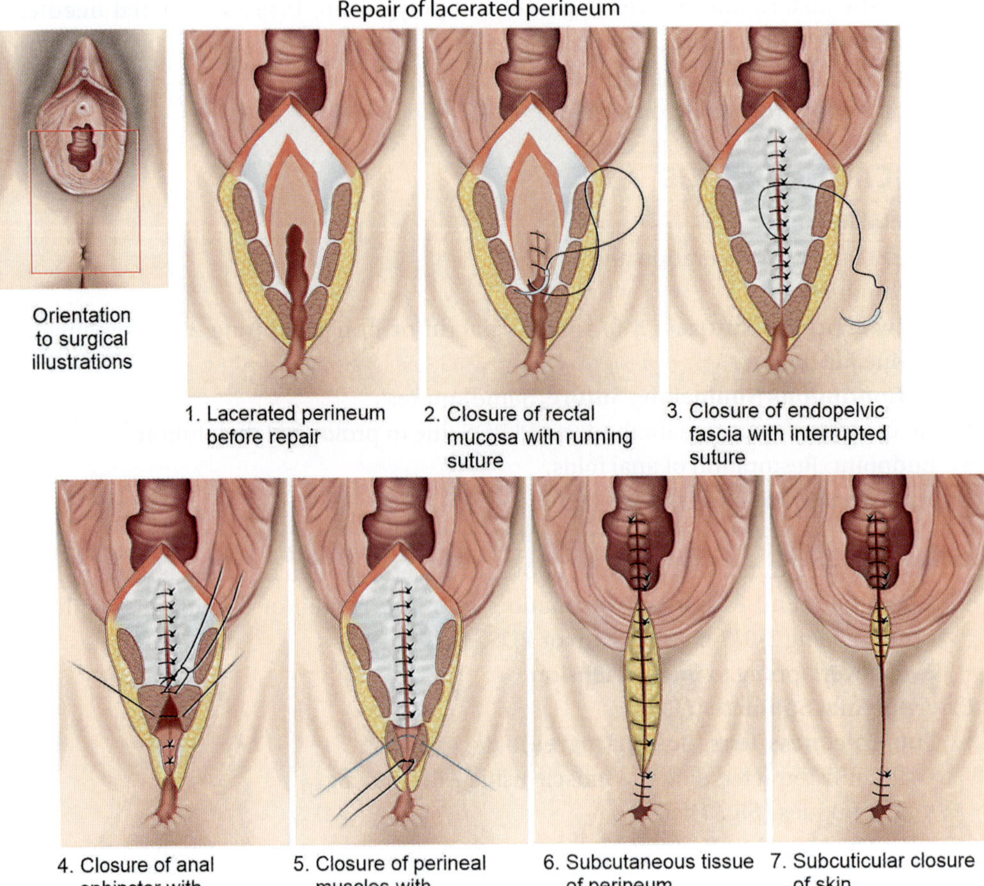

Fig. 3: Oasis repair.

Source: Jadav N, Bhalerao S. Prevention and Management of Perineal Tear Internet. FOGSI-ICOG Good Clinical Practice Recommendations. New Delhi: Federation of Obstetric and Gynaecological Societies of India (FOGSI) & Indian College of Obstetricians and Gynaecologists (ICOG). [online] Available from https://www.fogsi.org/wp-content/uploads/2024/08/Binder_Prevention-and-Management-of-Perineal-Tear.pdf [Last accessed December, 2025].

- **Bowel Care:**
  - Low-residue diet (e.g., white rice and bananas) for 7 days to reduce stool bulk.
  - Osmotic laxatives (lactulose 15 mL BID or PEG 17 g daily) to ease bowel movements.
  - Hydration (2–3 L/day).[4]
- **Bladder Care:** Remove catheter after ≥12 hours; check postvoid residual urine.[4]
- **Posture:** Supine/lateral positioning for 48 hours; avoid prolonged sitting; use towels under thighs.[4]
- **Pelvic Floor Exercises:** Start post-pain resolution (3–7 days); 10-second squeezes, 10 repetitions TID; consult physiotherapist.[12]
- **Wound Care:** Daily baths, frequent pad changes, perineal hygiene; inspect wound with mirror for breakdown signs.[4]

- **Debriefing:** Counsel on recovery, complications, and future delivery implications (e.g., cesarean for persistent incontinence).[4]

PROGNOSIS

- **Short-Term:** 20–25% risk of wound infection or breakdown within 6 weeks.[6]
- **Long-Term:** 60–80% asymptomatic at 1 year; 10–20% report anal incontinence, dyspareunia, or perineal pain.[2]
- **Future Pregnancies:** Cesarean is recommended if persistent anal incontinence.[4]

FOLLOW-UP

- **Timing:** 6–12 weeks postpartum to assess healing and complications.[4]
- **Advice:**
  - Delay intercourse until healing complete (~6 weeks).
  - Report warning signs (e.g., redness, discharge, and incontinence) immediately.[4]

CERVICAL TEARS

Clinical Features

- **Incidence:** ~1–2% of vaginal deliveries; higher with operative vaginal delivery (forceps: 5–10%) or precipitous labor.[3]
- **Types:**
  - **Simple Tears:** Superficial, often asymptomatic.
  - **Annular Detachment:** Complete circumferential tear, rare; associated with prolonged labor or long cervix.[3]
- **Signs:**
  - Excessive bleeding post-third stage despite contracted uterus.
  - Visible tear on cervical inspection.[3]

DIAGNOSIS

- **Exploration:**
  - Perform in lithotomy position under good lighting post-third stage, especially after operative delivery.
  - Use right-angled vaginal retractor anteriorly, Sims speculum posteriorly, and sponge holders to grasp cervical margin clockwise.[4]
  - Digital examination unreliable due to floppy postpartum cervix.[3]
- **Findings:** Bleeding tear or annular detachment; assess for lower uterine segment extension.[3]

MANAGEMENT

- **Indications for Repair:** Active bleeding or deep tears; superficial tears may heal spontaneously.[4]

- **Technique:**
  - **Setting:** Operating theatre under general anesthesia.
  - **Sutures:** Chromic catgut 0 or polyglactin 0 on round-bodied atraumatic needle; include full cervical thickness to secure retracted vessels.[4]
  - **Procedure:**
    - Start at tear apex; avoid excessive traction on friable cervix.
    - Assistant gently pushes fundus to access cervix.
    - If apex inaccessible:
      - **Step-Ladder Stitch:** Place stitch at visible tear top, hold long, and traction to reach higher levels until apex is sutured.[3]
      - **Laparotomy:** If tear extends to lower uterine segment (equivalent to uterine rupture), open lower segment as in cesarean, locate apex, and repair; avoid ureter injury.[4]
- **Post-Repair:** Oxytocin infusion to prevent PPH; antibiotics (e.g., cefazolin 1 g IV) for 24–48 hours.[4]

COMPLICATIONS (TABLE 2)

- **Early:**
  - PPH (major vessels involved).
  - Broad ligament hematoma.
  - Pelvic cellulitis/thrombosis.[3]
- **Late:**
  - Cervical ectropion.
  - Cervical incompetence (risk of preterm birth).[3]

RECENT ADVANCES AND GUIDELINES

- **RCOG Guidelines (2015, updated 2022):**[4]
  - Mandatory repair of third/fourth-degree tears by trained obstetricians in theatre.
  - Antibiotic prophylaxis and postoperative laxatives to reduce complications.
  - Routine cervical inspection postoperative vaginal delivery to detect tears.
- **NICE Guidelines (2017):**[5]
  - Emphasize informed consent, analgesia, and postoperative care for perineal tears.
  - Support pelvic floor exercises to reduce incontinence risk.
- **Intrapartum Ultrasound:** Endoanal ultrasound post-repair to confirm sphincter integrity (Level 2 evidence).[13]
- **Biofeedback Therapy:** Limited evidence for improving sphincter function post-repair.[12]
- **Tranexamic Acid:** Reduces PPH risk in severe perineal/cervical tears (RR 0.61).[14]

TABLE 2: Complications of cervical tears.[3,4]

Timing	*Complication*
Early	PPH, broad ligament hematoma, pelvic cellulitis, and thrombosis
Late	Cervical ectropion and cervical incompetence

KEY POINTS FOR POSTGRADUATE EDUCATION

- Perineal tears occur in ~50–80% of vaginal deliveries; third/fourth-degree tears affect 1–3%.
- Cervical tears occur in 1–2%, often with operative deliveries; annular detachment is rare.
- Third/fourth-degree perineal tears require immediate theatre repair under anesthesia by trained obstetricians.
- Layer-by-layer repair with absorbable sutures (polyglactin/PDS) minimizes complications.
- Overlapping EAS repair reduces fecal incontinence compared to end-to-end in full-thickness tears.
- Cervical tears with active bleeding need suturing; laparotomy for lower segment extension.
- Antibiotic prophylaxis and laxatives are standard postoperative care.
- Long-term risks include anal incontinence (10–20%) and cervical incompetence.
- RCOG/NICE guidelines advocate trained repair, consent, and follow-up at 6–12 weeks.
- Pelvic floor exercises and hygiene reduce complications; cesarean is recommended for future pregnancies with persistent incontinence.

REFERENCES

1. Sultan AH, et al. Third and fourth degree perineal tears: Management and outcomes. BJOG. 2017;124(4):618-25.
2. Frohlich J, et al. Incidence and risk factors for obstetric anal sphincter injuries. Acta Obstet Gynecol Scand. 2018;97(6):718-25.
3. Landy HJ, et al. Cervical lacerations: Incidence and management. Am J Obstet Gynecol. 2016;214(3):368.e1-368.e6.
4. Royal College of Obstetricians and Gynaecologists. (2015). Third- and fourth-degree perineal tears, Management. Green-top Guideline No. 29. [online] Available from https://www.rcog.org.uk/guidance/browse-all-guidance/green-top-guidelines/third-and-fourth-degree-perineal-tears-management-green-top-guideline-no-29/ [Last accessed December, 2025].
5. National Institute for Health and Care Excellence. (2017). Intrapartum care for healthy women and babies (CG190). [online] Available from https://www.nice.org.uk/guidance/cg190 [Last accessed December, 2025].
6. Gurol-Urganci I, et al. Risk factors for obstetric anal sphincter injury. Obstet Gynecol. 2018;132(4):998-1006.
7. Thiagamoorthy G, et al. Management of perineal trauma. Curr Opin Obstet Gynecol. 2019;31(5):334-40.
8. South Australian Perinatal Practice Guidelines. Perineal Trauma Repair. 2018.
9. Fitzpatrick M, et al. Suture materials for obstetric anal sphincter repair: A randomized trial. Obstet Gynecol. 2017;130(2):344-50.
10. Fernando RJ, Sultan AH, Kettle C, et al. Methods of repair for obstetric anal sphincter injuries. Cochrane Database Syst Rev. 2013;2013(12):CD002866.
11. Kettle C, et al. Perineal repair techniques for third- and fourth-degree tears. Cochrane Database Syst Rev. 2013;10:CD002866.
12. Woodley SJ, Lawrenson P, Boyle R, et al. Pelvic floor muscle training for preventing and treating urinary and faecal incontinence in antenatal and postnatal women. Cochrane Database Syst Rev. 2020;7:CD007471.
13. Walsh KA, et al. Endoanal ultrasound in the assessment of obstetric anal sphincter injuries. Ultrasound Obstet Gynecol. 2019;54(2):247-53.
14. Saccone G, Corte LD, D'Alessandro P, et al. Prophylactic use of tranexamic acid after vaginal delivery reduces the risk of primary postpartum hemorrhage. J Matern Fetal Neonatal Med. 2020;33(19):3368-74.

Episiotomy

Ruchika Garg

INTRODUCTION

Episiotomy is a surgical incision of the perineum and vaginal wall to facilitate vaginal delivery.[1] Once routine, its use has declined due to associated complications and evidence favoring a restrictive approach. This chapter provides a concise, evidence-based overview of episiotomy for medical postgraduate education, covering types, indications, techniques, complications, and current guidelines.

The World Health Organization (WHO) recommends a restrictive approach with a target episiotomy rate of 10%.[2]

BENEFITS

- **Maternal:**
  - Prevents perineal tears/lacerations.
  - Preserves pelvic floor integrity and reduce risk of urethral/anal dysfunction.
  - Facilitates operative vaginal delivery or shoulder dystocia management.[1]
- **Fetal:**
  - Expedites delivery in fetal distress.
  - Protects fetal head from trauma during delivery.[1]

TYPES

Four types exist, with midline and mediolateral being the most common **(Figs. 1 and 2** and **Table 1)**.

INDICATIONS

- **Maternal:**
  - Shortens second stage of labor.
  - Maternal exhaustion.
  - Facilitates instrumental delivery, vaginal breech, or shoulder dystocia.
  - Prevents severe perineal tears or manages prior perineal scarring.[1]
- **Fetal:**
  - Expedites delivery in fetal distress.
  - Facilitates face-to-pubis delivery or large fetus.[1]

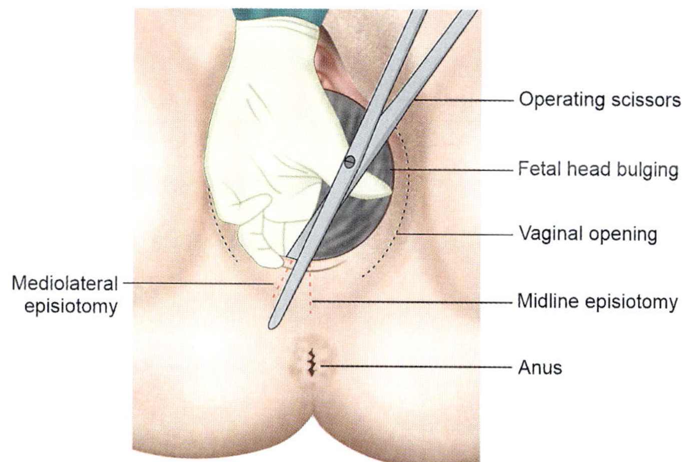

Fig. 1: Mediolateral and midline episiotomy.

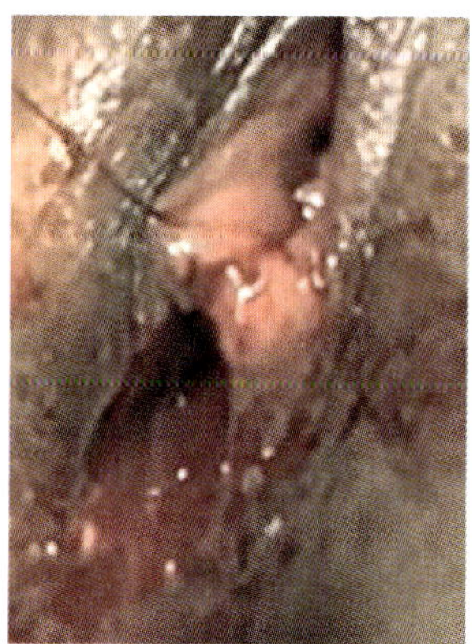

Fig. 2: Mediolateral episiotomy.

TABLE 1: Comparison of episiotomy types.

Type	*Description*	*Merits*	*Demerits*
Midline	Incision from vaginal fourchette toward anus, sparing anal sphincter[1]	Easy to perform, minimal blood loss, easy repair, less dyspareunia, and rare wound disruption	Higher risk of anal sphincter damage, more postoperative pain[3]
Mediolateral	Incision from fourchette at 45° toward ischial tuberosity, cutting multiple muscles[2]	Protects anal sphincter[2]	More painful, increased bleeding, difficult repair, and risk to Bartholin gland[3]
J-shaped	Midline for 1.5 cm, then curves at 5/7 o'clock to avoid sphincter[1]	Avoids anal sphincter	Not widely practiced, limited data[1]
Lateral	Incision from fourchette, straight or angled, now obsolete[1]	–	High complication risk, not recommended[1]

CONTRAINDICATIONS

- **Absolute:** Lack of patient consent.[2]
- **Relative:** Inflammatory bowel disease, severe perineal malformations.[1]
- Episiotomy is contraindicated if vaginal delivery is not feasible.[2]

STRUCTURES INVOLVED

The incision involves:

- Vaginal mucosa.
- Perineal body (superficial/deep transverse perineal muscles, bulbospongiosus, perineal membrane, and external anal sphincter fibers).
- Perineal skin.[1]

TIMING AND TECHNIQUE

- **Timing:** Perform at crowning (3–4 cm of fetal head visible) to minimize blood loss and complications.[2] For forceps delivery, incise after blade application.[1]
- **Prerequisites:**
  - Verbal patient consent.
  - Clear indication.
  - Adequate lighting and lithotomy position.
- **Instruments:**
  - Episiotomy scissors (angled, blunt tips).
  - Needle holder, absorbable sutures (e.g., Vicryl Rapide 2-0 and Polyglycolic acid).[3]
  - 1% lidocaine (10 mL), hemostatic/tissue forceps, syringes, gauze, sterile gloves, and surgical drape.

Technique:

- Clean perineum with antiseptic and infiltrate with 10 mL 1% lidocaine.
- Place two fingers between vagina and presenting part.
- Incise at peak of uterine contraction, ensuring adequate length.
- Control active bleeding with artery forceps.
- Postdelivery, inspect cervix, vagina, and perineum for tears/extensions before placental delivery.[2]

SUTURING

- **Principles:**
  - Use aseptic technique and ensure analgesia.
  - Close in layers: Vaginal mucosa, perineal muscles, and skin.
  - Start vaginal mucosa closure 1 cm above incision apex with absorbable sutures (e.g., Vicryl Rapide) to prevent hematoma.[3]
  - Reapproximate perineal muscles (continuous or interrupted sutures).
  - Close skin with continuous subcuticular sutures to reduce pain.[3,4]
- **Evidence:** Continuous suturing reduces short-term pain, analgesia need, and suture material use compared to interrupted suturing.[3,4]

TABLE 2: Complications of episiotomy.

Type	*Complications*
Immediate	Extension to rectum (common in midline), primary hemorrhage, vulvar hematoma, infection, wound disruption, rectal fistula, and necrotizing fasciitis (rare)[3]
Remote	Dyspareunia, persistent discharge (granulation tissue), poorly healed scar, and delayed recovery due to urinary retention[3]

Note: Risk of complications increases with operative vaginal delivery; midline episiotomy has higher rectal extension risk, mediolateral has more bleeding.[3]

- **Post-Repair:**
  - Inspect vagina for gaps, rectal stitches, or residual bleeding.
  - Perform rectal examination to confirm sphincter integrity.[2]

POSTNATAL CARE

- **Wound Care:** Clean and dry daily to prevent infection.[2]
- **Pain Management:**
  - Cooling treatments (ice packs and cool gel) reduce pain.[5]
  - Sitz baths or analgesics (paracetamol, ibuprofen, and diclofenac suppositories) are effective.[6]
- **Monitoring:** Assess for hematoma, infection, or wound disruption.

COMPLICATIONS

The complications of episiotomy are shown in Table 2.

ROUTINE VERSUS SELECTIVE EPISIOTOMY

- **Routine:** Performed in all vaginal deliveries, especially primigravida, to reduce tears.[1]
- **Selective:** Performed only when indicated (e.g., fetal distress and instrumental delivery).[2]
- **Evidence:**
  - Selective approach reduces episiotomy rates and complications.[7]
  - WHO recommends a 10% episiotomy rate, discouraging routine use.[2]
  - ACOG (2016) supports selective use for maternal/fetal indications.[1]
  - FIGO (2019) endorses restrictive policy.[8]
  - Systematic reviews find no benefit of routine episiotomy over selective.[9]

RECENT ADVANCES AND GUIDELINES

- **Suture Materials:** Vicryl Rapide reduces postoperative pain and dehiscence compared to chromic catgut.[3]
- **Continuous Suturing:** Preferred for less pain and material use.[3,4]
- **Pain Management:** Nonpharmacologic (cooling) and pharmacologic (NSAIDs) options improve outcomes.[5,6]

- **Guidelines:**
  - WHO (2018): Restrictive episiotomy policy.[2]
  - ACOG (2016): Selective use based on obstetrician judgment.[1]
  - FIGO (2019): Endorses restrictive approach.[8]

KEY POINTS

- Episiotomy facilitates vaginal delivery but is associated with complications.
- Mediolateral episiotomy is preferred globally; midline risks anal sphincter damage.
- Continuous suturing reduces postnatal pain and suture material use.
- Selective episiotomy is supported by WHO, ACOG, and FIGO, with a target rate of 10%.
- Proper timing (at crowning) and technique minimize complications.

REFERENCES

1. American College of Obstetricians and Gynecologists' Committee on Practice Bulletins—Obstetrics. Practice Bulletin No. 165: Prevention and Management of Obstetric Lacerations at Vaginal Delivery. Obstet Gynecol. 2016;128(1):e1-e15.
2. World Health Organization. (2018). WHO Recommendation on Episiotomy Policy. [online] Available from https://bestdoulas.com/wp-content/uploads/2020/06/epiguidelines.pdf. [Last accessed December, 2025].
3. Kettle C, Dowswell T, Ismail KM. Continuous and interrupted suturing techniques for repair of episiotomy or second-degree tears. Cochrane Database Syst Rev. 2012;11(1):CD000947.
4. Kettle C, Hills RK, Ismail KMK. Continuous versus interrupted sutures for repair of episiotomy or second-degree tears. Cochrane Database Syst Rev. 2007;(4):CD000947.
5. East CE, Df Dorward E, Whale RE, et al. Local cooling for relieving pain from perineal trauma sustained during childbirth. Cochrane Database Syst Rev. 2020;10(10):CD006304.
6. Chou D, Abalos E, Gyte GML, et al. Paracetamol/acetaminophen (single administration) for perineal pain in the early postpartum period. Cochrane Database Syst Rev. 2021;(1):CD008407.
7. Melo I, Katz L, Coutinho I, et al. Selective episiotomy vs. implementation of a non-episiotomy protocol: a randomized clinical trial. Reprod Health. 2014;11:66.
8. Nassar AH, Visser GHA, Ayres-de-Campos D, et al. FIGO Statement: Restrictive use rather than routine use of episiotomy. Int J Gynaecol Obstet. 2019;146(1):17-9.
9. Hartmann K, Viswanathan M, Palmieri R, et al. Outcomes of routine episiotomy: a systematic review. JAMA. 2015;293(17):2141-8.

Pregnancy with Previous Cesarean Delivery: VBAC and TOLAC

Ruchika Garg

INTRODUCTION

The global cesarean section (CS) rate has surged from 7% in 1990 to 21% in 2021, driven by medical, social, and legal factors.[1] Prior CS accounts for 60% of elective and 14% of emergency CS, posing challenges in subsequent pregnancies.[1] Historically, Cragin's 1916 dictum "once a cesarean, always a cesarean" reflected high risks of classical CS scars. Modern advances—lower segment CS, safe anesthesia, antibiotics, and blood transfusion—have made vaginal birth after cesarean (VBAC) via trial of labor after cesarean (TOLAC) a viable option, with success rates of 60–80%.[2] However, failed TOLAC increases the risks of uterine rupture (0.2–1.8%) and emergency CS morbidity.[3] In India, CS rates approach 30% in urban areas, necessitating evidence-based VBAC protocols.[4] This chapter outlines complications, uterine scar integrity, VBAC predictors, contraindications, management, and complications for postgraduate medical education.

TYPES OF UTERINE SCARS

- Transverse lower segment cesarean scar (most common and safer)
- Classical scar (vertical uterine incision with higher rupture risk)
- T-shaped or other atypical scars
- Myomectomy scars (increased risk of rupture depending on depth and location)

Maternal risk	*Neonatal risk*
Uterine rupture (0.3–1% after 1 CS, up to 1.8% after 2 CS)	Preterm birth due to indicated delivery
Placenta previa/accreta spectrum	Intrauterine Growth Restriction (IUGR)
Placenta accreta spectrum	Neonatal respiratory morbidity
Postpartum hemorrhage	Neonatal ICU admissions
Surgical complications	Perinatal mortality (rare but increased)

RISKS ASSOCIATED WITH PREGNANCY IN SCARRED UTERUS

Clinical Evaluation and Surveillance

- Detailed obstetric history emphasizing type and number of prior uterine surgeries.
- Ultrasonographic evaluation early to locate placenta and assess scar integrity.
- High-resolution TVS/MRI may be required for placental implantation abnormalities.

- Counseling on risks of vaginal birth after cesarean (VBAC) versus repeat cesarean delivery (CD).

NICE GUIDELINES (2023–2025) ON PREGNANCY FOLLOWING CESAREAN SECTION

After One Previous Cesarean Section

- Inform women about benefits/risks of VBAC versus elective repeat cesarean delivery (ERCD).
- Offer trial of labor after cesarean (TOLAC) if no contraindications (e.g., classical scar and uterine rupture history).
- Continuous fetal monitoring during labor mandatory.
- Immediate access to cesarean delivery is essential in case of emergency.
- Induction with caution; prostaglandins contraindicated for induction in VBAC candidates, but cautious use of oxytocin is permitted.
- In labor, monitor carefully for signs of uterine rupture (abnormal CTG and pain).
- If VBAC fails or rupture suspected, proceed urgently to cesarean.

After Two Previous Cesarean Sections

- ERCD is more commonly recommended due to increased rupture risk (~1.8%).
- VBAC may be considered in selected cases with stringent monitoring and experienced units.
- Place of birth should be a facility equipped for emergency surgery and neonatal care.

RCOG GUIDELINES (GREEN-TOP 2015, UPDATED 2024)

- VBAC success in carefully selected women is approximately 60–80%.
- Key factors predicting successful VBAC: Prior vaginal birth, nonrecurrent indication for previous CS, and spontaneous labor onset.
- Major concerns in two or more CS pregnancies include higher rates of uterine rupture, placenta previa/accreta, and surgical complications.
- Careful antenatal planning and individualized counseling are emphasized.
- Repeat cesarean at 39 weeks reduces risk of uterine rupture but must be balanced against preterm delivery risks.

LABOR AND DELIVERY MANAGEMENT

Aspect	*VBAC*	*ERCD*
Timing of delivery	Spontaneous labor preferred	Usually schedule at 39 weeks
Monitoring	Continuous CTG mandatory	Routine fetal monitoring
Induction	Avoid prostaglandins; cautious oxytocin	No labor induction
Uterine rupture risk	0.5–1% with one prior CS	Minimal, surgical risks present
Emergency readiness	Immediate surgical access required	Planned surgery with blood products

Algorithm: Management of Pregnancy with One Previous Cesarean

Pregnant woman with prior cesarean → assess obstetric/medical status
↓
Discuss mode of delivery, risks, and preferences (VBAC vs. ERCD)
↓
If VBAC chosen → monitor throughout pregnancy; plan hospital birth with surgical team on standby
↓
In labor → continuous monitoring, avoid prostaglandins, cautious oxytocin
↓
Signs of rupture → emergency cesarean
↓
If ERCD chosen → schedule cesarean at 39 weeks unless contraindications arise

Algorithm: Management After Two Previous Cesarean Sections

Assess maternal–fetal status and scar type
↓
Discussion regarding stronger recommendation for ERCD due to higher rupture risk
↓
If VBAC considered → restrict to highly selected cases in equipped units with continuous fetal monitoring
↓
Planned ERCD at or before 39 weeks most common approach
↓
Close surveillance for placenta previa/accreta is mandatory

COUNSELING POINTS

- VBAC offers lower maternal morbidity and fewer complications than multiple repeat cesareans but carries a risk of uterine rupture.
- Repeat cesarean avoids rupture risk but may have surgical and placental complication risks in subsequent pregnancies.
- Informed and shared decision-making essential involving explanation of all risks and benefits.
- Women advised to seek care at tertiary centers with multidisciplinary teams.

SUMMARY

- Pregnancy in the scarred uterus carries increased risks of obstetric complications, notably uterine rupture and abnormal placental implantation.
- Careful risk assessment, antenatal surveillance, and delivery planning per NICE and RCOG guidelines optimize safety for mother and baby.
- VBAC is safe and encouraged in appropriately selected women with one previous cesarean.
- Multiple previous CS necessitate individualized counseling and often planned repeat cesarean.
- Multidisciplinary care teams and appropriate birth settings are critical components of management.

COMPLICATIONS OF PREGNANCY AFTER CESAREAN DELIVERY

Prior CS increases risks in subsequent pregnancies across antenatal, intrapartum, and postpartum periods **(Table 1)**.[5]

- **Antenatal:**
  - Spontaneous abortion (OR 1.3, 95% CI 1.1–1.5).
  - Placenta previa (OR 2.0, 95% CI 1.6–2.5).
  - Placenta accreta spectrum (PAS): Risk with placenta previa rises from 3% (1st CS) to 67% (≥5 CS).[6]
  - Cesarean scar pregnancy (CSP; 1:1,800 pregnancies).
  - Abruptio placentae (OR 1.5, 95% CI 1.2–1.9).
- **Intrapartum:**
  - Uterine rupture: 0.2–0.9% (1 low transverse scar), 2–6% (prior rupture), 2–9% (classical scar).[7]
  - Preterm labor (OR 1.4, 95% CI 1.1–1.8).
  - Increased operative interventions: Emergency CS, manual placenta removal.
- **Postpartum:**
  - Postpartum hemorrhage (PPH; OR 1.7, 95% CI 1.4–2.1).
  - Emergency hysterectomy (14–33% in uterine rupture cases).
  - Endometritis (higher in failed TOLAC).

UTERINE SCAR INTEGRITY

Scar integrity influences TOLAC safety and VBAC success **(Table 2)**.[8]

- **Factors Affecting Scar Strength:**
  - **Apposition:** Poor alignment weakens scar.
  - **Hemostasis:** Hematomas impair healing.
  - **Nutrition:** Anemia, hypoproteinemia delay repair.
  - **Infection:** Sepsis increases rupture risk (OR 2.5, 95% CI 1.8–3.4).
  - **Suture Technique:** Single-layer closure may increase rupture risk (RR 0.32, 95% CI 0.17–0.61).[9]
  - **Scar Type:** Low transverse (0.2–0.9% rupture) versus classical (2–9%).[7]
  - **Interdelivery Interval:** <18 months increases rupture risk threefold.[10]
  - **Multiple CS:** Myometrial thickness decreases with each CS.
- **Assessment:**
  - Ultrasound: Lower uterine segment (LUS) thickness at 34–39 weeks:[11]

TABLE 1: Complications after previous cesarean delivery.[5-7]

Period	*Complication*	*Risk (OR, 95% CI)*
Antenatal	Placenta Previa	2.0 (1.6–2.5)
	PAS (with previa)	3–67% (by CS number)
Intrapartum	Uterine Rupture	0.2–9% (by scar type)
Postpartum	PPH	1.7 (1.4–2.1)

TABLE 2: Factors affecting uterine scar integrity.[7-11]

Factor	*Impact on scar*	*Rupture risk*
Single-Layer Closure	Possible weaker scar	RR 0.32 (0.17–0.61)
Classical Scar	High rupture risk	2–9%
Interdelivery <18 months	Impaired healing	3-fold increase
LUS Thickness <2 mm	High rupture risk	9% VBAC success

TABLE 3: Predictors of VBAC success.[7,12-16]

Factor	*VBAC success rate*	*Notes*
Prior Vaginal Birth	80–90%	Strongest predictor
Spontaneous Labor	75%	Vs. 60% with induction
BMI >40 kg/m^2	61%	Obesity reduces success
Macrosomia (>4 kg)	50%	Increased failure risk

- <2 mm: High rupture risk, 9% VBAC success.
- 2–2.4 mm: Intermediate risk, 42% success.
- ≥2.5 mm: Low risk, 61% success.

FACTORS PREDICTING VBAC SUCCESS

Vaginal birth after cesarean success rates are 60–80% (70.4% after 1 CS, 51.4% after ≥2 CS).[12] Predictors include **(Table 3)**:

- **Favorable Factors:**[13]
  - One/two low transverse CS (0.2–0.9% rupture vs. 0.9–1.8% with multiple).[7]
  - Prior vaginal delivery (OR 3.9, 95% CI 2.8–5.4).
  - Spontaneous labor (75% success vs. 60% with induction).[14]
  - Nonrecurrent CS indication (e.g., breech, 60–90% success vs. dystocia, 50%).[15]
  - Preterm pregnancy (<37 weeks).
  - Normal BMI (85% success vs. 61% if BMI >40 kg/m^2).[16]
  - Patient consent and counseling.
- **Unfavorable Factors:**[13]
  - Maternal age >30 years, single status.
  - Macrosomia (>4 kg; 50% success).
  - Obesity (BMI >40 kg/m^2; 61% success).
  - Overdistended uterus (multifetal, polyhydramnios).
  - Preeclampsia, gestational age >40 weeks.
  - Induced labor (0.2–1.5% rupture risk).[14]

CONTRAINDICATIONS TO VBAC (TABLE 4)

- Absolute:[17]
  - Classical/T-shaped scar.
  - Prior uterine rupture.

TABLE 4: Contraindications to VBAC.[17]

Type	Contraindication	Reason
Absolute	Classical Scar	2–9% rupture risk
Absolute	Prior Rupture	6–32% recurrence risk
Relative	≥3 Prior CS	Increased rupture risk

- Obstetric contraindications (e.g., placenta previa).
- Patient refusal.
- Inadequate facilities.

- Relative:[17]
  - ≥3 prior CS.
  - Short interdelivery interval (<18 months).
  - Breech presentation.
  - Low vertical scar (1–7% rupture risk).

CRITERIA FOR TOLAC (ACOG 2019)

- **Prior Incision:**[17]
  - One low transverse CS: Low rupture risk (0.2–0.9%).
  - Classical/T-shaped/preterm CS: 2-fold rupture risk; avoid TOLAC.
  - Low vertical scar: Assess upper extent; avoid if contractile portion involved.
- **Scar Number:** ≥2 CS increases rupture risk (1.8% vs. 0.9%) but not contraindicated if low transverse.[17]
- **LUS Thickness:** ≥2.5 mm preferred.[11]
- **Interdelivery Interval:** ≥18 months reduces rupture risk.[10]
- **Prior Vaginal Birth:** Increases VBAC success (80–90%).[13]
- **Fetal Factors:** Avoid TOLAC if macrosomia (>4 kg) or breech (ECV contraindicated).[17]
- **Maternal Factors:** Obesity, diabetes reduce success; twins not contraindicated (75–85% success).[16]

MANAGEMENT OF VBAC

- **Antenatal Counseling:**[18]
  - Discuss TOLAC vs. ERCD: Risks (uterine rupture and PAS) and benefits (shorter recovery and lower PAS risk).
  - Review prior CS details (incision, healing, and complications) via discharge summary.
  - Informed consent mandatory.
- **Monitoring:**
  - Ultrasound: Assess LUS thickness, placenta location, and PAS risk.[11]
- **Timing:**[17]
  - TOLAC: Await spontaneous labor; avoid delivery <39 weeks unless indicated.
  - ERCD: Plan at 39 weeks if fetus mature.

- **Intrapartum Care:**[17]
  - **Facilities**: Tertiary center with senior obstetrician, anesthesia, blood transfusion, and emergency CS capabilities.
  - **Monitoring:** Continuous cardiotocography (CTG) and partogram for labor progress.
  - **Anesthesia:** Epidural is safe but may mask rupture symptoms; maintain vigilance.
  - **Augmentation:** Oxytocin is titrated (<4 contractions/10 min); avoid misoprostol (PGE1).[14]
  - **Third Stage:** Active management of third stage labor (AMTSL) to prevent PPH; avoid early placenta delivery if no separation.
  - **Exploration:** Avoid routine scar exploration; perform if excessive bleeding/ hypovolemia.
- **Postnatal:** Counsel on contraception, interdelivery interval (>18 months).

UTERINE RUPTURE (TABLE 5)

- **Definition:** Complete/partial separation of uterine scar, with fetal/placental extrusion.[7]
- **Incidence:** 0.2–0.9% (1 low transverse CS), 1.8% (2 CS), 6–32% (prior rupture).[7]
- **Signs/Symptoms:**[7]
  - Nonreassuring FHR (variable decelerations and bradycardia).
  - Cessation of contractions.
  - Abdominal pain (may be masked by epidural).
  - Loss of station and uterine contour.
  - Vaginal bleeding.
- **Management:**[7]
  - **Complete Rupture**: Emergency laparotomy; hysterectomy (14–33%) or repair in select cases.
  - **Fetal Outcome:** 50–75% demise if placenta intact; prompt delivery (decision-to-delivery <18 min) improves survival.
- **Maternal Risks:** Bladder injury, transfusion, and maternal death (rare in tertiary settings).

COMPLICATIONS OF VBAC VERSUS ERCD (TABLE 6)

- **VBAC:**[19]
  - Morbidity: 5.5% (vs. 3.6% ERCD).
  - Uterine rupture: 0.2–0.7% (0% in ERCD).
  - Failed TOLAC: 14.1% morbidity (vs. 2.4% successful VBAC).
  - Endometritis: Higher in failed TOLAC.

TABLE 5: Uterine rupture risks and management.[7]

Scar type	*Rupture risk*	*Management*
Low Transverse (1 CS)	0.2–0.9%	Laparotomy, repair/hysterectomy
Classical	2–9%	Hysterectomy preferred
Prior Rupture	6–32%	Avoid TOLAC

TABLE 6: Complications of VBAC versus ERCD.[19,20]

Outcome	*VBAC*	*ERCD*
Morbidity	5.5%	3.6%
Uterine Rupture	0.2–0.7%	0%
Failed TOLAC Morbidity	14.1%	N/A

- **ERCD:**[19]
  - Increased PAS risk (3–67% with previa).
  - Longer recovery, higher surgical complications.
- **Long-Term:** VBAC may reduce pelvic floor dysfunction, but data are limited.[20]

CURRENT GUIDELINES

- **ACOG (2019):**[17] TOLAC is safe for 1–2 low transverse CS; avoid with classical scar, prior rupture; tertiary facilities are required.
- **RCOG (2021):**[21] Support TOLAC after 2 CS if low transverse; emphasize counseling, CTG monitoring.
- **FOGSI (2023):**[22] Advocate VBAC in India with LUS thickness assessment, spontaneous labor preference.
- **WHO (2018):**[23] Promote VBAC to reduce CS rates; ensure informed consent, skilled care.

COST CONSIDERATIONS

Vaginal birth after cesarean is cost-effective (30–40% lower than ERCD) due to shorter hospital stays and fewer surgical resources.[24] However, failed TOLAC increases costs due to emergency CS and complications. Decision-making should prioritize safety over cost.

CONCLUSION

The global cesarean section (CS) rate has risen from 7% in 1990 to 21% in 2021, with prior CS accounting for 60% of elective and 14% of emergency CS. VBAC via trial of labor after cesarean (TOLAC) offers a safe alternative to elective repeat cesarean delivery (ERCD) in selected cases, reducing risks like placenta accreta spectrum (PAS). VBAC success rates range from 60% to 80%, but failed TOLAC increases morbidity, including uterine rupture (0.2–1.8%). Advances in lower segment CS, antibiotics, and anesthesia have shifted the paradigm from "once a cesarean, always a cesarean" to "once a cesarean, always a hospital delivery." Prior vaginal delivery, spontaneous labor, and nonrecurrent CS indications predict success, while classical scars, short interdelivery intervals, and macrosomia increase risks. Prenatal counseling, LUS thickness assessment, and tertiary care delivery with continuous monitoring are critical. Individualized management optimize maternal and fetal outcomes, reducing the burden of rising CS rates.

REFERENCES

1. Betran AP, Ye J, Moller AB, et al. Trends and projections of caesarean section rates: global and regional estimates. BMJ Glob Health. 2021;6(6):e005671.

2. Guise JM, Eden K, Emeis C, et al. Vaginal birth after cesarean: new insights. Evid Rep Technol Assess (Full Rep). 2015;191:1-397.
3. Silver RM, Branch DW. Placenta accreta spectrum. N Engl J Med. 2018;378(16):1529-36.
4. Desai G, Anand A, Modi D, et al. Caesarean section rates in India: a cross-sectional analysis. J Obstet Gynaecol India. 2020;70(4):247-53.
5. Sandall J, Tribe RM, Avery L, et al. Short-term and long-term effects of caesarean section on the health of women and children. Lancet. 2018;392(10155):1349-57.
6. Jauniaux E, Chantraine F, Silver RM, et al. FIGO consensus guidelines on placenta accreta spectrum disorders: epidemiology. Int J Gynaecol Obstet. 2018;140(3):265-73.
7. Landon MB, Grobman WA. Uterine rupture in patients attempting vaginal birth after cesarean delivery. Clin Obstet Gynecol. 2016;59(2):320-8.
8. Lappen JR, Grobman WA. Induction of labor in women with a prior cesarean delivery. Semin Perinatol. 2015;39(6):458-63.
9. Jastrow N, Demers S, Chaillet N, et al. Lower uterine segment thickness to predict uterine rupture: a systematic review. Eur J Obstet Gynecol Reprod Biol. 2016;207:7-14.
10. Stamilio DM, DeFranco E, Paré E, et al. Short interpregnancy interval: risk of uterine rupture and complications of vaginal birth after cesarean delivery. Obstet Gynecol. 2017;130(5):1076-82.
11. Kok N, Wiersma IC, Opmeer BC, et al. Sonographic measurement of lower uterine segment thickness to predict uterine rupture during a trial of labor. Ultrasound Obstet Gynecol. 2018,51(5):609-15.
12. Metz TD, Stoddard GJ, Henry E, et al. Success of trial of labor after two prior cesarean deliveries. Am J Obstet Gynecol. 2017;216(3):293.e1-6.
13. Grobman WA, Lai Y, Landon MB, et al. Prediction of vaginal birth after cesarean delivery. Obstet Gynecol. 2018;131(5):801-10.
14. Palatnik A, Grobman WA. Induction of labor versus expectant management for women with a prior cesarean delivery. Am J Obstet Gynecol. 2015;212(3):358.e1-6.
15. Eden KB, McDonagh M, Denman MA, et al. New insights on vaginal birth after cesarean: can it be predicted? Obstet Gynecol. 2016;128(5):967-76.
16. Hibbard JU, Gilbert S, Landon MB, et al. Trial of labor or repeat cesarean delivery in women with morbid obesity. Obstet Gynecol. 2016;127(3):489-96.
17. American College of Obstetricians and Gynecologists. Vaginal birth after cesarean delivery. Practice Bulletin No. 205. Obstet Gynecol. 2019;133(2):e110-e127.
18. Cheng ER, Declercq ER, Belanoff C, et al. Counseling about vaginal birth after cesarean: a national survey. Birth. 2015;42(3):237-45.
19. Curtin SC, Gregory KD, Korst LM, et al. Maternal morbidity for vaginal and cesarean deliveries. Natl Vital Stat Rep. 2015;64(4):1-16.
20. Gyhagen M, Bullarbo M, Nielsen TF, et al. Pelvic floor dysfunction after vaginal birth and cesarean section. Int Urogynecol J. 2020;31(6):1119-27.
21. Royal College of Obstetricians and Gynaecologists. Birth after previous caesarean birth. Green-top Guideline No. 45. BJOG. 2021;128(5):e28-e54.
22. Federation of Obstetric and Gynaecological Societies of India. Guidelines on vaginal birth after cesarean. J Obstet Gynaecol India. 2023;73(Suppl 1):45-52.
23. World Health Organization. WHO recommendations: non-clinical interventions to reduce unnecessary caesarean sections. Geneva: WHO; 2018.
24. Gilbert SA, Grobman WA, Landon MB, et al. Cost-effectiveness of trial of labor after previous cesarean delivery. Obstet Gynecol. 2016;127(2):277-84.

Placenta Accreta Spectrum Disorders

Ruchika Garg

INTRODUCTION

Placenta accreta spectrum (PAS) disorders describe abnormal placental invasion into the uterine myometrium due to defective decidualization, encompassing placenta accreta (superficial attachment), increta (myometrial invasion), and percreta (serosal or pelvic organ invasion).[1] First described in 1950, PAS prevalence has risen with increasing cesarean deliveries, now estimated at 0.17% globally (range 0.01–1.2%).[2] PAS is a major cause of obstetric hemorrhage, with 60–70% maternal morbidity and historical mortality of 5–7%, though modern multidisciplinary care has lowered mortality to <1%.[3] Prenatal diagnosis and planned delivery in tertiary centers are critical to improving outcomes.[4] In India, PAS contributes to 10–15% of severe postpartum hemorrhage cases, necessitating standardized protocols.[5] This chapter outlines pathophysiology, risk factors, diagnosis, management, and complications of PAS for postgraduate medical education.

METHODS

A systematic literature search was conducted using PubMed and Google Scholar for articles published between January 2015 and June 2025. Search terms included *placenta accreta spectrum, obstetric hemorrhage, cesarean hysterectomy, prenatal diagnosis*, and *multidisciplinary care*. Inclusion criteria were: (1) Original research, reviews, or guidelines, (2) English language, (3) peer-reviewed, (4) relevant to obstetrics, and (5) full-text available. From 120 articles identified, 25 duplicates were removed, 70 irrelevant articles were excluded, and 25 were selected for review.

PATHOPHYSIOLOGY

Placenta accreta spectrum results from defective decidualization at the endometrium–myometrium interface, often at a uterine scar, leading to abnormal trophoblast invasion.[6]

- **Mechanism:**
  - Absent/scanty decidua prevents normal cleavage plane formation, allowing trophoblast attachment to myometrium.[6]
  - Avascular scar tissue promotes deep invasion under low oxygen tension.[7]
- **Subtypes:**[6]
  - **Placenta Accreta:** Villi attach to myometrium without invasion.
  - **Placenta Increta:** Villi penetrate deeply into myometrium.

TABLE 1: PAS Subtypes and pathological features.[6,7]

Subtype	*Description*	*Histopathology*
Placenta Accreta	Villi attach to myometrium	No decidua, villi on myometrial surface
Placenta Increta	Villi invade myometrium	Villi within myometrial fibers
Placenta Percreta	Villi penetrate serosa/pelvic organs	Villi beyond serosa, into adjacent structures

TABLE 2: Risk factors for PAS disorders.[9-12]

Risk factor	*Odds ratio (95% CI)*	*Notes*
Cesarean Delivery	3.0–6.7	Risk increases with number
Placenta Previa	3.0–67.0	Synergistic with cesareans
Uterine Surgery	2.0–4.0	Curettage, myomectomy, and ablation
ART	3.1 (1.5–6.4)	Limited evidence

  - **Placenta Percreta:** Villi invade through serosa, potentially into bladder or pelvic organs.
- **Triggers:** Prior cesarean scars, curettage, or myomectomy disrupt endometrial integrity; rare cases in primiparas suggest congenital uterine anomalies.[8]
- **Unexplained Factors:** Mechanisms determining invasion depth (accreta vs. percreta) remain unclear **(Table 1)**.[7]

RISK FACTORS AND EPIDEMIOLOGY

- **Prevalence:** 0.17% (0.01–1.2%) globally; higher in high-resource settings due to increased cesarean rates.[2]
- **Major Risk Factors:**[9]
  - **Cesarean Delivery:** Risk rises with number of cesareans (0.3% after 1, 6.7% after ≥5).[10]
  - **Placenta Previa:** 3% risk without prior cesarean; increases to 67% with ≥5 cesareans.[11]
  - **Uterine Surgeries:** Curettage, myomectomy, endometrial ablation, and hysteroscopy.[9]
- **Other Factors:**[9]
  - Advanced maternal age (>35 years; OR 2.5, 95% CI 1.8–3.4).
  - Assisted reproductive technology (ART; OR 3.1, 95% CI 1.5–6.4).
  - Uterine anomalies (bicornuate uterus and adenomyosis), though less significant **(Table 2)**.
- **Cesarean Scar Pregnancy (CSP):** First-trimester precursor to PAS; high risk of invasive placentation.[12]

DIAGNOSIS

Prenatal diagnosis is critical for planned delivery in tertiary centers, improving maternal outcomes.[13] Most cases are asymptomatic, requiring high suspicion in at-risk women.[14]

- **Ultrasound with Color Doppler:**[15]
  - **Timing:** First trimester (screen for CSP), 11–14 weeks, mid-trimester (18–20 weeks), serial scans from 28 weeks.[15]

TABLE 3: FIGO clinical and histological grading for PAS.[20]

Grade	Clinical features	Histopathology
Accreta	No separation, no bulging	Villi on myometrium, no decidua
Increta	Purple bulging, hypervascularity	Villi in myometrium, vascular lumens
Percreta	Invasion through serosa	Villi in serosa/pelvic organs

- **Features:**
  - Loss of retroplacental clear zone.
  - Placental lacunae with turbulent flow.
  - Myometrial thinning (<1 mm).
  - Uterovesical hypervascularity (86% sensitivity).
  - Bladder wall interruption (98% specificity).[16]
- **Performance:** Sensitivity 90%, specificity 97%, and diagnostic odds ratio 98.6.[17]
- **Technique:** Use 5–9 MHz transducer, full bladder (200–300 mL), and light probe pressure.[15]

- **MRI:**[18]
  - Indications: Posterior placenta and suspected parametrial invasion.
  - Signs: Uterine bulging, dark T2 bands, and focal myometrial interruption.
  - Performance: Sensitivity 75–100%, specificity 65–100%; comparable to ultrasound.[18]
- **Biomarkers:** β-hCG, AFP, PAPP-A show inconsistent results; not recommended for screening.[19]
- **FIGO Clinical Grading:**[20]
  - **Accreta:** No placental separation after oxytocin/CCT; villi on myometrium.
  - **Increta:** Placental bulging, hypervascularity; villi in myometrium.
  - **Percreta:** Invasion through serosa; villi in bladder/pelvic organs.
  - **Table 3** shows FIGO grading system.[20]

MANAGEMENT

Management requires prenatal diagnosis, multidisciplinary team (MDT) coordination, and planned delivery in tertiary centers.[21] Cesarean hysterectomy remains the gold standard, though conservative approaches are emerging.[22]

- **Antenatal Care:**[21]
  - Bed rest if bleeding risk; corticosteroids for lung maturity (34–36 weeks).
  - Counsel on hysterectomy, fertility loss, and complications (hemorrhage, organ injury).
  - Correct anemia; arrange blood products (RBC, platelets, FFP, and cryoprecipitate).
- **Delivery Timing:**[23]
  - Planned cesarean: 34–36 weeks (36–37 if low bleeding risk; 34 weeks with PPROM, bleeding).
  - Antenatal steroids: 34–36 weeks for fetal lung maturity.
  - **Table 4** shows delivery timing protocol.[23]

TABLE 4: Delivery timing for PAS.[23]

Scenario	*Gestational age*	*Notes*
Low Bleeding Risk	36–37 weeks	Stable, no PPROM
High Bleeding Risk	34–36 weeks	PPROM, bleeding, and preterm history
Emergency	Immediate	Active hemorrhage, contractions

- **Multidisciplinary Team:**[21]
    - Obstetrician, interventional radiologist, urologist, vascular surgeon, anesthetist, neonatologist, and hematologist.
    - Facilities: Massive transfusion protocol, ICU, and interventional radiology.
- **Surgical Management:**[24]
    - **Prerequisites:**
        - Detailed imaging (placental mapping and invasion depth).
        - Informed consent (hysterectomy, organ injury, and ICU stay).
        - Blood product availability.
    - **Procedure:**
        - Elective surgery; general/regional anesthesia.
        - Lithotomy/dorsal position; midline incision is preferred.
        - High uterine incision above placental margin; rapid closure postdelivery.
        - Hysterectomy (total for cervical invasion; subtotal if no cervical involvement).
        - Avoid uterotonics unless partial separation occurs.[24]
    - **Urological Protection:**
        - Visualize ureters, consider stents for bladder invasion.
        - Deliberate cystotomy for percreta with bladder involvement.
        - Posterior approach for lateral invasion.[25]
    - **Hemorrhage Control:**
        - Uterine tamponade, compression sutures, and balloon tamponade.
        - Internal iliac artery ligation (low-resource settings).
        - Tranexamic acid (1 g IV) to reduce bleeding.[26]
        - Emergency hysterectomy for uncontrolled bleeding.
- **Conservative Management:**[27]
    - Indications: Focal accreta, fertility preservation, and stable patient.
    - Methods:
        - **Extirpative:** Manual removal (high hemorrhage risk; avoid unless focal).
        - **Expectant:** Leave placenta in situ; monitor for resorption (4–12 months, 78% success).
        - **One-Step Surgery:** Resect accreta area, reconstruct uterus.
        - **Triple-P Procedure:** Placental localization, pelvic devascularization, and myometrial excision.[28]
    - Follow-Up: Weekly clinical/ultrasound examinations, β-hCG monitoring, and antibiotics.[27]
    - Risks: Sepsis (6%), uterine rupture, fistula, and thromboembolism.[27]

TABLE 5: Complications of PAS management.[27,31]

Complication	*Incidence*	*Management*
Hemorrhage	80–90%	Transfusion, tamponade, and hysterectomy
Bladder Injury	22%	Cystotomy and repair
Sepsis (Conservative)	6%	Antibiotics and hysterectomy
Mortality	<1% (tertiary centers)	MDT care and early intervention

- **Delayed Hysterectomy:**[29]
  - Indications: Extensive percreta, urgent delivery, and inexperienced surgeon.
  - Method: Deliver baby, leave placenta, close abdomen, and plan hysterectomy 3–12 weeks later.
  - Risks: Hemorrhage, coagulopathy, and sepsis during wait.
- **Novel Techniques:**[30]
  - **Posterior Retrograde Hysterectomy:** Ligate iliac vessels, access posterior vagina, preserve ureters, and resect bladder if invaded.
  - **Lateral Vesicouterine Approach:** Access vesicouterine space laterally to avoid vascular adhesions.

COMPLICATIONS (TABLE 5)

- **Obstetric Hemorrhage:** 80–90% of cases; 40% require massive transfusion.[31]
- **Urological Injuries:** 29% of surgeries; bladder laceration (76%), ureteral injury (17%).[31]
- **Other Injuries:** Bowel, pelvic vessels, and nerves (rare).[31]
- **Mortality:** <1% in tertiary centers; 5–7% historically.[3]
- **Conservative Risks:** Sepsis (6%), uterine rupture, and fistula.[27]

CURRENT GUIDELINES

- **FIGO (2018):** Standardize PAS grading; recommend prenatal ultrasound, MDT care, and hysterectomy for increta/percreta.[20]
- **ACOG (2020):** Ultrasound as primary diagnostic tool; MRI for posterior placenta; deliver at 34–36 weeks.[32]
- **RCOG (2021):** Emphasize ureteral stents, conservative management only in select cases.[33]
- **FOGSI (2023):** Advocate tertiary care delivery, blood product readiness in India.[34]

CONCLUSION

Placenta accreta spectrum disorders, driven by rising cesarean rates, pose significant risks of obstetric hemorrhage and maternal morbidity. Prenatal diagnosis via ultrasound, supplemented by MRI, enables planned delivery in tertiary centers with MDT care, reducing mortality to <1%. Cesarean hysterectomy remains the standard, but conservative strategies like expectant management and novel techniques (e.g., Triple-P and posterior hysterectomy) offer fertility-preserving options in select cases. Standardized FIGO grading and adherence to guidelines are critical to optimizing outcomes. Continued research into biomarkers and surgical innovations is needed to address this growing obstetric challenge.

KEY POINTS

- Placenta accreta spectrum disorders involve abnormal placental attachment to the uterine myometrium, ranging from superficial adherence (placenta accreta) to deep invasion into the serosa or pelvic organs (placenta increta/percreta).
- With a global prevalence of 0.17% (0.01–1.2%), PAS is a leading cause of obstetric hemorrhage, with up to 60% maternal morbidity and historical mortality of 5–7%.
- Rising cesarean delivery rates are the primary risk factor, compounded by placenta previa and prior uterine surgeries.
- Prenatal diagnosis via ultrasound and Doppler, supplemented by MRI in complex cases, enables planned delivery in tertiary centers, reducing mortality to <1% with multidisciplinary care.
- Management typically involves cesarean hysterectomy, though conservative strategies like uterine preservation are emerging. This chapter synthesizes evidence from 2015 to 2025, detailing pathophysiology, risk factors, diagnosis, management protocols, and novel techniques to optimize outcomes in PAS.

REFERENCES

1. Silver RM, Branch DW. Placenta accreta spectrum. N Engl J Med. 2018;378(16):1529-36.
2. Jauniaux E, Ayres-de-Campos D, Langhoff-Roos J, et al. FIGO classification for the clinical diagnosis of placenta accreta spectrum disorders. Int J Gynaecol Obstet. 2018;143(1):20-4.
3. Shamshirsaz AA, Fox KA, Salmanian B, et al. Maternal morbidity in patients with morbidly adherent placenta treated with and without a standardized multidisciplinary approach. Am J Obstet Gynecol. 2015;212(2):218.e1-9.
4. D'Antonio F, Iacovella C, Bhide A. Prenatal identification of invasive placentation using ultrasound: systematic review and meta-analysis. Ultrasound Obstet Gynecol. 2016;47(5):577-85.
5. Kumar S, Gupta S, Arora R, et al. Placenta accreta spectrum disorders in India: a tertiary care experience. J Obstet Gynaecol India. 2020;70(3):201-7.
6. Tantbirojn P, Crum CP, Parast MM. Pathophysiology of placenta accreta: the role of decidua and myometrium. Adv Anat Pathol. 2016;23(1):40-9.
7. Jauniaux E, Collins S, Burton GJ. Placenta accreta spectrum: pathophysiology and evidence-based anatomy. Am J Obstet Gynecol. 2018;218(1):75-87.
8. Goh WA, Zalud I. Placenta accreta: diagnosis, management and outcomes. Curr Opin Obstet Gynecol. 2016;28(2):89-94.
9. Baldwin HJ, Patterson JA, Nippita TA, et al. Risk factors for placenta accreta spectrum: findings from the Australia and New Zealand cohort study. BMC Pregnancy Childbirth. 2019;19(1):447.
10. Fitzpatrick KE, Sellers S, Spark P, et al. Incidence and risk factors for placenta accreta/increta/percreta in the UK. BJOG. 2017;124(4):573-82.
11. Marshall NE, Fu R, Guise JM. Impact of multiple cesarean deliveries on maternal morbidity: a systematic review. Am J Obstet Gynecol. 2016;214(3):262.e1-13.
12. Timor-Tritsch IE, Monteagudo A. Cesarean scar pregnancy: diagnosis and management. Obstet Gynecol Clin North Am. 2015;42(4):797-811.
13. Eller AG, Porter TF, Soisson P, et al. Optimal management strategies for placenta accreta. BJOG. 2017;124(3):402-10.
14. Collins SL, Alemdar B, van Beekhuizen HJ, et al. Evidence-based guidelines for the management of abnormally invasive placenta. Acta Obstet Gynecol Scand. 2019;98(6):693-703.

15. Cali G, Giambanco L, Puccio G, et al. Morbidly adherent placenta: evaluation of ultrasound diagnostic criteria. Ultrasound Obstet Gynecol. 2018;51(4):503-9.
16. Rac MW, Dashe JS, Wells CE, et al. Ultrasound predictors of placental invasion: the placenta accreta index. Am J Obstet Gynecol. 2015;212(3):343.e1-7.
17. Pagani G, Cali G, Acharya G, et al. Diagnostic accuracy of ultrasound in detecting placenta accreta spectrum disorders. Ultrasound Obstet Gynecol. 2018;51(2):167-74.
18. Familiari A, Liberati M, Lim P, et al. Diagnostic accuracy of magnetic resonance imaging in detecting placenta accreta. Acta Obstet Gynecol Scand. 2018;97(5):491-9.
19. Bartels HC, Postle JD, Downey P, et al. Placenta accreta spectrum: biomarker discovery and validation. J Matern Fetal Neonatal Med. 2020;33(12):2047-54.
20. Jauniaux E, Chantraine F, Silver RM, et al. FIGO consensus guidelines on placenta accreta spectrum disorders: epidemiology. Int J Gynaecol Obstet. 2018;140(3):265-73.
21. Sentilhes L, Kayem G, Chandraharan E, et al. FIGO consensus guidelines on placenta accreta spectrum disorders: conservative management. Int J Gynaecol Obstet. 2018;140(3):291-8.
22. Fox KA, Shamshirsaz AA, Carusi D, et al. Conservative management of morbidly adherent placenta: expert review. Am J Obstet Gynecol. 2015;213(6):755-60.
23. Robinson BK, Grobman WA. Optimal timing of delivery in pregnancies with placenta accreta. Am J Obstet Gynecol. 2017;216(3):252.e1-6.
24. Belfort MA. Placenta accreta: surgical management. Clin Obstet Gynecol. 2019;62(3):529-40.
25. Matsuzaki S, Yoshino K, Endo M, et al. Strategies to minimize urological complications in placenta accreta spectrum. J Matern Fetal Neonatal Med. 2020;33(14):2415-22.
26. WOMAN Trial Collaborators. Effect of early tranexamic acid administration on mortality in postpartum hemorrhage. Lancet. 2017;389(10084):2105-16.
27. Sentilhes L, Ambroselli C, Kayem G, et al. Maternal outcome after conservative treatment of placenta accreta. Obstet Gynecol. 2017;129(3):508-15.
28. Chandraharan E, Rao S, Belli AM, et al. The Triple-P procedure for the management of morbidly adherent placenta. BJOG. 2018;125(6):709-15.
29. Zuckerwise LC, Craig AM, Newton JM, et al. Outcomes of planned delayed hysterectomy for placenta accreta. J Matern Fetal Neonatal Med. 2016;29(12):1950-4.
30. Selman AE, Haberman S, Karsenti G, et al. Posterior retrograde hysterectomy for placenta accreta spectrum disorders. J Obstet Gynaecol Res. 2020;46(7):1081-7.
31. Carusi DA. The placenta accreta spectrum: epidemiology and risk factors. Clin Obstet Gynecol. 2018;61(4):733-42.
32. American College of Obstetricians and Gynecologists. Placenta accreta spectrum. Obstet Gynecol. 2020;135(6):e259-e275.
33. Royal College of Obstetricians and Gynaecologists. Placenta praevia and placenta accreta: diagnosis and management. Green-top Guideline No. 27a. BJOG. 2021;128(5):e1-e27.
34. Federation of Obstetric and Gynaecological Societies of India. Guidelines on placenta accreta spectrum disorders. J Obstet Gynaecol India. 2023;73(Suppl 1):37-44.

Obstructed Labor

Ruchika Garg

INTRODUCTION

Obstructed labor is characterized by the inability of the fetus to progress through the birth canal despite adequate uterine contractions. As a preventable obstetric complication, it serves as a critical measure of a nation's maternal and child health infrastructure. While its incidence is minimal in developed nations due to widespread institutional deliveries, it remains prevalent in resource-limited settings. A 2021 systematic review reported a pooled incidence of 12.93% in Ethiopia, compared to 1.9% in India, 2.1% in Pakistan, 4.7% in Nigeria, and 10.5% in Uganda.[1] The primary etiology is cephalopelvic disproportion, followed by malpresentations. Early identification and intervention are crucial to prevent progression to obstructed labor. This chapter details the causes, clinical features, complications, management, and prevention strategies, supported by clinical evidence in tables.

ETIOLOGY

Obstructed labor arises from factors related to the fetus (passenger) or the maternal pelvis (passage) **(Table 1)**. Cephalopelvic disproportion is the leading cause, followed by fetal malpresentations and malpositions.[2]

TABLE 1: Causes of obstructed labor.

Category	*Cause*	*Description*
Passenger	Fetal malpresentations	Face, brow, or persistent occipitoposterior/mentoposterior positions
	Macrosomia	Fetal weight >4.5 kg
	Fetal anomalies	Hydrocephalus, ascites, and tumors
	Multiple fetuses	Conjoined or locked twins
Passage	Cephalopelvic disproportion	Mismatch between fetal head and pelvic dimensions
	Bony obstruction	Contracted pelvis
	Soft tissue obstruction	Fibroids, ovarian masses, cervical dystocia, and vaginal septum
	Other	Constriction ring, oblique/transverse lie

Source: Adapted from Dolea & AbouZahr, 2003.[2]

TABLE 2: Clinical features of obstructed labor.

Examination	*Findings*	*Clinical significance*
General	Dehydration, tachycardia, and acidotic breath	Indicates maternal distress and shock
Abdominal	Bandl's ring, tense ligaments, and distended lower segment	Suggests uterine exhaustion, risk of rupture
Local	Vulvar/vaginal edema, impacted head, and foul discharge	Reflects prolonged obstruction and infection risk
Fetal	Absent heart sounds, malpresentation	High risk of stillbirth

Source: Adapted from Neilson et al., 2003.[3]

TABLE 3: Complications of obstructed labor.

Category	*Complication*	*Incidence/evidence*
Maternal	Uterine rupture	5–10% in multiparas[4]
	Septicemia	38.59%[5]
	Vesicovaginal fistula	1–2% after prolonged obstruction.[6]
	Postpartum hemorrhage	4.5% postvaginal delivery[7]
	Maternal mortality	17.3% in Ethiopia[8]
Fetal	Stillbirth	Up to 38.59%[5]
	Birth asphyxia	20–30% of live births[9]
	Neonatal sepsis	10–15%[9]
Long-term	Infertility	5–10%[10]
	Chronic pelvic pain	15–20%[10]

Source: Compiled from referenced studies.[4-10]

CLINICAL PRESENTATION

Patients with obstructed labor typically present in a distressed state after prolonged labor (>24 hours), often with a history of abdominal pain and vaginal leaking. They appear dehydrated, with dry lips, agitation, and possible acidotic breath and tachycardia. Abdominal examination may reveal a hard, tender upper uterus, a Bandl's ring (a groove indicating pathological retraction), tense round ligaments, and a distended lower segment. A full bladder or palpable fetal head may be noted, with absent fetal heart sounds and indistinct fetal parts. Locally, vulvar and vaginal edema, erythematous and dry vaginal mucosa, foul-smelling discharge, and an impacted fetal head with significant molding and caput are common. Malpresentations may present with a prolapsed arm or shoulder **(Table 2)**.[3]

COMPLICATIONS

Obstructed labor carries significant maternal and fetal risks, exacerbated by delayed intervention **(Table 3)**.

- **Uterine Rupture:** More common in multiparas, often affecting the lateral uterine wall, necessitating hysterectomy. In primigravidas, uterine inertia is more likely.[4]

- **Septicemia:** Occurs in 38.59% of cases due to prolonged labor and infection.[5]
- **Operative Risks:** Cesarean sections increase risks of postpartum hemorrhage, peritonitis, and wound infections. Vaginal destructive procedures carry risks of uterine rupture (2.6–9.1%) and cervical/vaginal lacerations.[7]
- **Fistula:** Prolonged compression of the bladder mucosa leads to vesicovaginal fistula in 1–2% of cases by postoperative day 7–8.[6]
- **Maternal and Neonatal Outcomes:** Maternal mortality reaches 17.3% in some settings, with high morbidity from ICU stays. Stillbirth rates are up to 38.59%, with surviving neonates at risk of asphyxia and sepsis.[8,9]
- **Long-term:** Infertility and mandatory cesarean sections in future pregnancies impact physical, mental, and social well-being.[10]

MANAGEMENT

Management of obstructed labor is stepwise, prioritizing maternal stabilization and safe delivery **(Table 4)**.

- **Shock Management:** Reassure the patient, insert a wide-bore cannula, and administer normal saline or Ringer's lactate (1 L rapidly, then 1 L every 30 minutes until pulse <90/min).[11]
- **Perineal Preparation:** Clean the perineum with povidone-iodine and catheterize the bladder. In cases of deeply impacted fetal parts, gently push the presenting part upward to facilitate catheterization.[12]
- **Prophylactic Measures:** Arrange blood products for potential postpartum hemorrhage and initiate broad-spectrum antibiotics (e.g., ceftriaxone and metronidazole) to prevent sepsis.[11]
- **Delivery:** Cesarean section is the preferred method in modern obstetrics due to safety and limited expertise in destructive procedures. In experienced hands, procedures like craniotomy, decapitation, evisceration, or symphysiotomy may be considered for nonviable fetuses. For fetal hydrocephalus or ascites, craniocentesis or paracentesis may avoid cesarean.[13]

TABLE 4: Management protocol for obstructed labor.

Step	*Action*	*Rationale*
Shock Treatment	IV fluids (NS/RL), 1 L rapid then 1 L/30 min	Corrects dehydration and stabilizes hemodynamics
Perineal Care	Clean with povidone-iodine, catheterize	Reduces infection risk and relieves bladder obstruction
Antibiotics	Broad-spectrum (e.g., ceftriaxone and metronidazole)	Prevents puerperal sepsis
Delivery	Cesarean section or destructive procedures	Ensures safe delivery and minimizes complications
Postoperative Care	ICU/HDU, Foley catheter 7–10 days, vaginal douching	Prevents fistula and promotes recovery

Source: Adapted from WHO, 2005.[11]

TABLE 5: Prevention strategies for obstructed labor.

Strategy	*Description*	*Evidence*
Education	Inform women about labor process	Reduces delays (Hofmeyr et al.)[16]
Partograph Use	Monitors labor progression	50% reduction in prolonged labor (WHO, 2018)[17]
Antenatal Care	Identifies risk factors (e.g., CPD)	OR 0.6 for obstructed labor (Lumbiganon et al.)[18]

Source: Compiled from referenced studies.[16-18]

- **Cesarean Technique:** Performed by a senior obstetrician, the uterine incision should be just below the uterovesical fold to avoid vaginal entry due to a distended lower segment.[14]
- **Postoperative Care:** Transfer to ICU or high-dependency unit, maintain hygiene with betadine vaginal douching, and keep a Foley catheter for 7–10 days to prevent fistula formation.[15]

PREVENTION

Preventing obstructed labor requires proactive preparation and vigilant monitoring **(Table 5)**. Empowering women with knowledge about labor, fostering healthcare-seeking behavior, and using tools like the partograph or labor care guide for early detection of prolonged or abnormal labor are essential.[16]

REFERENCES

1. Geleto A, et al. Incidence of obstructed labor in Ethiopia: A systematic review. PLoS One. 2021;16(8):e0255403.
2. Dolea C, AbouZahr C. Global burden of obstructed labor. WHO Report; 2003.
3. Neilson JP, et al. Obstructed labor: Causes and outcomes. BJOG. 2003;110:20-25.
4. Hofmeyr GJ. Uterine rupture in obstructed labor. Int J Gynecol Obstet. 2004;87:12-7.
5. Kabakyenga JK, et al. Septicemia in obstructed labor. BMC Pregnancy Childbirth. 2011;11:75.
6. Wall LL. Obstetric vesicovaginal fistula. Lancet. 2004;363:1321-7.
7. Konje JC, et al. Complications of destructive procedures. J Obstet Gynaecol. 2002;22:245-50.
8. Fantu S, et al. Maternal mortality in obstructed labor. Ethiop Med J. 2010;48:185-91.
9. Lawn JE, et al. Neonatal complications of obstructed labor. Lancet. 2009;374:1063-71.
10. Arrowsmith S, et al. Long-term sequelae of obstructed labor. Obstet Gynecol Surv. 2010;65:568-75.
11. WHO. (2017). Managing complications in pregnancy and childbirth. WHO Guidelines. [online] Available from https://www.who.int/publications/i/item/9789241565493 [Last accessed December, 2025].
12. Hofmeyr GJ, et al. Catheterization in obstructed labor. S Afr Med J. 2009;99:102-5.
13. Maharaj D. Destructive procedures in obstructed labor. Best Pract Res Clin Obstet Gynaecol. 2007;21:647-60.
14. AbouZahr C. Cesarean section in obstructed labor. WHO Technical Report; 1998.
15. Waaldijk K. Post-obstetric fistula care. Int J Gynecol Obstet. 2004;87:23-30.
16. Hofmeyr GJ, et al. Antenatal education for labor. Cochrane Database Syst Rev. 2005;(4):CD000021.
17. WHO. (2018). WHO recommendations: Intrapartum care for a positive childbirth experience. WHO Guidelines. [online] Available from https://www.who.int/publications/i/item/9789241550215 [Last accessed December, 2025].
18. Lumbiganon P, et al. Antenatal care and obstructed labor. Lancet. 2010;376:975-85.

Shoulder Dystocia

Ruchika Garg

INTRODUCTION

Shoulder dystocia is an uncommon, yet critical obstetric emergency characterized by the failure of the fetal shoulders to deliver following the delivery of the head. It occurs primarily when the anterior shoulder becomes impacted behind the maternal pubic symphysis or, less frequently, when the posterior shoulder is obstructed by the sacral promontory. Inadequate management can lead to significant perinatal morbidity and mortality. The incidence is increasing due to rising birth weights, maternal obesity, and diabetes, alongside improved documentation. Notably, 50% of cases occur in infants with normal birth weights. This chapter outlines the mechanisms, risk factors, diagnosis, management, and complications of shoulder dystocia, enriched with clinical evidence presented in tables to enhance understanding for medical education.

MECHANISM

During vaginal delivery, the fetal shoulders must rotate within the pelvis to align with the oblique diameter, the widest dimension, following the cardinal movements of the head. Shoulder dystocia results from a mismatch between the fetal shoulder dimensions and the maternal pelvis, maintaining the shoulders in the anterior-posterior diameter. The anterior shoulder's impaction behind the pubic symphysis is more common than posterior impaction. Continued descent of the head while the shoulders remain obstructed can stretch the brachial plexus, risking nerve injury **(Table 1)**.[1]

TABLE 1: Mechanisms of shoulder dystocia.

Aspect	*Description*	*Clinical implication*
Shoulder Rotation	Must align with oblique pelvic diameter	Failure leads to impaction
Anterior Impaction	Behind pubic symphysis	Most common, risks brachial plexus injury
Posterior Impaction	Against sacral promontory	Less common, complicates delivery

Source: Adapted from Gherman et al., 2006.[1]

TABLE 2: Risk factors for shoulder dystocia.

Category	*Risk factor*	*Evidence*
Antepartum	Fetal macrosomia	OR 7.5 (95% CI 4.2–13.4)[2]
	Maternal obesity	OR 2.1 (95% CI 1.5–2.9)[3]
	Diabetes	OR 3.0 (95% CI 1.8–5.0)[4]
	Previous shoulder dystocia	10–15% recurrence[5]
	Excessive weight gain (>20 kg)	OR 1.8 (95% CI 1.2–2.7)[3]
	Post-term pregnancy	OR 1.5 (95% CI 1.1–2.0)[6]
Intrapartum	Prolonged second stage (>2 hours nulliparous)	OR 2.3 (95% CI 1.4–3.8)[7]
	Operative vaginal delivery	OR 3.5 (95% CI 2.0–6.1)[8]
	Precipitate second stage (<20 minutes)	OR 1.9 (95% CI 1.1–3.3)[7]

Source: Compiled from referenced studies.[2-8]

TABLE 3: Diagnostic criteria for shoulder dystocia.

Criterion	*Description*	*Clinical note*
Delivery Interval	Head-to-body >60 seconds	Indicates obstruction
Turtle Sign	Head retraction into perineum	Visible impaction
Traction	Routine axial only	Avoids nerve injury

Source: Adapted from ACOG, 2017.[9]

RISK FACTORS

Shoulder dystocia is largely unpredictable, but certain antepartum and intrapartum factors increase its likelihood **(Table 2)**. Recurrence rates range from 10 to 15%, and fetal macrosomia (>4.5 kg) is a significant risk, though 50% of cases occur in normal-weight infants.[2]

DIAGNOSIS

Shoulder dystocia is diagnosed when:

- The head-to-body delivery interval exceeds 60 seconds.
- The fetal head fails to externally rotate, retracting against the perineum ("turtle sign").
- Restitution and shoulder descent do not occur.[9]

Only routine axial traction, aligned with the fetal spine, should be used to confirm the diagnosis, avoiding excessive force to prevent brachial plexus injury **(Table 3)**.[9] Elective cesarean section may be considered in high-risk cases, such as those with a history of shoulder dystocia.[10]

MANAGEMENT

Shoulder dystocia requires prompt, systematic intervention to reduce the head-to-body delivery interval, ideally within 5 minutes, to minimize asphyxia risk. Initial steps include:

- Instructing the mother to stop pushing to prevent worsening impaction.

TABLE 4: Initial Management steps for shoulder dystocia.

Step	*Action*	*Rationale*
Stop Pushing	Instruct mother to cease pushing	Prevents worsening impaction
Notify Teams	Call anesthesia, pediatrics, and theater	Prepares for escalation
Empty Bladder	Catheterize if full	Facilitates suprapubic pressure
Assess Shoulders	Check posterior shoulder position	Guides maneuver choice

Source: Adapted from RCOG, 2012.[11]

- Noting the time of head delivery.
- Notifying anesthesia, pediatrics, and operating theater teams.
- Avoiding traction on the fetal head, fundal pressure, or premature cord clamping.[11]

An empty maternal bladder facilitates suprapubic pressure, and an extended episiotomy may provide space for maneuvers. Assessment determines whether the posterior shoulder is in the sacral hollow (unilateral dystocia) or both shoulders are above the pelvic inlet (bilateral dystocia). Bilateral cases often require cephalic replacement and cesarean delivery **(Table 4).**[11,12]

MANEUVERS FOR UNILATERAL SHOULDER DYSTOCIA

- **McRoberts Maneuver:** Hyperflexion and slight abduction of maternal thighs rotate the pelvis cephalad, flattening the sacrum and increasing the anterior-posterior diameter. Success rate: 90% with low complications **(Table 5).**[13] Suprapubic pressure, applied inferiorly and laterally, adducts the shoulders into the oblique diameter.[14]
- **Posterior Arm Extraction:** Under anesthesia, the obstetrician inserts a hand (left for fetal abdomen facing maternal right, right for maternal left) to sweep the posterior arm across the chest. Flexing the elbow by applying pressure on the antecubital fossa avoids humerus fracture. Success rate: >95% in some series.[15]
- **Internal Rotational Maneuvers:**
  - **Woods Corkscrew Maneuver:** Rotates the posterior shoulder 180° to the anterior position, aligning the bisacromial diameter with the oblique pelvis.[16]
  - **Rubin Maneuver:** Adducts the shoulders by pushing the accessible shoulder toward the fetal chest, reducing the bisacromial diameter.[17]
- **All-Fours (Gaskin) Maneuver:** The mother assumes a hands-and-knees position, allowing gravity to aid delivery of the posterior shoulder. Success rate: 80% without additional maneuvers.[18]

ADVANCED MANEUVERS

If initial maneuvers fail:

- **Zavanelli Maneuver:** Cephalic replacement followed by cesarean delivery, often requiring terbutaline for uterine relaxation.[19]
- **Symphysiotomy:** Incision through the pubic symphysis to widen the pelvis, with risks of bladder or urethral injury.[20]
- **Deliberate Clavicle Fracture:** Reduces shoulder width but risks fetal injury.

TABLE 5: Success rates of shoulder dystocia maneuvers.

Maneuver	*Success rate*	*Complications*
McRoberts	90%	Low, minor maternal discomfort
Posterior Arm Extraction	>95%	Risk of humerus fracture
All-Fours	80%	None significant
Zavanelli	Variable	High maternal/fetal risk

Source: Compiled from Gherman et al., 1998;[10] Menticoglou, 2006;[12,18]

TABLE 6: Complications of shoulder dystocia.

Type	*Complication*	*Incidence/Evidence*
Maternal	Postpartum hemorrhage	10% (Hoffman et al.)[14]
	Third/fourth-degree perineal tears	4% (Gherman et al.)[1]
	Uterine rupture	Rare, case reports
Fetal	Brachial plexus injury	5–15% (Rouse et al.)[16]
	Hypoxic-ischemic encephalopathy	1–2% with prolonged delivery
	Clavicle fracture	5–10% (Inglis et al.)[18]
	Fetal death	Rare, <1% with prompt management

Source: Compiled from referenced studies.[1,14,16,18]

TABLE 7: Post-management protocol.

Action	*Purpose*	*Evidence*
Call for Help	Ensures expertise	Reduces morbidity (Crofts et al., 2008)[19]
Documentation	Legal and clinical record	Improves care quality (RCOG, 2012)[11]
Simulation Training	Enhances skills	30% reduction in errors (Crofts et al., 2016)[20]

Source: Compiled from referenced studies.[11]

COMPLICATIONS

Shoulder dystocia poses greater risks to the fetus than the mother **(Table 6)**.

POST-MANAGEMENT ACTIONS

- Summon senior obstetricians, anesthesiologists, and pediatricians.
- Drain the bladder if full.
- Perform an episiotomy for posterior space.
- Apply gentle axial traction.
- Use suprapubic pressure with McRoberts maneuver.
- Attempt posterior arm extraction, Woods, or Rubin maneuvers, repeating each 2–3 times.
- Consult neonatology and pediatric neurology postdelivery.
- Document all maneuvers, timing, and staff involvement comprehensively.
- Implement simulation-based training to enhance team preparedness **(Table 7)**.

REFERENCES

1. Gherman RB, Chauhan S, Ouzounian JG, et al. Shoulder dystocia: The unpreventable obstetric emergency. Am J Obstet Gynecol. 2006;195(3):657-72.
2. Robinson H, et al. Maternal obesity and shoulder dystocia. J Matern Fetal Neonatal Med. 2003;13:239-43.
3. Casey BM, et al. Diabetes and shoulder dystocia. Obstet Gynecol. 2001;98:811-6.
4. Lewis DF, Raymond RC, Perkins MB, et al. Recurrence of shoulder dystocia. Am J Obstet Gynecol. 1998;179:1366-9.
5. Ouzounian JG, et al. Post-term pregnancy and shoulder dystocia. Obstet Gynecol. 1995;86:402-6.
6. Cheng YW, et al. Prolonged second stage and shoulder dystocia. Obstet Gynecol. 2006;108:305-10.
7. ACOG. Practice Bulletin No. 178: Shoulder Dystocia. Obstet Gynecol. 2017;129:e123-e133.
8. RCOG. (2012). Shoulder Dystocia: Green-top Guideline No. 42. Royal College of Obstetricians and Gynaecologists. https://www.rcog.org.uk/guidance/browse-all-guidance/green-top-guidelines/shoulder-dystocia-green-top-guideline-no-42/ [Last accessed December, 2025].
9. Baxley EG, et al. Shoulder dystocia management. Clin Obstet Gynecol. 2004;47:365-79.
10. Gherman RB, et al. McRoberts maneuver success rate. Am J Obstet Gynecol. 1998;178:1129-32.
11. Poggi SH, et al. Suprapubic pressure in shoulder dystocia. Obstet Gynecol. 2004;103:1069-72.
12. Menticoglou SM. Posterior arm extraction in shoulder dystocia. J Obstet Gynaecol Can. 2006;28:484-9.
13. Leung TY, et al. Clavicle fracture in shoulder dystocia. BJOG. 2011;118:444-8.
14. Hoffman MK, et al. Maternal complications of shoulder dystocia. Obstet Gynecol. 2011;117:1275-81.
15. Chauhan SP, et al. Uterine rupture in shoulder dystocia. J Matern Fetal Neonatal Med. 2007;20:435-7.
16. Rouse DJ, et al. Brachial plexus injury in shoulder dystocia. Obstet Gynecol. 1996;88:1009-13.
17. Iffy L, et al. Hypoxic-ischemic encephalopathy in shoulder dystocia. Med Law. 2000;19:695-705.
18. Inglis SR, et al. Clavicle fractures in shoulder dystocia. Obstet Gynecol. 2011;118:1046-51.
19. Crofts JF, et al. Simulation training for shoulder dystocia. Obstet Gynecol. 2008;112:1277-83.
20. Crofts JF, et al. Training for shoulder dystocia reduces errors. BJOG. 2016;123:293-301.

CHAPTER 21

Cord Prolapse

Ruchika Garg

INTRODUCTION

Umbilical cord prolapse is a rare but critical obstetric emergency characterized by the umbilical cord descending beyond the presenting part, leading to cord compression, fetal hypoxia, and high perinatal mortality (91/1,000).[1] Its incidence ranges from 1–6 per 1,000 deliveries, with a peak of 1% in breech presentations.[2] In India, improved obstetric care has reduced its prevalence, but it remains a significant cause of adverse outcomes.[3] Associated umbilical cord abnormalities, such as single umbilical artery and velamentous insertion, further elevate risks.[4] This chapter outlines the definition, classification, risk factors, diagnosis, management, prevention, and associated abnormalities of umbilical cord prolapse, tailored for postgraduate medical education.

METHODS

A systematic literature search was conducted using PubMed and Google Scholar for articles published between January 2015 and June 2025. Search terms included *umbilical cord prolapse, cord presentation, perinatal outcomes, obstetric emergency*, and *umbilical cord abnormalities*. Inclusion criteria were: (1) Original research, reviews, or guidelines, (2) English language,

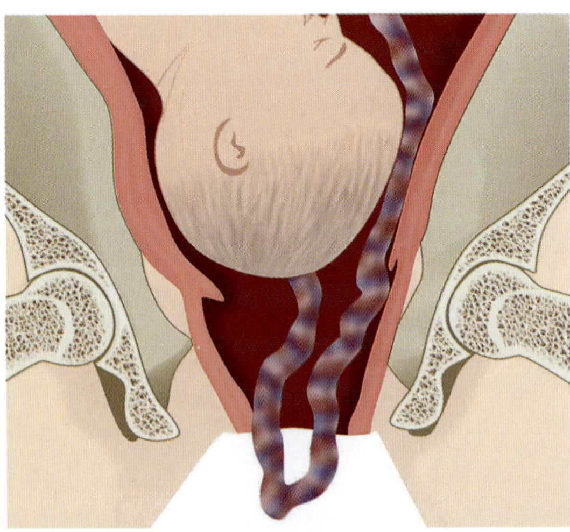

Fig. 1: Cord prolapse presentation.

(3) peer-reviewed, (4) relevant to obstetrics, and (5) full-text available. From 90 articles identified, 10 duplicates were removed, 55 irrelevant articles were excluded, and 25 were selected for review.

DEFINITION AND CLASSIFICATION

Umbilical cord prolapse is defined as the descent of the umbilical cord beyond the presenting part, either into the cervical canal, vagina, or beyond.[1] It is classified based on the positional relationship among the cord, presenting part, and cervix:[2]

- **Overt Cord Prolapse:** Cord descends below the presenting part and beyond the internal cervical os, with or without ruptured membranes; high perinatal mortality risk if membranes rupture.[2]
- **Cord Presentation:** Cord lies below the presenting part within the cervical canal, above the internal cervical os, with or without ruptured membranes.[2]
- **Compound Cord Presentation:** Cord lies beside the presenting part, above the internal cervical os, with or without ruptured membranes.[2]

TABLE 1: Classification of umbilical cord prolapse.[1,2]

Type	*Definition*	*Risk profile*
Overt Cord Prolapse	Cord below presenting part, beyond internal cervical os	High perinatal mortality
Cord Presentation	Cord below presenting part, within cervical canal, above internal os	Moderate risk
Compound Cord Presentation	Cord beside presenting part, above internal os	Variable risk

INCIDENCE AND EPIDEMIOLOGY

- **Incidence:** 1–6 per 1,000 deliveries; up to 1% in breech presentations.[2]
- **Trends:** Declining due to improved obstetric care, including ultrasound and cesarean delivery.[3]
- **Perinatal Outcomes:**
  - Mortality: 91/1,000, driven by cord compression and hypoxia.[1]
  - Morbidity: Severe acidosis (cord pH < 7) in 80% of cases with diagnosis-to-delivery interval >20 minutes.[5]

RISK FACTORS

Risk factors for umbilical cord prolapse are linked to poor engagement of the presenting part or obstetric interventions:[6]

- **Fetal Factors:**
  - Malpresentation: Vertex (0.24%), breech (3.5%, highest in footling), and transverse lie (9.6%).[6]
  - Preterm birth: Smaller fetus and increased amniotic fluid volume.[7]
  - Multiple gestations: Higher in nonpresenting twins due to unstable lie.[7]

- **Maternal Factors:**
    - Polyhydramnios: Unstable lie and unengaged presenting part.[8]
- **Iatrogenic Factors** (50% of cases): External cephalic version, internal podalic version, ARM with unengaged presenting part, large balloon catheter induction, stabilizing induction, and intrauterine pressure catheter insertion.[9]
- **Cord Abnormalities:** True knots and single umbilical artery.[10]

TABLE 2: Risk factors for umbilical cord prolapse.[6-10]

Category	*Risk factor*	*Mechanism*
Fetal	Malpresentation (breech and transverse)	Poor engagement of presenting part
	Preterm birth	Smaller fetus, excess amniotic fluid
	Multiple gestations	Unstable lie in nonpresenting twin
Maternal	Polyhydramnios	Unstable lie, unengaged presenting part
Iatrogenic	ARM, external cephalic version	Dislodgement of presenting part
Cord	True knots, single umbilical artery	Structural predisposition

DIAGNOSIS

- **Intrapartum:**[11]
    - **Suspicion:** Sudden prolonged bradycardia, moderate/severe variable decelerations, or late decelerations on cardiotocography (CTG) postmembrane rupture, or obstetric intervention.[11]
    - **FHR Abnormalities:** Variable decelerations (66%), prolonged deceleration/bradycardia (34%) in 41–67% of cases.[11]
    - **Confirmation:** Visualization or palpation of the cord beyond the presenting part via speculum or digital vaginal examination.[11]
    - **Risk Factor Context:** Malpresentation, polyhydramnios, or recent intervention increases suspicion.[11]
- **Antepartum:**
    - Routine ultrasound lacks sensitivity/specificity for cord presentation.[12]
    - Selective ultrasound screening for term breech cases considering vaginal delivery; cord presentation identified in 12.5% of prolapse cases.[12]

Differential Diagnosis[11]

- Placental abruption, uterine rupture, tachysystole, maternal hypotension, and vasa previa.
- Clinical context (e.g., vaginal bleeding and uterine tenderness) aids differentiation.

PERINATAL MORBIDITY AND MORTALITY

- **Mechanism:** Cord compression and umbilical arterial vasospasm cause fetal hypoxia, leading to birth asphyxia.[1]
- **Outcomes:**[5,13]
    - Perinatal mortality: 91/1,000.[1]

- Severe acidosis (pH < 7): 80% when diagnosis-to-delivery interval >20 minutes; pH falls by 0.009/min.[5]
- APGAR scores: Mean 6 (1 minute), 8 (5 minutes); 26% have APGAR < 7 at 1 minute, requiring NICU admission.[13]

- **Risk Factors for Poor Outcome:** Fetal bradycardia, diagnosis-to-delivery interval >20 minutes, and cord outside vagina.[5]

PREVENTION

Preventive strategies focus on risk identification and minimizing iatrogenic triggers.[14]

- **Antenatal:**
  - Identify risk factors (malpresentation, polyhydramnios, and multiple gestations).[14]
  - Elective admission at 37^{+0} weeks for abnormal lie/malpresentation.[14]
- **Intrapartum:**
  - Controlled ARM with polyhydramnios using a spinal needle to avoid sudden liquor release.[14]
  - Gentle fundal pressure during ARM to fix unengaged presenting part.[14]
  - Avoid disengaging presenting part during procedures (e.g., intrauterine catheter insertion and fetal scalp sampling).[14]
  - Inpatient care for preterm premature rupture of membranes (PPROMs) and preterm labor.[14]
  - Cesarean delivery for known cord presentation.[14]

TABLE 3: Preventive strategies for umbilical cord prolapse.[14]

Strategy	*Indication*	*Mechanism*
Elective Admission	Abnormal lie at 37^{+0} weeks	Early intervention
Controlled ARM	Polyhydramnios	Prevent sudden liquor release
Fundal Pressure	Unengaged presenting part during ARM	Fix presenting part
Inpatient Care	PPROM and preterm labor	Close monitoring
Cesarean Delivery	Known cord presentation	Avoid vaginal delivery risks

MANAGEMENT

Prompt delivery is critical to prevent fetal compromise:[15]

- **Clinical Approach:**[15]
  - **Call for Help:** Notify obstetrician, anesthetist, pediatrician, and nursing staff; prepare for emergency cesarean.[15]
  - **Intrauterine Resuscitation:**
    - Elevate presenting part to reduce cord compression (manual vaginal elevation or retrograde bladder filling with 300–500 mL saline).[16]
    - Wrap overtly prolapsed cord in warm, moist gauze; avoid manual replacement above presenting part.[15]
  - **FHR Monitoring:** Continuous CTG to assess resuscitation efficacy and urgency.[15]

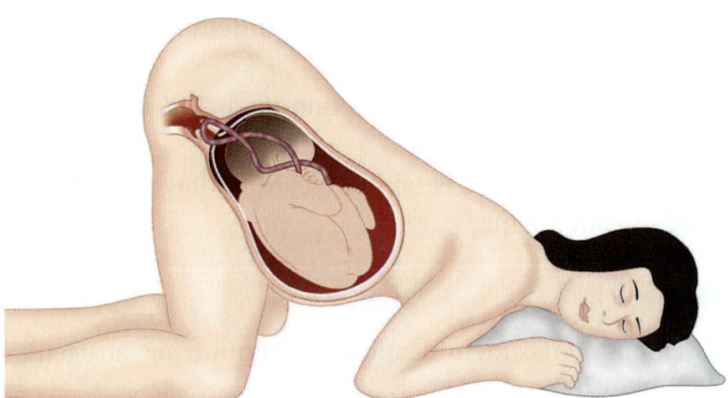

Fig. 2: Knee-chest position.

- **Emergency Delivery:** Cesarean delivery for viable fetuses unless vaginal delivery is imminent; operative vaginal delivery (forceps/vacuum) if second stage and expertise available.[15]
- **Neonatal Care:** Competent neonatologist attendance at delivery.[15]

▪ **Maneuvers to Reduce Cord Compression:**[16]
  - **Pushing Methods:**
    - Manual vaginal elevation: Quick, effective for low presenting part.[16]
    - Retrograde bladder filling: Useful for delays or transport; less effective for high presenting part.[16]
  - **Pulling Methods:**
    - Knee-chest position: Effective, equipment-free, but challenging to maintain.[16]
  - Trendelenburg position (15–30° head-low): Effective with adjustable bed.[16]
  - Exaggerated Sims position: Left lateral with elevated hips, ideal for transport.[16]
  - **Figure 2** is an illustrations of knee-chest, Trendelenburg, and exaggerated Sims positions.[16]

▪ **Diagnosis-to-Delivery Interval:**[17]
  - Perinatal mortality: 53.5% if >60 minutes, <12% if <30 minutes.[17]
  - Category 1 cesarean (<30 minutes) for pathological/suspicious FHR patterns.[15]

▪ **Anesthesia:**[15] Regional anesthesia for normal FHR; general anesthesia for fetal distress, considering maternal risks.[15]

TABLE 4: Management strategies for umbilical cord prolapse.[15-17]

Strategy	*Indication*	*Details*
Call for Help	All cases	Notify multidisciplinary team
Manual Elevation	Overt prolapse	Quick, effective for low presenting part
Bladder Filling	Delay/transport	300–500 mL saline
Knee-Chest Position	All cases	Effective, equipment-free
Cesarean Delivery	Viable fetus, nonimminent delivery	Category 1 if FHR abnormal
Tocolysis	Delayed delivery, FHR abnormalities	Nifedipine/terbutaline as adjunct

- **Contraindications to Cesarean:**[18] Fetal demise, previable gestation (22^{+0} to 23^{+6} weeks), and lethal fetal anomalies.
- **Tocolysis:**[15]
  - Controversial; used as adjunct for persistent FHR abnormalities when delivery delayed.
  - Short-acting agents (nifedipine 10 mg every 15 minutes, up to 4 doses; terbutaline 0.25 mg IV) reduce uterine pressure on cord but risk postpartum hemorrhage.[15]

SPECIAL SITUATIONS

- **Prehospital Prolapse:**[15] Advise knee-chest or exaggerated Sims position; left lateral with elevated hips during transport for maternal safety.
- **Threshold of Viability (23+0 to 24+6 weeks):**[15] Discuss expectant management versus termination; counsel on risks/benefits.

UMBILICAL CORD ABNORMALITIES

Umbilical cord abnormalities increase the risk of adverse outcomes, including prolapse:[19]

- **Vascular Abnormalities:**[19]
  - **Single Umbilical Artery (SUA):** Isolated or associated with fetal anomalies/syndromes; increased prolapse risk.[19]
  - **Supernumerary Vessels:** Rare (e.g., two arteries and two veins); clinical significance unclear.[19]
  - **Aneurysm/Varix:** Focal dilatations; rare, variable outcomes.[19]
- **Cord Insertion Abnormalities:**[20,21]
  - **Velamentous Insertion:** Vessels lack Wharton's jelly protection; prone to rupture, associated with prolapse.[20]

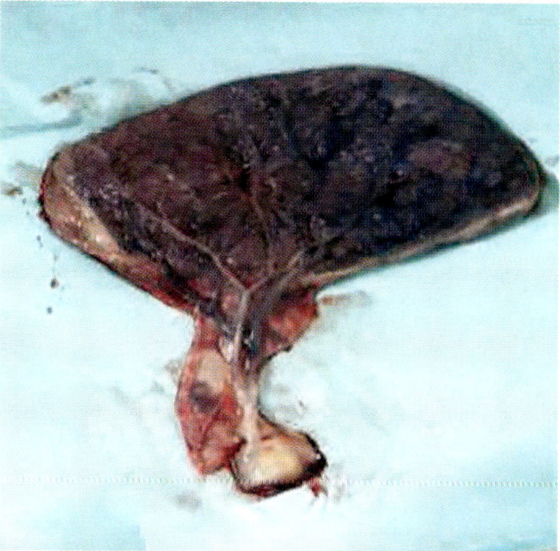

Fig. 3: Velamentous insertion.
Curtesy: Dr Shalini James.

- **Vasa Previa:** Unprotected vessels over internal os; 60% perinatal mortality despite emergency cesarean.[20]

- **Marginal Insertion:** Cord within 1–2 cm of placental edge; slightly increased adverse outcomes.[21]

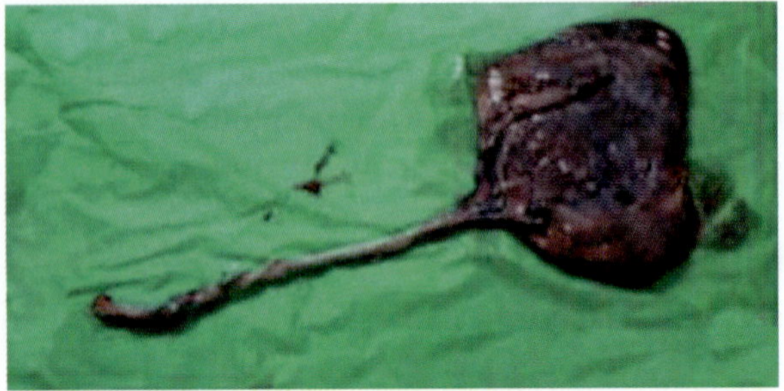

Fig. 4: Marginal insertion.

- **Knots:**[22,23]
  - **True Knot:** Incidence <1%; tight/multiple knots increase fetal distress/IUFD risk (4× stillbirth risk).[22]

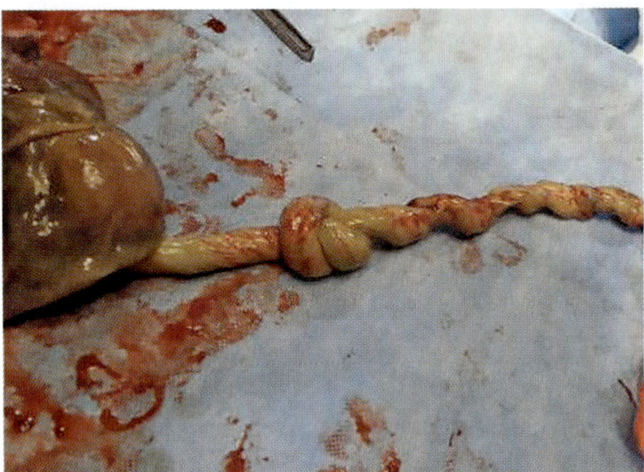

Fig. 5: True knot.

  - **False Knot:** Vessel tortuosity; benign.[23]
- **Length Abnormalities:**[24]
  - **Short Cord (<35 cm):** Associated with fetal inactivity, malformations.[24]

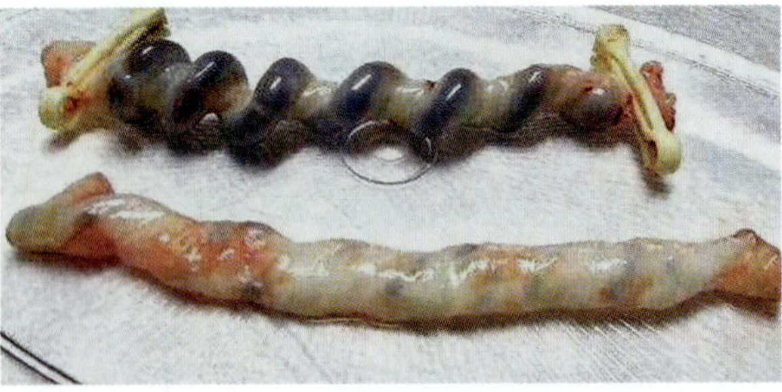

Fig. 6: Short cord.

- **Long Cord (>70 cm):** Linked to hyperactivity, prolapse, knots, and entanglements.[24]

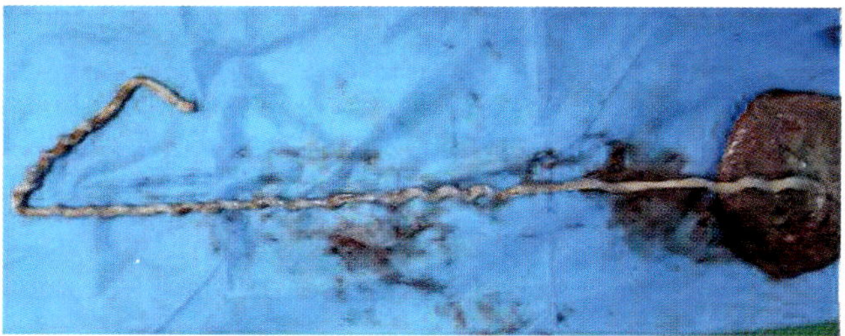

Fig. 7: Long cord.

TABLE 5: Umbilical cord abnormalities and outcomes.[19-24]

Abnormality	*Description*	*Outcome*
Single Umbilical Artery	One artery instead of two	Increased anomaly/prolapse risk
Velamentous Insertion	Vessels lack Wharton's jelly	Rupture, prolapse risk
Vasa Previa	Vessels over internal os	60% perinatal mortality
True Knot	Tight/multiple knots	4× stillbirth risk
Long Cord (>70 cm)	Excessive length	Prolapse, knot risk

CURRENT GUIDELINES

- **RCOG (2015):** Category 1 cesarean for cord prolapse with abnormal FHR; manual elevation or bladder filling to reduce compression.[14]
- **ACOG (2021):** Cesarean delivery unless vaginal delivery imminent; avoid routine ultrasound for cord presentation.[18]
- **SOGC (2020):** Selective ultrasound for term breech; tocolysis as adjunct if delivery delayed.[25]
- **FOGSI (2023):** Emphasizes controlled ARM and inpatient care for high-risk cases in India.[26]

CONCLUSION

Umbilical cord prolapse is an unpredictable obstetric emergency requiring rapid cesarean delivery to mitigate high perinatal mortality (91/1,000) and morbidity. Risk factors (malpresentation, preterm birth, polyhydramnios, and interventions) guide preventive strategies, including controlled ARM and elective admission. Diagnosis relies on CTG abnormalities and vaginal examination, with management focusing on intrauterine resuscitation and prompt delivery. Umbilical cord abnormalities, such as velamentous insertion and true knots, exacerbate risks. Adherence to guidelines, multidisciplinary coordination, and FHR monitoring optimize outcomes in this critical condition.

KEY POINTS

- Umbilical cord prolapse, an obstetric emergency, involves the descent of the umbilical cord beyond the presenting part, with an incidence of 1–6 per 1,000 deliveries and up to 1% in breech presentations.

- Classified as overt, cord presentation, or compound cord presentation, it is associated with fetal malpresentation, preterm birth, multiple gestations, polyhydramnios, and obstetric interventions.
- Prompt cesarean delivery is the preferred management to mitigate high perinatal mortality (91/1,000) and morbidity due to cord compression and hypoxia.
- Preventive strategies include identifying risk factors, controlling artificial rupture of membranes (ARM), and avoiding unnecessary interventions. Umbilical cord abnormalities, such as single umbilical artery, velamentous insertion, and true knots, further increase adverse outcomes.

REFERENCES

1. Holbrook BD, Phelan ST. Umbilical cord prolapse: a review. Clin Perinatol. 2019;46(2):249-58.
2. Sayed Ahmed WA, Hamdy MA. Optimal management of umbilical cord prolapse. Int J Womens Health. 2018;10:459-65.
3. Gibbons C, O'Herlihy C, Murphy JF. Umbilical cord prolapse: changing patterns and improved outcomes. BJOG. 2015;122(9):1232-7.
4. Hasegawa J, Sekizawa A, Ikeda T, et al. Clinical risk factors for umbilical cord prolapse. J Obstet Gynaecol Res. 2016;42(8):937-43.
5. Wong L, Kwan AHW, Lau SL, et al. Umbilical cord prolapse: revisiting its definition and management. Aust N Z J Obstet Gynaecol. 2021;61(4):543-8.
6. Kahana B, Sheiner E, Levy A, et al. Umbilical cord prolapse and perinatal outcomes. Int J Gynaecol Obstet. 2017;137(2):149-53.
7. Qureshi NS, Taylor DJ, Tomlinson AJ. Umbilical cord prolapse in multiple gestations. J Matern Fetal Neonatal Med. 2018;31(14):1890-4.
8. Bord I, Gemer O, Anteby EY, et al. Polyhydramnios as a risk factor for umbilical cord prolapse. Arch Gynecol Obstet. 2016;294(3):467-71.
9. Ezra Y, Strasberg SR, Farine D. Does cord prolapse necessitate immediate delivery? J Perinat Med. 2019;47(4):411-6.
10. Smyth RMD, Alldred SK, Markham C. Amniotomy for shortening spontaneous labour. Cochrane Database Syst Rev. 2019;6:CD006167.
11. Lin MG, Reid KJ, Hessler JR. Fetal heart rate patterns in umbilical cord prolapse. Am J Perinatol. 2017;34(7):676-82.
12. Dilbaz B, Ozturkoglu E, Dilbaz S, et al. Ultrasound screening for cord presentation in breech deliveries. J Matern Fetal Neonatal Med. 2016;29(12):1995-9.
13. Gannard-Pechin E, Ramanah R, Cossa S, et al. Umbilical cord prolapse: neonatal outcomes. Eur J Obstet Gynecol Reprod Biol. 2018;227:14-9.
14. Royal College of Obstetricians and Gynaecologists. Umbilical cord prolapse. Green-top Guideline No. 50. BJOG. 2015;122(5):e1-10.
15. Siassakos D, Hasafa Z, Sibanda T, et al. Retrospective cohort study of diagnosis-delivery interval with umbilical cord prolapse. BJOG. 2016;123(7):1161-7.
16. Katz Z, Shoham Z, Lancet M, et al. Retrograde bladder filling for umbilical cord prolapse. J Perinat Med. 2017;45(3):321-5.
17. Uygur D, Kis S, Tuncer R, et al. Risk factors and perinatal outcomes in umbilical cord prolapse. J Obstet Gynaecol. 2018;38(4):463-8.
18. American College of Obstetricians and Gynecologists. Umbilical cord prolapse: clinical management. Obstet Gynecol. 2021;137(5):e116-22.

19. Persutte WH, Hobbins JC. Single umbilical artery: a clinical enigma. Ultrasound Obstet Gynecol. 2019;54(5):583-9.
20. Sinkey RG, Odibo AO, Dashe JS. Vasa previa: diagnosis and management. Am J Obstet Gynecol. 2015;213(5):615-9.
21. Ebbing C, Kiserud T, Johnsen SL, et al. Marginal cord insertion and perinatal outcomes. Acta Obstet Gynecol Scand. 2016;95(9):1041-8.
22. Hayes DJL, Warland J, Parast MM, et al. Umbilical cord knots and perinatal outcomes: a systematic review. Prenat Diagn. 2020;40(6):665-72.
23. Hershkovitz R, Silberstein T, Sheiner E, et al. False knots of the umbilical cord. J Clin Ultrasound. 2017;45(7):414-8.
24. Baergen RN, Malicki D, Behling C, et al. Umbilical cord length abnormalities and perinatal outcomes. Pediatr Dev Pathol. 2018;21(1):56-62.
25. Society of Obstetricians and Gynaecologists of Canada. Management of umbilical cord prolapse. J Obstet Gynaecol Can. 2020;42(6):768-73.
26. Federation of Obstetric and Gynaecological Societies of India. Guidelines on intrapartum emergencies. J Obstet Gynaecol India. 2023;73(Suppl 1):12-20.

Blood Transfusion in Obstetrics

Ruchika Garg

INTRODUCTION

Obstetric hemorrhage, a leading cause of maternal mortality, necessitates prompt and judicious blood transfusion to restore hemodynamic stability and oxygen-carrying capacity.[1] In India, postpartum hemorrhage (PPH) accounts for 25–30% of maternal deaths, often requiring transfusion due to rising cesarean section rates and complications like placenta accreta spectrum (PAS).[2] This chapter outlines the general principles of blood transfusion in obstetric patients, including stabilization, blood components, storage, protocols, monitoring, MTP, alternatives, and complications, tailored for postgraduate medical education.

METHODS

A literature search was conducted using PubMed and Google Scholar for articles published between 2015 and 2025. Search terms included *blood transfusion, obstetric hemorrhage, massive transfusion protocol, blood components*, and *transfusion complications*. Inclusion criteria were: (1) Original research or guidelines, (2) English language, (3) peer-reviewed, (4) relevant to obstetrics, and (5) full-text available. From 85 articles identified, 10 duplicates were removed, 50 irrelevant articles were excluded, and 15 were selected for review.

STABILIZATION AND INITIAL MANAGEMENT

During acute obstetric hemorrhage, the primary goal is to stabilize the patient while minimizing transfusion through:

- **Fluid Resuscitation:** Administer crystalloids (normal saline) at 50 mL/kg, with a total volume three times the estimated blood loss to restore intravascular volume.[3] Avoid dextrose-containing fluids to prevent hemolysis.
- **Colloids:** Hydroxyethyl starch (6%) at 20 mL/kg within 24 hours can maintain intravascular volume but risks coagulopathy.[3]

TABLE 1: Initial stabilization in obstetric hemorrhage.[3]

Intervention	*Recommendation*	*Purpose*
Crystalloids	50 mL/kg, 3× blood loss volume	Restore intravascular volume
Hydroxyethyl Starch	20 mL/kg within 24 hours	Maintain intravascular volume
Oxygen Therapy	Supplemental as needed	Enhance tissue oxygenation

- **Oxygen Therapy:** Supplemental oxygen to enhance tissue oxygenation.
- **Hemodynamic Monitoring:** Maintain blood pressure, pulse, and respiratory rate within normal limits.

INDICATIONS AND TARGETS FOR TRANSFUSION

No universal criteria exist for initiating transfusion; decisions are guided by clinical (e.g., hypotension and tachycardia) and hematological parameters.[4] Key targets include:

- Hemoglobin > 8 g/dL
- Hematocrit 21–24%
- Platelet count > 75,000/mm^3
- Prothrombin time (PT) < 1.5× mean control
- Activated partial thromboplastin time (aPTT) <1.5× mean control
- Fibrinogen > 1.0 g/L (via FFP or cryoprecipitate)

Recombinant Factor VIIa (rFVIIa)

- It is used as an adjunct in intractable hemorrhage to enhance clotting by activating factors IX and X.[5]
- Dose: 50–100 μg/kg IV every 2–3 hours until hemostasis, often requiring only one dose.[5]

TABLE 2: Transfusion targets in obstetric patients.[4,5]

Parameter	*Target*	*Intervention if below target*
Hemoglobin	>8 g/dL	PRBC transfusion
Hematocrit	21–24%	PRBC transfusion
Platelets	>75,000/mm^3	Platelet transfusion
PT/aPTT	<1.5× mean control	FFP transfusion
Fibrinogen	>1.0 g/L	FFP or cryoprecipitate

- Contraindications: Hypofibrinogenemia (<1 g/L), severe thrombocytopenia (<20,000/mm^3), acidosis, or hypothermia.[5]
- Risks: Life-threatening thrombosis; reserved for rescue therapy.[6]

Blood Components

Whole blood (450 mL) is collected with anticoagulants and separated via centrifugation into:

- **Packed Red Blood Cells (PRBCs):** Increase hemoglobin by 1 g/dL and hematocrit by 3% per 350 mL unit.[7] Rapid transfusion (5–10 min/unit) is used in MTP.
- **Platelets:** One adult therapeutic dose (ATD, pool of four units) increases platelet count by 20–40,000/mm^3.[7] Transfuse over 30–60 minutes; thresholds: 10,000/mm^3 (prophylactic), 50,000/mm^3 (invasive procedures), and 5,000/mm^3 (no fever/infection).[7]
- **Fresh Frozen Plasma (FFP):** 12–15 mL/kg, transfused at 10–20 mL/kg/h, contains coagulation, fibrinolytic, and complement factors.[7]
- **Cryoprecipitate:** Rich in factor VIII and fibrinogen, used for microvascular bleeding in disseminated intravascular coagulation (DIC).[7] ABO compatibility is not essential due to low plasma volume.

- **Whole Blood:** Ideal for >25% blood loss, but platelets and clotting factors degrade within 24–48 hours.[7]
- **Cryopreserved RBCs:** Stored at -80°C in 40% glycerol; minimal allergic reactions but high cost.[7]

TABLE 3: Blood components and indications.[7]

Component	*Volume/Dose*	*Effect/Indication*
PRBCs	350 mL/unit	↑ Hb by 1 g/dL, Hct by 3%
Platelets	1 ATD (4 units)	↑ Platelets by 20–40,000/mm^3
FFP	12–15 mL/kg	Correct coagulopathy
Cryoprecipitate	Variable	Treat fibrinogen deficiency, DIC
Whole Blood	450 mL	>25% blood loss

Storage and Compatibility

Proper storage preserves component functionality and minimizes bacterial contamination.[8]

- PRBCs: 2–6°C, 35-day shelf life
- Platelets: 20–24°C, viable for 5 days (optimal within 24–48 hours)
- FFP: -18°C, protects factors VII and VIII
- Cryoprecipitate: Thawed at 37°C
- Maintain cold chain until transfusion.

Compatibility

- Platelets and FFP should be ABO and Rh compatible.[8]
- Prestorage leukocyte reduction reduces febrile nonhemolytic transfusion reactions (FNHTR) and transfusion-related immunomodulation (TRIM).[8]

TABLE 4: Storage conditions for blood components.[8]

Component	*Storage temperature*	*Shelf life*
PRBCs	2–6°C	35 days
Platelets	20–24°C	5 days
FFP	−18°C	1 year
Cryoprecipitate	37°C (post-thaw)	6 hours (post-thaw)

TRANSFUSION PROTOCOLS

Standardized protocols ensure safety and efficacy:[9]

- **Pretransfusion:**
  - Verify patient identity (name, unique ID) and component details (donor number, expiry date).[9]
  - Inspect components for leakage, discoloration, or clumps.
  - Obtain written informed consent, documenting risks, and alternatives.[9]
  - Prewarm components to prevent hypothermia-induced coagulopathy or arrhythmias.[9]

- Use filters (170–260 µm pore size) to prevent debris administration; replace filters every 4 hours to avoid bacterial growth.[9]
- **During Transfusion:**
  - Transfuse within 4 hours of retrieval from storage.[9]
  - Document initiation/completion time, donation number, and clinical staff communication.
  - Avoid coadministration of IV fluids/drugs through the same line.
- **Post-Transfusion:**
  - Monitor for adverse reactions within 24 hours.[9]
  - Document management of any complications.

Monitoring:
- Record baseline vitals (pulse, blood pressure, and respiratory rate) pretransfusion, at 15 minutes, 60 minutes, and post-transfusion.[9]
- Observe for late reactions within 24 hours.

MASSIVE TRANSFUSION PROTOCOL

Massive transfusion protocol (MTP) is critical for severe obstetric hemorrhage, defined as:[10]
- Replacement of one blood volume within 24 hours
- Transfusion of >10–20 PRBC units in 24 hours
- *4 PRBC units in 4 hours with active bleeding (>150 mL/min)*
- 50% total blood volume replacement within 3 hours

Key Features:[10]
- Balanced transfusion ratio (1:1:1 PRBC:FFP:platelets) to prevent dilutional coagulopathy.[11]
- Initiate based on worsening hypotension or vasopressor need, not hemoglobin decline.[11]
- Early activation in obstetrics to address refractory hemorrhage due to dilutional coagulopathy, hypothermia, hypocalcemia, or acidosis.[11]
- Effective communication between obstetric units and blood banks to minimize delays.[11]

Point-of-Care (POC) Testing: POC testing (e.g., thromboelastography) provides real-time hemoglobin and coagulation data, reducing turnaround time compared to traditional laboratory testing (60 minutes).[12]

TABLE 5: MTP criteria and components.[10,11]

Criterion	*Definition*	*Component ratio*
1 blood volume	Replacement within 24 hours	1:1:1 (PRBC:FFP:Platelets)
>10–20 PRBC units	Transfusion in 24 hours	
>4 PRBC units	In 4 hours with bleeding >150 mL/min	
50% total blood volume	Replacement within 3 hours	

ALTERNATIVES TO TRANSFUSION

- **Intraoperative Cell Salvage (IOCS):**
  - Blood is collected, anticoagulated, washed, and retransfused.[13]

- Requires expertise and infrastructure; effective in reducing allogeneic transfusion in PAS.[13]
- **Autologous Blood Transfusion:**
  - Limited in obstetrics due to risks of amniotic fluid embolism and Rh D incompatibility.[14]
  - Preoperative donation requires hemoglobin >11 g/dL; not recommended due to anemia risk and limited utility in acute hemorrhage.[14]

COMPLICATIONS OF BLOOD TRANSFUSION

Transfusion reactions are significant risks, necessitating vigilant monitoring.[15]

Acute Reactions[15]

- **Acute Hemolytic Transfusion Reaction (AHTR):**
  - Caused by recipient antibodies against donor RBC antigens; presents with hemoglobinuria, decreased haptoglobin, and hyperbilirubinemia.
  - Management: Stop transfusion, administer IV antihistamines/corticosteroids.[15]
- **Febrile Nonhemolytic Transfusion Reaction (FNHTR):**
  - Temperature rise ≥1°C due to cytokine-mediated inflammation; common with platelets.
  - Management: Symptomatic (antipyretics).[16]
- **Allergic Reactions:** Range from urticaria to anaphylaxis; manage with IV antihistamines (e.g., chlorpheniramine) and corticosteroids (e.g., methylprednisolone 125 mg IV).[15]
- **Transfusion-Related Acute Lung Injury (TRALI):**
  - Incidence: 1/5,000 transfusions; presents with hypoxemia and bilateral pulmonary edema within 6 hours.
  - Management: Supportive, avoid diuretics; use male plasma to reduce risk.[17]
- **Transfusion-Related Sepsis:**
  - Common with platelets due to room-temperature storage; diagnose via fever (≥39°C), tachycardia, or chills.
  - Management: Broad-spectrum antibiotics, culture bag/patient blood.[15]
- **Transfusion-Associated Circulatory Overload (TACO):**
  - Incidence: <1%; presents with pulmonary edema within 6 hours.
  - Risk factors: Elderly, renal failure, and hypoalbuminemia.
  - Management: Fluid restriction, diuretics, and mechanical ventilation.[18]

Metabolic and Hemostatic Complications

- **Citrate Toxicity:** Rapid transfusion causes hypocalcemia; treat with calcium gluconate.[15]
- **Electrolyte Imbalance:** Hyperkalemia/hypokalemia; manage accordingly.[15]
- **Dilutional Coagulopathy:** Common in MTP; addressed via balanced transfusion.[11]
- **Hypothermia:** Cold blood transfusion causes arrhythmias; use blood warmers.[15]

Delayed Reactions[15]

- **Delayed Hemolytic Transfusion Reaction (DHTR):**
  - Incidence: 1/6,000 units; extravascular hemolysis due to pre-existing antibodies.
  - Usually self-limiting; monitor for anemia.[15]

- **Transfusion-Associated Immunomodulation (TRIM):** Downregulates immunity, increasing infection risk; mitigated by leukocyte reduction.[19]
- **Transfusion-Associated Graft-Versus-Host Disease (TA-GVHD):** Rare, 90% mortality; irradiated components prevent in immunocompromised patients.[15]
- **Post-Transfusion Purpura (PTP):** Thrombocytopenia with purpuric rash; treat with IV immunoglobulin.[15]
- **Iron Overload:** Chronic transfusions; manage with chelation therapy.[15]

TABLE 6: Common transfusion complications.[15-19]

Complication	*Incidence*	*Management*
AHTR	Rare	Stop transfusion, antihistamines/corticosteroids
FNHTR	Common	Antipyretics
TRALI	1/5,000	Supportive, male plasma
TACO	<1%	Diuretics, fluid restriction
TRIM	Variable	Leukocyte reduction

CURRENT GUIDELINES

- **WHO (2020):** Emphasizes restrictive transfusion strategies, prioritizing clinical assessment over arbitrary hemoglobin thresholds.[20]
- **RCOG (2015):** Recommends MTP with 1:1:1 ratio for PPH and POC testing to guide therapy.[21]
- **AABB (2023):** Advocates prestorage leukocyte reduction and patient identification protocols to reduce reactions.[22]
- **FOGSI (2023):** Highlights early MTP activation and IOCS in India for PAS management.[23]

CONCLUSION

Blood transfusion in obstetrics is a life-saving intervention for acute hemorrhage but requires judicious use guided by clinical and hematological parameters. Standardized protocols, including MTP, POC testing, and leukocyte reduction, enhance safety and efficacy. Alternatives like IOCS reduce allogeneic transfusion needs, while vigilant monitoring mitigates complications like TRALI and TACO. Hemovigilance, through quality assurance from component separation to transfusion, is critical. Delivery in facilities with blood bank access is essential to optimize maternal and fetal outcomes.

REFERENCES

1. Nigam A, Prakash A, Saxena P. Blood transfusion in obstetrics. Kathmandu Univ Med J. 2015;13(52):355-9.
2. Munoz M, Stensballe J, Ducloy-Bouthors AS, et al. Patient blood management in obstetrics: prevention and treatment of postpartum haemorrhage. Blood Transfus. 2019;17(2):112-36.
3. Shields LE, Goffman D, Caughey AB. ACOG Practice Bulletin No. 183: Postpartum Hemorrhage. Obstet Gynecol. 2017;130(4):e168-86.

4. Patterson JA, Roberts CL, Bowen JR, et al. Blood transfusion during pregnancy, birth, and the postnatal period. Obstet Gynecol. 2019;133(1):132-9.
5. Franchini M, Lippi G, Favaloro EJ. Recombinant factor VIIa in postpartum hemorrhage: a systematic review. Thromb Res. 2016;141:92-7.
6. Levi M, Toh CH, Thachil J, et al. Guidelines for the diagnosis and management of disseminated intravascular coagulation. Br J Haematol. 2018;180(3):341-58.
7. Carson JL, Stanworth SJ, Dennis JA, et al. Transfusion thresholds for guiding red blood cell transfusion. Cochrane Database Syst Rev. 2021;12:CD002042.
8. Callum JL, Pinkerton PH, Lima A, et al. Blood component storage and handling. Transfus Med Rev. 2019;33(3):151-7.
9. Kaufman RM, Djulbegovic B, Gernsheimer T, et al. Platelet transfusion: a clinical practice guideline from the AABB. Ann Intern Med. 2015;162(3):205-13.
10. Holcomb JB, Tilley BC, Baraniuk S, et al. Transfusion of plasma, platelets, and red blood cells in a 1:1:1 vs a 1:1:2 ratio and mortality in patients with severe trauma. JAMA. 2015;313(5):471-82.
11. Green L, Knight M, Seeney FM, et al. The management of major obstetric haemorrhage: a UK national survey. Transfus Med. 2017;27(5):341-9.
12. Wikkelsø AJ, Edwards HM, Afshari A, et al. Pre-emptive treatment with fibrinogen concentrate for postpartum haemorrhage. Br J Anaesth. 2015;114(4):623-33.
13. Sullivan IJ, Ralph CJ. Obstetric intra-operative cell salvage: a review of an established service. Transfus Med. 2019;29(3):161-8.
14. Liumbruno GM, Liumbruno C, Rafanelli D. Autologous blood transfusion in obstetrics: where are we going? Blood Transfus. 2016;14(2):121-7.
15. Delaney M, Wendel S, Bercovitz RS, et al. Transfusion reactions: prevention, diagnosis, and treatment. Lancet. 2016;388(10061):2825-36.
16. Goel R, Tobian AAR, Shaz BH. Non-infectious transfusion-associated adverse events and their mitigation. Transfus Med Rev. 2019;33(4):201-7.
17. Vlaar APJ, Juffermans NP. Transfusion-related acute lung injury: a clinical review. Crit Care. 2015;19:177.
18. Alam A, Huang S, Alam M, et al. Transfusion-associated circulatory overload: a review. Transfus Med. 2020;30(4):282-91.
19. Vamvakas EC, Blajchman MA. Transfusion-related immunomodulation (TRIM): an update. Blood Rev. 2018;32(6):449-59.
20. World Health Organization. Clinical transfusion practice guidelines. Reprinted 2009. Geneva: World Health Organization; 2001. Available from: https://cdn.who.int/media/docs/default-source/blood-transfusion-safety/guidelines-and-principles-for-safe-blood-transfudion-practice.pdf
21. Royal College of Obstetricians and Gynaecologists. Green-top guideline no. 52: prevention and management of postpartum haemorrhage. BJOG. 2015;122(5):e1-40.
22. AABB. Standards for Blood Banks and Transfusion Services, 33rd edition. Bethesda: AABB; 2023.
23. Federation of Obstetric and Gynaecological Societies of India. Guidelines on postpartum hemorrhage management. J Obstet Gynaecol India. 2023;73(Suppl 1):45-52.

Preterm Labor

Ruchika Garg

DEFINITION AND CLASSIFICATION

Preterm labor (PTL) is the occurrence of regular uterine contractions accompanied by cervical changes (dilatation ≥2 cm and/or effacement ≥80% or progressive changes) before 37^{+0} weeks gestation.

WHO CLASSIFICATION (2022–2025)

Category	*Gestational age range*
Extremely preterm	$<28^{+0}$ weeks
Very preterm	28^{+0} to 31^{+6} weeks
Moderate to late preterm	32^{+0} to 36^{+6} weeks

Subcategories

- Spontaneous preterm labor (60–70%)
- Preterm prelabor rupture of membranes (PPROM) (25–30%)
- Provider-initiated (iatrogenic) preterm birth (10–15%)[1]

EPIDEMIOLOGY

- Global preterm birth rate approximately 11.1% (~13.4 million births annually).[2]
- India: Highest absolute numbers with 13.0–13.5% incidence (~3.6 million/year).
- Survival without major morbidity improves with gestational age:
- 24 weeks: 60–70%
- 28 weeks: >90%
- 34 weeks: >98% (in tertiary centers)

RISK FACTORS FOR PRETERM LABOR

Strong risk factors (or > 3)	*Moderate risk factors (or 1.5–3)*	*Emerging/modifiable risks*
Previous spontaneous PTL	Multiple pregnancy	Periodontal disease
PPROM in current pregnancy	Short cervical length (<25 mm)	Air pollution (PM2.5 exposure)

Contd...

Contd...

Strong risk factors (or > 3)	*Moderate risk factors (or 1.5–3)*	*Emerging/modifiable risks*
Cervical surgery (LLETZ/cone)	Bacterial vaginosis	Maternal stress/depression
Uterine anomalies	Extremes of BMI (<18.5 kg/m^2 or ≥30 kg/m^2)	SARS-CoV-2 infection during pregnancy
Smoking/substance abuse	Suboptimal weight gain	Low socioeconomic status
	Anemia (Hb < 10 g/dL)	

PATHOPHYSIOLOGY

Four overlapping mechanisms contribute to preterm labor:

1. Infection/Inflammation (30–40%): Ascending genital tract infections trigger cytokine storms leading to prostaglandin release and uterine contractions.

Strategy	*Target population*	*Efficacy (recent data)*	*Recommendation*
Universal cervical length screening	Singleton pregnancies at 18–24 weeks	CL <25 mm → 55–60% risk PTB <34 weeks	Strongly recommended (FIGO and SMFM)
Vaginal progesterone[3]	Singleton with short cervix	40–45% reduction in PTB <34 weeks	Grade A
Cervical cerclage	History (≥3 PTBs) or CL <25 mm + prior PTB	30–40% reduction in PTB < 34 weeks	Grade A
Arabin pessary	Singleton with short cervix	Conflicting data	Not recommended (SMFM 2024)
17-OH progesterone caproate (17OHP-C)	Prior spontaneous PTB	No benefit; withdrawn from markets	Withdrawn
Aspirin (150 mg)	High-risk preeclampsia	Modest PTB reduction via PE prevention	Recommended (for PE prevention)
Periodontal therapy	Active periodontal disease	40–60% reduction in PTB (RCT 2024)	Encouraged
Smoking cessation + progesterone	Smokers with short cervix	Synergistic effect (2025 trial)	Strongly encouraged

2. Decidual hemorrhage/abruption: Causes uterine irritability and preterm contractions.
3. Maternal-fetal hypothalamic-pituitary-adrenal (HPA) axis activation: Stress stimulates corticotropin-releasing hormone and cortisol affecting uterine activity.
4. Pathological uterine distension: Due to polyhydramnios or multiples prompting early myometrial activation.

Key biochemical molecules implicated: IL-6, TNF-α, MMP-8, fetal fibronectin, and phosphorylated IGFBP-1.

PREDICTION AND PREVENTION STRATEGIES[4]

Diagnosis of Preterm Labor

Clinical Triad (all not always present)

- Regular painful contractions (≥4/20 min or ≥8/60 min)
- Cervical dilatation ≥2 cm or ≥80% effacement
- Progressive cervical change on repeated examinations (digital or TVUS)

Biomarkers

Biomarker	*Utility*
Fetal fibronectin (fFN)	Negative predictive value >98% between 22 and 35 weeks
Phosphorylated IGFBP-1 (Actim Partus)	Used adjunctively
Placental alpha macroglobulin-1 (PAMG-1/Amnisure)	Highest specificity
Combined CL + fFN	Best predictive performance

Acute Tocolysis

Drug	*Dose regimen*	*Duration*	*Advantages*	*Disadvantages/ contraindications*
Nifedipine	20 mg oral stat → 10–20 mg q30 min ×3, then 10–20 mg q4–6h	≤48 hours	Oral administration, good safety	Maternal tachycardia, hypotension
Atosiban	IV bolus 6.75 mg → 18 mg/h ×3 h → 6 mg/h	≤48 hours	Minimal maternal/ fetal side effects	Costly, less efficacy
Indomethacin	50 mg rectal → 25 mg q6h	≤48 hours	Potent before 32 weeks	Fetal ductus closure risk >48 hours or ≥32 weeks
Betamimetics (ritodrine/ terbutaline)	Largely abandoned	–	–	Maternal pulmonary edema, hyperglycemia

Note: No evidence that tocolytics improve survival beyond 7 days.

Corticosteroids for Fetal Lung Maturity

- Betamethasone 12 mg IM 24 hours apart ×2 doses OR dexamethasone 6 mg IM 12 hours apart ×4 doses
- Indicated: 24^{+0} to 34^{+6} weeks regardless of delivery mode
- Rescue dose allowed if <34 weeks, previous treatment >14 days prior, and new risk occurs
- Late preterm (34^{+0} to 36^{+6} weeks): Single course if delivery anticipated within 7 days (ALPS 2024 follow-up)

Magnesium Sulphate for Neuroprotection

- Loading: 4–6 g IV over 20–30 minutes
- Maintenance: 1–2 g/h for 12–24 hours (stop if delivery not imminent)
- Indication: Predicted preterm birth <32^{+0} weeks
- Number needed to treat (NNT) to prevent one case of cerebral palsy: 46–63

Management of Preterm Labor[5]

- Confirm diagnosis: Contractions + cervical change
- Exclude contraindications: Chorioamnionitis, placental abruption, fetal distress, and severe preeclampsia
- Transfer to NICU-equipped center if <32–34 weeks
- Initiate tocolytics (≤48 hours) for steroid administration window
- Administer antenatal corticosteroids
- Magnesium sulfate neuroprotection if <32 weeks
- Group B *Streptococcus* prophylaxis if unknown/positive (penicillin)
- Do not delay delivery beyond 34 weeks solely for lung maturity

MANAGEMENT OF PPROM AND PTL

Gestational age	*Management approach*
34–36^{+6} weeks	Expectant or induce labor
24–33^{+6} weeks	Expectant, antibiotics (erythromycin 250 mg q6h ×10 days), corticosteroids, magnesium sulfate
<24 weeks	Individualized counseling based on fetal viability and risks

LONG-TERM OUTCOMES OF PRETERM INFANTS (2024 DATA)

- 24 weeks: 65–70% intact survival in high-resource settings
- 28 weeks: >90% survival with 80–85% free of major disability
- Late preterm infants have increased risk of neurodevelopmental disorders (ADHD, autism, cerebral palsy) with relative risk 1.3–1.8

KEY EXAMINATION TAKEAWAYS FOR POSTGRADUATES

- Vaginal progesterone plus cervical length screening is the cost-effective prevention strategy in singleton pregnancies.[3]
- 17-OH progesterone caproate is now obsolete.
- Nifedipine is preferred tocolytic globally.
- Antenatal corticosteroids is beneficial up to 36^{+6} weeks if delivery imminent.
- Magnesium sulphate for neuroprotection only <32 weeks.
- Periodontal disease and air pollution are modifiable emerging risks for PTL.
- No evidence supports maintenance tocolysis, bed rest, or hydration.

REFERENCES

1. WHO. (2023). Preterm Birth Fact Sheet, 2023. [online] Available from https://www.who.int/newsroom/fact-sheets/detail/preterm-birth [Last accessed December, 2025].
2. Chawanpaiboon S, Vogel JP, Moller AB, et al. Global, regional, and national estimates of levels of preterm birth in 2014: a systematic review and modelling analysis. Lancet Glob Health. 2019;7:E37-46.
3. Norman JE, Marlow N, Messow CM, Shennan A, Bennett PR, Thornton S, et al.; OPPTIMUM study group. Vaginal progesterone prophylaxis for preterm birth (the OPPTIMUM study): a multicentre, randomised, double-blind trial. Lancet. 2016;387(10033):2106-16.
4. Medley N, Vogel JP, Care A, et al. Interventions to prevent preterm birth: network meta-analysis. Cochrane. 2023;CD012865.
5. Joseph Biggio; Society for Maternal-Fetal Medicine (SMFM). SMFM Consult Series #70: Management of short cervix in individuals without a history of spontaneous preterm birth. Am J Obstet Gynecol. 2024;231:B2-B17.

CHAPTER 24

Postpartum Collapse

Ruchika Garg

INTRODUCTION

Postpartum collapse is a critical obstetric emergency characterized by sudden loss of consciousness or reduced consciousness due to multiorgan system involvement within 6 weeks postpartum. It is a leading cause of maternal morbidity and mortality, necessitating prompt recognition and multidisciplinary management.

Causes of Postpartum Collapse

The causes are categorized by organ systems and linked to the "4H/4T/E" framework for reversible factors.

TABLE 1: Causes of postpartum collapse.[1]

S. No.	*Organ system*	*Direct causes*	*Indirect causes*	*4h/4T/E association*
1	Central Nervous System	Eclampsia	Intracranial hemorrhage	Hypoxia and eclampsia
2	Respiratory System	Amniotic fluid embolism	Pulmonary embolism and trauma	Thromboembolism and tension pneumothorax
3	Cardiovascular System	Postpartum cardiomyopathy	Congestive cardiac failure, arrhythmias, myocardial infarction/ischemia, cardiomyopathy, and trauma	Hypoxia and tamponade
4	Digestive System	Mendelson's syndrome (aspiration pneumonitis)	Splenic artery rupture and hepatic rupture	Hypoxia and hypovolemia
5	Reproductive System	Postpartum hemorrhage and acute uterine inversion	-	Hypovolemia
6	Miscellaneous	Puerperal sepsis	Anaphylaxis, Drug overdose (e.g., Magnesium sulphate and Oxytocin)[2]	Hypovolemia, toxicity, hypo/hyperkalemia, and hyponatremia

PHYSIOLOGICAL CHANGES IN PREGNANCY

Pregnancy induces significant physiological adaptations that predispose women to complications and challenge resuscitation:

- **Cardiovascular System:**
  - Hemodilution: Plasma volume increases by 50%, RBC volume by 20-30%, leading to anemia.
  - Cardiac output rises by 40%, with 10% directed to uterine blood flow at term.
  - Reduced venous return due to aortocaval compression and lower vascular resistance.
  - Susceptibility to hypovolemia, supine hypotension, and pulmonary edema.
- **Respiratory System:**
  - Reduced functional residual capacity due to diaphragmatic splinting.
  - Increased oxygen consumption and compensated respiratory alkalosis.
  - Risk of rapid hypoxia, difficult intubation due to laryngeal edema, and breast hypertrophy.
- **Digestive System:** Reduced gastric motility and esophageal sphincter tone increase aspiration risk (Mendelson's syndrome).
- **Hematological System:** Hypercoagulable state due to elevated fibrinogen and clotting factors (II, VII, and X), predisposing to thrombotic events.

EARLY IDENTIFICATION AND SCREENING

Early detection is critical to improve outcomes. Obstetric warning scores identify at-risk patients:

- **Modified Early Obstetric Warning Score (MEOWS):**[3]
- Monitors pulse, blood pressure, respiratory rate, temperature, consciousness (AVPU), urine output, and lochia.
- Triggers: Two yellow alerts (score >4) or one red alert (score >3) prompt urgent evaluation.
- Sensitivity: 89%; Specificity: 79%; Positive predictive value: 39%.

TABLE 2: Modified early obstetric warning score (MEOWS).

Score	*Conscious level (AVPU)*	*Temperature (°C)*	*Pulse rate (beats/min)*	*Respiratory rate (breaths/min)*	*Systolic BP (mm Hg)*	*Diastolic BP (mm Hg)*	*Urine output (mL)*	*Lochia*
3	Unconscious, respond to pain	<35, >38	<40, >120	<10, >30	<90, >160	>100	<10	Abnormal
2	Respond to voice	35–36	40–50, 100–120	21–30	150–160	90–100	<30	–
1	–	–	–	–	–	–	–	–
0	Alert	36.1–37.2	61–100	12–20	110–140	60–90	>30	Normal

- **Maternal Early Warning Trigger (MEWT):**[4]
- Includes diagnostic and management pathways for hemorrhage, sepsis, hypertensive disorders, and cardiopulmonary issues.
- Triggers: One red or two yellow sustained parameters (over 20 minutes) require provider evaluation.
- Reduces severe maternal morbidity; screen-positive rate: 2.3%.[5]

TABLE 3: Maternal early warning trigger (MEWT).

Parameter	*Yellow triggers*	*Red triggers*
Mental status	Altered	–
Oxygen saturation (% on room air)	90–93	<90
Systolic BP (mm Hg)	<80 or 156–160	>160
Diastolic BP (mm Hg)	<45 or 106–110	>110
Heart rate (beats/min)	<50 or 111–130	>130
Respiratory rate (breaths/min)	<12 or 25–30	>30
Temperature (°C)	≤36	≤38
Mean arterial pressure (mm Hg)	–	<55
Nursing concern	Clinically uncomfortable	–

CLINICAL APPROACH TO POSTPARTUM COLLAPSE

Management requires a multidisciplinary team, including obstetricians, neonatologists, anesthesiologists, intensivists, hematologists, and radiologists.

Initial Management

Resuscitation is modified due to pregnancy-related physiological changes:

- **Call for Help:** Activate code blue team.
- **Assess Consciousness:** Use AVPU (Alert, Verbal, Pain, Unresponsive) to evaluate sensorium.
- **Prevent Hypoxemia:** Administer 100% oxygen at 10–15 L/min via face mask.
- **IV Access:** Use ≥16-gauge cannula; consider central venous, intraosseous, or venous cut-down if needed. IV access above diaphragm to bypass aortocaval compression.
- **Circulation:**
  - Initiate chest compressions if no cardiac output: rate ≥100/min, depth ≥5 cm, minimal interruptions (<10 seconds).
  - Compression-to-ventilation ratio: 30:2.
  - Aggressive fluid replacement for hemorrhage; monitor for volume overload.
  - Defibrillation for ventricular fibrillation/pulseless ventricular tachycardia: 120–200 J biphasic shock, use adhesive pads.
- **Airway:**
  - Risk of aspiration and difficult intubation; use 6–7 mm cuffed endotracheal tube.
  - Prepare for failed intubation with supraglottic devices (e.g., laryngeal mask airway).
  - Confirm tube position with waveform capnography.

- **Breathing:**
  - Use bag-mask ventilation or supraglottic devices until intubation.
  - Ensure visible chest rise; continue high-flow oxygen (10–15 L/min).
- **Drugs:**
  - Follow ACLS protocols: Epinephrine, adenosine, amiodarone, atropine, etc.
  - Epinephrine is preferred over vasopressin; amiodarone for refractory ventricular fibrillation/tachycardia.
- **Treat Reversible Causes:** Address 4H/4T/E (Hypovolemia, Hypoxia, Hypo/Hyperkalemia, Hypothermia, Thromboembolism, Toxicity, Tension pneumothorax, Tamponade, Eclampsia) during resuscitation.

Illustrates CAB (Circulation, Airway, and Breathing) or ABCDE approach, AVPU assessment, CPR, and defibrillation steps.

TABLE 4: Crash/resuscitation cart contents.

Category	*Items*
Medicines	Epinephrine, norepinephrine (cardiac arrest);[6] Ketamine, rocuronium, etomidate (rapid sequence intubation); Aspirin (myocardial infarction); Nitroglycerine, $MgSO_4$ (hypertensive crisis); Amiodarone, adenosine, metoprolol (refractory VF/VT); Atropine (bradycardia); Calcium gluconate ($MgSO_4$ toxicity); Sodium bicarbonate (metabolic acidosis); Hydrocortisone (endotoxic shock); Chlorpheniramine, hydrocortisone (anaphylaxis)
Equipment	Laryngoscope; Cuffed ET tubes (6–7 mm essential); Bag and mask; IV cannulas (14/16 gauge essential); CV catheter; NG tube; Defibrillator

Management by Specific Cause

- **Postpartum Hemorrhage (PPH):**[7]
  - Leading cause of obstetric ICU admission; incidence in India: 5.7/1,000 live births; 25% of global maternal deaths (WHO).[8]
  - Definition: Primary PPH (≥500 mL blood loss within 24 hours); secondary PPH (24 hours to 12 weeks).
  - Types: Minor (500–1,000 mL), Major (moderate: 1,000–2,000 mL; severe: >2,000 mL).
  - Causes: 4T's (Tone, Trauma, Tissue, Thrombin); atonic PPH most common.
  - Risk Factors (PARTUM): Prolonged labor, Polyhydramnios, Previous C-section, Antepartum hemorrhage, Recent bleeding, Twins, Uterine fibroids, and Multiparity.
- **Management:**
  - Insert two 14/16-gauge IV cannulas; cross-match 4 units packed RBCs.
  - Send blood for CBC, coagulation, fibrinogen, renal, and liver function tests.
  - Administer 2 L crystalloids, then 1.5 L colloids until blood is available.
  - Use HAEMOSTASIS algorithm: HAEMO (pharmacological: oxytocin, methergin, PGF2α, PGE1, tranexamic acid 1 g IV); STASIS (surgical: conservative to hysterectomy).
  - Targets: Central venous pressure 4–8 cmH_2O, urine output >0.5 mL/kg/h.
  - Ultrasound for concealed hemorrhage.

TABLE 5: PPH kit contents.

Category	*Items*
Oxytocics	**First Line:** Oxytocin (10 ampoules, 5U/ampule)
	Second Line: Methyl ergometrine (5 ampoules, 0.2 mg/ampule); 15-methyl PGF2α (8 ampoules, 250 μg/ampule); PGE1 (5 tablets, 200 μg/tablet); Tranexamic acid (4 ampoules, 0.5 g/ampule)
For EUA and Tamponade	Sims speculum, Anterior vaginal retractor, three sponge-holding forceps, Needle holder, 2 artery forceps, Scissors, Vicryl No. 1, Toothed forceps, Curette; Tamponade: 2 condoms, silk thread, 16-gauge Foley's catheter, Normal saline with IV set, and Vaginal pack

- **Septic Shock/Severe Sepsis:**[9]
  - Second leading cause of maternal mortality in India; originates from genital tract (puerperal sepsis) or elsewhere (e.g., pyelonephritis and pneumonia).
  - Puerperal Sepsis: Infection of reproductive tract from labor/rupture of membranes to 6 weeks postpartum; criteria: fever (>38.5°C), pelvic pain, abnormal discharge, and uterine subinvolution.
  - Pathogens: Group A/B Streptococcus, *E. coli*, *S. aureus*, and MRSA.
- **Management:**
  - Send CBC, liver/kidney function tests, cultures, blood sugar, electrolytes, urine, ABG, and radiology.
  - Biomarkers: C-reactive protein, procalcitonin, and cytokines (IL-6 and TNF-α).
  - Follow Surviving Sepsis Campaign: Initiate care bundle within 6 hours.
  - Antibiotics (within 1 hour): Piperacillin-tazobactam 4.5 g IV 6-hourly + Clindamycin 900 mg IV 8-hourly; add Vancomycin 500 mg IV 6-hourly or Linezolid 600 mg IV 12-hourly for MRSA.
  - Fluid: 30 mL/kg crystalloids over 3 hours; vasopressors (adrenaline/noradrenaline) or inotropes (dobutamine) if needed; low-dose steroids (<300 mg) for refractory hypotension.
  - ICU transfer for multiorgan dysfunction.
- **Eclampsia:** Generalized tonic-clonic convulsions or coma in preeclampsia patients, typically within 48 hours postpartum.
  - **Management:**
    - Tests: CBC, liver/kidney function, coagulation, urinary proteins, ECG, and fundus.
    - Anticonvulsant: Magnesium sulphate (Pritchard regimen): 14 g loading (4 g IV 20%, 10 g IM 50%), then 5 g IM 50% 4-hourly for 24 hours postdelivery or last convulsion.[2]
    - Monitor: Deep tendon reflexes, respiratory rate, and urine output.
    - Recurrence: 2 g $MgSO_4$ IV bolus; if refractory, phenobarbital 300 mg IV or intubation.
    - Antihypertensives: Labetalol (20 mg IV, then 40–80 mg every 10–15 min, maximum 300 mg); Nitroglycerine infusion for uncontrolled BP/pulmonary edema.
    - Diuretic: Furosemide 20-40 mg IV for pulmonary edema.
    - Terminate pregnancy if indicated.

- **Amniotic Fluid Embolism (AFE):**[10]
  - Rare (1.7/100,000 pregnancies) but fatal (67/1,000 births); amniotic fluid or fetal debris enters maternal pulmonary circulation.
  - Triad: Hypotension, hypoxia, and coagulopathy within 30 minutes postpartum.
  - **Management:**
    - Supportive: High-quality CPR in ICU.
    - Correct coagulopathy with fresh frozen plasma; reserve recombinant factor VIIa for massive transfusion failure.
    - Biomarkers: Serum tryptase and Sialyl Tn (STN) may aid diagnosis.
    - **Latest Insight:** No specific diagnostic test; focus on rapid supportive care.[10]
- **Pulmonary Thromboembolism (PE):**
  - Incidence: 2–6%; symptoms: dyspnea, chest pain, tachycardia, hemoptysis, and shock.
  - **Management:**
    - Tests: Compression duplex ultrasound for DVT; chest X-ray, V/Q scan, or CTPA for PE.
    - Massive PE: Unfractionated heparin (80 mg/kg IV loading, 18 mg/kg infusion, and target APTT 1.5–2.5× normal).
    - Less severe: LMWH (enoxaparin 1.5 mg/kg daily, dalteparin 10,000–18,000 units daily, and tinzaparin 175 units/kg daily) for 3 months.
    - Consider IVC filter for recurrence.

Uterine Inversion:

- Incidence: 1/8,000 to 1/28,000 deliveries
- **Management:**
  - Immediate manual reposition (Johnson maneuver) without anesthesia if needed.
  - Delayed cases: Resuscitate, use O'Sullivan's hydrostatic method (5 L saline) or surgical approaches (Huntington's, Haultain's).
  - Post-procedure: Uterotonics for 24 hours, broad-spectrum antibiotics.
- **Postpartum Cardiomyopathy (PPCM):**
  - New-onset heart failure from last month of pregnancy to 5 months postpartum; incidence: 1/1,500 to 1/4,000.
  - **Management:**
    - Tests: ECG, echocardiography, cardiac enzymes, BNP, and CRP.
    - Treatment: Diuretics (furosemide), vasodilators (hydralazine), beta-blockers, and LMWH.
    - Cardiology consultation for MI or aortic dissection.
- **Mendelson's Syndrome:**
  - Aspiration of gastric contents; symptoms: respiratory compromise, pulmonary edema.
  - **Management:** Intubation by senior anesthesiologist, suction, and symptomatic treatment.
- **Anaphylaxis:**
  - Incidence: 1–3.5/10,000 pregnancies; criteria: sudden onset, airway/breathing/circulation issues, skin/mucosal changes.

- **Management:**
  - Epinephrine 0.5 mg IM (1:1,000), repeat every 5–15 min.
  - Oxygen, 1–2 L normal saline, inhalational steroids, and salbutamol.
  - Refractory: Epinephrine infusion, chlorpheniramine 10 mg IM, and hydrocortisone 200 mg IM.

- **Drug Toxicity:**
  - $MgSO_4$ toxicity: Levels >10 mEq/L cause reflex loss, respiratory paralysis.
  - **Management:** Stop drug; 10 mL 10% calcium gluconate IV over 10 minutes; intralipid 20% for local anesthetic toxicity.

DEBRIEFING AND DOCUMENTATION

- Regularly update family on maternal condition and prognosis.
- Obtain written informed consent.
- Document all resuscitative measures.

PREVENTION

- **High-Risk Monitoring:** Strict observation for early complication detection.
- **Warning Scores:** Routine use of MEOWS/MEWT for early intervention.
- **Audits:** Review Maternal Near Miss cases to refine protocols.
- **Training:** Conduct obstetric drills, use simulation, and display algorithm charts.
- **Quality Initiatives:** Implement programs in labor rooms and wards.

REFERENCES

1. Chu J, Johnston TA, Geoghegan J. Maternal collapse in pregnancy and the puerperium. BJOG. 2020;127:e14-e52.
2. Pritchard JA, et al. Magnesium sulfate in eclampsia: The Pritchard regimen revisited. Am J Obstet Gynecol. 2018;218:S2–S3.
3. Singh A, et al. Validation of the Modified Early Obstetric Warning Score (MEOWS) in a tertiary care hospital. J Obstet Gynaecol India. 2016;66:314-9.
4. Shields LE, Wiesner S, Klein C, et al. Maternal early warning trigger tool reduces maternal morbidity. Am J Obstet Gynecol. 2016;214:527.e1-527.e6.
5. Knight M, Bunch K, Tuffnell, et al. Saving Lives, Improving Mothers' Care: Lessons learned to inform maternity care from the UK and Ireland Confidential Enquiries into Maternal Deaths and Morbidity 2014–16. Oxford: NPEU; 2018.
6. Jeejeebhoy FM, Zelop CM, Lipman S, et al. Cardiac arrest in pregnancy: A scientific statement from the American Heart Association. Circulation. 2015;132(18):1747-73.
7. ACOG Practice Bulletin No. 183: Postpartum hemorrhage. Obstet Gynecol. 2017;130:e168-e186.
8. Say L, Chou D, Gemmill A, et al. Global causes of maternal death: A WHO systematic analysis. Lancet Glob Health. 2014;2(6):e323-33.
9. Dellinger RP, et al. Surviving Sepsis Campaign: International guidelines for management of sepsis and septic shock. Crit Care Med. 2017;45:486-552.
10. Clark SL, Hankins GD, Dudley DA, et al. Amniotic fluid embolism: analysis of the national registry. Am J Obstet Gynecol. 1995;172(4 Pt 1):1158-67; discussion 1167-9.

Prolonged Pregnancy and Post-term Pregnancy

Ruchika Garg

INTRODUCTION

Post-term pregnancy, defined by the American College of Obstetricians and Gynecologists (ACOG) as gestation ≥42 0/7 weeks, poses increased maternal and fetal risks, including stillbirth, macrosomia, and cesarean delivery. Accurate gestational dating is essential for diagnosis and management. This comprehensive chapter, tailored for postgraduate medical examinations, provides an evidence-based overview of epidemiology, pathophysiology, risks, diagnosis, management, and a clinical case scenario, incorporating recent data (2015–2025), RCOG/NICE guidelines, and Indian examination relevance.

EPIDEMIOLOGY

Global incidence of post-term pregnancy is 4–14%, with 2–7% reaching ≥43 weeks.[1] In India, prevalence is 5–10%, reduced to ~1.5% with ultrasound vs. last menstrual period (LMP).[2] US data (2022) reports 5.8%.[3]

PATHOPHYSIOLOGY

Labor initiation involves maternal (cervical ripening, prostaglandin surge, and oxytocin receptor sensitivity), fetal [corticotropin-releasing hormone (CRH), adrenocorticotropic hormone (ACTH), cortisol, and dehydroepiandrosterone (DHEA)], and placental factors.[4] Disruptions, such as anencephaly or placental sulfatase deficiency, delay labor by impairing the hypothalamic-pituitary-adrenal axis.[5]

RISK FACTORS[6]

- Genetic: 23–30% heritability; 15% recurrence risk.
- Race: South Asians (39 weeks) versus Caucasians (40 weeks).
- Maternal: Primiparity, age > 35 years, obesity (BMI ≥ 30 kg/m^2: 37–52% risk).
- Fetal: Male fetus, anencephaly, and adrenal disorders.
- **Obstetric: Prior post-term pregnancy (3 × risk).**

Women who were themselves products of a prolonged pregnancy are at higher risk of post-term pregnancy. Women with prior prolonged pregnancy have an increased risk of subsequent post-term pregnancy (27% with one prior prolonged pregnancy and 39% with two prior prolonged pregnancies). Twin studies also support a genetic predisposition, increased in women whose twin sister has had a previous post-term birth, especially in monozygotic than in dizygotic twins.

PATERNAL ROLE IN RECURRENCE RISK

The risk of recurrence of post-term pregnancy was reduced from 19.9% to 15.4% when the father of the baby changed between the first and second pregnancy.[6]

MATERNAL AND FETAL RISKS

Maternal[7]

- Cesarean section (CS): ~22% in induced post-term versus 10% term.
- Prolonged labor, lacerations, chorioamnionitis, and postpartum hemorrhage.
- Anxiety beyond 41 weeks, higher in nulliparas.

Fetal/Neonatal[8]

- Uteroplacental insufficiency
- Oligohydramnios
- Intrauterine growth restriction (IUGR; 3.8% vs. 2.2%)
- Meconium-stained amniotic fluid (MSAF; 29%), stillbirth (3.2/1,000 at 42 weeks).
- Macrosomia: 2× risk; shoulder dystocia and neurological injuries.
- Postmaturity syndrome: 10–20%; wrinkled skin, meconium staining (Clifford Stages I–III).
- Long-term: Infections, epilepsy, and delayed milestones.

DIAGNOSIS

First-trimester ultrasound (crown-rump length, ±5–7 days) is most accurate; LMP overestimates post-term rates (9.5% vs. 1.5%).[9] In vitro fertilization (IVF) uses embryo age/transfer date. Pregnancies without ultrasound before 22 0/7 weeks are poorly dated.[10]

MANAGEMENT

Prevention

- Ultrasound dating: Reduces misdiagnosis by 50–70%[11]
- Membrane sweeping (≥39 weeks): Decreases IOL need by 20–30%; causes discomfort.[12]

Expectant Management

- Low-risk pregnancies with consent; twice-weekly surveillance [cardiotocography (CTG) and amniotic fluid index (AFI)] at 41–42 weeks.[13]
- Risks: Stillbirth (3/1,000), CS.
- Counseling: Perinatal risks and surveillance limitations.

Induction of Labor (IOL)

- **Timing:**
  - NICE (2021): IOL at 41 weeks.[14]
  - ACOG (2020): 42 0/7–42 6/7 weeks; consider 41–42 weeks or 39 weeks (nulliparas, ARRIVE).[15]
  - WHO (2018): IOL at 41 weeks.[16]
- **Methods:**
  - Bishop's score <6: Dinoprostone or Foley catheter; nitric oxide donors ineffective.[17]
  - MAGPOP Trial (2023): Balloon catheters versus dinoprostone; no CS rate difference, less analgesia with balloons.[18]
- **Outcomes:**
  - ARRIVE (2018): 39-week IOL reduced CS (18.6% vs. 22.2%), perinatal issues (4.3% vs. 5.4%).[19]
  - INDEX (2022): 41-week IOL lowered perinatal risks (1.7% vs. 3.1%).[20]
  - SWEPIS (2019): Halted due to expectant group mortality.[21]
  - Cochrane (2020): IOL reduced perinatal deaths, CS, and NICU admissions.[22]

Ultrasound: Cervical length (<25 mm) predicts labor/IOL success.[23]

RCOG/NICE Guidelines:[24,25]

- RCOG (2023): IOL at 41 weeks; sweeps at 39 weeks.
- NICE (2021): Sweeps at 39 weeks; IOL at 41 weeks; earlier for high-risk.

Postmaturity, postmaturity syndrome and dysmaturity are not synonymous terms to post-term pregnancy. They are often used to describe the features of a neonate who appears to have been in utero longer than 42 weeks of gestation. They describe the effects of intrauterine growth restriction (IUGR) secondary to uteroplacental insufficiency encountered in a post-term pregnancy.

DYSMATURITY: POSTMATURITY SYNDROME

Incidence: 20%; increase with association of oligohydramnios

Stage 1: Alert facial expression; recent weight loss with decreased subcutaneous fat and muscle mass

Stage 2: Green meconium staining of skin and umbilicus, fetal distress, and hypoxia

Stage 3: Yellow staining of nails, skin, and umbilicus, indicative of prolonged passage of meconium

Criteria to Establish the Diagnosis of Postmaturity Retrospectively

General appearance: Baby looks thin and old. Skin is wrinkled. There is absence of vernix caseosa. Body and the cord are stained with greenish yellow color. Head is hard without much evidence of molding. Nails are protruding beyond the nail beds.

Weight often more than 3 kg and length is about **54 cm. Both are variable and even an IUGR baby may be born.**

Complication

Post-term pregnancies is associated **with increased fetal morbidity:** Meconium aspiration syndrome, neonatal academia as demonstrated by low umbilical cord pH levels, low 5-minute APGAR scores, neonatal encephalopathy, admission to neonatal intensive care unit (NICU), fetal macrosomia, shoulder dystocia, clavicular fractures, and higher infant deaths in the first year of life.[3,8]

Post-term pregnancy is associated with **significant risks to the mothe**r, which include: Labor dystocia (9–12% vs. 2–7% at term), severe perineal lacerations (third and fourth degree tears), related to macrosomia (3.3% vs. 2.6% at term), operative vaginal delivery, doubling in cesarean section (CS) rates, the attendant complications (14% vs. 7% at term), and maternal anxiety.[8]

Management

Accurate Pregnancy Dating

Last menstrual period has traditionally been used to calculate the expected date of delivery (EDD). But many inaccuracies could exist because of cycle irregularity, recent use of hormonal contraception or because of bleeding early in pregnancy.

Routine ultrasound examination for pregnancy dating demonstrated a reduction in the rate of false positive diagnosis and thereby the overall rate of post-term pregnancy from 10% to 15% to approximately 2–5%, and thereby minimized unnecessary intervention. When using ultrasound for dating, it is necessary to understand the margin of error reported at various times during gestation. The variation by ultrasonography generally is ± 7 days up to 20 weeks of gestation, ± 14 days between 20 and 30 weeks of gestation, and ± 21 days beyond 30 weeks of gestation (ACOG, 2004).

PREVENTION OF POST-TERM PREGNANCY

Induction of labor at term is the most decisive way of prevention. However, clinicians and patients alike are concerned about risks associated with induction of labor including an increased cesarean section rate.

MANAGEMENT OF POST-TERM PREGNANCIES BY ACOG 2014

The incidence of post-term pregnancies may vary by population, in part as a result of differences in regional management practices for pregnancies that go beyond the estimated date of delivery. Accurate determination of gestational age is essential to accurate diagnosis and appropriate management of late-term and post-term pregnancies. Antepartum fetal surveillance and induction of labor have been evaluated as strategies to decrease the risks of perinatal morbidity and mortality associated with late-term and post-term pregnancies.

NICE recommends induction between 41^{+0} and 42^{+0} weeks. The committee considered it would be cost effective to offer continuous cardiotocography as they were aware of evidence of an increased risk of stillbirth or neonatal death after 42 weeks of pregnancy.

The offer should be preceded by a full discussion of the benefits and risks to the woman and her baby. The committee was aware that ultrasound is used antenatally for monitoring amniotic fluid volume after 42 weeks of pregnancy, and they sought evidence about the effectiveness of ultrasound for measuring amniotic fluid volume for women in labor after 42 weeks of pregnancy. No evidence was identified and the committee agreed not to make a recommendation about the use of ultrasound for measuring amniotic fluid volume for women in labor after 42 weeks of pregnancy.

A Cochrane review found that "sweeping of the membranes, performed as a general policy in women at term, was associated with reduced duration of pregnancy and reduced frequency of pregnancy continuing beyond 41 weeks (RR: 0.59; 95% CI: 0.46–0.74) and 42 weeks (RR: 0.28; 95% CI: 0.15–0.50)". However, clinicians are advised to consider the balance of maternal discomfort over avoidance of other induction methods.[22]

A Cochrane review found no difference between nonstress testing (NSTs) and biophysical profiles (BPP), though the latter may be associated with a higher cesarean delivery rate, albeit based on limited numbers of patients evaluated. There is limited evidence suggesting that twice-weekly testing might be superior to once-weekly testing in post-term gestations, but no firm recommendation is made. Given the link between oligohydramnios and post-term pregnancies and the former's association with increased perinatal morbidity and mortality, ACOG opines that ultrasonographic assessment of amniotic fluid volume to detect oligohydramnios is warranted. The latter studies should use the deepest vertical pocket of amniotic fluid of 2 cm or less as the appropriate diagnostic criteria. Thus, the use of either BPP or a modified BPP (NST plus amniotic fluid assessment) twice weekly beginning at or beyond 41 0/7 weeks seems warranted.

A recent Cochrane registry report suggests that induction of labor at 41 completed weeks' gestation is associated with fewer perinatal deaths, risk ratio (RR) of 0.31 (95% CI: 0.12–0.88) and significantly fewer cesarean deliveries (RR: 0.89; 95% CI: 0.81–0.97) compared with expectant management.[3] The number needed to treat to prevent one perinatal death was 410 (95% CI: 322–1492). Other benefits of induction include fewer cases of meconium aspiration syndrome. The ACOG concludes that "Induction of labor between 41 0/7 and 42 0/7 weeks *can be* considered" and "Induction of labor after 42 0/7 weeks and by 42 6/7 weeks of gestation *is recommended*, given evidence of an increase in perinatal morbidity and mortality."

One trial, the SWEPIS trial, was stopped early due to a significantly higher perinatal mortality rate in the expectant group. It was a multicenter open-label randomized superiority trial of 2,760 women with low-risk uncomplicated singleton pregnancies, which compared outcomes between induction of labor at 41 weeks versus expectant management until 42 weeks. It concluded that induction of labor at 41 weeks is associated with decreased risk of perinatal mortality compared to at 42 weeks.[24]

ANTEPARTUM FETAL SURVEILLANCE

Women who reached 42 weeks gestation and opt to continue their pregnancy with conservative management should undergo antenatal fetal surveillance. Despite the fact that there is no evidence to suggest that antepartum fetal surveillance in post-term pregnancies decreases perinatal mortality, antenatal fetal surveillance has become a common practice in these cases on the basis of universal acceptance. The reasons are:

- Data suggest a gradual increase in perinatal morbidity and mortality during this period.
- There is no evidence that antenatal fetal monitoring adversely affects post-term women.
- The published studies are of insufficient power to demonstrate benefit of monitoring in these cases.
- Because of ethical and medicolegal considerations, no studies have included post-term patients who were not monitored, and it is unlikely that any future studies will do so. Umbilical artery Doppler velocimetry has no proven benefit in monitoring the post-term fetus and is not recommended for this indication. The frequency of antenatal surveillance among post-term women, it seems that twice-weekly testing is widely acceptable by many clinicians (ACOG, 2004). Using CTG and AF volume assessment constitutes an acceptable standard by many clinicians.

INDUCTION OF LABOR

Induction of labor is indicated when the benefits of delivery outweighs the risks associated with induction. The main concern around induction of labor in post-term low risk pregnancies is related to uterine overstimulation, fetal distress, failure of induction, and increase in cesarean section rates. There are also risks associated with induction in particular groups of patients with specific risk factors such as risk of uterine rupture in women with previous cesarean section. Induction of labor is more likely to succeed when the cervix is favorable. To assess cervix, we have various techniques from digital cervical examination (Bishop score), ultrasound assessment of cervical length, and more recently biochemical markers (estriol/estradiol ratio).

The risk of adverse pregnancy outcome increases with advancing maternal age. Women aged ≥40 years have an increased risk of adverse perinatal and maternal outcome when pregnancy goes beyond 41 weeks *(https://pubmed.ncbi.nlm.nih.gov/32072610/)*.

Special Consideration

Induction of labor in women with unfavorable cervical score: As such lower doses (e.g., 25 μg intravaginal misoprostol) are preferable to 50 μg. When PG is used, fetal heart rate monitoring should be performed routinely to assess fetal well-being because of the risk of uterine hyperstimulation. Elective induction resulted in a lower cesarean delivery rate, primarily related to fewer surgeries performed for nonreassuring fetal heart rate tracings. Patient satisfaction was significantly higher in women randomly assigned to labor induction. Although not universally accepted, most of the data suggest that routine induction at 41 weeks of gestation has fetal benefit without incurring the additional maternal risks of a higher rate of cesarean delivery.

Flowchart 1: Management of post-term pregnancy.

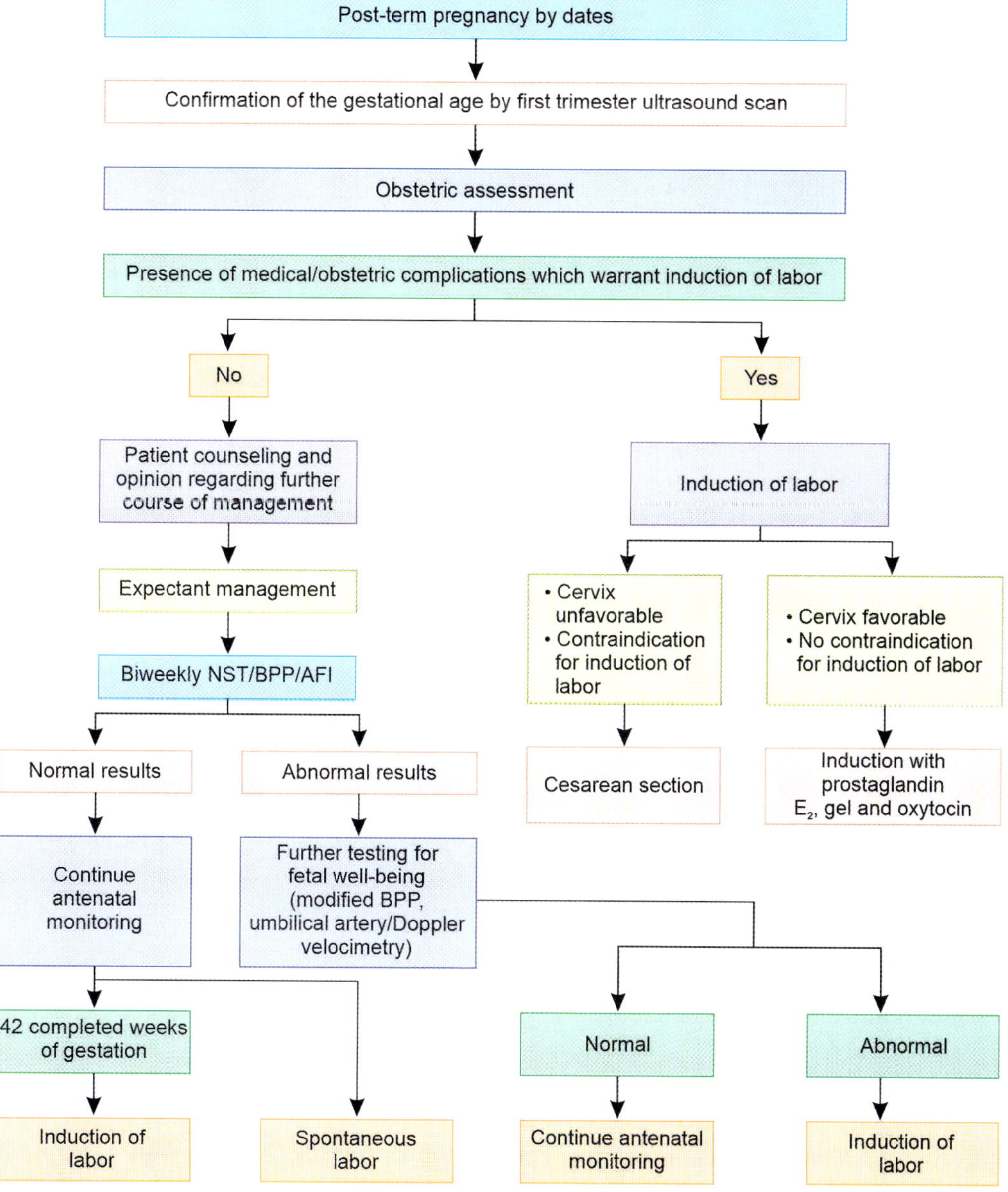

CLINICAL CASE SCENARIO

Case: A 30-year-old primigravida at 41 3/7 weeks (ultrasound-dated) presents without labor. Her BMI is 31 kg/m^2, and has family history of post-term delivery. AFI 5.5 cm, CTG reactive, cervical length 28 mm, and Bishop's score 4.

Flowchart 2: Approach to post-term pregnancy.

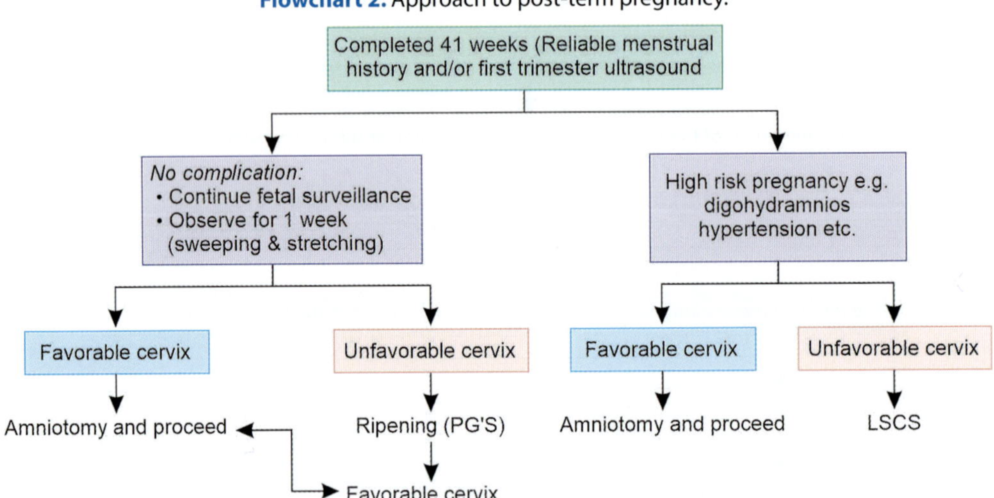

TABLE 1: Post-term pregnancy prevalence.[1-3]

Region	*Prevalence (%)*	*Notes*
Global	4–14	2–7% ≥43 weeks
India	5–10	Ultrasound: ~1.5%
US (2022)	5.8	CDC data

Questions:
- **Next step?**
- **Risks of expectant management?**

Answers:
- Offer IOL (NICE 2021). Perform membrane sweeping, start dinoprostone, and monitor for MSAF/fetal distress.
- Stillbirth (3/1,000), oligohydramnios, MSAF (29%), CS (~22%), and anxiety. Discussion: Obesity and family history increase risk; low AFI warrants IOL.

FUTURE RESEARCH

- Universal IOL feasibility in low-resource settings.
- Long-term neonatal outcomes of early IOL.
- Genetic markers for post-term risk.

Appeared in DNB (2019, Paper-3), NEET-PG (2022). Focus: Risks, IOL timing, surveillance. Challenges: LMP reliance and limited rural ultrasound (30% access).

KEY POINTS

- Prevalence: 5–10% (India); ultrasound reduces to ~1.5% **(Table 1)**.
- Risks: CS (~22%), stillbirth (3.2/1000), and postmaturity (10–20%) **(Table 2)**.

TABLE 2: Maternal and fetal risks.[7,8]

Category	*Risks*	*Incidence*
Maternal	CS, lacerations	CS: ~22%
Fetal	Stillbirth, MSAF	Stillbirth: 3.2/1,000
Neonatal	Postmaturity	10–20%

TABLE 3: Diagnostic methods.[9,10]

Method	*Accuracy*	*Limitations*
Ultrasound (CRL)	±5–7 days	Rural access limited
LMP	±14–21 days	Recall errors
IVF	Exact	IVF-specific

TABLE 4: Management options.[14-22]

Strategy	*Indications*	*Benefits*	*Risks*
Sweeping	≥39 weeks	Reduces IOL	Discomfort
Expectant	Low risk	Avoids intervention	Stillbirth
IOL (41 weeks)	Singletons	Lower CS, risks	Resource-intensive
Ripening	Bishop's <6	Improves IOL	Hyperstimulation

- Diagnosis: Ultrasound critical; LMP unreliable **(Table 3)**.
- Management: Sweeps at 39 weeks; IOL at 41 weeks; ARRIVE/INDEX support early IOL **(Table 4)**.
- RCOG/NICE: Early sweeps, IOL at 41 weeks.
- India: Address ultrasound access, cultural barriers.

REFERENCES

1. Muglu J, et al. BMJ. 2019;364:l416.
2. Chawla S, et al. J Obstet Gynaecol India. 2018;68(5):345-50.
3. CDC. NCHS; 2023.
4. Norwitz ER, et al. Am J Obstet Gynecol. 2017;216(1):15-28.
5. Smith R, et al. Placenta. 2018;71:50-6.
6. Olesen AW, et al. Epidemiology. 2019;30(3):433-9.
7. Kortekaas JC, et al. Acta Obstet Gynecol Scand. 2020;99(5):627-34.
8. Eden RD, et al. Am J Perinatol. 2017;34(7):678-84.
9. Gardosi J, et al. Ultrasound Obstet Gynecol. 2018;51(2):211-7.
10. ACOG. Obstet Gynecol. 2020;136(4):e48-e69.
11. Crowther CA, et al. Lancet. 2016;387(10025):1161-9.
12. Finucane EM, et al. Cochrane Database Syst Rev. 2020;4:CD000451.
13. Divon MY, et al. Am J Obstet Gynecol. 2018;218(2):S119-25.
14. NICE. NG207. 2021.
15. ACOG. Obstet Gynecol. 2019;133(2):e156-e165.
16. WHO. Induction of Labour Guidelines. 2018.
17. Chanrachakul B, et al. Eur J Obstet Gynecol Reprod Biol. 2017;210:343-8.

18. Diguisto C, et al. BJOG. 2023;130(4):356-64.
19. Grobman WA, et al. N Engl J Med. 2018;379(6):513-23.
20. Alkmark M, et al. BMJ. 2022;376:e066907.
21. Wennerholm UB, et al. BMJ. 2019;367:l6131.
22. Middleton P, et al. Cochrane Database Syst Rev. 2020;3:CD004945.
23. Ramanathan G, et al. Ultrasound Obstet Gynecol. 2020;55(3):396-402.
24. RCOG. Green-top No. 81. 2023.
25. NICE. NG207. 2021.

Antenatal Care

Ruchika Garg

INTRODUCTION

Antenatal care (ANC) is critical for optimizing maternal and fetal outcomes through health promotion, risk assessment, and timely interventions. The Focused Antenatal Care (FANC) model, endorsed by WHO in 2002, recommended four targeted visits for low-risk pregnancies but was associated with higher perinatal mortality compared to models with ≥8 contacts.[1] In 2016, WHO updated guidelines to advocate ≥8 contacts, emphasizing a "positive pregnancy experience" encompassing physical health, sociocultural normality, and emotional well-being.[2] The inverted pyramid of ANC, proposed by Kypros Nicolaides, prioritizes first-trimester screening to identify high-risk pregnancies early, enabling personalized care.[3] In India, ANC coverage remains suboptimal, with only 50% of women receiving ≥8 visits, underscoring the need for effective models.[4] This chapter outlines ANC schedules, interventions, first-trimester screening, Leopold maneuvers, and fundal height measurement for postgraduate medical education.

METHODS

A systematic literature search was conducted using PubMed and Google Scholar for articles published between January 2015 and June 2025. Search terms included *antenatal care, focused antenatal care, inverted pyramid, first-trimester screening,* and *Leopold maneuvers.* Inclusion criteria were: (1) Original research, reviews, or guidelines, (2) English language, (3) peer-reviewed, (4) relevant to obstetrics, and (5) full-text available. From 110 articles identified, 20 duplicates were removed, 65 irrelevant articles were excluded, and 25 were selected for review.

FOCUSED ANTENATAL CARE (FANC) AND WHO 2016 GUIDELINES

- **FANC (2002):**[1]
  - Recommended four targeted visits for low-risk pregnancies.
  - Interventions: Nutritional counseling, risk assessment, preventive measures (e.g., tetanus toxoid), and management of physiological symptoms.
  - Drawbacks: Not tested in high-mortality settings; associated with increased perinatal mortality (RR: 1.15, 95% CI: 1.02–1.30).[5]
- **WHO 2016 Guidelines:**[2]
  - ≥8 contacts to reduce perinatal mortality and enhance maternal satisfaction.
  - "Contact" emphasizes active engagement between pregnant women and providers.

- Goals: Maintain healthy pregnancy, ensure positive labor/birth, and promote maternal autonomy.
- Key Areas:
  - **Nutritional Interventions:** Iron-folic acid and calcium supplementation.
  - **Maternal/Fetal Assessment:** Ultrasound and biochemical screening.
  - **Preventive Measures:** Tetanus toxoid and malaria prophylaxis.
  - **Physiological Symptoms:** Manage nausea, heartburn, and pelvic pain.
  - **Health Systems:** Improve ANC utilization and quality.

TABLE 1: Comparison of FANC and WHO 2016 ANC models.[1,2,5]

Model	*Visits/Contacts*	*Focus*	*Outcomes*
FANC (2002)	4 visits	Targeted interventions, low-risk pregnancies	Higher perinatal mortality
WHO 2016	≥8 contacts	Positive pregnancy experience, risk detection	Reduced perinatal mortality, higher satisfaction

INVERTED PYRAMID OF ANTENATAL CARE

- **Concept:**[3]
  - Shifts focus to first-trimester screening ($11–13^{+6}$ weeks) to identify high-risk pregnancies.
  - High-risk cases receive intensified monitoring; low-risk cases require fewer visits.
  - Enabled by advances in ultrasound and biochemical screening.
- **Rationale:**
  - Many complications (e.g., preeclampsia and fetal growth restriction) originate in first trimester due to placental dysfunction.[6]
  - Early intervention (e.g., aspirin for preeclampsia) is most effective before 16 weeks.[7]
- **Traditional versus Inverted Pyramid:**
  - **Traditional:** Increased visits in late pregnancy (weekly from 36 weeks).
  - **Inverted:** Intensive first-trimester evaluation, tailored subsequent care.

First-Trimester Screening

First-trimester screening ($11–13^{+6}$ weeks) identifies risks for aneuploidies, structural defects, and fetomaternal complications.[8]

- **Fetal Aneuploidy Screening:**[8]
  - **Combined test:** Maternal age, nuchal translucency (NT), PAPP-A, and free β-hCG.
    - Detection rate: 90% for trisomy 21, 95% for trisomies 18/13; false-positive rate 5%.[8]
  - **Additional Markers:** Placental growth factor (PlGF), alpha-fetoprotein (AFP), nasal bone, ductus venosus (DV) flow, and tricuspid regurgitation (TR).
    - Detection rate: 93–96% for trisomy 21 (false-positive rate 2.5%).[8]
  - **Contingent Protocol:**
    - High risk (>1:50): Offer invasive testing (CVS/amniocentesis).
    - Intermediate risk (1:51–1:1,000): Additional markers; invasive test if risk ≥1:100.
    - Low risk (<1:1,000): Reassure.[8]

- **Congenital Structural Defects:**[9]
  - Increased NT (>3.5 mm): Associated with diaphragmatic hernia, omphalocele, cardiac defects, and genetic syndromes (e.g., Noonan syndrome); 50% anomaly risk if NT ≥ 6.5 mm.[9]
  - Open neural tube defects: Detected via intracranial translucency (IT), brainstem size, frontomaxillary angle; 51–65% detection rate with transabdominal/transvaginal ultrasound.[9]
  - Cardiac defects: NT > 99th percentile, TR, and abnormal DV flow; 52% detection rate.[9]
- **Multiple Gestations:**[10]
  - Assess chorionicity, amnionicity, and risks [e.g., twin-twin transfusion syndrome (TTTS)].
  - NT discordance or abnormal DV flow predicts TTTS risk.[10]
- **Fetomaternal Complications:**[11]
  - **Preeclampsia (PE):** Maternal blood pressure, uterine artery pulsatility index (PI), PAPP-A, and PlGF.
    - Detection rate: 90% (historical factors, BP, and PI); 96% with PAPP-A/PlGF.[11]
  - **Fetal Growth Restriction (FGR):** PAPP-A, PlGF, and maternal characteristics; 60% detection for preterm SGA.[11]
  - **Preterm Birth**: Transvaginal cervical length; high-risk cases benefit from progesterone.[12]
  - **Gestational Diabetes Mellitus (GDM):** Adiponectin, sex hormone-binding globulin, and maternal characteristics; 75% detection.[13]
  - **Macrosomia:** Increased NT, free β-hCG, and low adiponectin.[13]

TABLE 2: First-trimester screening targets and detection rates.[8-13]

Target	*Markers*	*Detection rate*
Trisomy 21	NT, PAPP-A, β-hCG, PlGF, and nasal bone	93–96% (2.5% FPR)
Structural Defects	NT, IT, and frontomaxillary angle	51–65%
Preeclampsia	BP, uterine artery PI, PAPP-A, and PlGF	96%
FGR	PAPP-A, PlGF, and maternal factors	60% (preterm SGA)
Preterm Birth	Cervical length	Identifies high-risk cases

ANTENATAL CARE SCHEDULE AND INTERVENTIONS

- **WHO/NICE 2021 Schedule:**[14]
  - **Nulliparous:** 10 contacts (12, 20, 26, 30, 34, 36, 38, 40, 41, and 42 weeks).
  - **Parous:** 7 contacts (12, 25, 31, 34, 36, 38, and 40 weeks).
- **Key Interventions:**[2,14]
  - **First Contact (<12 weeks):**
    - Detailed history, physical examination, blood tests (FBC, blood group, Rhesus status, HIV, syphilis, hepatitis B, and thyroid), urine dipstick, and ultrasound (gestational age and aneuploidy screening).
    - Counseling: Diet, exercise, smoking cessation, and minor ailments.
    - Supplements: Folic acid (400 μg/day) and iron (30–60 mg/day).

- **Subsequent Contacts:**
    - Monitor blood pressure, symphysis-fundal height (SFH), and fetal movements.
    - Screen for preeclampsia, GDM (GCT at 24–28 weeks), and fetal anomalies (18–20^{+6} weeks).
    - Discuss birth preferences, postnatal care, and mental health.
- **Complications Management:**[14]
    - **Hypertension:** Refer if BP ≥ 160/110 mm Hg; aspirin for preeclampsia risk.
    - **Nausea/Vomiting:** Ginger, doxylamine/pyridoxine for mild cases; IV fluids for hyperemesis.
    - **Vaginal Discharge:** Investigate/treat infections (e.g., clotrimazole for candidiasis).
    - **Pelvic Pain:** Physiotherapy and lumbopelvic belt.

TABLE 3: WHO/NICE ANC Schedule (2021).[14]

Visit	*Timing (weeks)*	*Nulliparous*	*Parous*	*Key interventions*
1	<12	Yes	Yes	History, ultrasound, and blood tests
2	20	Yes	25	GCT and anomaly scan
3	26	Yes	31	BP, SFH, and fetal movements
4	30	Yes	34	Ultrasound (BPP if needed)
5	34	Yes	36	Discuss birth plan
6	36	Yes	38	Check for breech
7	38	Yes	40	Discuss prolonged pregnancy
8	40	Yes	–	Monitor fetal well-being
9	41	Yes	–	Plan induction
10	42	Yes	–	Induction if undelivered

ANTENATAL EXAMINATION

- **Components:**[15]
    - **History:** Demographic details, obstetric history (gravida, parity, and complications), menstrual history, past medical/surgical history, and family history.
    - **Physical Examination:**
        - General: Vital signs (BP, pulse, and temperature), BMI, and head-to-toe assessment (skin, eyes, mouth, thyroid, and breasts).
        - Systemic: Cardiorespiratory, gastrointestinal, genitourinary, and musculoskeletal.
        - Obstetric: Abdominal examination (fundal height, fetal lie, and presentation), Leopold maneuvers, and auscultation (FHR).
    - **Investigations:** Blood tests, urine dipstick, ultrasound, and GCT.
- **Antenatal Record:** Single record for each mother, documenting all findings for continuity of care.[15]

TABLE 4: Physical examination parameters in ANC.[15]

Parameter	*Normal values*	*Notes*
Blood Pressure	120/80 mm Hg	Validate device for pregnancy
Pulse	60–90 beats/min	Monitor for tachycardia
BMI (Asia-Pacific)	Normal: 18.5–22.9	Adjust for ethnicity
Fundal Height	Matches gestational age (cm)	Plot on gravidogram

Leopold Maneuvers

- **Purpose:** Determine fetal position, presentation, and engagement in third trimester.[16]
- **Preparation:**[16]
  - Wash hands, explain procedure, and obtain consent.
  - Empty maternal bladder, position supine with 15° left tilt.
  - Expose abdomen from xiphisternum to pubic symphysis.
- **Technique:**[16]
  - **First Maneuver (Fundal Grip):** Palpate fundus to identify fetal pole (head: hard, ballotable; breech: soft, nodular). Assess gestational age via fundal height.
  - **Second Maneuver (Umbilical Grip):** Palpate lateral uterine walls to determine fetal lie (longitudinal, transverse) and back position.
  - **Third Maneuver (Pawlik Grip):** Grasp lower uterus to confirm presenting part and engagement.
  - **Fourth Maneuver:** Palpate lower uterus to assess head flexion and descent into pelvis.
  - **Fifth Maneuver (Zagenmeister):** Estimate head engagement using rule of fifths (2 cm per fifth above pelvic brim).
- **Findings:**
  - FHR (120–160 beats/min) best heard over fetal back.
  - Cephalic presentation: FHR below umbilicus; breech: near umbilicus.

FUNDAL HEIGHT MEASUREMENT

- **Purpose:** Assess gestational age, fetal growth, and amniotic fluid volume.[17]
- **Method:**[17]
  - Position mother supine, empty bladder.
  - Centralize uterus, place ulnar border of left hand on fundus.
  - Measure from pubic symphysis to fundus using a tape measure (cm).
  - Plot on gravidogram to monitor growth serially.
- **Interpretation:**[17]
  - Matches gestational age (±2 cm) in second/third trimesters.
  - **Large SFH:** Multiple gestation, polyhydramnios, macrosomia, and incorrect dates.
  - **Small SFH:** FGR, oligohydramnios, IUD, and transverse lie.
- **McDonald's Rule:** Fundal height (cm) ≈ gestational age (weeks) after 20 weeks.[17]

TABLE 5: Fundal height by gestational age.[17]

Weeks	*Fundal height*	*Landmark*
12	Pubic symphysis	Just palpable
20	1–2 cm below umbilicus	Umbilical plane
36	Xiphoid process	Peak height
40	Slightly below 36 weeks	Lightening occurs

CURRENT GUIDELINES

- **WHO (2016):** ≥8 ANC contacts; first contact <12 weeks; ultrasound before 24 weeks.[2]
- **NICE (2021):** 10 contacts for nulliparous, 7 for parous; screen for GDM, preeclampsia, and fetal anomalies.[14]
- **FOGSI (2023):** Emphasizes first-trimester screening, GCT at booking, and community-based ANC in India.[18]
- **ISUOG (2020):** First-trimester ultrasound for aneuploidy, anomalies, and risk prediction.[19]

CONCLUSION

The evolution from FANC to WHO's 2016 ≥8-contact model reflects the need for comprehensive ANC to reduce perinatal mortality and enhance maternal satisfaction. The inverted pyramid approach, leveraging first-trimester ultrasound and biochemical screening, enables early risk stratification and personalized care, particularly for aneuploidies, structural defects, and fetomaternal complications. Standardized schedules, Leopold maneuvers, and fundal height measurement ensure consistent monitoring. Adherence to WHO/NICE guidelines, integration of community-based care, and investment in data collection are critical to optimizing maternal and fetal outcomes globally.

KEY POINTS

- Antenatal care (ANC) aims to ensure a positive pregnancy experience through health promotion, risk detection, and disease management.
- The Focused Antenatal Care (FANC) model, recommended by WHO in 2002, proposed four targeted visits for low-risk pregnancies but faced criticism for increased perinatal mortality compared to models with ≥8 contacts.
- In 2016, WHO updated guidelines to recommend ≥8 contacts, emphasizing a positive pregnancy experience defined by physical, sociocultural, and emotional well-being.
- The inverted pyramid of ANC, proposed by Kypros Nicolaides, shifts focus to first-trimester screening to identify high-risk pregnancies early using ultrasound and biochemical markers, enabling personalized care.

REFERENCES

1. Vogel JP, Habib NA, Souza JP, et al. Antenatal care packages with reduced visits and perinatal mortality: a secondary analysis. BJOG. 2015;122(6):771-80.

2. World Health Organization. (2016). WHO recommendations on antenatal care for a positive pregnancy experience. [online] Available from https://www.who.int/publications/i/item/9789241549912 [Last accessed December, 2025].
3. Nicolaides KH. Turning the pyramid of prenatal care. Fetal Diagn Ther. 2016;40(1):1-6.
4. Kumar G, Choudhary TS, Srivastava A, et al. Antenatal care coverage in India: a national survey. J Matern Fetal Neonatal Med. 2020;33(15):2567-73.
5. Dowswell T, Carroli G, Duley L, et al. Alternative versus standard packages of antenatal care for low-risk pregnancy. Cochrane Database Syst Rev. 2015;7:CD000934.
6. Rolnik DL, Wright D, Poon LC, et al. Aspirin versus placebo in pregnancies at high risk for preterm preeclampsia. N Engl J Med. 2017;377(7):613-22.
7. Bujold E, Roberge S, Lacasse Y, et al. Prevention of preeclampsia with low-dose aspirin in high-risk pregnancies. Obstet Gynecol. 2016;128(3):402-8.
8. Gil MM, Accurti V, Santacruz B, et al. First-trimester screening for trisomies 21, 18, and 13. Ultrasound Obstet Gynecol. 2017;50(3):293-301.
9. Syngelaki A, Chelemen T, Dagklis T, et al. First-trimester screening for fetal abnormalities. Ultrasound Obstet Gynecol. 2015;46(4):396-405.
10. Khalil A, Rodgers M, Baschat A, et al. ISUOG practice guidelines: role of ultrasound in twin pregnancy. Ultrasound Obstet Gynecol. 2016;47(2):247-63.
11. Poon LC, Shrivastava V, Tan MY, et al. First-trimester prediction of preeclampsia. Am J Obstet Gynecol. 2019;221(2):112.e1-112.e18.
12. Romero R, Nicolaides KH, Conde-Agudelo A, et al. Vaginal progesterone for preventing preterm birth. Am J Obstet Gynecol. 2018;218(3):291-304.
13. Sweeting AN, Wong J, Appelblom H, et al. First-trimester biomarkers for gestational diabetes mellitus. Diabetes Res Clin Pract. 2020;164:108189.
14. National Institute for Health and Care Excellence. (2021). Antenatal care (NG201). [online] Available from https://www.nice.org.uk/guidance/ng201 [Last accessed December, 2025].
15. American College of Obstetricians and Gynecologists. Routine prenatal care. Obstet Gynecol. 2020;136(4):e81-e93.
16. Simkin P, Ancheta R. Leopold maneuvers: a critical review. J Perinat Educ. 2017;26(2):67-73.
17. Papageorghiou AT, Ohuma EO, Altman DG, et al. International standards for symphysis-fundal height. Lancet Glob Health. 2016;4(12):e853-e860.
18. Federation of Obstetric and Gynaecological Societies of India. Guidelines on antenatal care. J Obstet Gynaecol India. 2023;73(Suppl 1):29-36.
19. Salomon LJ, Alfirevic Z, Berghella V, et al. ISUOG practice guidelines: performance of first-trimester fetal ultrasound scan. Ultrasound Obstet Gynecol. 2020;56(1):106-20.

Clinical Approach to First Trimester Bleeding in Pregnancy

Ruchika Garg

INTRODUCTION

Vaginal bleeding in the first trimester affects 20–40% of pregnant women, typically originating from maternal sources.[1] It is associated with a 1.6-fold increased risk of adverse outcomes, including preterm labor (PTL), preterm premature rupture of membranes (PPROM), and intrauterine growth restriction (IUGR).[2] Persistent or recurrent bleeding heightens these risks, and second-trimester bleeding correlates with perinatal mortality, amniotic fluid disorders, premature rupture of membranes (PROM), preterm delivery, low birth weight, and low neonatal Apgar scores.[3,4] While 50% of women with early bleeding achieve normal pregnancies,[2] accurate diagnosis and management are critical to address life-threatening conditions such as ectopic pregnancy or miscarriage. This chapter outlines a systematic clinical approach to first trimester bleeding, integrating history, examination, investigations, and management, supported by evidence-based tables.

CAUSES OF FIRST TRIMESTER BLEEDING

First trimester bleeding may stem from obstetric, gynecological, or adjacent structural causes **(Table 1)**. Major obstetric causes include miscarriage (10–20% of clinical pregnancies), ectopic pregnancy (1–2%), and molar pregnancy.[5] Implantation bleeding, subchorionic hemorrhage, or idiopathic bleeding in viable pregnancies are also common. Gynecological causes involve cervical or vaginal pathology (e.g., infections and malignancies), while adjacent structures such as the bladder or anus may contribute [e.g., urinary tract infections (UTIs) and hemorrhoids].[6]

TABLE 1: Causes of first trimester bleeding.

Category	*Causes*
Obstetric	Implantation bleeding, miscarriage, ectopic pregnancy, molar pregnancy, subchorionic hemorrhage, and idiopathic bleeding in viable pregnancy
Gynecological (Cervix/Vagina/ Vulva)	Infections (e.g., chlamydia), trauma, malignancy, ruptured varicose veins, and cervical abnormalities (e.g., polyps and ectropion)
Adjacent Structures (Bladder/ Anus)	Hemorrhoids, urinary tract infection (UTI), schistosomiasis, trauma, infection, and malignancy

Source: Adapted from Breeze C. Early pregnancy bleeding. Aust Fam Physician. 2016;45(5):283-6.[6]

CLINICAL ASSESSMENT

Prompt evaluation of vaginal bleeding in early pregnancy is essential to identify life-threatening conditions (e.g., ectopic pregnancy, septic abortion, or massive hemorrhage). The approach begins with assessing hemodynamic stability, followed by a detailed history, physical examination, and targeted investigations.

Initial Assessment

- **Hemodynamic Stability:** Young women may lose significant blood before showing instability.[6] In unstable patients, suspect:
  - Ruptured ectopic pregnancy (acute abdominal pain and shoulder tip pain)
  - Incomplete miscarriage with cervical shock (hypotension, bradycardia due to products in cervical os)
  - Massive hemorrhage from miscarriage or molar pregnancy[6]

    Action: Perform speculum examination to remove products of conception (POC) from the cervical os and consider urgent surgical intervention (e.g., suction curettage, laparoscopy, or laparotomy).[6]
- **Stable Patients:** Proceed with comprehensive evaluation, including history, examination, and imaging.[6]

History

A thorough history guides diagnosis and risk assessment:

- **Menstrual and Pregnancy Details:** Last menstrual period (LMP), cycle regularity, pregnancy confirmation, and estimated gestational age.
- **Bleeding Characteristics:** Onset, frequency, volume (compared to normal menstruation), color (fresh red vs. dark brown). Minimal bleeding may still indicate ectopic pregnancy.[6]
- **Precipitating Factors:** Bleeding post-intercourse or defecation suggests cervical pathology (e.g., infection and malignancy) or hemorrhoids.[6]
- **Associated Symptoms:**
  - Abdominal pain/cramps (acute, localized, or generalized).
  - Shoulder tip pain, nausea, or fainting (suggests intra-abdominal bleeding from ectopic pregnancy).
  - Syncope, chest pain, or dyspnea (indicates significant blood loss/anemia).
  - Passage of tissue (incomplete miscarriage).
  - Fever (septic abortion, infection like malaria).[7]
  - Dysuria or hematuria (UTI and schistosomiasis).[6]
  - Vaginal discharge [sexually transmitted infections (STIs) like chlamydia].[6]
- **Medical/Obstetric History:** Diabetes, thyroid disorders, prior miscarriages, pelvic inflammatory disease (PID), or nonsterile procedures increase miscarriage or ectopic risk.[8]
- **Medications/Toxins:** Anticoagulants, non-steroidal anti-inflammatory drugs (NSAIDs), misoprostol, or toxins (e.g., lead and mercury) elevate miscarriage risk.[9]
- **Trauma/Sexual Assault:** May cause vaginal or perigenital lacerations.[6]
- **Pre-pregnancy Bleeding:** Suggests cervical/vaginal lesions.[6]

Physical Examination

- **Vital Signs:** Assess blood pressure, pulse, temperature, and respiratory rate for instability or infection.[6]
- **Abdominal Examination:** Check for tenderness, distension, guarding, or rigidity. The fundus is palpable above the pubic symphysis at ~12 weeks, earlier in multiple pregnancies or gestational trophoblastic disease (GTD).[6]
- **Perineal Inspection:** Evaluate bleeding volume, trauma, or lesions.[6]
- **Speculum Examination:**
    - Localize bleeding (vagina, cervix, and uterus).
    - Assess bleeding amount and cervical os (open/closed).
    - Identify polyps, ulcers, or tissue in the os (remove and send for histopathology to confirm POC).[6]
- **Bimanual Examination:** Assess uterine size, shape, consistency, and adnexal masses/tenderness. Avoid vigorous manipulation if ectopic pregnancy is suspected to prevent rupture.[6]
    - **Closed Os:** Suggests threatened miscarriage, complete miscarriage, missed abortion, or ectopic pregnancy.
    - **Open Os:** Indicates inevitable or incomplete miscarriage.[6]

INVESTIGATIONS

Diagnosis relies on ultrasound and serum β-human chorionic gonadotropin (β-hCG) to determine pregnancy location and viability **(Table 2)**.

- **Ultrasound:** Transvaginal ultrasound (TVS) is the gold standard. Key findings:
    - Gestational sac visible from ~4 weeks + 3 days (assuming regular cycles).[10]
    - Nonviable pregnancy: Mean sac diameter (MSD) >25 mm without a fetus, or crown-rump length (CRL) > 7 mm without fetal heart activity (confirm after 7-day rescan).[10]
    - Ectopic pregnancy: Adnexal mass (>88% of cases), free fluid in the pouch of Douglas (ruptured ectopic).[11]
- **Serum β-hCG:**
    - Rises exponentially until 6–7 weeks, doubling (≥66%) every 48 hours in viable pregnancies.[12]

TABLE 2: Diagnostic criteria for first trimester bleeding.

Condition	*Ultrasound findings*	*β-hCG pattern*
Viable IUP	Gestational sac and fetal heart activity	Doubles every 48 hours
Nonviable IUP	MSD >25 mm, no fetus; CRL >7 mm, no heart activity	Falling or plateaued
Ectopic	Adnexal mass and free fluid	Slow rise (<50% in 48 hours) or normal in 21%
PUL	No intra-/extrauterine pregnancy	Variable; requires serial monitoring

Source: Adapted from Barnhart KT, Sammel MD, Rinaudo PF, et al. Symptomatic patients with an early viable intrauterine pregnancy: HCG curves redefined. Obstet Gynecol. 2004;104(1):50-5; Dogra V, Paspulati RM, Bhatt S. First trimester bleeding evaluation. Ultrasound Q. 2005;21(2):69-85; quiz 149-50, 153-4.[11,12]

    - Falling β-hCG suggests nonviable pregnancy (intrauterine or ectopic).
    - Plateaued or slow-rising β-hCG (<50% in 48 hours) indicates ectopic or nonviable intrauterine pregnancy, though 21% of ectopics show normal rise.[3]
    - Discriminatory zone (1,500–2,000 IU/L): Gestational sac should be visible on TVS; absence suggests ectopic or early pregnancy.[7]
- **Other Tests:**
    - Blood group/antibody status (Rh D immunoglobulin need).
    - Hemoglobin, crossmatching (severe bleeding/ectopic).
    - Erythrocyte sedimentation rate (ESR)/leukocytes (infection).
    - Urine pregnancy test (confirm pregnancy).
    - Midstream urine analysis (UTI).
    - Culdocentesis (if ultrasound unavailable) to detect blood/pus in the pouch of Douglas.[4]

PREGNANCY OF UNKNOWN LOCATION

Pregnancy of unknown location (PUL) occurs when a positive urine pregnancy test shows no intrauterine or ectopic pregnancy on TVS, and no retained POC are visible.[10] Possible scenarios:

- Early intrauterine pregnancy
- Complete miscarriage
- Ectopic pregnancy
- Spontaneously resolving pregnancy[10]

    Management: Serial β-hCG measurements (0 and 48 hours) and repeat ultrasound. Monitor symptoms closely, as ectopic pregnancy remains a risk. Hospital admission may be needed if symptoms worsen.[10]

MANAGEMENT OF SPECIFIC CONDITIONS

Miscarriage

Miscarriage, defined as pregnancy loss before 20 weeks or fetal weight <500 g, is the leading cause of first trimester bleeding (10–20% of pregnancies).[13,14] Subtypes are outlined in **Table 3.**

- **Threatened Miscarriage:**
    - **Management:** Expectant, with 50% progressing to viable pregnancies. Progestogens may reduce miscarriage risk (Cochrane Review), but evidence on congenital anomalies is limited.[15]
    - **Risks:** 2.6-fold increased miscarriage risk later; 17% develop complications (e.g., PTL and IUGR).[11]
- **Complete Miscarriage:** Confirm closed cervix and no retained POC via TVS. Monitor ongoing bleeding.[6]
- **Inevitable/Incomplete/Missed Miscarriage:** Options include:
    - **Expectant:** 60% of incomplete miscarriages resolve in 2 weeks, 90% by 6–8 weeks; missed miscarriages take longer. Monitor with serial β-hCG and ultrasound.[16]
    - **Medical:** Misoprostol (vaginal/oral) is highly effective for uterine evacuation.[17]

TABLE 3: Miscarriage subtypes.

Type	*Definition*
Threatened	Bleeding before 20 weeks, closed cervix
Inevitable	POC passage imminent, open cervix
Incomplete	Retained POC, nonviable IUP
Missed	Nonviable IUP without bleeding
Septic	Miscarriage with uterine infection
Recurrent	≥3 consecutive miscarriages
Complete	Full POC expulsion

Sources: American College of Obstetricians and Gynecologists' Committee on Practice Bulletins—Gynecology. ACOG Practice Bulletin No. 200: Early Pregnancy Loss. Obstet Gynecol. 2018;132(5):e197-e207.

- **Surgical:** Manual vacuum aspiration (MVA) or suction curettage for hemorrhage, sepsis, or patient preference. Risks include perforation, hemorrhage, and endometritis.[6]
- **MIST Trial:** Compared management options, showing similar efficacy but higher unplanned admissions with expectant (49%) and medical (18%) versus surgical (8%).[18]

- **Septic Abortion:** Characterized by fever, uterine tenderness, and foul discharge, often from incomplete miscarriage or unsterile procedures. Risks include septic shock (25–50% mortality).[19]
  - **Management:** Fluid resuscitation, broad-spectrum IV antibiotics (e.g., ampicillin, gentamicin, and metronidazole). Perform MVA after 12–24 hours of antibiotics if no septic shock; check for perforation or foreign bodies.[20]

Ectopic Pregnancy

Ectopic pregnancies, 95% tubal, are life-threatening if ruptured.[21] Management depends on stability and eligibility **(Table 4)**.

- **Surgical:** Indicated for unstable patients, ruptured ectopic, failed medical management, or methotrexate contraindications. Laparoscopic salpingectomy is preferred; salpingostomy may require follow-up methotrexate (4–15% failure rate).[22,23]
- **Medical:** Methotrexate (50 mg/m^2 IM, single dose) for stable patients with β-hCG < 5,000 IU/L, adnexal mass < 3.5 cm, and no fetal cardiac activity. Success rate: ~85%. Up to 15% require surgery.[16,24]

TABLE 4: Ectopic pregnancy management.

Approach	*Criteria*	*Success rate*
Surgical	Unstable, ruptured, failed medical	>95% (salpingectomy)[22]
Medical (Methotrexate)	Stable, β-hCG < 5,000 IU/L, mass < 3.5 cm	~85%[16]
Expectant	Asymptomatic, declining β-hCG	Variable[24]

Source: Hajenius PJ, Mol F, Mol BW, et al. Interventions for tubal ectopic pregnancy. Cochrane Database Syst Rev. 2007;2007(1):CD000324; 24. Menon S, Colins J, Barnhart KT. Establishing a human chorionic gonadotropin cutoff to guide methotrexate treatment of ectopic pregnancy: a systematic review. Fertil Steril. 2007;87(3):481-4.[22,24]

- **Expectant:** Limited to asymptomatic, stable patients with low, declining β-hCG.[24]
- **Fertility Outcomes:** Similar across methotrexate, salpingostomy, and salpingectomy.[24]

Molar Pregnancy (Gestational Trophoblastic Disease)

Molar pregnancies present with irregular bleeding, hyperemesis, excessive uterine enlargement, or vesicle passage. β-hCG may be markedly elevated (>100,000 IU/mL) or normal in partial moles.[25]

- **Diagnosis:** Histopathology confirms hydropic villi and trophoblastic hyperplasia.[25]
- **Management:**
  - Suction evacuation (preferred for complete/partial moles). Avoid oxytocin before evacuation to prevent tumor embolization.[25]
  - Anti-D prophylaxis post-evacuation.
  - Histological examination of POC from repeat evacuations to detect persistent trophoblastic neoplasia.[25]
- **Follow-Up:** Monitor β-hCG every 1–2 weeks. If normal within 56 days, follow for 6 months post-evacuation; otherwise, 6 months from normalization.[25]

INCIDENTAL CAUSES

- **Cervical Malignancy:** Common in developing countries, presenting with post-coital or recurrent bleeding. Diagnosed via speculum and bimanual examination (solid mass).[26]
- **Infections:** Chlamydia, gonorrhea, or schistosomiasis may cause bleeding. UTIs (cystitis and pyelonephritis) require antibiotics.[6]
- **Cervical Polyps:** Often benign (99%), bleeding post-intercourse. Managed conservatively or via polypectomy if symptomatic.[6]
- **Cervical Ectropion:** Hormonal changes cause endocervical eversion, leading to contact bleeding. Resolves post-delivery; no treatment needed.[6]
- **Subchorionic/Idiopathic Bleeding:** Diagnosed after excluding serious causes. Subchorionic hematomas may cause contractions or miscarriage (10% recurrence).[27] Reassurance is key.
- **Hemorrhoids:** Mistaken for vaginal bleeding; managed conservatively with laxatives and analgesics.[6]

BLEEDING IN LATE PREGNANCY

Late pregnancy bleeding may result from placenta previa, placental abruption, ruptured vasa previa, uterine scar disruption, or benign causes (e.g., cervical polyps, bloody show). The first four are life-threatening and require urgent management.[6]

CONCLUSION

First trimester bleeding, affecting 20–40% of pregnancies, causes significant distress and requires sensitive, evidence-based management.[1] A systematic approach—history, examination, ultrasound, and β-hCG—ensures accurate diagnosis of miscarriage, ectopic pregnancy, or molar pregnancy. Incidental causes should only be considered after ruling out serious conditions. Management options (expectant, medical, and surgical) are tailored to the patient's condition, preferences, and stability, with close follow-up to optimize outcomes and support emotional well-being.

KEY POINTS

- Bleeding occurs in 20–40% of first trimester pregnancies.[1]
- Always exclude ectopic pregnancy due to its life-threatening potential.[6]
- History, physical examination, and ultrasound are critical for diagnosis.[6]
- Miscarriage management includes expectant, medical, or surgical options.[16-18]
- Septic abortion requires urgent antibiotics and MVA.[20]
- Ectopic pregnancy management includes surgery, methotrexate, or expectant care.[22,24]
- Molar pregnancy requires suction evacuation and β-hCG monitoring.[25]
- Incidental causes (e.g., polyps and ectropion) are diagnosed after excluding serious conditions.[6]

REFERENCES

1. Queensland Clinical Guidelines. Early pregnancy loss. Guideline No. MN22.29-V8-R27 Queensland Health. 2025. Available from: http://www.health.qld.gov.au/qcg.
2. Snell BJ. Assessment and Management of Bleeding in the First Trimester of Pregnancy. J Midwifery Womens Health. 2009;54:483-91.
3. Hossain R, Harris T, Lohsoonthorn V, et al. Risk of preterm delivery in relation to vaginal bleeding in early pregnancy. Eur J Obstet Gynecol Reprod Biol. 2007;135(2):158-63.
4. Koifman A, Levy A, Zaulan Y, et al. The clinical significance of bleeding during the second trimester of pregnancy. Arch Gynecol Obstet. 2008;278(1):47-51.
5. King Edward Memorial Hospital. Clinical guidelines – Ectopic pregnancy. Subiaco, WA: Department of Health, 2014.
6. Breeze C. Early pregnancy bleeding. Aust Fam Physician. 2016;45(5):283-6.
7. National Collaborating Centre for Women's and Children's Health (UK). Ectopic Pregnancy and Miscarriage: Diagnosis and Initial Management in Early Pregnancy of Ectopic Pregnancy and Miscarriage (NICE Clinical Guidelines, No. 154). London: RCOG Press; 2012.
8. Early pregnancy bleeding. Aust J Gen Pract. 2016 May;45(5):283–286. Available from: https://www.racgp.org.au/afp/2016/may/early-pregnancy-bleeding.
9. Duff P, Edwards RK, Davis JD, et al. Obstetrics and Gynecology: Just the Facts. New York: McGraw-Hill; 2004.
10. Australasian Society for Ultrasound in Medicine. Guidelines for the performance of first trimester ultrasound. Sydney: ASUM, 2014.
11. Dogra V, Paspulati RM, Bhatt S. First trimester bleeding evaluation. Ultrasound Q. 2005;21(2):69-85; quiz 149-50, 153-4.
12. Barnhart KT, Sammel MD, Rinaudo PF, et al. Symptomatic patients with an early viable intrauterine pregnancy: HCG curves redefined. Obstet Gynecol. 2004;104(1):50-5.
13. American College of Obstetricians and Gynecologists' Committee on Practice Bulletins—Gynecology. ACOG Practice Bulletin No. 200: Early Pregnancy Loss. Obstet Gynecol. 2018;132(5):e197-e207.
14. Alberman E. Spontaneous abortion: epidemiology. In: Stabile S, Grudzinkas G, Chard T (Eds). Spontaneous Abortion: Diagnosis and Treatment. London: Springer Verlag, 1992. pp. 9-20.
15. Wahabi HA, Fayed AA, Esmaeil SA, et al. Progestogen for treating threatened miscarriage. Cochrane Database Syst Rev. 2011;(12):CD005943. Update in: Cochrane Database Syst Rev. 2018;8:CD005943.

16. Nanda K, Lopez LM, Grimes DA, et al. Expectant care versus surgical treatment for miscarriage. Cochrane Database Syst Rev. 2012;2012(3):CD003518.
17. Neilson JP, Gyte GM, Hickey M, et al. Medical treatments for incomplete miscarriage (less than 24 weeks). Cochrane Database Syst Rev. 2010;(1):CD007223. Update in: Cochrane Database Syst Rev. 2013;28(3):CD007223.
18. Trinder J, Brocklehurst P, Porter R, et al. Management of miscarriage: expectant, medical, or surgical? Results of randomised controlled trial (miscarriage treatment (MIST) trial). BMJ. 2006;332(7552):1235-40.
19. Kumar V, Abbas AK, Aster JC. Robbins Basic Pathology. Philadelphia, PA: Elsevier Saunders; 2007.
20. Stubblefield PG, Averbach SH, Grimes DA. Septic abortion: prevention and management. Glob. libr. women's med. (ISSN: 1756-2228), 2008 (updated 2012).
21. Farquhar CM. Ectopic pregnancy. Lancet. 2005;366(9485):583-91.
22. Hajenius PJ, Mol F, Mol BW, et al. Interventions for tubal ectopic pregnancy. Cochrane Database Syst Rev. 2007;2007(1):CD000324.
23. Fernandez H, Capmas P, Lucot JP, et al. Fertility after ectopic pregnancy: the DEMETER randomized trial. Hum Reprod. 2013;28(5):1247-53.
24. Menon S, Colins J, Barnhart KT. Establishing a human chorionic gonadotropin cutoff to guide methotrexate treatment of ectopic pregnancy: a systematic review. Fertil Steril. 2007;87(3):481-4.
25. RCOG. (2010). Gestational Trophoblastic Disease (Green top Guideline No. 38). [online] Available from https://www.rcog.org.uk/guidance/browse-all-guidance/green-top-guidelines/gestational-trophoblastic-disease-green-top-guideline-no-38/ [Last accessed December, 2025].
26. Onwudiegwu U, Bako A, Oyewumi A. Cervical cancer--a neglected health tragedy. J Obstet Gynaecol. 1999;19(1):61-4.
27. Jager B. Vaginal bleeding in the first trimester of pregnancy. In: Beekhuizen H, Unkels R (Eds). Gynecology for Less-Resourced Locations. Meadowbank, London: Sapiens Publishing Ltd.; 2012.

CHAPTER 28

Ectopic Pregnancy

Ruchika Garg, Geetanjali Sharma

INTRODUCTION

Ectopic pregnancy is a life-threatening condition where a fertilized ovum implants outside the endometrial lining of the uterus, most commonly in the fallopian tube (90–95% of cases). It occurs in approximately 1–2% of pregnancies, with an incidence of 1:80 or higher in some populations. Early diagnosis is critical to prevent severe complications such as massive intraperitoneal hemorrhage, which contributes to 10–11.5% of maternal mortality. This response addresses the causes, symptoms, signs, diagnosis, and management of ectopic pregnancy, with a focus on chronic ectopic pregnancy, and answers the self-assessment questions provided. Ectopic pregnancy occurs due to factors that disrupt the normal migration of the fertilized ovum to the uterine cavity or create a favorable environment for implantation outside the uterus **(Fig. 1)**.

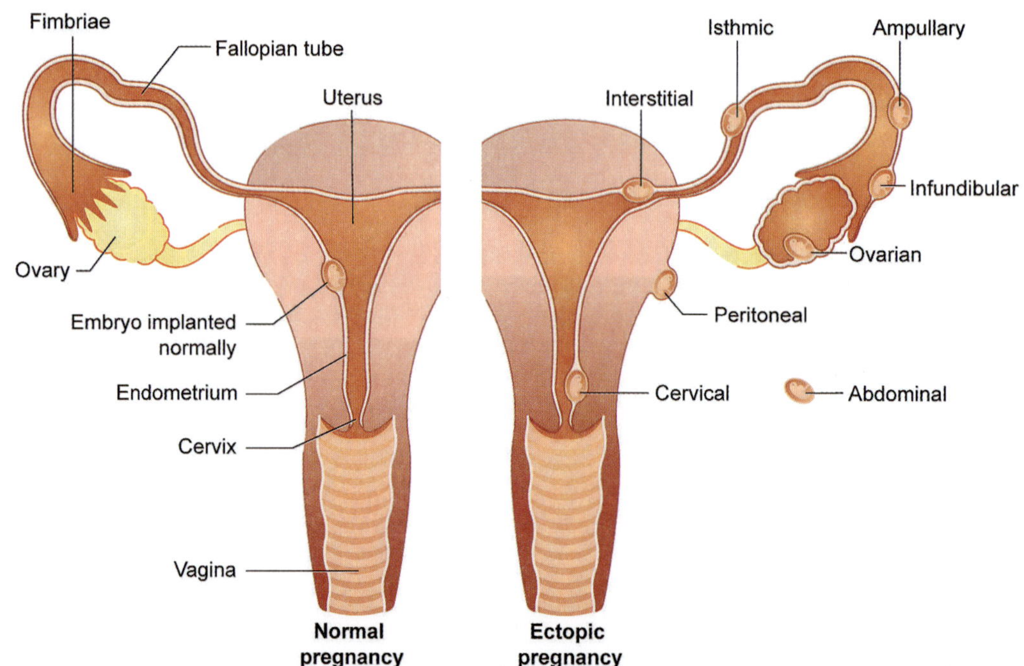

Fig. 1: Normal pregnancy and ectopic pregnancy.

CAUSES

Key causes include tubal factors: pelvic inflammatory disease (PID): Ascending infections, particularly *Chlamydia trachomatis* and gonorrhea, cause tubal damage, increasing ectopic risk. *Chlamydia* is a major contributor due to subclinical damage. PID increases the risk sevenfold after one episode, with tubal blockage rates rising from 12.8% after one episode to 75% after three.

Previous Tubal Surgery: Procedures such as tubectomy, tubal reanastomosis, or surgery for prior ectopic pregnancy increase risk due to scarring or partial stenosis.

Genital Tuberculosis: Common in India, it causes tubal damage and is a leading cause of ectopic pregnancy (FOGSI GCPR).

Congenital Tubal Abnormalities: Accessory ostia, diverticula, or salpingitis isthmic nodosum can trap the ovum.

Contraceptive Use: Intrauterine contraceptive devices (IUCDs)—while IUCDs reduce overall pregnancy risk, 53% of pregnancies with an IUCD in situ are ectopic. Progestogen-containing IUCDs decrease tubal motility, increasing risk.

Progestogen-Only Pills (POP): These reduce tubal peristalsis, favoring ectopic implantation.

Assisted Reproductive Technology (ART): ART, particularly in vitro fertilization (IVF), increases ectopic risk (2.1–8.6% vs. 2% in natural conception) due to multiple embryo transfers, fresh embryo transfers, or excessive fluid medium during transfer.

Other Factors: Endometriosis and pelvic adhesions—these distort tubal anatomy, impairing ovum transport.

Smoking: Increases risk by affecting tubal ciliary function.

Previous Ectopic Pregnancy: Recurrence risk is 10% after one ectopic and >25% after two.

Transperitoneal Ovum Migration: Ovum migration to the contralateral tube increases ectopic risk (reported in 8–41.38% of cases).

Age > 35 Years: Older maternal age is associated with higher risk.

Infertility: Prolonged infertility or irregular contraceptive use increases risk.

Half of ectopic pregnancy cases have no identifiable risk factors. Symptoms and signs of chronic ectopic pregnancy (or subacute) refers to a less acute presentation where the ectopic gestation forms a tubal mole, peritubal hematoma, or pelvic hematocele, often without immediate rupture. It is characterized by:

SYMPTOMS

Amenorrhea: Typically short (2–6 weeks), present in 75% of cases.

Abdominal Pain: Recurrent, vague, or mild pain in the lower abdomen or iliac fossa, less severe than in acute rupture.

Vaginal Bleeding: Slight, intermittent, or continuous dark or blood-stained discharge due to decidual shedding. A decidual cast (smooth inner surface, no chorionic villi) may be passed, which is pathognomonic.

Retention of Urine: Caused by a pelvic hematocele pressing the cervix against the bladder neck.

Fever: Rare, mild if present, due to secondary infection of a hematocele (temperature rarely exceeds 99.4°F).

SIGNS

General Examination

- Mild tachycardia proportional to anemia from localized bleeding.
- No high-grade fever (distinguishing from pyosalpinx).
- Breast changes of early pregnancy may be present.

Abdominal Examination

- Tenderness in one or both iliac fossae.
- Distension or a palpable irregular mass (hematocele) in the lower abdomen.

Pelvic Examination

- Soft cervix and slightly enlarged uterus.
- Brownish vaginal bleeding.
- Irregular, tender swelling in the posterior fornix or pouch of Douglas with variable consistency (neither solid nor cystic).
- Retort-shaped swelling (tubal mole or hematocele) may displace the uterus to the opposite side.
- Gentle vaginal examination is crucial to avoid rupturing an unruptured ectopic.

DIFFERENTIAL DIAGNOSIS

Chronic ectopic pregnancy mimics several conditions:

- Pyosalpinx: High-grade fever, vaginal discharge, bilateral pelvic masses, and absence of amenorrhea.
- Septic Abortion: History of pregnancy termination, high fever, offensive discharge, and leukocytosis.
- Pelvic Abscess: Fever and culdocentesis revealing pus.
- Twisted Ovarian Cyst: Acute pain, no amenorrhea, confirmed by ultrasound.
- Ruptured Chocolate Cyst: Rare, mimics shock, but no amenorrhea and negative β-hCG.
- Uterine Fibroid: Pain from torsion or red degeneration, diagnosed by ultrasound.

MANAGEMENT OF CHRONIC ECTOPIC PREGNANCY

The management of chronic ectopic pregnancy depends on the patient's hemodynamic stability, β-hCG levels, ultrasound findings, and fertility desires. Options include expectant, medical, or surgical approaches **(Flowchart 1)**.

Diagnostic Approach

- Urine Pregnancy Test: Positive in most cases but cannot rule out ectopic if negative.
- Serum β-hCG: Levels $<$ 6,500 mIU/mL suggest ectopic or missed abortion.

Flowchart 1: Approach for management of ectopic pregnancy.

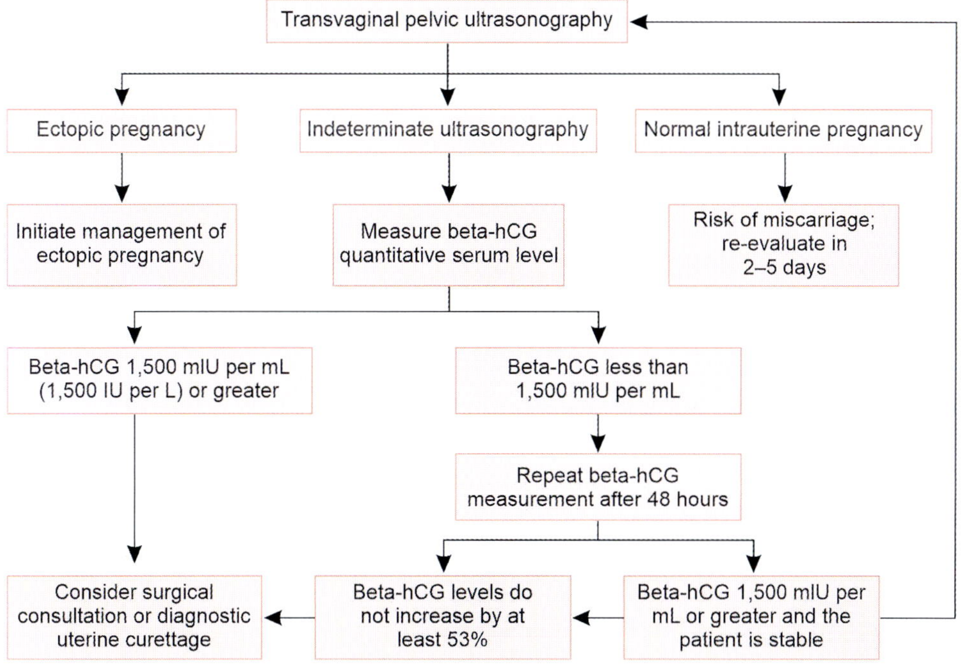

- Slow rise (<66% increase in 48 hours) or plateauing levels indicate ectopic pregnancy.
- Serial β-hCG monitoring is critical for stable patients.
- Transvaginal Ultrasound (TVS): Gold standard for diagnosis.
- Findings: Empty uterine cavity, adnexal mass (50–60% of cases), gestational sac (5–40%), or free fluid in the pouch of Douglas.
- Specific Signs: Blob sign (blood clot with trophoblast), bagel sign (empty tubal sac), or ring of fire on Doppler (increased vascularity) **(Figs. 2 to 4)**.
- Laparoscopy: Used when diagnosis is uncertain despite ultrasound and β-hCG, allowing both diagnosis and treatment **(Fig. 5)**.

Expectant Management

Criteria: Hemodynamically stable, no significant pain.

- Tubal ectopic <35 mm, no fetal cardiac activity on TVS.
- β-hCG ≤ 1,000 IU/L (or up to 1,500 IU/L in some cases).
- Patient compliance with follow-up.

Protocol: Monitor β-hCG on days 2, 4, and 7.

- If β-hCG declines by ≥15%, continue weekly monitoring until undetectable.
- If β-hCG rises or declines <15%, reassess for medical or surgical intervention.

Suitability: Best for small, unruptured ectopic with low β-hCG, but prolonged follow-up may be impractical.

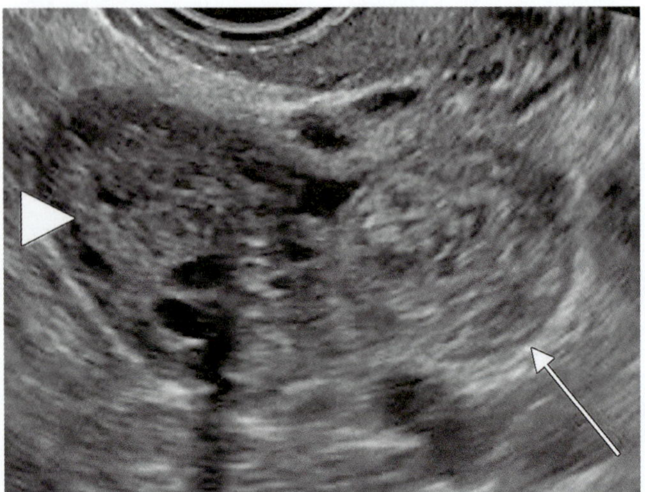

Fig. 2: Blob sign on TVS.

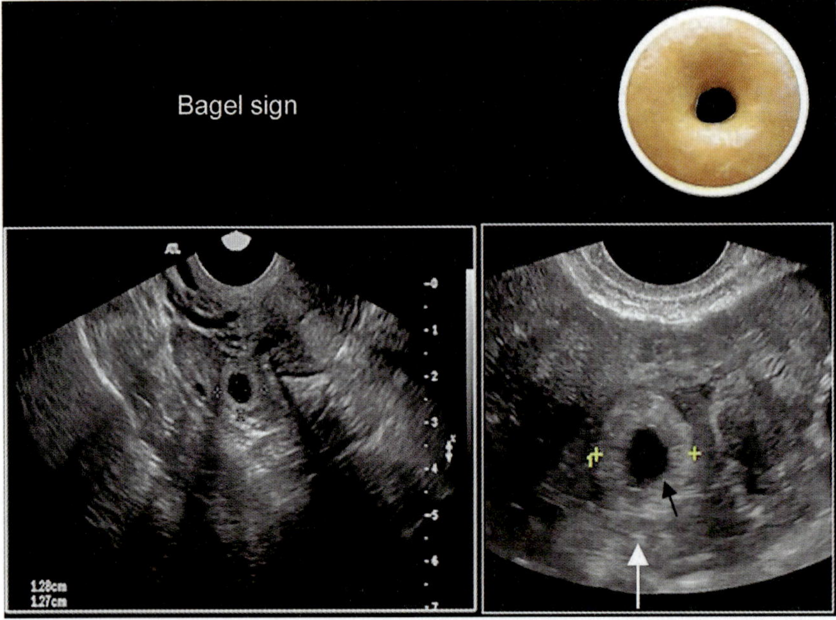

Fig. 3: Bagel sign on TVS of ectopic pregnancy.

Medical Management

Methotrexate (MTX)

Mechanism: Folate antagonist inhibiting DNA/RNA synthesis in trophoblastic tissue.

Criteria: Hemodynamically stable, unruptured ectopic.

- β-hCG <1,500–5,000 IU/L.
- Gestational sac <3.5 cm, no fetal cardiac activity.

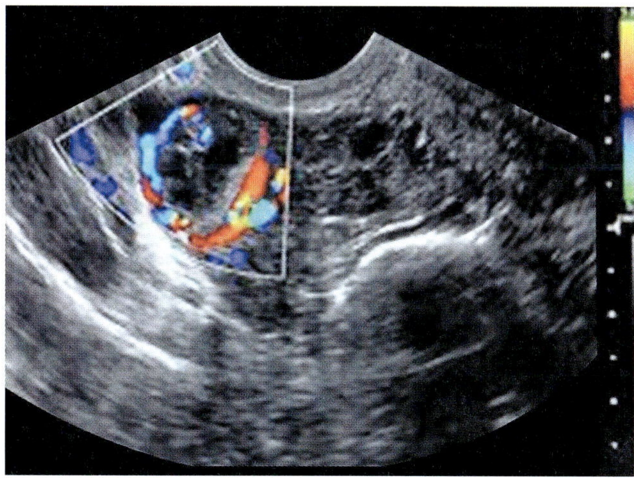

Fig. 4: Ring of fire appearance on Doppler of ectopic pregnancy.

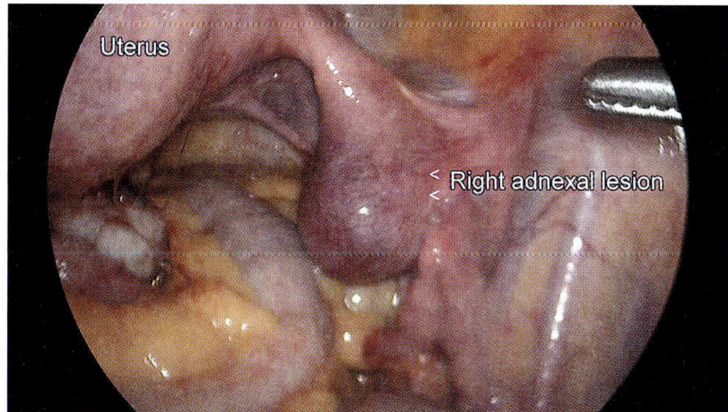

Fig. 5: Laparoscopic image of ectopic pregnancy.

- No contraindications (e.g., liver/renal dysfunction, anemia, and immunodeficiency).
- Desire for future fertility and willingness for follow-up.

Protocol: Single dose—50 mg/m^2 intramuscularly.

- Monitor β-hCG on days 4 and 7; ≥15% decline indicates success.
- Weekly β-hCG until <15 IU/L.
- If inadequate decline, repeat TVS, consider second MTX dose or surgery.

Success Rate: 65–95%, with 4% requiring a second dose.

Side Effects: Flatulence, bloating, elevated liver enzymes, stomatitis, rarely bone marrow suppression or alopecia.

Contraindications: Renal impairment (creatinine >1.3 mg%), liver dysfunction (SGOT/SGPT >50 IU/L), low hemoglobin, or drug allergy.

Post-Treatment: Avoid alcohol and pregnancy for 3 months (teratogenic risk).

Other Drugs: Local injection of MTX, KCl, or prostaglandins under ultrasound/laparoscopic guidance (less common).

Surgical Management

Laparoscopy: Preferred for stable patients due to faster recovery, less pain, and shorter hospital stay.

Salpingectomy: Indicated for gestational sac >4 cm, damaged tube, or healthy contralateral tube.

- Lower risk of persistent trophoblast (1%) and recurrent ectopic (5%).
- Involves clamping mesosalpinx, removing the tube, and transfixing pedicles.

Salpingotomy: Preferred for infertility, prior ectopic, or contralateral tubal damage.

- Incision on antimesenteric border, removal of conceptus, and optional suturing.
- Higher risk of persistent trophoblast (7%) and recurrent ectopic (8%).
- Requires β-hCG follow-up and possible MTX for persistent trophoblast.

Laparotomy: Reserved for hemodynamically unstable patients or when laparoscopy is unavailable.

Followup

- Weekly β-hCG monitoring until undetectable.
- Contraception (e.g., barrier methods) for 3–6 months to allow recovery and avoid teratogenic effects of MTX.
- Assess contralateral tube during surgery to evaluate future fertility prognosis.

Rh-Negative Patients

Administer 100–150 µg anti-D immunoglobulin post-surgery or MTX to prevent Rh isoimmunization.

CASE-BASED MANAGEMENT SCENARIOS CASE 3

A 24-year-old woman, 2 months amenorrhea, Positive Pregnancy Test, Empty Uterus on Ultrasound Approach: Diagnosis: Suspect ectopic pregnancy (pregnancy of unknown location, PUL).

Investigations: Measure serum β-hCG; repeat after 48 hours to assess doubling time.

- If β-hCG <1,500 IU/L and stable, repeat TVS in 1–2 weeks.
- If β-hCG >1,500 IU/L with empty uterus, high suspicion of ectopic.

Management: If stable (no pain, no free fluid); Expectant management if β-hCG <1,000 IU/L, no fetal cardiac activity, and sac < 35 mm.

MTX (50 mg/m^2) if β-hCG 1,000–5,000 IU/L, unruptured ectopic confirmed, and no contraindications.

If Unstable or Diagnostic Uncertainty: Laparoscopy to confirm and treat (salpingectomy or salpingotomy based on fertility desires and contralateral tube status).

Follow-Up: Weekly β-hCG until undetectable; contraception for 3–6 months.

SUGGESTED READING

1. Committee on Practice Bulletins—Gynecology. Tubal ectopic pregnancy. *ACOG Practice Bulletin No. 193*. Obstet Gynecol. 2018;131(3):e91-e108. doi:10.1097/AOG.0000000000002560[1][2]
2. Hendriks E, Rosenberg R, Prine L. Ectopic pregnancy: diagnosis and management. *Am Fam Physician*. 2020;101(10):599-606. PMID: 32463525[6]
3. National Institute for Health and Care Excellence. Ectopic pregnancy and miscarriage: diagnosis and initial management. NICE guideline [NG126]. London: NICE; 2023. Available from: https://www.nice.org.uk/guidance/ng126.[4][5]
4. Royal College of Obstetricians and Gynaecologists. Diagnosis and management of ectopic pregnancy. Green-top Guideline No. 21. BJOG. 2016;124(3):e95-e116. doi:10.1111/1471-0528.14189[3]
5. (https://www.guidelinecentral.com/guideline/308463/)
6. (https://www.fertilehealthexpert.com/wp-content/uploads/2021/11/Ectopic-Pregnancy-ACOG.pdf)
7. (https://www.rcog.org.uk/guidance/browse-all-guidance/green-top-guidelines/diagnosis-and-management-of-ectopic-pregnancy-green-top-guideline-no-21/)
8. (https://www.nice.org.uk/guidance/NG126)
9. (https://www.nice.org.uk/guidance/ng126)
10. (https://www.ncbi.nlm.nih.gov/books/NBK539860/)
11. (https://ppl-ai-file-upload.s3.amazonaws.com/web/direct-files/attachments/129115750/6a3ad322-19ea-4fb0-85b9-91dba739ea56/15-c.pdf)
12. (https://www.hse.ie/eng/about/who/acute-hospitals-division/woman-infants/clinical-guidelines/the-diagnosis-and-management-of-ectopic-pregnancy-2024-.pdf)
13. (https://bridgetotreatment.org/wp-content/uploads/ACCESS_BRIDGE_-PROTOCOL_Ectopic_Pregnancy_in_the_ED_Restricted.pdf)
14. (https://pmc.ncbi.nlm.nih.gov/articles/PMC10071153/)
15. (https://moh.gov.om/media/bjwmnavh/guidelines-of-ectopic-pregnancy.pdf)
16. (https://www.aafp.org/pubs/afp/issues/1999/0415/p2365.html)
17. (https://www.bmj.com/content/345/bmj.e8136/rapid-responses)
18. (https://www.peninsulahealth.org.au/wp-content/uploads/Investigation-and-Management-of-Ectopic-Pregnancy.pdf)
19. (https://www.ectopicpregnancy.co.uk/for-professionals/nice-guidance/)
20. (https://www.fogsi.org/wp-content/uploads/gcpr/Ectopic-Pregnancy.pdf)
21. (https://www.bmj.com/content/367/bmj.l6283)
22. (https://www.acog.org/womens-health/faqs/ectopic-pregnancy)
23. (https://about.openlibhums.org/Download_PDFS/publication/KnuGX1/Acog_Practice_Bullet_In_Tubal_Ectopic_Pregnancy.pdf)
24. (https://www.rcog.org.uk/for-the-public/browse-our-patient-information/ectopic-pregnancy/)
25. (https://www.nice.org.uk/guidance/ng126/resources/ectopic-pregnancy-and-miscarriage-diagnosis-and-initial-management-pdf-66141662244037)

Cesarean Scar Ectopic Pregnancy and Isthmocele

Ruchika Garg

INTRODUCTION

Cesarean scar ectopic pregnancy (CSEP) and isthmocele are rare but significant complications of prior cesarean delivery (CD). CSEP involves implantation of a pregnancy within the myometrial scar of a previous CD, while isthmocele is a defect or niche at the scar site, often leading to symptoms or secondary complications. This chapter provides a concise overview of their epidemiology, pathophysiology, diagnosis, and management for postgraduate medical education, incorporating recent data (2015–2025) and RCOG/NICE guidelines.

EPIDEMIOLOGY

Cesarean scar ectopic pregnancy incidence ranges from 1:1,800 to 1:2,500 pregnancies, comprising ~6% of ectopic pregnancies in women with prior CD, with rising rates due to increasing CD prevalence. Isthmocele occurs in 19–84% of women post-CD, detected via imaging, though only 20–30% are symptomatic. Risk factors for both include multiple CDs, retroflexed uterus, and surgical techniques (e.g., single-layer closure).

PATHOPHYSIOLOGY

Cesarean scar ectopic pregnancy: Implantation occurs in the myometrial defect of the cesarean scar, often due to poor scar healing or thin myometrium. The embryo may grow toward the bladder (type 1, endogenic) or uterine cavity (type 2, exogenic), increasing risks of rupture, hemorrhage, or placenta accreta spectrum (PAS).

Isthmocele: A niche forms from incomplete myometrial healing, creating a fluid-filled pouch at the scar site. This defect disrupts uterine contractility, leading to postmenstrual spotting, dysmenorrhea, infertility, or obstetric complications (e.g., CSEP and PAS) **(Table 1).**

TABLE 1: Key features of CSEP and Isthmocele.

Condition	*Pathology*	*Complications*	*Prevalence*
CSEP	Implantation in scar	Rupture, hemorrhage, PAS	1:1,800–1:2,500
Isthmocele	Myometrial defect	Spotting, infertility, and CSEP	19–84%

DIAGNOSIS

Cesarean Scar Ectopic Pregnancy

- **Clinical:** Amenorrhea, vaginal bleeding, or pain; often asymptomatic early.
- **Imaging:** Transvaginal ultrasound (TVUS) is first line, showing a gestational sac in the scar, empty uterus/cervix, thin myometrium (<2 mm), or vascularity on Doppler. MRI confirms complex cases.
- **Criteria:** Sac in anterior lower uterine segment, no intrauterine pregnancy, thin/absent myometrium between sac and bladder.

Isthmocele

- **Clinical:** Postmenstrual spotting, pelvic pain, and infertility.
- **Imaging:** TVUS detects a hypoechoic niche; saline infusion sonohysterography or hysteroscopy enhances visualization. MRI for surgical planning **(Figs. 1 and 2)**.

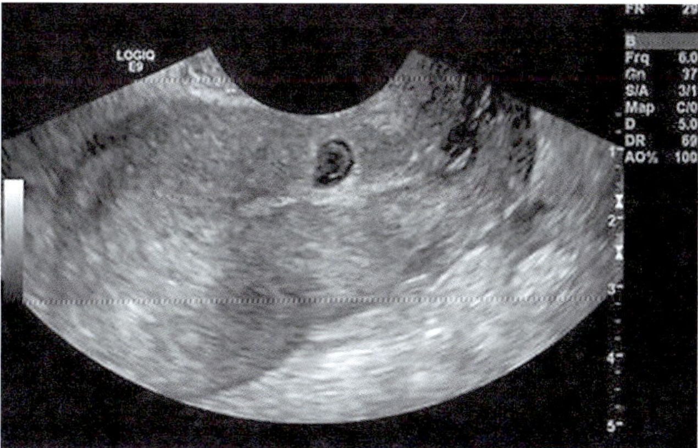

Fig. 1: Ultrasound features of CSEP.

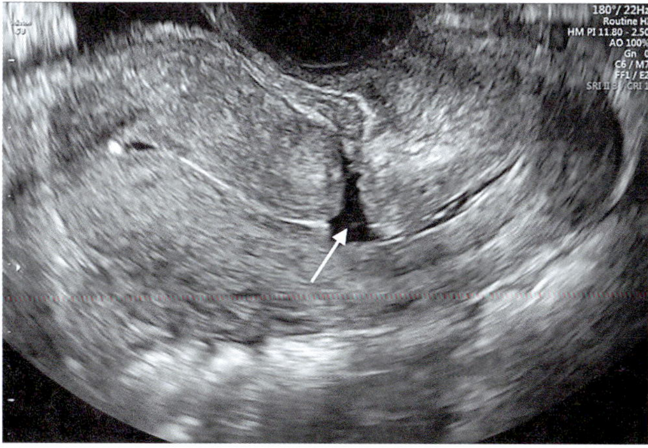

Fig. 2: Ultrasound features of isthmocele.

MANAGEMENT

Cesarean Scar Ectopic Pregnancy

- **Expectant:** Rarely used due to high rupture risk (30–40%); suitable for asymptomatic, small sacs with declining β-hCG.
- **Medical:** Systemic methotrexate (50 mg/m^2) for stable patients, sac <3 cm, β-hCG <5,000 IU/L; success rate 70–80%. Local methotrexate injection under ultrasound guidance improves outcomes.
- **Surgical:** Suction curettage for type 2 CSEP
- Laparoscopic/hysteroscopic resection for larger or symptomatic cases. Hysterectomy for life-threatening hemorrhage or PAS.
- **Uterine Artery Embolization (UAE):** Adjunct for bleeding control.

Isthmocele

- **Conservative:** Hormonal therapy (e.g., combined oral contraceptives) for mild symptoms; success rate 50%.
- **Surgical:** Hysteroscopic resection for small niches (<50% myometrial thickness); laparoscopic/vaginal repair for larger defects or infertility. Success rate 80–90% for symptom relief.

RCOG/NICE GUIDELINES

- **RCOG Green-top Guideline No. 21 (2023):** Recommends TVUS for CSEP diagnosis, methotrexate for stable cases, and surgical resection for complications.
- **NICE NG201 (2021):** Advises hysteroscopy for symptomatic isthmocele; laparoscopic repair for fertility concerns.

KEY POINTS

- CSEP (1:1,800–1:2,500) and isthmocele (19–84%) are rising with CD rates.
- CSEP risks rupture and PAS
- Isthmocele causes spotting and infertility.
- TVUS is diagnostic; methotrexate and surgical resection are key for CSEP; hysteroscopy/laparoscopy for isthmocele.
- RCOG/NICE emphasize early diagnosis and tailored management.

SUGGESTED READING

1. Dominguez JA, Devine KM, Huddleston AJ, et al. Diagnosis and management of isthmocele (Cesarean scar defect): a State-of-the-Art Review. Ultrasound Obstet Gynecol. 2023;62(4):452-464. doi:10.1002/uog.26171
2. Kennedy A, Jha P, Yuan J, et al. Cesarean scar ectopic pregnancy: a do-not-miss diagnosis. Radiographics. 2024;44(4):e230199. doi:10.1148/rg.230199
3. Lin R, Littner Y. Cesarean scar ectopic pregnancy: nuances in diagnosis, management, and future fertility. Best Pract Res Clin Obstet Gynaecol. 2024;95:102507. doi:10.1016/j.bpobgyn.2023.102507
4. National Institute for Health and Care Excellence. Ectopic pregnancy and miscarriage: diagnosis and initial management. NICE guideline [NG126]. London: NICE; 2023. Available from: https://www.nice.org.uk/guidance/ng126
5. Royal College of Obstetricians and Gynaecologists. Diagnosis and management of ectopic pregnancy. Green-top Guideline No. 21. BJOG. 2023. doi:10.1111/1471-0528.17602

Gestational Trophoblastic Disease and Neoplasia

Ruchika Garg

DEFINITION AND CLASSIFICATION

Gestational trophoblastic disease (GTD) encompasses a spectrum of disorders from abnormal trophoblast proliferation, ranging from benign hydatidiform moles to malignant gestational trophoblastic neoplasia (GTN).

- **Modified WHO Classification (2020):**
  - **Molar Pregnancies:**
    - Hydatidiform mole (complete and partial) **(Fig. 1)**
    - Invasive mole

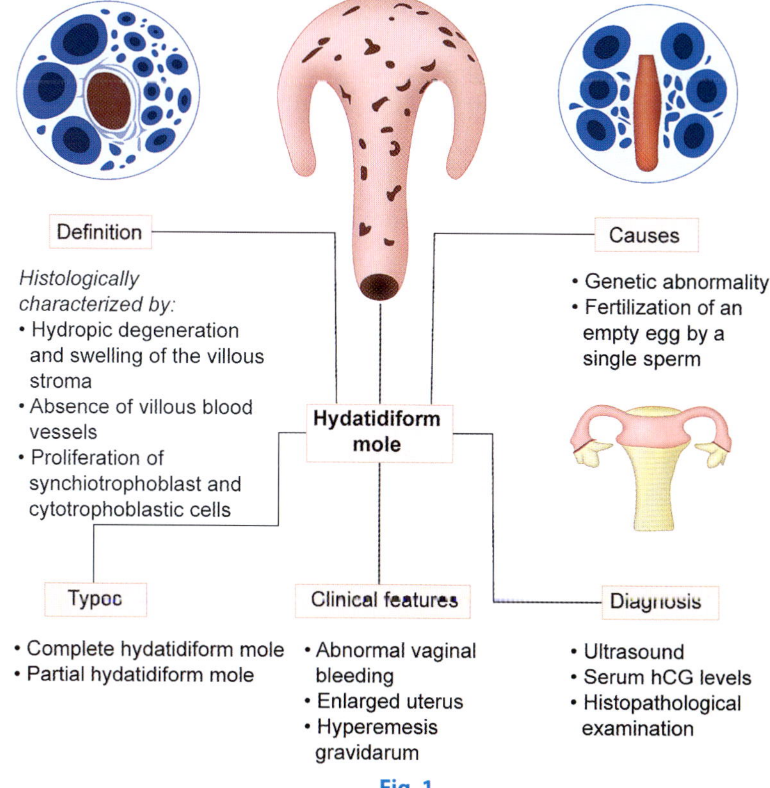

Fig. 1

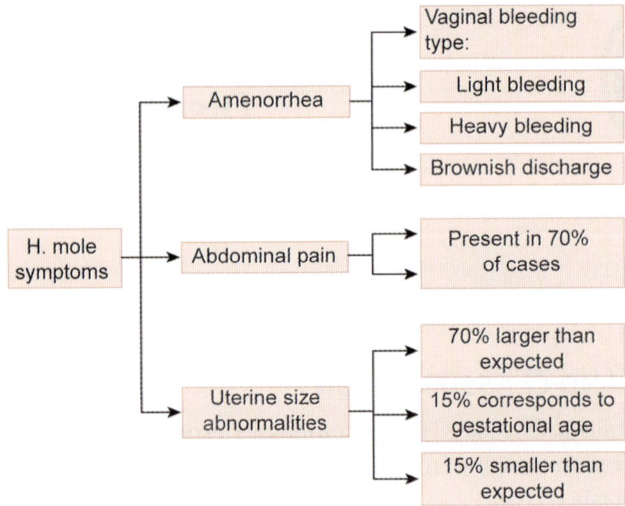

Fig. 1: Hydatidiform mole and clinical symptoms.
Source: Ngan HYS, Seckl MJ, Berkowitz RS, et al. Diagnosis and management of gestational trophoblastic disease: 2021 update. Int J Gynaecol Obstet. 2021;155 Suppl 1:86-93. doi:10.1002/ijgo.13877

- **Trophoblastic Tumors:**
    - Invasive mole
    - Choriocarcinoma
    - Placental site trophoblastic tumor (PSTT)
    - Epithelioid trophoblastic tumor (ETT)

EPIDEMIOLOGY

- **Global Incidence:** 0.6–2.3 per 1,000 pregnancies; higher in Asian/African populations (India: ~1 in 160 pregnancies).
- **Developed Countries:** Complete mole: 1–3 per 1,000; partial mole: ~3 per 1,000 pregnancies.
- **Complete Mole:**
    - Fertilization of an empty ovum by a single sperm (46,XX, paternal origin) or two sperms (46,XX/XY, 5–10%). Complete hydatidiform moles typically result from the fertilization of an empty egg (an egg where the nuclear material is lost or inactivated) by a single haploid sperm (23,X chromosomes). This haploid set of chromosomes then duplicates to form 46,XX chromosomes, making the complete mole homozygous and of paternal origin. In 5–10% cases, the empty egg is fertilized by two separate sperms, resulting in either a 46,XX or 46,XY heterozygous chromosomal constitution. Complete moles are the most common type of molar pregnancy.
    - No fetal tissue; higher malignant potential.
- **Partial Mole:**
    - Triploidy (69,XXY/XXX) from dispermic fertilization or paternal chromosome reduplication **(Figs. 2A and B)**. Partial hydatidiform mole contains one set of maternal chromosomes along with two sets of paternal chromosomes, leading to triploidy.

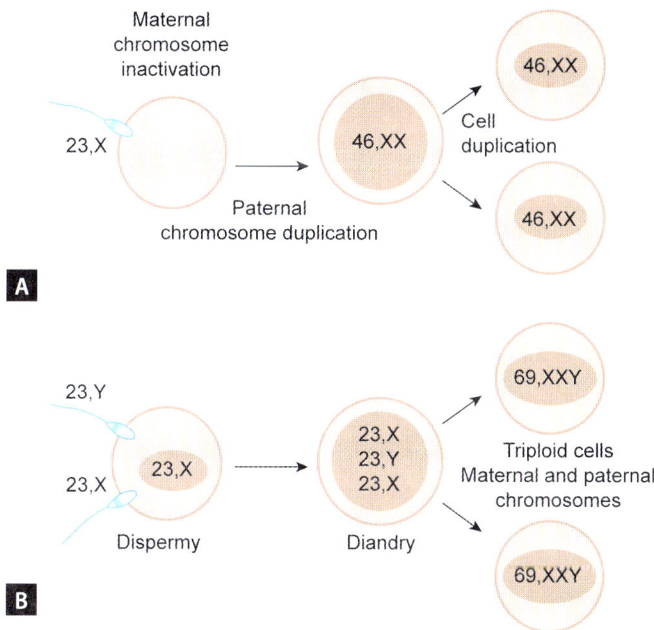

Figs. 2A and B: Pathogenesis of complete and partial mole.
Source: Berkowitz RS, Goldstein DP. Molar pregnancy. N Engl J Med. 2009;360(16):1639-45. doi:10.1056/NEJMcp0900696

- Fetal tissue present; lower malignant risk **(Table 1)**.

- **Key Genetic Marker:** p57 expression absent in complete moles (no maternal genome) but present in partial moles.

RISK FACTORS

- Extremes of maternal age (<21, >35; 7.5× risk >40).
- Prior molar pregnancy (10x risk; 15–20% after two moles).
- Ethnicity (Asian/African higher risk).
- Dietary deficiencies (carotene and animal fats), smoking.
- Genetic mutations (NLRP7 and KHDC3L) in recurrent moles.

CLINICAL FEATURES

- **Common:** Vaginal bleeding (60%), passage of grape-like vesicles, first trimester.
- **Less Common:** Hyperemesis, uterine size-date discrepancy (larger in complete, smaller in partial), early preeclampsia, hyperthyroidism, and theca lutein cysts.
- **Rare:** Hemoptysis/seizures from lung/brain metastases.

DIAGNOSIS

- **Serum hCG:**
  - In complete moles, hCG levels are much higher for the corresponding gestational age, typically above 100,000 IU/L. These high values can erroneously give false-negative

TABLE 1: Differentiating features between complete and partial hydatidiform mole.

Feature	*Complete mole*	*Partial mole*
Chromosomal Origin	Paternal (46,XX; rarely 46,XY); fertilization of empty ovum by single (90%) or two sperms (5–10%)	Triploid (69,XXY/XXX); one maternal + two paternal sets (dispermic or reduplicated)
Karyotype	Diploid (46,XX or XY)	Triploid (69,XXY/XXX; rarely XYY)
Fetal Tissue	Absent (fetus resorbs early)	Present (fetal parts, amnion, or vessels with fetal RBCs)
p57 Expression	Absent (no maternal genome)	Present (maternal genome present)
Uterine Size	Larger than gestational age	Smaller or appropriate for gestational age
hCG Levels	Markedly elevated (>100,000 mIU/L); risk of Hook effect	Elevated, often within normal range for gestation
Ultrasound Findings	"Snowstorm" or "bunch of grapes" appearance; no fetus/amniotic fluid	"Swiss cheese" placenta; fetal parts/ amniotic fluid present
Theca Lutein Cysts	More common (25–30%)	Less common
Malignant Potential (GTN)	Higher (~5% risk of persistent trophoblastic disease)	Lower (<1% risk of persistent trophoblastic disease)
Histopathology	Diffuse villous edema, trophoblastic hyperplasia, no fetal tissue	Focal villous edema, partial trophoblastic hyperplasia, fetal tissue present
Clinical Presentation	Heavy bleeding, hyperemesis, early preeclampsia, hyperthyroidism more frequent	Milder symptoms; bleeding common, other features less frequent

Source: Royal College of Obstetricians and Gynaecologists. Gestational trophoblastic disease. Green-top Guideline No. 38. BJOG. 2021;128(2):e150-e172. doi:10.1111/1471-0528.16500.[1,2]

urine pregnancy test results due to oversaturation of assay's target antibodies. This is termed as the "Hook effect". Hence, serum estimation of hCG is preferred over urine.
- Partial mole: Elevated but often within normal range.

- **Ultrasound:**
  - Complete: complex, Echogenic intrauterine mass is seen containing multiple small cystic spaces that correspond to the hydropic villi on gross pathology ***"Snowstorm"/"bunch of grapes"*** appearance, no fetus/amniotic fluid.
  - Partial: Fetal parts seen enlarged, thickened placenta "Swiss cheese" placenta.
- **Other Tests:** Blood group (Rh typing), CBC, LFT/RFT/TFT, and coagulation profile.
- **Definitive Diagnosis:** Histopathology of products of conception.
- **Metastatic Workup:** Chest X-ray/CT, abdominopelvic/brain CT/MRI.

DIFFERENTIAL DIAGNOSIS (TABLE 2)

- Androgenetic/biparental mosaic conceptions, hydropic abortus, hyperemesis gravidarum, and placental mesenchymal dysplasia.

TABLE 2: Differential diagnosis of H. Mole.

Condition	*Key features*
Threatened Abortion	• Vaginal bleeding (slight) • No uterine enlargement • Closed cervical os • No fetal parts palpable • USG: Empty uterus
Multiple Pregnancy	• Enlarged uterus greater than expected for dates • USG: Multiple gestational sacs/fetuses
Fibroid with Pregnancy	• Irregularly enlarged uterus • Clinical: Firm areas seen within uterus • USG: Fibroid masses
Mistaken Dates	• Discrepancy in dates (clinical vs. USG) • USG shows less advanced gestation

MANAGEMENT OF MOLAR PREGNANCY

- **Suction Curettage:** Mainstay for complete/partial moles; ultrasound-guided for large uteri.
  - Avoid routine prostaglandin cervical preparation; use osmotic dilators if needed.
  - Post-evacuation: Oxytocics for bleeding; rarely embolization/hysterectomy.
- **Hysterectomy:** Considered in women >40 with complete family (>50% GTN risk reduction).
- **Rh-Negative Cases:** Anti-D immunoglobulin for partial moles; In cases of complete mole with poor vascularization of the chorionic villi and absence of the D antigen by trophoblast cells, anti-D is not needed, and may be given for complete moles if diagnosis delayed >72 hours.
- **Twin with Coexisting Mole:**
  - Termination: Suction curettage or medical methods if large uterus.
  - If patient opts for continuation of pregnancy: Refer to fetal medicine/GTD center for karyotyping.

Post-Evacuation Surveillance (RCOG 2020 Guidelines)

- **Complete Mole:**
  - Weekly hCG until normal for 3 weeks.
  - If normal within 56 days: Monthly hCG for 6 months from evacuation.
  - If not normal within 56 days: Monthly hCG for 6 months post-normalization.
- **Partial Mole:** Weekly hCG until normal, recheck at 4 weeks.
- **Contraception:** Advised until follow-up complete; 1 year if chemotherapy used.
- **Risk of Persistent Trophoblastic Disease (PTD):** ~5% (complete), <1% (partial).
- **Diagnosis Confirmation:**
  - Laboratory tests: CBC, LFT/RFT/TFT, and coagulation profile.
  - Imaging: Chest CT, brain MRI, and Doppler pelvic ultrasound.

TABLE 3: Risk factors for GTN.

Risk factor	*Details*
Timing Postevacuation	Greatest risk within 12 months, especially first 6 months post-molar evacuation
hCG Trend	Persistent, plateaued, or rising hCG during postevacuation surveillance
Persistent Vaginal Bleeding	Bleeding >8 weeks after pregnancy event
Maternal Age	Higher risk with advanced maternal age (e.g., >35 years)
Pre-evacuation hCG Levels	Levels >100,000 mIU/mL
Uterine Size	Larger than expected for gestational age
Theca Lutein Cysts	Cysts >6 cm

- **Treatment:** Low-risk GTN (score 4):
  - **Single-Agent Chemotherapy:**
    - Methotrexate: 1 mg/kg IM days 1, 3, 5, and 7 with folinic acid 0.1 mg/kg days 2, 4, 6, and 8, repeat every 14 days.
    - Alternative: Actinomycin-D (1.25 mg/m^2 IV every 2 weeks or 0.5 mg IV daily × 5 days every 2 weeks).
  - Continue until hCG <5 mIU/L for 3 weeks + 2–3 consolidation cycles.
  - If hCG plateaus/rises: Re-evaluate, switch to alternative single-agent; consider multiagent (EMA-CO) or hysterectomy if resistant.
- **Supportive Care:** Monitor theca lutein cysts (resolve post-treatment) and manage bleeding with oxytocics.
- **Surveillance:** Weekly hCG until normal for 3 weeks, then monthly for 12 months.
- **Contraception:** Oral preferred for 1-year postremission.
- **Future Pregnancies:** Early ultrasound, postdelivery hCG/placental histology (1–2% recurrent mole risk).
- **Prognosis:** ~100% cure rate, <5% recurrence.

Q2: MANAGEMENT OF GTN (SHORT ANSWER)

These tumors, in most cases, develop with or after some form of recognized pregnancy. In 50% cases, the develops after hydatidiform mole. In 25% cases, it develops after a miscarriage or tubal pregnancy, and in remaining cases, it develops after a preterm or term pregnancy. Although these tumors are histologically distinct, but they are usually diagnosed mainly by persistently elevated serum β-hCG levels because tissue is rarely available for study **(Table 3)**.

Gestational Trophoblastic Neoplasia: Risk Factors and Diagnostic Criteria

Diagnostic Criteria for GTN

- **Clinical Presentation:**
  - Irregular vaginal bleeding postpregnancy with uterine subinvolution.
  - Myometrial perforation: May cause intraperitoneal hemorrhage.

TABLE 4: FIGO/WHO Prognostic Scoring System for Gestational Trophoblastic Neoplasia (GTN).

Prognostic factor	*Score 0*	*Score 1*	*Score 2*	*Score 4*
Age (years)	<40	≥40	-	-
Antecedent Pregnancy	Mole	Abortion	Term	-
Interval from Index Pregnancy (months)	<4	4–6	7–12	>12
Pretreatment hCG (mIU/mL)	$<10^3$	10^3–10^4	10^4–10^5	$>10^5$
Largest Tumor Size (cm)	<3	3–5	>5	-
Site of Metastases	Lung	Spleen, Kidney	Gastrointestinal	Brain, Liver
Number of Metastases	0	1–4	5–8	>8
Prior Chemotherapy	None	-	Single agent	≥2 agents

- Metastatic signs: Bluish vaginal masses (lower genital tract metastases), cough, chest pain, hemoptysis, dyspnea (lung metastases), or seizures/paralysis (brain metastases).

- **Diagnostic Approach:**
  - **Serum hCG Estimation:** Prompt measurement for any irregular bleeding post-pregnancy; persistently elevated hCG suggests malignant transformation.
  - **Avoid Biopsy:** Tissue biopsy of vaginal metastases contraindicated due to high bleeding risk.
  - **Baseline Investigations:**
    - Hemogram, liver function tests (LFT), renal function tests (RFT).
    - Imaging:
      - Transvaginal ultrasound (to assess uterine involvement).
      - Chest X-ray or CT (to detect lung metastases).
      - Abdominopelvic and brain CT/MRI (to evaluate for distant metastases) **(Table 4)**.

The International Federation of Gynecology and Obstetrics (FIGO) and World Health Organization (WHO) prognostic scoring system (2009) is used to assess the risk of GTN and guide treatment. The total score determines whether the disease is low-risk (≤6) or high-risk (≥7).

Risk Categories

- **Low-Risk:** Total score 0–6 → Managed with single-agent chemotherapy (e.g., methotrexate or actinomycin-D).
- **High-Risk:** Total score ≥7 → Managed with multiagent chemotherapy (e.g., EMA-CO), with or without surgery or adjuvant radiotherapy. It includes combinations of Etoposide, Methotrexate, Actinomycin D, Cyclophosphamide, and Oncovin (vincristine).
- Ultra-High-Risk: Score ≥13 → May require low-dose induction chemotherapy (etoposide + cisplatin) before standard multiagent therapy to prevent complications like tumor collapse **(Fig. 3)**.
- Higher scores indicate increased risk of treatment resistance and worse prognosis.

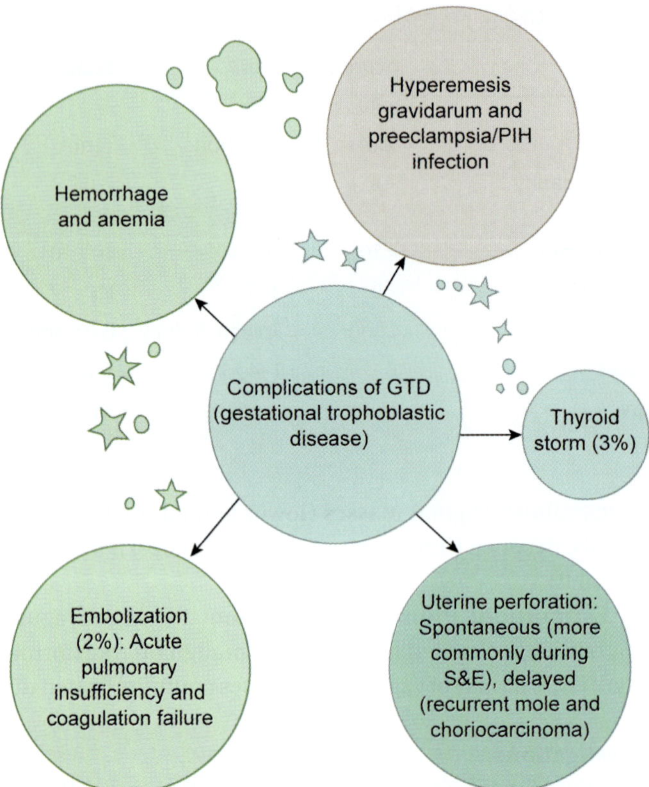

Fig. 3: Complications of GTD.
Source: Horowitz NS, Eskander RN, Adelman MR, Burke WM. Society of Gynecologic Oncology recommendations for the diagnosis and treatment of gestational trophoblastic disease. Gynecol Oncol. 2021;162(3):764-71. doi:10.1016/j.ygyno.2021.06.010

- Management should be guided by a specialized GTN center, with hCG surveillance post-treatment to monitor for recurrence.

Invasive Mole: This invasion in myometrium can result into uterine perforation and extension to adjacent organs like parametrium or vaginal vault.

Diagnostic Workup

- Persistent/rising hCG postpregnancy.
- Imaging: Pelvic ultrasound, chest CT, abdominopelvic/brain CT/MRI.
- Laboratory tests: CBC, LFT/RFT/TFT, and coagulation profile.
- Avoid vaginal lesion biopsy (bleeding risk).

Treatment by Risk Category

- **Low-Risk (FIGO/WHO Score 0–6):**
  - Single-agent chemotherapy (methotrexate or actinomycin-D).
  - Continue until hCG normal + 2–3 consolidation cycles.

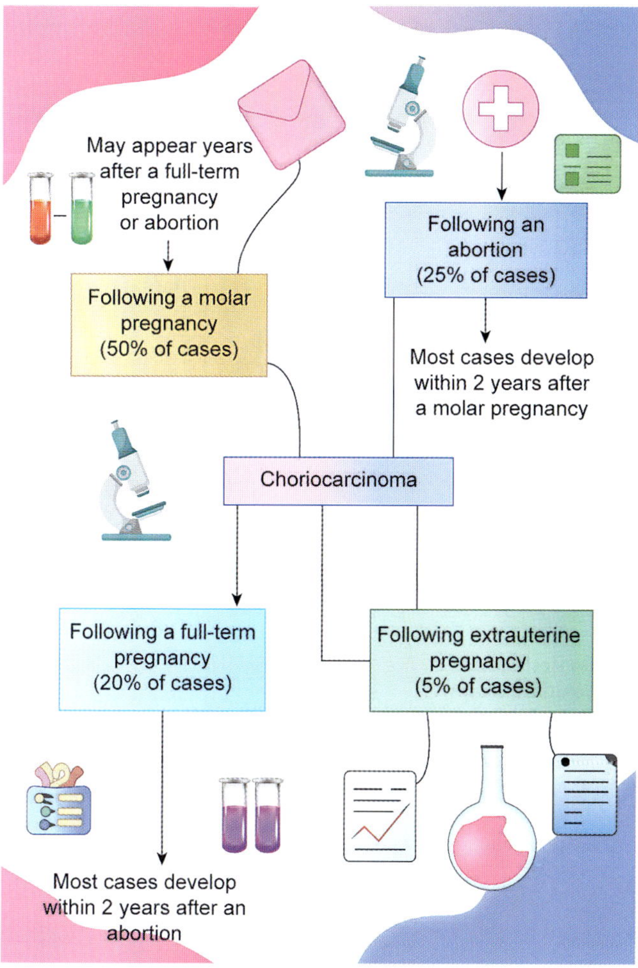

Fig. 4: Causes and common origins of choriocarcinoma.

- Switch agents if resistant; multiagent or hysterectomy if refractory.
- Cure rate: ~100%.

- **High-Risk (Score ≥7):**
  - EMA-CO (etoposide, methotrexate, actinomycin-D, cyclophosphamide, vincristine) every 2 weeks.
  - Ultra-high-risk (score ≥13): Low-dose etoposide + cisplatin induction, then EMA-CO.
  - Adjuvant surgery/radiotherapy if needed.
  - Cure rate: ~95%.
- **PSTT/ETT:**
  - Hysterectomy (mainstay); fertility-preserving curettage/chemotherapy (EMA/EP, paclitaxel-cisplatin) if desired.
  - MRI surveillance (hCG less reliable).

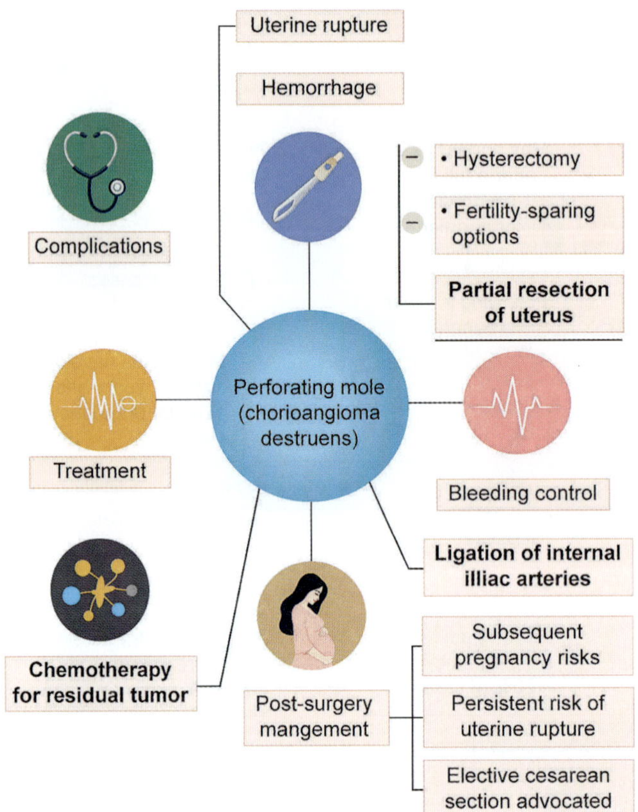

Fig. 5: Postsurgery management in perforating mole (chorioangioma destruens).
Source: Same as **Fig 1.**

- **Gestational Choriocarcinoma:** This is the most common, rapid growing, malignant GTN arising from abnormal trophoblastic cells undergoing hyperplasia and anaplasia. It invades myometrium and blood vessels causing hemorrhage and necrosis **(Fig. 4)**.

  Early spread to fallopian tubes, ovaries, and vagina with distant metastasis in the lung, liver, spleen, kidney, bowel, or brain.

  This most commonly follows a term pregnancy or a miscarriage, and only 25% cases follow a molar pregnancy. Myometrial tumor may spread outward and become visible on the uterine surface as dark, irregular nodules **(Fig. 5)**.

  Grossly, the tumor appears bulky with hemorrhagic and necrotic areas. Histologically, it shows absence of chorionic villi and presence of abnormal intermediate trophoblast and cytotrophoblast, rimmed with syncytiotrophoblasts.
- **Resistant/Recurrent GTN:**
  - Multiagent chemotherapy (e.g., EMA-CO, EMA/EP, cisplatin-based).
  - Salvage surgery or high-dose chemotherapy with stem cell rescue **(Fig. 6)**.
  - Emerging: PD-L1 inhibitors (pembrolizumab and avelumab).

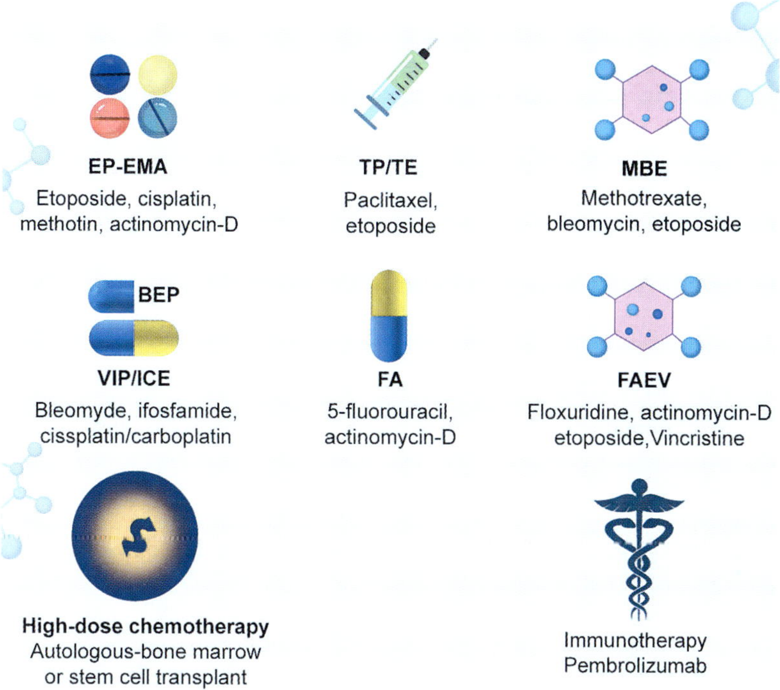

Fig. 6: Salvage Therapy in gestational trophoblastic disease (GTD).
Source: Barcellos M, et al. Pembrolizumab in gestational trophoblastic neoplasia. Gynecol Oncol Rep. 2025;51:101307. doi:10.1016/j.gore.2024.101307

Surveillance

- Low/High-Risk: hCG every 2 weeks for 3 months, then monthly for 12 months; high-risk may need longer.
- Ultra-High-Risk: 24 months; PSTT/ETT: 6-monthly MRIs for 5 years.
- Contraception: 1-year postremission.

Subsequent Pregnancies

- 1–2% recurrent mole risk; early ultrasound, postdelivery hCG/placental histology.
- No increased abortion/congenital anomaly risk.

RECENT LITERATURE UPDATES (2023–2025)

- **Immunotherapy:** Pembrolizumab shows promise in chemoresistant GTN (case reports, 2023).
- **Genetic Insights:** NLRP7/KHDC3L mutations linked to recurrent moles; genetic screening recommended in such cases.
- **hCG Assays:** Improved sensitivity reduces Hook effect errors; serum hCG remains gold standard.

- **RCOG 2023 Update:** Emphasizes GTD center registration, streamlined hCG surveillance protocols.

KEY POINTS FOR POSTGRADUATES

- **FIGO/WHO Scoring:** Critical for risk stratification and treatment planning.
- **Chemotherapy:** Single-agent for low-risk; EMA-CO for high-risk; hysterectomy for PSTT/ETT.
- **Surveillance:** Rigorous hCG/MRI monitoring to detect recurrence.
- **Contraception:** Essential to avoid hCG misinterpretation.
- **Prognosis:** Excellent with appropriate management; recurrence rare.

SUGGESTED READING

1. Baas IO, et al. Immunotherapy for gestational trophoblastic neoplasia: a new paradigm. Best Pract Res Clin Obstet Gynaecol. 2024;94:102486. doi:10.1016/j.bpobgyn.2023.102486
2. Berkowitz RS, Goldstein DP. Molar pregnancy. N Engl J Med. 2009;360(16):1639-45. doi:10.1056/NEJMcp0900696
3. FIGO. (2021). FIGO Cancer Report 2021. [online] Available from https://www.figo.org/figo-cancer-report-2021 [Last accessed December, 2025].
4. Horowitz NS, et al. Society of Gynecologic Oncology recommendations for gestational trophoblastic disease. Gynecol Oncol. 2021;162(3):764-771. doi:10.1016/j.ygyno.2021.06.010
5. RCOG. Gestational Trophoblastic Disease (Green-top Guideline No. 38). [online] Available from https://www.rcog.org.uk/guidance/browse-all-guidance/green-top-guidelines/gestational-trophoblastic-disease-green-top-guideline-no-38/ [Last accessed December, 2025].
6. Royal College of Obstetricians and Gynaecologists. Gestational trophoblastic disease. Green-top Guideline No. 38. BJOG. 2021;128(2):e150-e172. doi:10.1111/1471-0528.16500
7. International Federation of Gynecology and Obstetrics. FIGO Cancer Report 2021. Int J Gynaecol Obstet. 2021;155 Suppl 1:45-93

Invasive Prenatal Diagnostic Procedures

Ruchika Garg

OVERVIEW

Invasive prenatal testing remains the gold standard for definitive fetal diagnosis despite widespread use of NIPT. All procedures must be performed under continuous ultrasound guidance by trained fetal medicine specialists.[1]

SUMMARY TABLE

Procedure	*Gestational age*	*Sample obtained*	*Diagnostic yield*	*Procedure-related fetal loss rate**	*Main specific complication*
Amniocentesis[2]	≥15^{+0} weeks	Amniotic fluid (AFC)	Karyotype, microarray, PCR, infections	0.1–0.5%	Amniotic fluid leakage, chorioamnionitis
Chorionic Villus Sampling	10^{+0} to 13^{+6} weeks	Chorionic villi	Karyotype, microarray, single-gene tests	0.5–1.0%	Limb reduction defect (<10 weeks), vaginal bleeding
Cordocentesis (PUBS/FBS)	≥18 weeks	Fetal blood (umbilical vein)	Rapid karyotype, anemia, thrombocytopenia, infections	1–2% (up to 5–7% if hydrops/ IUGR)	Cord hematoma, bradycardia, fetal exsanguination

*Fetal loss rates are background-corrected (2020–2025 meta-analyses)

KEY TECHNICAL POINTS

Amniocentesis

- Needle: 20–22 G spinal needle
- Volume: 15–30 mL (discard first 2–3 mL)
- Approach: Avoid transplacental route in Rh-negative unless unavoidable
- High maternal cell contamination risk: Bloody tap, transplacental pass, ≥2 attempts, inexperienced operator
- Culture failure: <0.5%; mosaicism: 0.1–0.3%

Chorionic Villus Sampling

- Never perform <10^{+0} weeks → risk of limb reduction defects and oromandibular hypoplasia
- Minimum villi required: 5–10 mg (dry weight)
- Transabdominal preferred over transcervical (lower infection and bleeding risk)
- Placental mosaicism (CPM): 1–2% → confirm by amniocentesis if abnormal
- Operator standard: <1:100 loss rate and <5% sampling failure for competence

Cordocentesis

- Preferred site: Placental cord insertion >> free loop >> intrahepatic vein
- Target: Umbilical vein only (artery → spasm and bradycardia)
- Highest risk procedure; reserved for: – Rapid karyotype when mosaicism suspected – Fetal anemia (MCA-PSV >1.5 MoM) – Thrombocytopenia, infections, metabolic disorders

INDICATIONS (2025)

Strong indications	*Relative/Controversial indications*
Positive NIPT (high chance)	Advanced maternal age alone (>35 or >40)—not accepted in most guidelines[3]
Abnormal first/second trimester screening[4]	IVF without PGT
Major fetal structural anomaly on ultrasound	Previous aneuploidy without recurrence risk
Known parental translocation/balanced rearrangement	
Monogenic disorder with known mutation	
Suspected fetal infection (CMV, toxoplasma, and parvovirus)	
Nonimmune hydrops/severe early IUGR	

PRE- AND POSTPROCEDURE PROTOCOL

- Confirm fetal viability, GA, placental site, and liquor volume
- Rh status → Anti-D 300 µg IM within 72 hours if Rh-negative and unsensitized
- No routine antibiotic prophylaxis
- No routine tocolysis
- Postprocedure USG: Fetal heart, placental hematoma, and liquor volume
- Written report: Indication, approach, punctures, sample appearance, and fetal viability

GENETIC TESTING OPTIONS ON INVASIVE SAMPLES5

Test	*Turnaround time*	*Detects*
QF-PCR/FISH	1–3 days	Aneuploidies (13, 18, 21, X, Y)
Conventional karyotype	10–14 days	Numerical + large structural abnormalities
Chromosomal microarray (CMA/aCGH)	7–14 days	CNVs >50–100 kb, microdeletion/duplication
Exome/Genome sequencing[6]	2–6 weeks	Single-gene disorders, de-novo mutations

Chromosomal microarray analysis (CMA) is now recommended as first-line over karyotype when structural anomalies are present (ISUOG/ACOG 2020–2025).

KEY EXAMINATION-ORIENTED POINTS

- Only amniocentesis can reliably diagnose open neural tube defects (AF-AFP + AChE)
- Chorionic villus sampling (CVS) cannot diagnose NTDs
- Confined placental mosaicism → next step is amniocentesis.
- Highest risk procedure = cordocentesis
- Limb reduction defects are specific to CVS <10 weeks
- Procedure-related loss drops dramatically after operator performs >100 cases/year

REFERENCES

1. ISUOG Practice Guidelines (updated): performance of 11–14-week ultrasound scan. Ultrasound Obstet Gynecol. 2023;61:127-43. doi:10.1002/uog.26106.
2. Akolekar R, Beta J, Picciarelli G, et al. Procedure-related risk of miscarriage following amniocentesis and chorionic villus sampling: a systematic review and meta-analysis. Ultrasound Obstet Gynecol. 2015;45(1):16-26.
3. Ghi T, Sotiriadis A, Calda P, et al. ISUOG Practice Guidelines: invasive procedures for prenatal diagnosis. Ultrasound Obstet Gynecol. 2016;48(2):256-68.
4. Wulff CB, Gerds TA, Rode L, et al. Risk of fetal loss associated with invasive testing following combined first-trimester screening for Down syndrome: a national cohort of 147,987 singleton pregnancies. Ultrasound Obstet Gynecol. 2016;47(1):381-44.
5. American College of Obstetricians and Gynecologists' Committee on Practice Bulletins—Obstetrics; Committee on Genetics; Society for Maternal-Fetal Medicine. Screening for Fetal Chromosomal Abnormalities: ACOG Practice Bulletin, Number 226. Obstet Gynecol. 2020 Oct;136(4):e48-e69.
6. Lord J, Bateman M, et al. Prenatal exome sequencing analysis in fetal structural anomalies detected by ultrasonography (PAGE): a cohort study. Lancet. 2019;393(10173):747-57.

Medical Termination of Pregnancy

Ruchika Garg

DEFINITION

- Medical termination of pregnancy (MTP) is the intentional and lawful termination of pregnancy before fetal viability.
- In India, governed by the Medical Termination of Pregnancy Act (1971, implemented 1972), updated in 2021 extending legal limits to 24 weeks with exceptions.
- Enacted to reduce maternal mortality from unsafe abortions.
- MTP includes both medical and surgical termination methods.

OBJECTIVES OF MEDICAL TERMINATION OF PREGNANCY ACT

- Provide legal framework for safe abortion services.
- Reduce maternal deaths from unsafe abortions.
- Empower women to make reproductive choices.
- Address pregnancies from contraceptive failure, sexual violence, or health risks.

LEGAL GESTATIONAL LIMITS

Gestation age	*MTP permissible conditions*
Up to 20 weeks	Termination allowed broadly
20–24 weeks	Allowed for rape, fetal anomalies, and decided by medical board
Beyond 24 weeks	Permitted only for severe fetal anomalies certified by medical board (rare)

INDICATIONS FOR MEDICAL TERMINATION OF PREGNANCY

Indication category	*Examples*
Medical grounds	High maternal risk—severe cardiac disease, hypertension, diabetes, malignancy, and psychiatric illness
Eugenic grounds	Serious fetal anomalies—congenital malformations, genetic disorders, teratogenic exposure, and Rh sensitization
Humanitarian grounds	Pregnancy following rape and incest
Social grounds	Socioeconomic hardship and contraceptive failure (irrespective of marital status as per 2021 amendment)

Legal and consent requirements:

- Informed written consent from woman mandatory
- For minors or mentally incapacitated, guardian consent required
- Confidentiality strictly enforced by law

Authorized personnel and facilities:

- Only registered medical practitioners trained and approved can perform MTP.
- MTP must be conducted in approved health facilities meeting safety standards.
- *For ≤12 weeks:* Single doctor's approval is sufficient.
- *For 13–24 weeks:* Approval by two doctors is required, with adherence to legal criteria.

METHODS OF TERMINATION

First Trimester (≤12 weeks)

Method	*Description*	*Advantages*	*Limitations*
Manual vacuum aspiration (MVA)	Outpatient procedure using suction cannula	Quick, less invasive, and safe	Limited efficacy >12 weeks
Suction evacuation	Vacuum suction with electric pump	Minimal bleeding, outpatient suitable	Requires electricity and equipment
Medical abortion	Mifepristone + misoprostol	Effective and nonsurgical	Requires compliance and observing side effects

Second Trimester (13–20 weeks)

Method	*Description*	*Comments*
Dilatation and evacuation (D and E)	Surgical evacuation under ultrasound guidance	Less preferred due to higher complication rate
Prostaglandin regimens	Misoprostol or carboprost via multiple routes	Highly effective and commonly used
Hysterotomy	Rarely done classical cesarean section	Reserved for selected cases with contraindications to medical methods

Manual Vacuum Aspiration Syringe

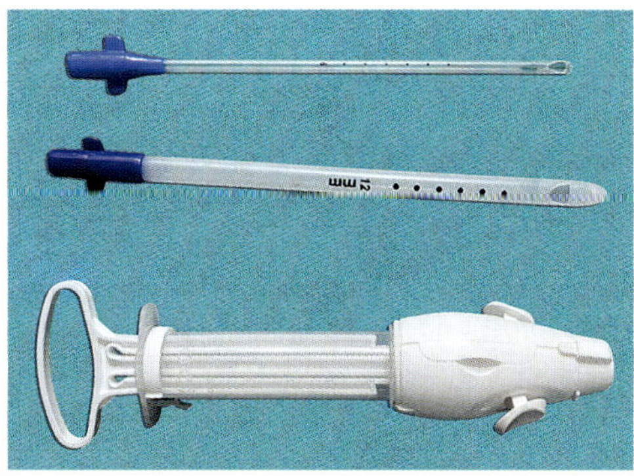

Medical Abortion Protocol

- *Day 1:* 200 mg mifepristone orally (Rh negative receive anti-D)
- Day 3: 800 μg misoprostol vaginally/orally every 3–4 hours (up to 5 doses)
- Follow-up at 2 and 4 weeks to confirm completion
- Success 90–98%, failure in 1–3%

Postprocedural Care and Follow-up

- Monitor vital signs, bleeding, and pain.
- Antibiotics prophylaxis as indicated
- Anti-D immunoglobulin for Rh-negative women
- Analgesics (tramadol and NSAIDs) as needed
- Follow-up ultrasound and β-hCG monitoring to confirm complete abortion
- Contraceptive counseling to prevent subsequent unintended pregnancies

COMPLICATIONS

Early (within 24 hours)	*Delayed (up to 2 weeks)*
Hemorrhage (0.3–1%)	Postabortal bleeding—incomplete evacuation
Uterine perforation (0.13–0.3%)	Infection and sepsis
Shock	Subinvolution and dysfunctional uterine bleeding
Cervical laceration	Infertility from cornual blockage or Asherman's syndrome
Thrombosis/embolism	Trophoblastic disease

KEY 2021 MTP AMENDMENT HIGHLIGHTS

- Gestational limit extended to 24 weeks for rape survivors, minors, and differently abled women
- Contraceptive failure clause extended to all women regardless of marital status
- Medical boards regulate MTP beyond 24 weeks for severe fetal defects.
- Identity confidentiality strictly mandated

MEDICAL TERMINATION OF PREGNANCY METHODS AND INDICATIONS

Trimester	*Medical methods*	*Surgical methods*	*Typical gestation*
First (≤12 weeks)	Mifepristone + misoprostol	Manual vacuum aspiration and suction evacuation	Up to 12 weeks
Second (13–20 weeks)	Prostaglandins (misoprostol and carboprost) and methotrexate combos	Dilatation and evacuation and hysterotomy (rare)	13–20 weeks

SUMMARY

- MTP is a legally regulated procedure aimed at safe pregnancy termination, reducing unsafe abortion-related mortality.
- Indications span medical, fetal, humanitarian, and social grounds
- Early pregnancy terminations mostly use medical or minimally invasive surgical methods; second trimester relies more on prostaglandins.
- Proper counseling, informed consent, skilled providers, and follow-up are essential to ensure safety and minimize complications.

Abortions

Ruchika Garg, Shaifali Singh

INTRODUCTION

Vaginal bleeding in the first trimester affects 15–25% of pregnancies and is a common cause of anxiety for patients and clinicians.[1] While some cases resolve with a healthy pregnancy, others may lead to adverse outcomes such as miscarriage or ectopic pregnancy. Accurate diagnosis, using clinical history, examination, and investigations like transvaginal ultrasound (TVS) and serum beta-human chorionic gonadotropin (β-hCG), is crucial for effective management. This chapter addresses the causes and management of first-trimester bleeding, focusing on spontaneous abortion, and incorporates RCOG and NICE guidelines for postgraduate medical education.

LONG QUESTION: CAUSES OF BLEEDING IN FIRST TRIMESTER AND MANAGEMENT OF SPONTANEOUS ABORTION

Causes of Bleeding in First Trimester

First-trimester bleeding may result from obstetric or nonobstetric causes, with varying implications for pregnancy outcome **(Table 1)**.

- **Risks:** Bleeding increases the risk of miscarriage (30–50% with heavy bleeding), preterm delivery, and preterm premature rupture of membranes (PPROM).[3]
- **Diagnosis Challenges:** Urine pregnancy tests may yield false positives (e.g., chemical pregnancy) or false negatives (e.g., early ectopic); correlation with β-hCG and TVS is essential.[4]

Management of Spontaneous Abortion in First Trimester

Spontaneous abortion (miscarriage) is defined as pregnancy loss before 20 weeks, with most occurring in the first trimester. Management depends on the type of abortion (threatened, inevitable, incomplete, complete, or missed), clinical stability, and patient preference, guided by RCOG Green-top Guideline No. 25 (2023) and NICE NG126 (2023).[5,6]

Evaluation

- **History:**
  - **Menstrual History:** Last menstrual period (LMP), cycle regularity.
  - **Contraception:** Recent use of combined oral contraceptives (COCs).

TABLE 1: Causes of bleeding in first trimester.[2]

Cause	*Description*	*Prevalence*
Implantation bleeding	Light bleeding due to embryo implantation in endometrium (3–5 days postfertilization)	20–30%
Threatened abortion	Bleeding with viable intrauterine pregnancy; cervix closed	10–15%
Inevitable abortion	Bleeding with open cervix; pregnancy loss imminent	5–10%
Incomplete abortion	Partial expulsion of products of conception (POC)	5–10%
Complete abortion	Full expulsion of POC; uterus empty	5–10%
Missed abortion	Nonviable pregnancy with retained POC; no bleeding/pain	2–5%
Gestational trophoblastic neoplasia (GTN)	Abnormal trophoblastic proliferation (e.g., hydatidiform mole)	<1%
Ectopic Pregnancy	Implantation outside uterus (e.g., fallopian tube)	1–2%
Local causes	Cervical/vaginal lesions (e.g., polyps, erosion, cervicitis, and trauma)	1–3%
Subchorionic hematoma	Blood collection between chorion and myometrium	5–10%

- **Bleeding:** Flow (light/moderate/heavy), color (red/brown/dark), clots, or POC passage.
- **Pain:** Abdominal cramps and low backache.
- **Associated Factors:** Sexual activity, vomiting, and heavy exertion.[7]

- **Examination:**
  - **Systemic:** Pulse, blood pressure (BP), respiratory rate (RR), pallor, and abdominal tenderness.
  - **Pelvic:**
    - Uterine size (correlate with gestational age).
    - Cervix: Os open (inevitable/incomplete) or closed (threatened/missed).
    - Adnexal mass/tenderness (rule out ectopic).
  - **Speculum:** Gentle examination to identify local causes (e.g., cervical polyp and erosion).[8]
- **Investigations (Table 2):**
  - **Biochemical:** Complete hemogram, blood group, β-hCG (serial if needed), blood sugar, creatinine, and thyroid-stimulating hormone (TSH).
  - **Ultrasound:** TVS preferred for intrauterine pregnancy (IUP) confirmation, fetal viability, subchorionic hematoma, or ectopic pregnancy.
  - **β-hCG Correlation:** Guides diagnosis when TVS is inconclusive.[9]

Classification and Management

Based on TVS findings, patients are categorized into three groups for management **(Table 3)**.

Specific Management of Spontaneous Abortion

- **Threatened Abortion:**
  - **Definition:** Bleeding with closed cervix, viable IUP on TVS (fetal cardiac activity present).

TABLE 2: β-hCG and TVS correlation for pregnancy diagnosis.[9]

Structure	*Gestational age*	*β-hCG level (mIU/mL)*	*TVS/TAS threshold*
Gestational sac	4–5 weeks	1,000–1,800	TVS: 1,000; TAS: 1,800
Yolk sac	5–6 weeks	1,000–7,200	TVS
Fetal pole	5–7 weeks	7,200–10,800	TVS
Cardiac activity	7 weeks	>10,800	TVS

TABLE 3: Management of first-trimester bleeding based on TVS findings.[5]

TVS finding	*Diagnosis*	*Management*
Viable IUP	Threatened abortion	Conservative (progesterone rest)
Nonviable IUP	Inevitable/incomplete/missed abortion, and GTN	Medical (misoprostol) or surgical (D&C)
Empty uterus	Complete abortion and ectopic pregnancy	Observation (complete); β-hCG monitoring, and medical/surgical (ectopic)

- **Management:**
  - **Rest:** Bedrest not mandatory but advised for heavy bleeding.
  - **Progesterone:**
    - **Natural Micronized Progesterone (NMP):** Vaginal (200–400 mg daily) or oral (100–300 mg sustained-release) until 12 weeks. Injectable NMP (100 mg IM daily) for acute bleeding, then oral/vaginal maintenance.
    - **Dydrogesterone:** Oral 40 mg stat, then 10 mg twice/thrice daily until 12 weeks. No androgenic or cardiovascular side effects.[10]
  - **Tranexamic Acid:** 500–1,000 mg oral/IV for heavy bleeding (off-label use).
  - **Discontinue Aspirin:** If patient is on low-dose aspirin, stop until bleeding resolves.
  - **Monitoring:** Weekly TVS and β-hCG if bleeding persists. Repeat TVS in 2 weeks if cardiac activity absent by 7 weeks but sac present.[11]
- **Outcome:** 50–70% continue to term; risk of miscarriage increases with heavy bleeding or subchorionic hematoma.[12]

- **Inevitable/Incomplete/Missed Abortion:**
  - **Definition:**
    - **Inevitable:** Open cervix, heavy bleeding, and imminent loss.
    - **Incomplete:** Partial POC expulsion, open cervix.
    - **Missed:** Nonviable IUP with retained POC, closed cervix.
  - **Management Options:**
    - **Medical** (Gestational age <7 weeks)**:**
      - **Misoprostol:** 400–800 mcg vaginally/orally, single or repeat dose after 3 hours. Antiemetic (e.g., ondansetron) advised. Success rate: 80–90%.[13]
      - Contraindications: Hemodynamic instability, infection, and allergy to misoprostol.

- **Surgical:**
  - **Dilatation and Curettage (D&C):** Preferred for heavy bleeding, infection, or patient preference. Performed under anesthesia; success rate: 95–99%.[14]
  - Risks: Uterine perforation (<1%), infection (2–5%).
- **Expectant:**
  - Suitable for stable patients without infection, preferring noninvasive approach.
  - Monitor with weekly TVS, coagulation profile, and symptoms. Most expulsions occur within 2 weeks (success rate: 50–70%).[15]
  - Risks: Prolonged bleeding, infection (1–3%).

- **USG Criteria for Nonviability (<10 Weeks):**
  - Gestational sac ≥25 mm, no embryo/yolk sac.
  - Crown-rump length (CRL) ≥7 mm, no cardiac activity.
  - Gestational sac <5 mm.
  - Fetal bradycardia <80 bpm.[16]
- **Complete Abortion:**
  - **Definition:** Full POC expulsion, empty uterus on TVS, closed cervix.
  - **Management:**
    - Confirm with TVS and declining β-hCG.
    - Observation; no intervention unless bleeding persists.
    - Antibiotics (e.g., doxycycline) if infection suspected.[17]
- **Postabortion Care:**
  - **Antibiotics:** Doxycycline 100 mg twice daily for 5–7 days to prevent infection.
  - **Contraception:** Initiate immediately (e.g., oral contraceptives, IUD); advise 3-month delay before next pregnancy.
  - **Rh Prophylaxis:** Anti-D immunoglobulin (50–100 mcg IM) within 72 hours for Rh-negative women.[18]

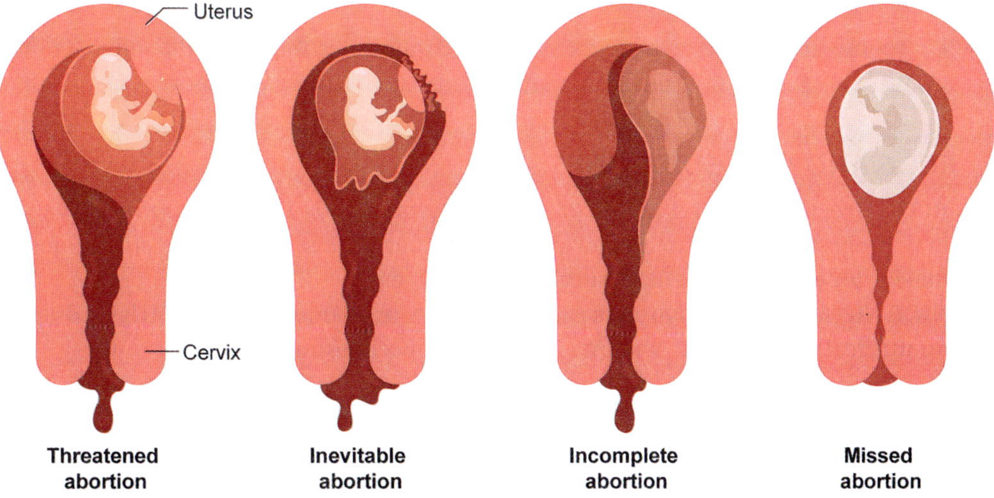

Fig. 1: Different types of abortion.

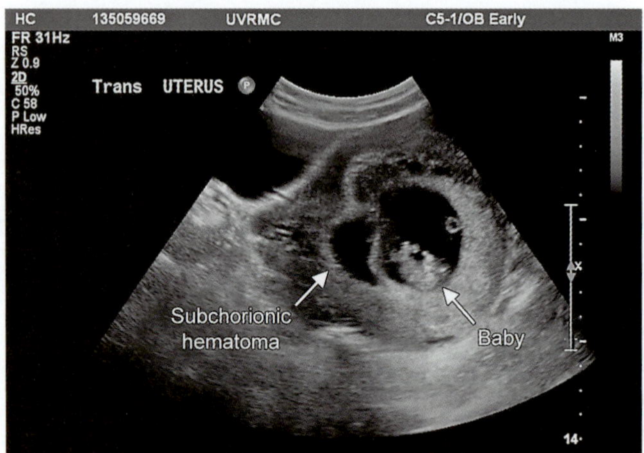

Fig. 2: Subchorionic hematoma.

- **Investigation for Recurrent Loss:** Karyotyping of POC (if ≥2 losses), parental karyotyping if POC not available, screen for antiphospholipid syndrome (APLA), thyroid disorders, diabetes.[19]
- **Counseling:** Address psychological impact; refer to support groups if needed.

- **Subchorionic Hematoma:**
  - **Definition:** Blood collection between chorion and myometrium, seen in 5–10% of pregnancies.
  - **Risks:** Increased miscarriage risk (20–30%) if behind placenta or large (>50% of sac).[20]
  - **Management:** Same as threatened abortion (progesterone, rest). Monitor with TVS every 1–2 weeks.
- **Local Causes:**
  - **Evaluation:** Gentle speculum examination to identify cervical/vaginal lesions (e.g., polyp, erosion, cervicitis).
  - **Management:** Treat specific cause (e.g., antibiotics for cervicitis, polypectomy for bleeding polyp). Rule out malignancy in persistent cases.[21]

RCOG AND NICE GUIDELINES

- **RCOG Green-top Guideline No. 25 (2023):** Recommends TVS as the primary diagnostic tool, progesterone for threatened abortion with prior miscarriage, and shared decision-making for expectant/medical/surgical management.[5]
- **NICE NG126 (2023):** Advocates early pregnancy assessment units (EPAUs), misoprostol for medical management, and psychological support postmiscarriage.[6]

KEY POINTS FOR SPONTANEOUS ABORTION

- Incidence of first-trimester bleeding: 15–25%; miscarriage risk: 30–50% with heavy bleeding.
- Causes include implantation bleeding, abortions (threatened, inevitable, incomplete, complete, and missed), GTN, ectopic pregnancy, and local lesions.

- Diagnosis relies on history, pelvic exam, TVS, and β-hCG.
- Threatened abortion: Progesterone (NMP or dydrogesterone), rest, and monitoring.
- Inevitable/incomplete/missed abortion: Medical (misoprostol <7 weeks), surgical (D&C), or expectant management.
- Post-abortion care: Antibiotics, contraception, Rh prophylaxis, and investigation for recurrent loss.
- RCOG/NICE emphasize patient-centered care and early assessment.

SHORT QUESTION

Gestational Trophoblastic Neoplasia

- **Definition:** A spectrum of trophoblastic disorders, including hydatidiform mole (complete/partial), invasive mole, and choriocarcinoma. Incidence: 1–2 per 1,000 pregnancies.[22]
- **Classification (Table 4):**
  - **Complete Mole:** No fetal tissue, diploid (46XX, paternal origin).
  - **Partial Mole:** Fetal tissue present, triploid (69XXX/XXY).
  - **Invasive Mole/Choriocarcinoma:** Malignant, invasive forms.
- **Management:**
  - **Baseline Evaluation:** β-hCG, chest X-ray, complete blood count, thyroid function, and liver/renal function.
  - **Suction Evacuation:** Preferred for molar pregnancy, regardless of uterine size. Risks: Embolization (1–2%) and thyroid storm (<1%).[23]
  - **Monitoring:** Weekly β-hCG until three consecutive normal values, then monthly for 6–12 months.
  - **Chemotherapy:** Methotrexate or actinomycin-D for persistent β-hCG or malignant GTN (FIGO staging). Success rate: 90–95%.[24]
  - **Contraception:** Barrier methods or oral contraceptives for 6–12 months postnormalization of β-hCG.
  - **Rare Cases:** Twin pregnancy with mole and normal fetus may continue with amniocentesis for fetal karyotyping if maternal status stable.[25]

TABLE 4: Features of GTN.[22]

Type	*Clinical Features*	*USG Findings*	*β-hCG Levels*
Complete mole	Large uterus, bleeding, vesicles, hyperemesis, and hyperthyroidism	Snowstorm appearance and theca lutein cysts	>100,000 mIU/mL
Partial mole	Bleeding and absent fetal heart	Partial molar tissue and fetus	10,000–100,000 mIU/mL
Choriocarcinoma	Metastases (lung and brain) and bleeding	Heterogeneous mass	Variable and high

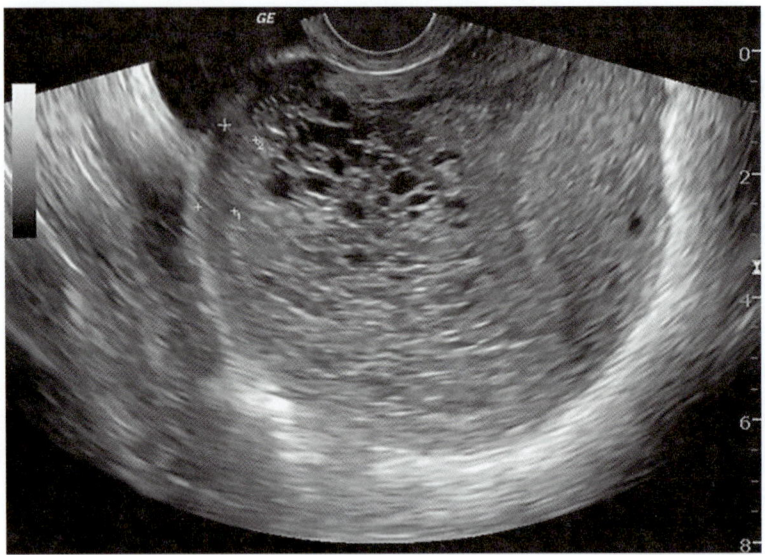

Fig. 3: Snowstorm appearance of complete molar pregnancy.

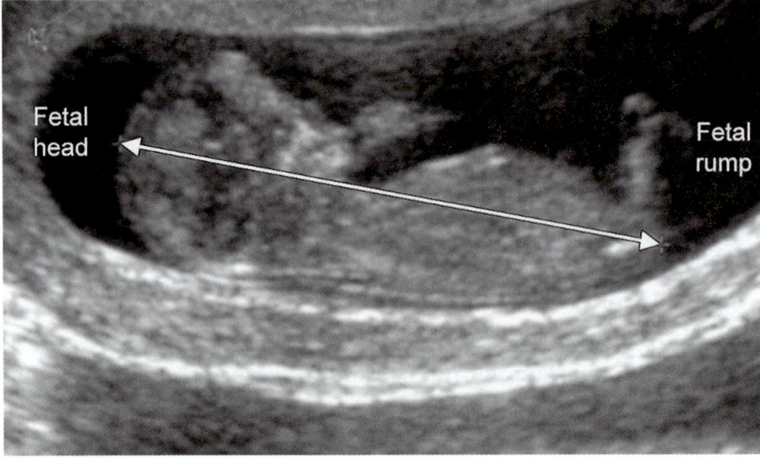

Fig. 4: CRL measurement.

Importance of Ultrasound in First-trimester Bleeding

- **Role:** TVS is the gold standard for diagnosing first-trimester bleeding, distinguishing viable from nonviable pregnancies and identifying causes **(Table 5)**.
- **CRL Measurement**
- **Key Findings:**
    - **Gestational Sac:** Seen at 4.4–4.6 weeks, grows 1 mm/day, double-ring sign.
    - **Yolk Sac:** Appears at 5–6 weeks; irregular shape suggests aneuploidy.

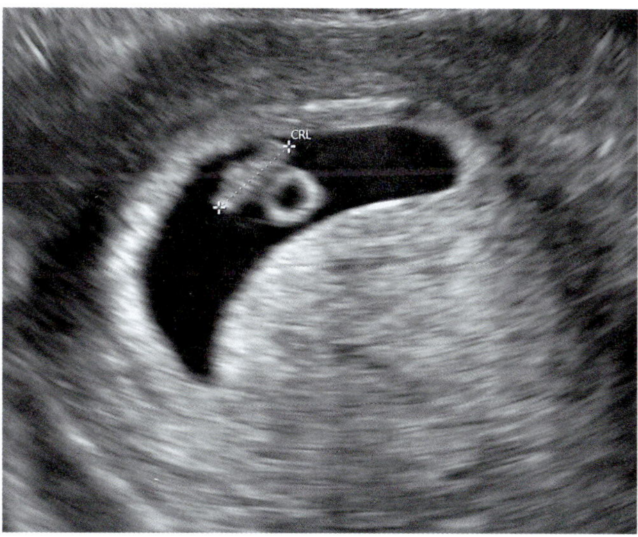

Fig. 5: Fetal pole.

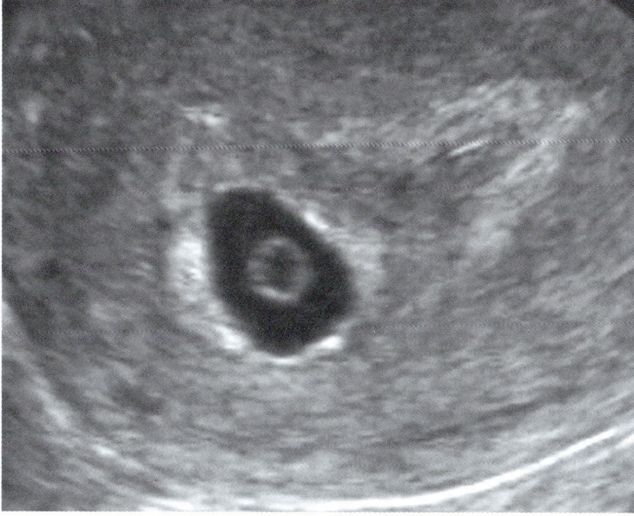

Fig. 6: Pregnancy failure.

- **Fetal Pole:** CRL ≥5 mm with cardiac activity by 7 weeks indicates viability.
- **Subchorionic Hematoma:** Assess size and location.
- Pregnancy Failure

- **Criteria for Poor Outcome (<10 Weeks):**
  - Gestational sac >20 mm, no embryo/yolk sac.
  - CRL <6 mm, no cardiac activity.
  - Sac diameter <5 mm.
  - Fetal bradycardia <80 bpm.[26]

TABLE 5: TVS Findings in first-trimester bleeding.[26]

Finding	*Implication*	*Management*
Viable IUP	Threatened abortion	Progesterone, monitoring
Nonviable IUP	Missed/inevitable abortion	Medical/surgical
Empty uterus	Complete abortion/ectopic	β-hCG, medical/surgical
Snowstorm	GTN	Suction evacuation

TABLE 6: Progesterone preparations for first-trimester bleeding.[29]

Type	*Route*	*Dose*	*Advantages*	*Side effects*
NMP	Vaginal	200–400 mg/day	High endometrial concentration	Minimal
NMP	Oral	100–300 mg/day	Convenient	Nausea, sedation
NMP	IM	100 mg/day	Rapid onset	Pain, rare abscess
Dydrogesterone	Oral	10–40 mg/day	No androgenic effects	None significant

- **Follow-up:** Repeat TVS in 7 days if inconclusive; nuchal translucency scan at 11–14 weeks for aneuploidy risk.[27]

Role of Progesterone in First-trimester Bleeding

- **Function:** Progesterone supports implantation, endometrial growth, and pregnancy maintenance. Levels <6–10 ng/mL at 6 weeks suggest nonviable pregnancy.[28]
- **Indications:** Threatened abortion, recurrent miscarriage, and luteal phase defect.
- **Preparations (Table 6):**
  - **NMP:** Vaginal (200–400 mg daily), oral (100–300 mg sustained-release), or injectable (100 mg IM daily for acute bleeding).
  - **Dydrogesterone:** Oral 40 mg stat, then 10 mg twice/thrice daily; no androgenic effects.
- **Administration:**
  - Vaginal: First uterine pass effect, high endometrial concentration, and minimal systemic side effects.
  - Oral: Convenient, but sedative effects (e.g., nausea and headache).
  - Injectable: Rapid onset, used for acute bleeding; rarely causes abscess.
- **Duration:** Continue until 12–14 weeks (placental takeover).
- **Evidence:** Reduces miscarriage risk in threatened abortion (30–40%) and recurrent loss (50–60%).[29]
- **Side Effects:** Minimal with NMP/dydrogesterone; no fetal cardiovascular risks.[30]

Recurrent Pregnancy Loss in First-trimester

- **Definition:** ≥2 consecutive pregnancy losses before 20 weeks, documented by USG or histopathology. Evaluation may start after two losses in high-risk cases (e.g., maternal age >40).[31]

TABLE 7: Causes and investigations for RPL.[31]

Cause	*Investigations*	*Treatment*
Genetic	POC/parental karyotyping and PGD	ART with PGD
Endocrine	TSH, HbA1c, and prolactin	Correct disorder
Thrombophilia	APLA and thrombophilia profile	LMWH + aspirin
Uterine	3D USG and hysteroscopy	Surgical correction
Unexplained	Lifestyle modification	Progesterone prophylaxis

- **Causes (Table 7):**
  - **Genetic:** Aneuploidy (50–60%) and parental translocations (<5%).
  - **Endocrine:** Diabetes, thyroid disorders, hyperprolactinemia, and PCOS.
  - **Thrombophilia:** Antiphospholipid syndrome (APLA), inherited thrombophilias.
  - **Uterine:** Anomalies (e.g., septum) and fibroids.
  - **Lifestyle:** Smoking, alcohol, BMI >25, and heavy exertion.
  - **Unexplained:** 30–40% of cases.

- **Management:**
  - **Lifestyle:** Smoking cessation, alcohol avoidance, and weight optimization (BMI 18.5–24.9).
  - **Investigations:** TSH, HbA1c, prolactin, APLA, thrombophilia profile, 3D USG, and parental karyotyping. POC karyotyping after ≥3 losses; consider immunological tests (e.g., ANA) in rare cases.
  - **Treatment:**
    - **Genetic:** Preimplantation genetic diagnosis (PGD) via ART.
    - **APLA:** Low-molecular-weight heparin (LMWH) + low-dose aspirin.
    - **Endocrine:** Correct thyroid/diabetes/PCOS.
    - **Uterine:** Surgical correction (e.g., septoplasty).
    - **Unexplained:** Progesterone (NMP or dydrogesterone) from conception to 12 weeks; psychological support.[32]
  - **Prognosis:** 60–70% live birth rate with appropriate management.[33]

Key Points

- First-trimester bleeding (15–25%) may indicate implantation, abortion, GTN, ectopic, or local causes.
- TVS and β-hCG are critical for diagnosis; TVS identifies viable vs. nonviable pregnancies.
- Threatened abortion: Progesterone (NMP/dydrogesterone) reduces miscarriage risk.
- Inevitable/incomplete/missed abortion: Medical (misoprostol), surgical (D&C), or expectant management.
- GTN: Suction evacuation, β-hCG monitoring, and chemotherapy for persistent disease.
- RPL: Investigate after ≥2 losses; treat genetic, endocrine, thrombophilic, or uterine causes.
- RCOG/NICE guidelines emphasize early assessment, patient choice, and psychological support.

REFERENCES

1. Everett C. Incidence and outcome of bleeding before 20 weeks. BMJ 2015;351:h3518.
2. Hasan R, Baird DD, et al. Patterns of vaginal bleeding in early pregnancy. Obstet Gynecol 2017;130(2):433-41.
3. Breeze C, Lees C. Bleeding in early pregnancy: Risks. BJOG. 2019;126(5):604-10.
4. Barnhart KT. Diagnostic tests for early pregnancy bleeding. N Engl J Med. 2016;375(8):757-64.
5. Royal College of Obstetricians and Gynaecologists. Green-top Guideline No. 25: Early Pregnancy Loss; 2023.
6. National Institute for Health and Care Excellence. NG126: Ectopic Pregnancy and Miscarriage; 2023.
7. Farquharson RG, Jauniaux E. Clinical assessment of early pregnancy bleeding. Hum Reprod Update. 2015;21(6):832-41.
8. Jurkovic D, Overton C. Pelvic examination in early pregnancy. Ultrasound Obstet Gynecol. 2018;51(3):287-93.
9. Doubilet PM, Benson CB. β-hCG and ultrasound in early pregnancy. Radiology. 2016;280(2):349-57.
10. Coomarasamy A, Devall AJ, et al. Progesterone for threatened miscarriage. N Engl J Med 2020;382(23):2234-44.
11. NICE. Progesterone in early pregnancy bleeding. BJOG. 2021;128(8):1033-9.
12. Tuuli MG, Norman SM. Subchorionic hematoma and pregnancy outcome. Am J Obstet Gynecol. 2016;215(4):515.e1-8.
13. Zhang J, Gilles JM, et al. Misoprostol for early pregnancy loss. N Engl J Med 2015;372(11):1028-35.
14. Tulandi T, Al-Fozan HM. Surgical management of miscarriage. Clin Obstet Gynecol. 2018;61(3):514-21.
15. Elson CJ, Salim R. Expectant management of miscarriage. Lancet. 2017;389(10076):1351-8.
16. Doubilet PM, Benson CB. Ultrasound criteria for pregnancy failure. Ultrasound Q 2019;35(2):114-20.
17. ACOG. Post-abortion care. Obstet Gynecol. 2018;132(5):e194-200.
18. RCOG. Rh prophylaxis in early pregnancy. BJOG. 2016;123(8):1255-61.
19. Practice Committee of ASRM. Evaluation of recurrent pregnancy loss. Fertil Steril. 2017;108(6):933-41.
20. Johns J, Jauniaux E. Subchorionic hematoma and miscarriage risk. Ultrasound Obstet Gynecol. 2015;46(6):652-8.
21. Lumsden MA, Norman JE. Cervical causes of bleeding in pregnancy. BJOG. 2017;124(9):1305-11.
22. Seckl MJ, Sebire NJ. Gestational trophoblastic disease. Lancet. 2016;388(10057):1803-12.
23. Lurain JR. Management of molar pregnancy. J Reprod Med. 2015;60(5-6):194-200.
24. Alazzam M, Tidy J, et al. Chemotherapy for GTN. Cochrane Database Syst Rev. 2016;5:CD008528.
25. Suksai M, Suwanrath C. Twin pregnancy with molar pregnancy. J Perinat Med. 2018;46(7):785-90.
26. Bottomley C, Bourne T. Ultrasound in early pregnancy bleeding. Best Pract Res Clin Obstet Gynaecol. 2016;34:79-89.
27. Nicolaides KH. First-trimester screening for aneuploidy. N Engl J Med. 2015;373(17):1649-58.
28. Yovich JL, Conceicao JL. Progesterone in early pregnancy. Hum Reprod. 2016;31(8):1641-8.
29. Devall AJ, Papadopoulou A. Progesterone for miscarriage prevention. BJOG. 2021;128(7):1115-22.
30. Wahabi HA, Fayed AA. Dydrogesterone in threatened abortion. Cochrane Database Syst Rev. 2017;10:CD013697.
31. ESHRE. Recurrent pregnancy loss: Guideline. Hum Reprod Open. 2018;2018(2):hoy004.
32. Bender Atik R, Christiansen OB. Management of RPL. Lancet 2020;395(10222):601-12.
33. Coomarasamy A, Dhillon-Smith RK. RPL: Outcomes. N Engl J Med. 2021;385(12):1132-40.

Recurrent Pregnancy Loss

Ruchika Garg

MULTIPLE CHOICE QUESTIONS

1. **What percentage of recurrent miscarriage is due to antiphospholipid syndrome?**
   a. 5%
   b. 15%
   c. 20%
   d. 30%

2. **What is the incidence of recurrent pregnancy loss?**
   a. 1%
   b. 5%
   c. 10%
   d. 15%

3. **After three first-trimester miscarriages, the chance of a future successful pregnancy is:**
   a. 50%
   b. 60%
   c. 70%
   d. 80%

4. **The most common congenital uterine anomaly in recurrent miscarriage patients is:**
   a. Unicornuate
   b. Septate
   c. Bicornuate
   d. Arcuate

5. **Which of the following is not a diagnostic criterion for APS?**
   a. Recurrent thrombosis
   b. Pregnancy morbidity
   c. Positive APKL antibody on two occasions
   d. Positive ds-DNA antibody

6. **The best treatment for unexplained recurrent first-trimester miscarriage is:**
   a. Aspirin
   b. Aspirin + LMWH
   c. Progesterone
   d. Reassurance and support

7. **Chances of having a healthy baby in parental balanced translocation is:**
   a. 20%
   b. 40%
   c. 60%
   d. 80%

8. **Which of the following is an acquired thrombophilia?**
   a. Protein S deficiency
   b. Protein C deficiency
   c. APLA syndrome
   d. Factor V Leiden mutation

9. **Cytogenetic analysis of pregnancy tissue is to be done in all, *except*:**
   a. First miscarriage
   b. Third miscarriage
   c. Beyond third miscarriage
   d. Second trimester loss

10. The first-line investigation for suspected congenital uterine anomaly in recurrent miscarriage is:

a. Hysterosalpingogram
b. 3D USG
c. MRI
d. Laparoscopy

11. The recommended endocrine test in a woman with recurrent miscarriage is:

a. Thyroid function test
b. Prolactin
c. HbA1C
d. Progesterone

12. The following are risk factors for recurrent miscarriage, *except*:

a. Smoking
b. Advanced maternal age
c. Advanced paternal age
d. Consanguinity

Explanations

Ans. 1 b. 15%

Ans. 2 a. 1%

Ans. 3 b. 60%

Ans. 4 b. Septate

Ans. 5 d. Positive ds-DNA antibody

Ans. 6 d. Reassurance and support

Ans. 7 c. 60%

Ans. 8 c. APLA syndrome

Ans. 9 a. First miscarriage

Ans. 10 b. 3D USG

Ans. 11 a. Thyroid function test

Ans. 12 d. Consanguinity

SHORT QUESTIONS AND ANSWERS

1. Write a short note on antiphospholipid syndrome. ***(MGRMU, oct 2018)***

Ans. The antiphospholipid syndrome is an immunological condition with autoantibodies against the phospholipid binding proteins. It is characterized by unexplained thrombosis and pregnancy-related complications. Treatment is variable depending on the clinical presentation.

Diagnosis is by the revised "Sapporo's criteria", which requires at least one clinical and laboratory criterion to be positive.

Clinical Criteria

- One or more unexplained fetal deaths of a morphologically normal fetus at gestation >10 weeks
- One or more preterm births of morphologically normal neonates before 34 weeks of gestation, secondary to eclampsia, severe preeclampsia, or placental insufficiency

Three or more consecutive spontaneous pregnancy losses <10 weeks after excluding anatomic and hormonal abnormalities in the mother and parental chromosomal abnormalities.

Laboratory Criteria

- Detection of anticardiolipin antibody IgG and IgM
- Detection of lupus anticoagulant
- Detection of β2 glycoprotein antibody IgG or IgM. These tests are to be done twice 6 weeks apart, because a low positive level due to any viral illness may revert to normal.

Management

- Women with APLA should avoid estrogen-containing hormonal contraceptives.
- Low-dose aspirin 75 mg orally and unfractionated heparin or LMWH 40 mg subcutaneously from a positive pregnancy test till at least 34 weeks of gestation
- Antenatal surveillance is required to prevent any complications.
- Heparin to be stopped before the labor to minimize the risk of bleeding
- Aspirin can be stopped any time after 36 weeks of gestation at least 7–10 days before delivery.
- Anticoagulant prophylaxis is also recommended in the postpartum period to prevent deep vein thrombosis and cortical venous thrombosis.

2. Write a short note on the cervical encerclage. ***(MS, MGRMU)***

Ans. Cervical cerclage is a surgical method of reinforcing a weak or incompetent cervix with a suture, in an attempt to prolong the pregnancy. It is typically done after 12 weeks of gestation but not later than 24 weeks, benefits being improved pregnancy outcome in up to 80–90% cases.

Indications

- History of recurrent second-trimester losses or preterm births due to cervical insufficiency
- Short cervical length >25 mm before 24 weeks
- Previous cervical surgery such as Cone biopsy, LEEP, forcible dilatation of cervix, and amputation of the cervix in Manchester operation done for the collapse

Prerequisites

- Confirm the viability of pregnancy.
- Exclude major congenital anomalies.
- Any infection should be treated.

Procedure

Cerclage is done under regional or general anesthesia:

- McDonald's suture: A No. 2 monofilament nonabsorbable purse string suture is placed above the external os and the knot is tied posterior to the cervix, thereby tightening the internal os.
- Shirodkar's stitch: It is a more complex stitch involving dissecting the bladder away.
- Emergency/rescue cerclage: It is done with cervical dilation and bulging bag of membranes, benefits being controversial. Trendelenburg's position and filling the bladder with saline helps in containing the BOM. The techniques need high expertise, and there is an increased risk of rupture of membranes and chorioamnionitis.

Complications

The risks with cerclage are inadvertent cervical injury, rupture of membranes, chorioamnionitis and preterm labor. When complications occur or if the uterine contraction starts, the stitch has to be cut immediately. If not, the suture is removed at 36–37 weeks.

In conclusion, cervical encerclage is a vital intervention in a woman with cervical insufficiency to achieve a successful pregnancy outcome.

3. What is the basis of genetic testing in couple with recurrent pregnancy losses?

(Manipal University)

Ans. Chromosomal abnormalities in pregnancy are the most common cause of recurrent miscarriage, contributing to over 50% of first-trimester losses, and becoming less prevalent in second-trimester losses. The most common chromosomal abnormality detected at karyotyping is "numerical" termed "aneuploidy", occurring as a result of the nondisjunction of chromosomes during meiosis. The most commonly encountered aberration is trisomy (51%) followed by polyploidy (18%), and monosomy (15%), while structural chromosomal abnormalities contribute to around 6.5%. Most often, these aneuploidies occur due to some error in gametogenesis namely nondisjunction, translocations, duplications, deletions, or insertions of a segment of chromosome. Hence, as a result of numerical or structural imbalance in the oocyte or sperm, an abnormal embryo is formed, thereby increasing the risk of miscarriage. Parental chromosomal rearrangements can also lead to embryonic aneuploidy (2% –5% of recurrent miscarriage). Gene mutations in women have also been implicated with loci identified on chromosome 9. An increase in maternal and paternal age has also been shown to have a strong association with an increased risk of miscarriage.

Cytogenetic analysis of the pregnancy tissue should be done in the third and subsequent miscarriage and in any second-trimester miscarriage, in combination with other routine investigations. Whenever this detects an unbalanced chromosomal abnormality, parental peripheral blood karyotyping has to be performed. Karyotyping of products of conception can give inconclusive or false negative results due to a lack of fetal cells or contamination with maternal cells. In such situations, or whenever the pregnancy tissue is not available for testing, then parental karyotyping should be offered. If there is an abnormal karyotype, genetic counseling, IVF with preimplantation genetic testing (PGT), and familial chromosomal studies are to be offered. The various techniques used are FISH, array comparative genomic hybridization (array CGH), single nucleotide polymorphism (SNP) assay, and next-generation sequencing (NGS). Genetic testing in recurrent miscarriage is an area with plenty of scope for research, which may enable targeted interventions to help couples achieve a successful pregnancy outcome.

LONG QUESTIONS AND ANSWERS

1. (A) Define recurrent pregnancy loss and discuss etiological factors?
(B) How will you evaluate a couple with recurrent pregnancy loss?

(DNB April, Dec 2016)

Ans. (A) Recurrent miscarriage, also known as recurrent pregnancy loss, is typically defined as the occurrence of three or more consecutive pregnancy losses before 24 weeks of gestation

(RCOG, 2023). This condition affects 1% of women. It can be emotionally challenging for couples trying to conceive.

The definitions are varied and clinicians have to use their clinical discretion if they want to evaluate the couple after 2 losses. The ASRM (American Society of Reproductive Medicine) has recommended evaluation after 2 first trimester clinical pregnancy losses (Those documented by ultrasound or histopathological examination). Also, the ESHRE 2017 guidelines (European Society for Human Reproduction and Embryology) have come up with a definition of 2 or more pregnancy losses.

Etiology

Recurrent pregnancy loss is characterized by multifactorial etiology.

- *Epidemiological factors:* Advanced maternal age, advanced paternal age, number of previous miscarriages, black ethnicity smoking, excessive alcohol consumption, excess caffeine intake, and women with BMI <19 or >25 kg/m^2.
- *Autoimmune:*
    - Acquired thrombophilia: Antiphospholipid antibody syndrome, defined as the association between aPL antibodies—lupus anticoagulant (LAC), anticardiolipin antibodies (IgM and IgG) and β2 glycoprotein antibodies with adverse pregnancy outcome and recurrent vascular thrombosis.
    - Inherited thrombophilia: Factor V Leiden mutation, protein C and S deficiency, antithrombin III deficiency and prothrombin gene mutation have been implicated as a cause of recurrent miscarriage. The underlying pathology is thrombosis of the utero placental circulation, which is detrimental to the fetus. Second trimester miscarriages are more common with this condition than first trimester losses.
- *Genetic:*
    - Parental chromosomal abnormalities, the most common being reciprocal translocation.
    - Fetal chromosomal abnormalities, trisomy being the most common followed by aneuploidy.
- *Anatomic:*
    - Most common congenital uterine anomaly implied in recurrent 1st trimester miscarriage is the canalization defects (septate) followed by unification defects (bicornuate and unicornuate). There has also been an association with increased 2nd trimester miscarriages.
    - Cervical insufficiency is another proven cause of 2nd trimester miscarriages. Other acquired causes for 2nd trimester losses are adenomyosis, fibroids, uterine synechiae, and polyps.
- *Endocrine:* Hyperprolactinemia, uncontrolled diabetes mellitus, thyroid dysfunction, polycystic ovarian disease and luteal phase defects have been shown to have some association with recurrent miscarriages.
- *Infections:* Bacterial vaginosis and chlamydia
- Male factors like ↑sperm DNA fragmentation
- *Environmental factors:* Cigarette smoking is suggested to affect trophoblastic function and is linked to recurrent pregnancy loss. Other lifestyle habits such as excessive alcohol and caffeine consumption, cocaine use may also play a causative role.

(B) History and examination

A detailed history has to be obtained including a full medical, surgical, and menstrual history. Lifestyle habits such as smoking, alcohol, and drugs have to be noted. Personal and family history of thrombosis is a clue to an underlying thrombophilia.

All details of the previous pregnancy losses to be noted namely the gestational age, the pattern of loss, and the treatment offered. Any history of surgical evacuation in the past is important as excessive dilatation and curettage can predispose to cervical incompetence or Asherman's syndrome.

A complete physical examination is also to be done including a general and a pelvic examination.

Investigations

This depends on the pattern of the previous pregnancy losses, namely the gestation at which each loss occurred and if the fetus as viable or not.

Medical comorbidities

- Tests to rule out diabetes mellitus, thyroid dysfunction, and hyperprolactinemia
- Genetic testing
- Karyotype assessment of the couple to detect underlying translocations.
- Immunological workup
- Testing for antiphospholipid antibodies—lupus anticoagulant (LAC), anticardiolipin antibodies (ACL IgG and IgM), and anti β2 glycoprotein antibodies.
- Evaluation of products of consumption
- Recommended in two or more pregnancy losses (RCOG and ASRM)
- Assessment of uterine anomalies
- 3D pelvic ultrasound, hysterosalpingogram (HSG), saline infusion sonohysterography (SISH), Hysteroscopy, and MRI.

Investigations not of proven value and are not recommended routinely are serum progesterone levels, endometrial biopsy, TORCH serology, tests for syphilis, and routine vaginal/cervical cultures for chlamydia, gonorrhea, and bacterial vaginosis.

Pre-pregnancy counseling should be given based on the results of the investigations. Advice regarding lifestyle changes has to be given namely optimization of body weight, cessation of smoking, alcohol, and drugs. Any treatable medical comorbidities need to be addressed. Once the pregnancy is confirmed, the woman should get booked into a dedicated "recurrent pregnancy loss clinic" for close antenatal surveillance and further management.

2. (A) Define Cervical incompetence and add a note on its diagnosis.
(B) Management of cervical incompetence. ***(MS MGRMU, May 2022)***

Ans. (A) Cervical incompetence or insufficiency is the inability of the cervix to retain the fetus in the absence of uterine contractions or labor, owing to a functional or structural defect in the cervix.

It is characterized by a mid-trimester painless cervical dilatation, resulting in expulsion of usually a live fetus. The causes could be a congenital or structural abnormality in the cervix leading to weakness or acquired causes such as a previous cervical surgery such as cone biopsy or loop electrosurgical excision procedure (LEEP), forcible dilation of the cervix, and amputation of the cervix in Manchester's operation.

The diagnosis of cervical incompetence is possible by a good history and clinical examination. It occurs typically in early mid-trimester, and the woman usually has no pain with some reporting a pelvic pressure or backache with an excessive vaginal discharge. The speculum examination reveals a shortened cervix (an effacement ≥80%) and dilated to 2 cm or more with or without bulging membranes. There is also a possibility of an asymptomatic patient with a transvaginal scan finding showing a short cervix ≤2.5 cm or funneling in which there is ballooning of membranes into a dilated internal os, with a closed external os (ultrasound diagnosis).

There are no reliable tests to predict cervical incompetence in a nonpregnant woman.

The diagnosis is often made retrospectively if she has a history of recurrent mid-trimester losses, consistent with the features of cervical insufficiency (history-based diagnosis). However, certain investigations such as a transvaginal ultrasound or MRI can help identify congenital uterine malformations which may be associated with an anatomical or structural abnormality of the cervix and could lead to an incompetent cervix in pregnancy. A hysterosalpingogram (HSG) in the premenstrual phase has also been used as a diagnostic test. One other test described in the past is a passage of a number 6–8 Hegar's dilator beyond the internal os without any resistance and absence of internal os snap on withdrawal. Balloon elastance test in which the ability of cervix to hold an inflated foley's balloon has also been described, but these tests are not validated.

(B) Nonsurgical methods such as bed rest, activity restriction, and vaginal pessary have been tried but not evidence based. The goal standard treatment is surgical where a suture is tied at the cervicovaginal junction to tighten the cervix. This procedure is called "cervical encerclage", and the procedure can be done transvaginally or transabdominally. The cerclage can be offered to a pregnant woman in 3 scenarios, namely,

1. Clinical features of cervical incompetence in the mid-trimester
2. History indicated
3. Ultrasound indicated

McDonald's stitch is the most commonly performed procedure, where using a number 2 monofilament suture, 4–5 bites are taken as high as possible in the cervix, taking care to avoid injury to the bladder or the rectum. The knot is tied anteriorly to facilitate removal at term or when patient goes to labor earlier. The Shirodkar's stitch involves the dissection of the vesicocervical mucosa, separating the bladder away and placing a nonabsorbable suture as close to the internal os as possible. Care is taken to dissect away both the bladder and rectum cephalad to avoid injury and after the knot is tied; the mucosa is replaced over the knot. In a patient with bulging membranes, an emergency cerclage called the "rescue cerclage" may be applied. Techniques to reduce the bulging membranes are placing the patient in a Trendelenburg's position and by gently placing a foley's catheter with a 30 mL balloon through the cervix and inflating it. As the cerclage is tightened, the foley's bulb is deflated and is gradually removed, while the knot is secured. A sponge on a holder can also be used to gently reduce the bulging membranes as the stitch is being taken.

Transabdominal cerclage is reserved for selected cases with previous failed transvaginal cerclage or a damaged very short cervix. This can be done by an open or laparoscopic approach. It can be offered prior to conception or can be done in early pregnancy if the expertise is available.

Certain prerequisites for cerclage are confirming the viability of the pregnancy, exclusion of major congenital anomalies in the fetus and ruling out any active infection. The possible complications are accidental rupture of membranes, chorioamnitis, cervical injury and preterm labor. When complications occur or if the uterine contractions start, the stitch has to be cut immediately. If not, the suture is to be removed at 36–37 weeks. To conclude, cervical encerclage is an intervention of paramount importance in women with cervical insufficiency to achieve a successful pregnancy outcome.

SUGGESTED READING

1. Balkawade N, Raghu AK, Pai HD (Eds). FOGSI Focus on Recurrent Pregnancy loss (2024). New Delhi: Evangel Publishing; 2024.
2. Cunningham F, Leveno KJ, Dashe JS, et al. (Eds). Williams Obstetrics, 26th edition. New York, NY: McGraw Hill; 2022.
3. Dutta DC. DC Dutta's Textbook of Obstetrics Including Perinatology and Contraception, 8th edition. New Delhi: Jaypee Brothers Medical Publisher's Ltd.; 2015.
4. ESHRE. (2023). Guideline on the management of recurrent pregnancy loss—an update. [online] Available from https://www.eshre.eu/guidelines-and-legal/guidelines/recurrent-pregnancy-loss [Last accessed December, 2025].
5. Melo P, Dhillon-Smith R, Islam MA, et al. Genetic causes of sporadic and recurrent miscarriage. Fertil Steril. 2023;120(5):940-4.
6. Prabhu TRB (Ed). Mudaliar and Menon's Clinical Obstetrics, 13th edition. Hyderabad: University Press; 2023.
7. Royal College of Obstetricians and Gynaecologists. (2023). Recurrent miscarriage (Green-top Guideline No. 17). [online] Available from https://www.rcog.org.uk/guidance/browse-all-guidance/green-top-guidelines/recurrent-miscarriage-green-top-guideline-no-17/ [Last accessed December, 2025].

Maternal Anatomy and Physiology

Ruchika Garg

INTRODUCTION

Pregnancy induces profound physiological adaptations to support maternal health and fetal development. These changes begin early in gestation, peak in the third trimester, and generally resolve by 6–12 weeks postpartum. Understanding these adaptations is critical for postgraduate medical students to differentiate normal physiology from pathological conditions in pregnancy. This chapter outlines changes in the **cardiovascular**, **respiratory**, **renal**, and **endocrine** systems, presented in tables and bullet points for quick reference.

1. CARDIOVASCULAR SYSTEM

Pregnancy increases cardiovascular demand to meet the metabolic needs of the mother and fetus. Adaptations ensure adequate uteroplacental perfusion while maintaining maternal hemodynamic stability **(Table 1)**.

Key Points:

- **Hemodynamic Changes**:
  - CO increases due to HR and SV rise, peaking in the third trimester.
  - SVR decreases due to progesterone-mediated vasodilation and placental low-resistance circulation.
  - BP drops in the second trimester, with diastolic falling more than systolic.
- **Physiological Anemia**:
  - Disproportionate plasma volume increase dilutes red cell mass, lowering hemoglobin.
  - Hematocrit decreases to 32–34%; values <10.5 g/dL warrant investigation.
- **Clinical Implications**:
  - Normal findings: Soft systolic flow murmur (90% of pregnant women), S3 gallop, and mild cardiomegaly on imaging
  - Pathological signs: Diastolic murmurs, severe tachycardia, or heart failure symptoms require urgent evaluation.
  - **ACOG (2024)**: Pregnant women with preexisting cardiac conditions (e.g., valvular disease) need multidisciplinary care.
- **Labor and Postpartum**:
  - Labor increases CO by 60–80% due to autotransfusion and pain.
  - Postpartum, CO normalizes within 2–6 weeks as plasma volume decreases.

TABLE 1: Cardiovascular changes in pregnancy.

Parameter	*Change*	*Magnitude*	*Clinical relevance*
Cardiac output (CO)	Increases	+30–50% (peaks at 28–32 weeks)	Enhances uteroplacental perfusion; CO rises further in labor (+60–80%)
Heart rate (HR)	Increases	+10–20 bpm (15–25%)	Contributes to CO increase; tachycardia (>100 bpm) may suggest pathology
Stroke volume (SV)	Increases	+20–30%	Early rise in SV drives CO increase in first trimester
Systemic vascular resistance (SVR)	Decreases	–20–30%	Due to vasodilation from progesterone and nitric oxide; lowers blood pressure
Blood pressure (BP)	Decreases (mid-trimester), then normalizes	Systolic: –5–10 mm Hg Diastolic: –10–15 mm Hg	Nadir at 20–24 weeks; returns to pre-pregnancy levels by term
Plasma volume	Increases	+40–50% (1–1.5 L)	Supports CO and prevents hypovolemia; peaks at 32 weeks
Red blood cell mass	Increases	+20–30%	Less than plasma increase, causing physiological anemia (Hb 10.5–11 g/dL)
Left ventricular mass	Increases	+10–20%	Reflects cardiac remodeling; reverses postpartum.
Aortocaval compression	Occurs (late pregnancy)	Supine position	Reduces venous return and CO by 10–30%; managed by left lateral tilt.

2. RESPIRATORY SYSTEM

Respiratory adaptations in pregnancy enhance oxygen delivery to the fetus and remove carbon dioxide, compensating for increased maternal metabolic demands **(Table 2)**.

Key Points:

- **Ventilatory Changes**:
  - Progesterone increases respiratory drive, raising tidal volume and minute ventilation.
  - $PaCO_2$ decreases, causing compensated respiratory alkalosis (bicarbonate falls to 18–22 mEq/L).
- **Mechanical Changes**:
  - Diaphragm elevates by 4–5 cm due to gravid uterus, reducing FRC and RV.
  - Chest wall compliance increases, preserving TLC.
- **Clinical Implications**:
  - Dyspnea of pregnancy (60–70% of women) is normal, attributed to increased ventilatory drive.
  - Pathological dyspnea: Consider pulmonary edema, embolism, or asthma exacerbation.
  - **RCOG (2022)**: Pregnant women with respiratory conditions (e.g., asthma) require optimized management to prevent hypoxia.

TABLE 2: Respiratory changes in pregnancy.

Parameter	*Change*	*Magnitude*	*Clinical relevance*
Minute ventilation	Increases	+40–50%	Driven by progesterone-stimulated hyperventilation; starts in first trimester
Tidal volume (TV)	Increases	+30–40%	Main contributor to increased minute ventilation
Respiratory rate (RR)	Minimal change	±0–10%	Remains stable; tachypnea (>20 breaths/min) may indicate pathology.
$PaCO_2$ (arterial CO_2)	Decreases	28–32 mmHg (from 40 mmHg)	Compensated respiratory alkalosis (pH 7.40–7.45) due to hyperventilation
PaO_2 (arterial O_2)	Increases slightly	100–105 mm Hg	Enhances oxygen delivery to fetus
Functional residual capacity (FRC)	Decreases	−20–25%	Due to diaphragmatic elevation by gravid uterus
Residual volume (RV)	Decreases	−15–20%	Contributes to reduced FRC
Total lung capacity (TLC)	Minimal change	−0–5%	Preserved due to increased chest wall compliance
Oxygen consumption	Increases	+20–30%	Reflects higher metabolic demands of mother and fetus

- **Anesthesia Considerations**:
  - Reduced FRC and increased oxygen consumption increase risk of hypoxia during intubation
  - **ACOG (2025)**: Preoxygenation is critical for safe general anesthesia in CS.

3. RENAL SYSTEM

Renal adaptations in pregnancy support increased plasma volume, waste excretion, and fluid-electrolyte balance, driven by hormonal and hemodynamic changes **(Table 3)**.

Key Points:

- **Renal Hemodynamics**:
  - Increased CO and decreased SVR drive higher RPF and GFR, peaking by 16–20 weeks.
  - Reduced serum creatinine and urea are normal; elevated levels suggest pathology.
- **Tubular Function**:
  - Glycosuria occurs due to increased GFR exceeding glucose reabsorption capacity.
  - Mild proteinuria is normal; significant proteinuria (>300 mg/24 h) warrants preeclampsia evaluation.
- **Anatomical Changes**:
  - Progesterone relaxes ureteral smooth muscle, causing dilatation (right > left due to uterine dextrorotation).
  - Hydronephrosis increases risk of urinary stasis and infections (UTIs in 5–10% of pregnancies).

TABLE 3: Renal changes in pregnancy.

Parameter	*Change*	*Magnitude*	*Clinical relevance*
Glomerular filtration rate (GFR)	Increases	+40–60%	Peaks in second trimester; enhances clearance of waste products
Renal plasma flow (RPF)	Increases	+50–80%	Driven by increased CO and vasodilation; peaks in mid-pregnancy
Serum creatinine	Decreases	0.4–0.8 mg/dL (0.8–1.2)	Normal pregnancy value; levels >0.8 mg/dL suggest renal impairment
Serum urea	Decreases	2–4 mg/dL (4–7)	Reflects increased GFR and hemodilution
Proteinuria	Increases slightly	Up to 300 mg/24 h	Levels >300 mg/24 h suggest preeclampsia or renal disease.
Urine glucose	Increases (glycosuria)	Variable	Due to reduced tubular reabsorption; not indicative of diabetes unless persistent
Kidney size	Increases	+1–1.5 cm	Due to hypertrophy and increased blood flow; resolves postpartum
Ureteral dilatation	Occurs (hydronephrosis)	Right > left	Progesterone and uterine compression; increases UTI risk
Sodium reabsorption	Increases	+900 mEq total	Maintains plasma volume; aldosterone driven

- **Clinical Implications**:
  - **NICE (2024)**: Routine urinalysis is recommended to detect asymptomatic bacteriuria, treated to prevent pyelonephritis.
  - Preeclampsia monitoring: Persistent proteinuria, hypertension, or rising creatinine require urgent evaluation.
- **Fluid Balance**:
  - Increased sodium reabsorption (via aldosterone) supports plasma volume expansion.
  - Edema in 80% of pregnancies is normal; sudden onset suggests pathology.

4. ENDOCRINE SYSTEM

Endocrine adaptations in pregnancy regulate metabolism, growth, and parturition, driven by placental hormones and maternal glandular changes **(Table 4)**.

Key Points:

- **Thyroid Function**:
  - hCG mimics TSH, suppressing TSH and increasing fT4 in the first trimester.
  - TBG rises due to estrogen, increasing total T4/T3; fT4 remains stable.
  - **ACOG (2024)**: Use trimester-specific TSH and fT4 ranges to diagnose thyroid disorders (e.g., hypothyroidism: TSH >4 mIU/L).

TABLE 4: Endocrine changes in pregnancy.

Parameter	*Change*	*Magnitude*	*Clinical relevance*
Thyroid-stimulating hormone (TSH)	Decreases (1st trimester), then stabilizes	–20–50% (1st trimester)	Due to hCG stimulation; normalizes by 2nd trimester
Free T4 (fT4)	Minimal change	Within normal range	Maintains maternal and fetal metabolism; trimester-specific ranges needed
Total T4 and T3	Increases	+50%	Due to increased thyroid-binding globulin (TBG) from estrogen
Cortisol	Increases	+200–300%	Driven by placental CRH; free cortisol rises, mimicking Cushingoid state
Insulin sensitivity	Decreases (2nd–3rd trimester)	–50%	Due to placental hormones (hPL, cortisol); increases gestational diabetes risk
Human placental lactogen (hPL)	Increases	Peaks at term	Promotes insulin resistance and nutrient availability for fetus.
Prolactin	Increases	+10-fold	Prepares breasts for lactation; driven by estrogen and progesterone
Parathyroid hormone (PTH)	Decreases slightly	–10–20%	Calcium transfer to fetus increases maternal absorption; calcitriol rises.
Estrogen	Increases	+1000-fold	Drives uterine growth, TBG increase, and vascular changes; placental production
Progesterone	Increases	+10-fold	Maintains pregnancy, relaxes smooth muscle, and reduces uterine contractility

- **Adrenal Function**:
  - Placental corticotropin-releasing hormone (CRH) increases cortisol, supporting fetal lung maturation.
  - Cortisol binding globulin rises, but free cortisol doubles, causing mild hypercortisolism.
- **Glucose Metabolism**:
  - Placental hormones (hPL, cortisol, and progesterone) induce insulin resistance, peaking in the third trimester.
  - **NICE (2024)**: Screen for gestational diabetes mellitus (GDM) at 24–28 weeks with oral glucose tolerance test (OGTT).
- **Calcium Metabolism**:
  - Increased calcitriol (1,25-dihydroxyvitamin D) enhances maternal calcium absorption for fetal bone development.
  - PTH decreases slightly, but ionized calcium remains stable.

- **Placental Hormones**:
  - Estrogen and progesterone, produced by the placenta, support uterine growth and prevent preterm labor.
  - hPL ensures fetal nutrient supply by promoting maternal lipolysis and insulin resistance.
- **Clinical Implications**:
  - Thyroid disorders (e.g., hypothyroidism) affect 2–3% of pregnancies; untreated cases increase miscarriage risk.
  - GDM affects 5–10% of pregnancies; untreated GDM increases macrosomia and neonatal hypoglycemia risk.
  - **RCOG (2022)**: Hyperemesis gravidarum may mimic hyperthyroidism due to elevated hCG.

Clinical Considerations for Postgraduate Students:

- **Differentiating Normal versus Pathological Changes**:
  - Cardiovascular: Systolic murmurs are normal; diastolic murmurs or heart failure symptoms are not.
  - Respiratory: Dyspnea is common, but hypoxia or tachypnea suggests pathology.
  - Renal: Mild proteinuria is normal; levels >300 mg/24 h indicate preeclampsia.
  - Endocrine: Mild hypercortisolism is normal; overt Cushing's syndrome requires investigation.
- **Management Principles**:
  - Use pregnancy-specific reference ranges for laboratory tests (e.g., TSH, creatinine, and hemoglobin).
  - Monitor high-risk patients (e.g., cardiac or renal disease) with multidisciplinary teams.
  - **ACOG (2025)**: Tailor anesthesia and labor management to account for physiological changes (e.g., reduced FRC and aortocaval compression).
- **Postpartum Reversal**:
  - Most changes resolve by 6–12 weeks postpartum; persistent abnormalities (e.g., hypertension and proteinuria) warrant follow-up.
  - Lactation maintains prolactin elevation and may delay thyroid normalization.

CONCLUSION

Pregnancy induces dynamic physiological adaptations in the cardiovascular, respiratory, renal, and endocrine systems to support maternal and fetal demands. Cardiovascular changes increase CO and plasma volume, respiratory adaptations enhance ventilation, renal changes boost GFR, and endocrine shifts regulate metabolism and pregnancy maintenance. Postgraduate medical students must recognize these normal adaptations to identify pathological conditions promptly. Familiarity with pregnancy-specific reference ranges and guideline recommendations (e.g., ACOG, NICE, and RCOG) is essential for effective obstetric care.

Placental Development—Structure and Abnormalities

Ruchika Garg

DEVELOPMENT OF THE PLACENTA

Placental formation occurs in a stepwise process, completed by the 12th week of gestation.[1]

- **Trophectoderm Differentiation** (Days 6–8 postfertilization):
  - Trophectoderm forms the trophoblast, encircling the blastocyst.
  - Blastocyst implants into the uterine wall (decidua) by day 6–7.
  - By day 8, trophoblast differentiates into:
    - Outer multinucleated syncytiotrophoblast.
    - Inner mononuclear cytotrophoblast.[2]
- **Chorionic Villi Formation**:
  - **Primary Villus** (Days 12–13): Syncytiotrophoblast grows, forming lacunae (intervillous spaces) filled with maternal blood via endometrial vessel erosion. Cytotrophoblast forms a core within syncytial trabeculae.[3]
  - **Secondary Villus** (Day 16): Extraembryonic mesoderm invades primary villi.
  - **Tertiary Villus** (Day 21): Fetal blood vessels develop in mesoderm, forming an arterio-capillary-venous system; fetal blood circulates in villi, maternal blood in intervillous spaces.[4]
- **Cytotrophoblastic Shell**: Cytotrophoblast cells emerge through syncytium, forming a continuous layer isolating syncytium from decidua.[5]
- **Chorion Development**:
  - Villi contacting decidua basalis proliferate, forming chorion frondosum (leafy chorion).
  - Villi abutting decidua parietalis regress, forming avascular chorion laeve (smooth chorion).[6]
- **Anchoring Villi**: Connect fetal mesoderm to maternal cytotrophoblastic shell.[7]
- **Maternal Cotyledons**: Placenta divides into 15–20 lobes by maternal septa.[8]
- **Definitive Placenta**: Forms by week 6, completes by week 12 with fusion of decidua parietalis and capsularis.[9]

STRUCTURE OF PLACENTA AT TERM

- **Gross Anatomy**:
  - Discoid, weighs ~500 g (1/6th fetal weight), 15-20 cm diameter, 2.5 cm thick, and 500 mL volume.

TABLE 1: Layers of the mature placenta.[11]

Layer	*Components*
Amniotic Membrane	Single-layered cubical epithelium
Chorionic Plate	Syncytiotrophoblast, cytotrophoblast, extraembryonic mesoderm with umbilical vessels
Basal Plate	Decidua (compact/spongy), Nitabuch layer (fibrinoid degeneration), cytotrophoblastic shell, and syncytiotrophoblast
Intervillous Space	Branch villi from stem villi, filled with maternal blood
Stem (Anchoring) Villi	Arise from chorionic plate, extend to basal plate; 60–100 villi form fetal cotyledons (3–5 per maternal cotyledon)

 - 80% fetal origin, 20% maternal (decidua basalis, intervillous blood).[10]
- **Layers** are shown in **Table 1**.

PLACENTAL CIRCULATION

- **Uteroplacental Circulation** (700–900 mL/min at term):
  - **Arterial**: 100–200 spiral arteries deliver blood to intervillous space after trophoblastic invasion (by 12–16 weeks), converting them to low-resistance uteroplacental arteries.[12]
  - **Intervillous Space**: Blood disperses laterally, migrates to basal plate; replaced every 15–20 seconds.[13]
  - **Venous Drainage**: Uterine veins drain intervillous blood; closed during contractions, open during relaxation. Fibrinolytic enzymes prevent clotting.[14]
- **Fetoplacental Circulation**:
  - Two umbilical arteries carry deoxygenated fetal blood to placenta, branching into villous vessels.
  - Umbilical vein returns oxygenated blood to fetus, with countercurrent flow enhancing exchange.[15]

SHORT NOTE AND LONG ANSWER

Development of Placenta

Abnormalities of the Placenta

Classified into shape/size, implantation, degenerative lesions, circulatory disturbances, tumors, and cord insertion anomalies.[16]

- **Abnormal shape and size are shown in Table 2.**
- **Abnormal Implantation**:
  - **Placenta Previa**:
    - Definition: Placenta partially/completely covers cervical os; increases risk of placenta accreta spectrum (PAS).[18]
    - Risk Factors: Advanced maternal age, multiparity, smoking, uterine leiomyoma, prior cesarean, elevated maternal serum alpha-fetoprotein, and ART.[19]

TABLE 2: Abnormal placental shapes and sizes.[17]

Type	*Description*	*Clinical importance*
Bipartite/Bilobate	Partly divided into two lobes	Risk of lobe retention, postpartum hemorrhage (PPH)
Duplex	Completely divided into two lobes	Similar risks as bipartite
Tripartite/Triplex	Divided into three lobes	Retention risk
Multilobate	>3 lobes	Increased PPH risk
Succenturiate	Accessory lobe(s) in membranes, connected by vessels	Retention, PPH; placenta spuria (no vascular connection) possible
Ring-Shaped	Annular shape	Antepartum hemorrhage (APH), fetal growth restriction (FGR), and PPH
Membranous (Diffusa)	Chorion covered by functioning villi, thin on ultrasound	High PPH risk, placenta accreta, previa; difficult manual removal
Fenestrated	Hole/defect in placenta	May mimic missing lobe, no vessels
Extrachorial (Circumvallate)	Chorionic plate smaller than basal plate; amnion/chorion folded, forming a ring	Risks: Miscarriage, malformations, APH, preterm labor, FGR, and retention
Placenta Marginata	Thin fibrous ring at chorionic plate margin	Minimal clinical impact

- Clinical Features: Painless, profuse, and recurrent vaginal bleeding (maternal origin).[20]
- Treatment: Cesarean delivery for active bleeding; expectant management if bleeding subsides (<36 weeks); elective cesarean at 36–37 weeks.[21]

- **Placenta Accreta**:
  - Definition: Abnormal trophoblast invasion into myometrium.[22]
  - Risk Factors: Prior cesarean (0.3% risk with 1, 6.74% with ≥5), multiparity, uterine surgery, Asherman's syndrome, and placenta previa.[23]
  - Diagnosis: Ultrasound (vascular lacunae, loss of hypoechoic zone, and reduced myometrial thickness); MRI for confirmation.[24]
  - Treatment: Bedrest, hemoglobin optimization, cesarean hysterectomy at 34–35 weeks, and ICU monitoring postdelivery.[25]
- **Degenerative Lesions**: Include placental infarction, subchorionic/perivillous fibrin deposition, hematomas, and calcification.[26]
- **Circulatory Disturbances**:
  - **Placental Infarction**: Due to reduced maternal blood supply; extensive infarction causes placental insufficiency.[27]
  - **Fibrin Deposition**: Affects >25% of villi, linked to FGR and adverse neonatal outcomes.[28]
  - **Hematomas**: Retroplacental, marginal, subamnionic, and subchorial; associated with bleeding risks.[29]
  - **Calcification**: Common on basal plate, increases with gestation, smoking, and maternal hypercalcemia.[30]

- **Placental Tumors**:
  - **Chorioangioma**: Benign hamartoma (1% incidence); large tumors (>4 cm) cause hydramnios, APH, fetal heart failure, and hydrops. Management: Surveillance, intrauterine transfusion, steroids, or fetal surgery.[31]
  - **Metastatic Tumors**: Rare (melanomas, leukemias, and breast cancer); confined to intervillous space, rarely affect fetus.[32]
- **Cord Insertion Anomalies**:
  - **Battledore Placenta**: Marginal cord insertion; risks cord prolapse/compression in low-lying placenta.[33]
  - **Velamentous Cord Insertion**: Cord inserts into membranes (1% incidence); risks preterm labor, FGR, fetal distress, and vasa previa. Management: Steroids and elective cesarean at 34–37 weeks for vasa previa.[34]

SHORT QUESTIONS AND ANSWERS

1. Discuss the indications and Benefits of Pathological Examination of Placenta.[35]

Ans.

- **Indications**: Maternal (e.g., diabetes and hypertension), fetal (e.g., FGR and stillbirth), and placental abnormalities (e.g., previa and accreta).
- **Benefits**:
  - Clarifies causes of preterm delivery, FGR, and neurodevelopmental damage.
  - Aids diagnosis of gestational trophoblastic diseases (e.g., choriocarcinoma and PSTT).
  - Enhances understanding of pregnancy complications and prevention strategies.

2. Discuss the Functions of the Placenta.[36]

Ans.

- **Respiratory**: Oxygen delivery (8 mL/kg/min) and CO_2 removal via diffusion.
- **Nutritive**: Transfers glucose (facilitated diffusion via GLUT-1/GLUT-3), amino acids (active transport), lipids, water, and electrolytes.
- **Excretory**: Removes urea, uric acid, and creatinine via diffusion.
- **Immunological**: Protects against paternal antigens.
- **Endocrine**: Produces estrogen, progesterone, hPL, and hCG; minimal transfer of maternal hormones.
- **Enzymatic**: Inactivates oxytocin (oxytocinase), pressor amines (diamine oxidase); synthesizes prostaglandins.
- **Barrier**: Limits transfer of high-molecular-weight (>500 Da) substances (e.g., insulin and heparin); allows IgG, certain viruses/parasites.
- **Heat Transfer**: Maintains fetal temperature (0.5°C above maternal) via umbilical blood flow.

3. Vasa Previa: Definition, Types, and Management.[37]

Ans.

- **Definition**: Umbilical vessels overlie the cervical os within membranes, at the risk of rupture or compression.

TABLE 3: Management of vasa previa.[40]

Intervention	*Details*
Antenatal Steroids	Administer at 28–32 weeks for lung maturity
Hospitalization	Consider at 30–34 weeks for surveillance
Cesarean Delivery	Plan at 34–36 weeks; avoid delayed cord clamping
Emergency Delivery	Expedite if vessels lacerated during hysterotomy

- **Incidence**: ~1% singleton and 6% twin pregnancies.[38]
- **Types**:
  - Type 1: Associated with velamentous cord insertion.
  - Type 2: Vessels span bilobate/succenturiate placenta lobes.
  - **Screening**: Midtrimester ultrasound with transvaginal color Doppler; up to 39% resolve spontaneously.[39]
  - **Management** is mentioned in **Table 3**.

MULTIPLE CHOICE QUESTIONS

Placental Development

1. **At what gestational age is the definitive placenta fully formed, according to the provided content?**
   a. 6 weeks
   b. 8 weeks
   c. 12 weeks
   d. 16 weeks
2. **Which cell layer differentiates into the syncytiotrophoblast by day 8 postfertilization?**
   a. Inner cell mass
   b. Trophectoderm
   c. Endoderm
   d. Mesoderm
3. **What is the primary function of the cytotrophoblastic shell in placental development?**
   a. Forms fetal blood vessels
   b. Isolates syncytium from decidua
   c. Secretes hCG
   d. Facilitates maternal blood flow
4. **On which day postfertilization do primary villi, consisting of syncytiotrophoblast and cytotrophoblast, form?**
   a. Days 6–7
   b. Days 8–10
   c. Days 12–13
   d. Days 16–18
5. **What structure invades primary villi to form secondary villi by day 16?**
   a. Fetal blood vessels
   b. Extraembryonic mesoderm
   c. Maternal spiral arteries
   d. Amniotic epithelium
6. **Which part of the chorion regresses to form the avascular chorion laeve?**
   a. Chorion frondosum
   b. Decidua basalis
   c. Decidua parietalis
   d. Cytotrophoblastic shell

7. How many maternal cotyledons typically form in the mature placenta?

a. 5–10
b. 10–15
c. 15–20
d. 20–25

8. What is the role of trabeculae in early placental development?

a. Form fetal capillaries
b. Separate lacunar spaces
c. Secrete progesterone
d. Anchor villi to decidua

Placental Structure

9. What is the approximate weight of the mature placenta at term?

a. 250 g
b. 500 g
c. 750 g
d. 1,000 g

10. Which layer of the placenta contains the Nitabuch layer?

a. Amniotic membrane
b. Chorionic plate
c. Basal plate
d. Intervillous space

11. How many stem (anchoring) villi typically persist in the human placenta?

a. 20–40
b. 40–60
c. 60–100
d. 100–120

12. What is the primary fetal component of the chorionic plate?

a. Decidua basalis
b. Syncytiotrophoblast
c. Umbilical vessels
d. Nitabuch layer

13. What is the volume of the mature placenta at term?

a. 250 mL
b. 500 mL
c. 750 mL
d. 1,000 mL

14. Which structure connects the fetal mesoderm to the maternal cytotrophoblastic shell?

a. Intervillous space
b. Anchoring villi
c. Chorion laeve
d. Basal plate

Placental Circulation

15. What is the approximate maternal blood flow rate in uteroplacental circulation at term?

a. 200–400 mL/min
b. 400–600 mL/min
c. 700–900 mL/min
d. 1,000–1,200 mL/min

16. What prevents clotting in the intervillous space?

a. Maternal heparin
b. Trophoblastic fibrinolytic enzymes
c. Fetal anticoagulants
d. Uterine contractions

17. By what gestational age is the second trophoblastic invasion of spiral arteries completed?

a. 8–10 weeks
b. 12–16 weeks
c. 16–20 weeks
d. 20–24 weeks

18. Which vessels carry deoxygenated blood to the placenta in fetoplacental circulation?

a. Umbilical vein
b. Umbilical arteries
c. Spiral arteries
d. Uterine veins

19. How often is maternal blood in the intervillous space replaced?
a. Every 5–10 seconds
b. Every 15–20 seconds
c. Every 30–40 seconds
d. Every 60 seconds

20. What enhances gaseous exchange in fetoplacental circulation?
a. Parallel blood flow
b. Countercurrent flow
c. Pulsatile flow
d. Intermittent flow

Placental Abnormalities

21. Which placental abnormality is associated with the highest risk of postpartum hemorrhage?
a. Bipartite placenta
b. Membranous placenta
c. Fenestrated placenta
d. Placenta marginata

22. What is the primary clinical concern with a succenturiate placenta?
a. Fetal growth restriction
b. Retention of accessory lobe
c. Umbilical cord prolapse
d. Placental infarction

23. Which ultrasound finding is diagnostic for placenta accreta?
a. Increased myometrial thickness
b. Loss of hypoechoic zone
c. Reduced vascular lacunae
d. Intact uterine serosa

24. What is the incidence of chorioangioma in placentas?
a. 0.1%
b. 1%
c. 5%
d. 10%

25. Which condition is a risk factor for placenta previa?
a. Primiparity
b. Prior cesarean delivery
c. Young maternal age
d. Normal AFP levels

26. What is the recommended gestational age for cesarean delivery in placenta previa with stable bleeding?
a. 32–34 weeks
b. 34–36 weeks
c. 36–37 weeks
d. 38–39 weeks

27. Which placental abnormality is characterized by a thin fibrous ring at the chorionic plate margin?
a. Circumvallate placenta
b. Placenta marginata
c. Bipartite placenta
d. Membranous placenta

28. What is the primary management for large chorioangiomas (>4 cm) causing fetal hydrops?
a. Expectant management
b. Intrauterine transfusion
c. Cesarean delivery at term
d. Antibiotics

29. Which cord insertion anomaly is associated with vasa previa?
a. Battledore placenta
b. Velamentous cord insertion
c. Central cord insertion
d. Marginal cord insertion

30. What is the risk of placenta accreta with five or more prior cesarean deliveries?
a. 0.3%
b. 1.5%
c. 3.0%
d. 6.74%

Placental Functions and Pathology

31. Which placental function involves the transfer of glucose via GLUT-1/GLUT-3 transporters?
a. Respiratory
b. Nutritive
c. Excretory
d. Immunological

32. What is the primary barrier function of the placenta?
a. Allows all maternal hormones
b. Limits substances >500 Da
c. Prevents IgG transfer
d. Blocks all pathogens

33. Which enzyme in the placenta inactivates oxytocin?
a. Diamine oxidase
b. Oxytocinase
c. Phospholipase A
d. Lactogen synthase

34. What is the approximate oxygen delivery rate to the fetus via the placenta?
a. 4 mL/kg/min
b. 8 mL/kg/min
c. 12 mL/kg/min
d. 16 mL/kg/min

35. Which maternal condition is an indication for placental pathological examination?
a. Normal vaginal delivery
b. Gestational diabetes
c. Term pregnancy
d. Uncomplicated labor

36. What is the incidence of vasa previa in twin pregnancies?
a. 1%
b. 3%
c. 6%
d. 10%

37. Which pathogen can cross the placental barrier to affect the fetus?
a. *Escherichia coli*
b. Rubella virus
c. *Staphylococcus aureus*
d. *Clostridium difficile*

38. What is the primary benefit of placental pathological examination in gestational trophoblastic disease?
a. Predicts maternal weight gain
b. Aids early diagnosis
c. Assesses fetal heart rate
d. Monitors labor progress

39. Which type of vasa previa involves vessels spanning bilobate or succenturiate placenta lobes?
a. Type 1
b. Type 2
c. Type 3
d. Type 4

40. What is the fetal temperature maintained by placental heat transfer relative to maternal temperature?
a. 0.2°C lower
b. Equal
c. 0.5°C higher
d. 1.0°C higher

Explanations

Ans. 1 c. 12 weeks

The definitive placenta is fully formed by the 12th week of gestation, with fusion of decidua parietalis and capsularis, completing development.[9]

Ans. 2 b. Trophectoderm

The trophectoderm differentiates into the trophoblast, which by day 8 forms the outer syncytiotrophoblast and inner cytotrophoblast.[2]

Ans. 3 b. Isolates syncytium from decidua

The cytotrophoblastic shell forms a continuous layer, isolating the syncytiotrophoblast from the maternal decidua, ensuring structural integrity.[5]

Ans. 4 c. Days 12–13

Primary villi, consisting of syncytiotrophoblast with a cytotrophoblast core, form on days 12–13, marking the start of villous development.[3]

Ans. 5 b. Extraembryonic mesoderm

Extraembryonic mesoderm invades primary villi by day 16, forming secondary villi, a precursor to vascularized tertiary villi.[4]

Ans. 6 c. Decidua parietalis

Villi abutting the decidua parietalis regress, forming the avascular chorion laeve (smooth chorion), while decidua basalis forms chorion frondosum.[6]

Ans. 7 c. 15–20

The placenta typically divides into 15–20 maternal cotyledons by maternal septa, organizing the intervillous space.[8]

Ans. 8 b. Separate lacunar spaces

Trabeculae are syncytial partitions that separate lacunar spaces (later intervillous spaces) in the syncytiotrophoblast during early development.[3]

Ans. 9 b. 500 g

The mature placenta weighs approximately 500 g, about one-sixth of fetal weight, at term.[10]

Ans. 10 c. Basal plate

The basal plate contains the Nitabuch layer, formed by fibrinoid degeneration of syncytiotrophoblast, anchoring the placenta to the decidua.[11]

Ans. 11 c. 60–100

Approximately 60–100 stem (anchoring) villi persist, forming fetal cotyledons (3–5 per maternal cotyledon).[11]

Ans. 12 c. Umbilical vessels

The chorionic plate includes extraembryonic mesoderm with branches of umbilical vessels, a key fetal component.[11]

Ans. 13 b. 500 mL

The mature placenta has a volume of approximately 500 mL at term, consistent with its size and function.[10]

Ans. 14 b. Anchoring villi

Anchoring villi connect fetal mesoderm to the maternal cytotrophoblastic shell, stabilizing the placenta.[7]

Ans. 15 c. 700–900 mL/min

Uteroplacental circulation delivers 700–900 mL/min of maternal blood to the intervillous space at term.[12]

Ans. 16 b. Trophoblastic fibrinolytic enzymes

Trophoblastic fibrinolytic enzymes prevent clotting in the intervillous space, ensuring continuous blood flow.[14]

Ans. 17 b. 12–16 weeks

The second trophoblastic invasion of spiral arteries, extending to radial arteries, is completed by 12–16 weeks, forming low-resistance vessels.[12]

Ans. 18 b. Umbilical arteries

Two umbilical arteries carry deoxygenated fetal blood to the placenta in fetoplacental circulation.[15]

Ans. 19 b. Every 15–20 seconds

Maternal blood in the intervillous space is replaced every 15–20 seconds, ensuring efficient exchange. [13]

Ans. 20 b. Countercurrent flow

Countercurrent flow between fetal and maternal blood enhances gaseous and nutrient exchange in fetoplacental circulation.[15]

Ans. 21 b. Membranous placenta

Membranous placenta has the highest PPH risk due to its thin structure, association with accreta/previa, and difficult manual removal.[17]

Ans. 22 b. Retention of accessory lobe

Succenturiate placenta risks retention of the accessory lobe, leading to PPH if not identified postdelivery.[17]

Ans. 23 b. Loss of hypoechoic zone

Loss of the hypoechoic zone between placenta and myometrium on ultrasound is a key diagnostic feature of placenta accreta.[24]

Ans. 24. b. 1%

Chorioangioma, a benign placental hamartoma, has an incidence of approximately 1%.[31]

Ans. 25 b. Prior cesarean delivery

Prior cesarean delivery is a major risk factor for placenta previa, increasing the likelihood of abnormal implantation.[19]

Ans. 26 c. 36–37 weeks

ACOG recommends elective cesarean at 36–37 weeks for placenta previa with stable bleeding to balance maternal and fetal risks.[21]

Ans. 27 b. Placenta marginata

Placenta marginata is characterized by a thin fibrous ring at the chorionic plate margin, with minimal clinical impact.[17]

Ans. 28 b. Intrauterine transfusion

Large chorioangiomas (>4 cm) causing fetal hydrops are managed with intrauterine transfusion, steroids, or fetal surgery to address complications.[31]

Ans. 29 b. Velamentous cord insertion

Velamentous cord insertion is associated with vasa previa, where vessels cross the cervical os, risking rupture.[34]

Ans. 30 d. 6.74%

The risk of placenta accreta increases to 6.74% with five or more prior cesarean deliveries, due to myometrial scarring.[23]

Ans. 31 b. Nutritive

Glucose transfer via GLUT-1/GLUT-3 transporters is a key nutritive function of the placenta, supporting fetal growth.[36]

Ans. 32 b. Limits substances >500 Da

The placenta limits transfer of substances >500 Da (e.g., insulin and heparin), acting as a selective barrier.[36]

Ans. 33 b. Oxytocinase

Oxytocinase, an enzyme in the placenta, inactivates oxytocin, regulating uterine activity.[36]

Ans. 34 b. 8 mL/kg/min

The placenta delivers approximately 8 mL/kg/min of oxygen to the fetus, supporting metabolic needs.[36]

Ans. 35 b. Gestational diabetes

Maternal conditions like gestational diabetes are the indications for placental pathological examination to assess complications.[35]

Ans. 36 c. 6%

Vasa previa has an incidence of approximately 6% in twin pregnancies, higher than in singletons (1%).[38]

Ans. 37 b. Rubella virus

The rubella virus can cross the placental barrier, causing congenital infections, unlike most bacteria.[36]

Ans. 38 b. Aids early diagnosis

Pathological examination aids early diagnosis of gestational trophoblastic diseases (e.g., choriocarcinoma), improving outcomes.[35]

Ans. 39 b. Type 2

Type 2 vasa previa involves vessels spanning bilobate or succenturiate placenta lobes, increasing rupture risk.[37]

Ans. 40 c. 0.5°C higher

The placenta maintains fetal temperature 0.5°C higher than maternal temperature via umbilical blood flow.[36]

REFERENCES

1. Benirschke K, Burton GJ, Baergen RN (Eds). Pathology of the Human Placenta, 6th edition. Springer; 2012.
2. Gude NM, et al. Placenta. 2004;25(10):763-74.

3. Burton GJ, Yung HW, Cindrova-Davies T, et al. Placenta. 2009;30(Suppl A):S43-8.
4. Kingdom J, et al. Placenta. 2000;21(Suppl A):S113-21.
5. Kaufmann P, Mayhew TM, Charnock-Jones DS, et al. Aspects of human fetoplacental vasculogenesis and angiogenesis. II. Changes during normal pregnancy. Placenta. 2004;25(2-3):114-26.
6. Moore KL, Persaud TVN, Torchia MG, et al. The Developing Human, 10th edition. Elsevier; 2016.
7. Huppertz B. Placenta. 2008;29(Suppl A):S10-5.
8. Cunningham FG, Leveno KJ, Bloom SL, et al. (Eds). Williams Obstetrics, 25th edition. McGraw-Hill Education, London; 2018.
9. Baergen RN. Manual of Pathology of the Human Placenta, 2nd edition. Springer; 2011.
10. Wang Y, et al. Placenta. 2010;31(8):631-8.
11. Redline RW. Placental pathology: a systematic approach with clinical correlations. Placenta. 2008;29(Suppl A):S86-91.
12. Brosens I, Pijnenborg R, Vercruysse L, et al. The "Great Obstetrical Syndromes" are associated with disorders of deep placentation. Am J Obstet Gynecol. 2011;204(3):193-201.
13. Ramsey EM, et al. Am J Anat. 1976;147(2):159-83.
14. Burton GJ, Watson AL, Hempstock J, et al. Uterine glands provide histiotrophic nutrition for the human fetus during the first trimester of pregnancy. J Clin Endocrinol Metab. 2002;87(6):2954-9.
15. Schneider H. Placenta. 1991;12(1):1-13.
16. Fox H, Sebire N (Eds). Pathology of the Placenta, 3rd edition. Elsevier; 2007.
17. Baergen RN, et al. Placenta. 2017;54:2-14.
18. Silver RM. Abnormal placentation: Placenta previa, vasa previa and placenta accreta. Obstet Gynecol. 2015;126(3):654-68.
19. Ananth CV, et al. Obstet Gynecol. 1997;90(6):935-40.
20. Oyelese Y, Smulian J. Placenta Previa, Placenta Accreta, and Vasa Previa. Obstet Gynecol. 2006;107(4):927-41.
21. ACOG Practice Bulletin No. 192. Obstet Gynecol. 2018;131(3):e78-90.
22. Jauniaux E, Collins S, Burton GJ, et al. Placenta accreta spectrum: pathophysiology and evidence-based anatomy for prenatal ultrasound imaging. Am J Obstet Gynecol. 2018;218(1):75-87.
23. Bowman ZS, et al. Clin Obstet Gynecol. 2014;57(2):372-86.
24. D'Antonio F, et al. Ultrasound Obstet Gynecol. 2014;44(5):503-9.
25. ACOG Committee Opinion No. 764. Obstet Gynecol. 2019;133(2):e110-27.
26. Redline RW, et al. Hum Pathol. 2004;35(12):1496-502.
27. Fitzgerald B, et al. Placenta. 2011;32(10):767-74.
28. Salafia CM, et al. Am J Perinatol. 1995;12(6):435-40.
29. Katz D, et al. Placenta. 2011;32(12):958-62.
30. Stanek J. Placenta. 2013;34(8):656-62.
31. Zanardini C, et al. Fetal Diagn Ther. 2010;28(2):87-93.
32. Al-Adnani M, et al. Pediatr Dev Pathol. 2007;10(5):397-401.
33. Benirschke K, et al. Placenta. 2000;21(7):645-52.
34. SMFM Consult Series #44. Am J Obstet Gynecol. 2015;213(5):604-10.
35. Langston C, Kaplan CG, Macpherson T, et al. Practice guideline for examination of the placenta: Developed by the Placental Pathology Practice Guideline Development Task Force of the College of American Pathologists. Arch Pathol Lab Med. 1997;121(5):449-76.
36. Sadler TW (Ed). Langman's Medical Embryology, 14th edition. Wolters Kluwer; 2019.
37. Matsuzaki S, et al. Placenta. 2019;84:54-60.
38. Ebbing C, et al. Ultrasound Obstet Gynecol. 2023;61(1):26-34.
39. Erfani H, et al. Am J Obstet Gynecol. 2020;223(5):739.e1-9.
40. ACOG Practice Bulletin No. 231. Obstet Gynecol. 2021;137(6):e128-44.

Medical Disorders in Pregnancy

37. **Hemoglobinopathies**
Ruchika Garg

38. **Gestational Diabetes Mellitus**
Ruchika Garg

39. **Hypertensive Disorders in Pregnancy**
Ruchika Garg

40. **Epilepsy and Antiepileptic Drugs in Pregnancy**
Ruchika Garg

41. **Anemia in Pregnancy**
Kalpana Kumari, Vandana Verma

42. **Cardiac Disease in Pregnancy**
Ruchika Garg

43. **Liver Disorders in Pregnancy**
Ruchika Garg

44. **Thrombocytopenia in Pregnancy**
Ruchika Garg

45. **Thyroid Disorders in Pregnancy**
Ruchika Garg

46. **Venous Thromboembolism in Pregnancy and Puerperium**
Ruchika Garg

47. **Renal Disorders in Pregnancy**
Prabhat Agrawal, Pavika Lal

48. **Psychiatric Disorders in Pregnancy and Postpartum**
Ruchika Garg

49. **Placenta Accreta Spectrum**
Ruchika Garg

Hemoglobinopathies

Ruchika Garg

INTRODUCTION

Hemoglobinopathies encompass a group of inherited disorders caused by quantitative or qualitative abnormalities in hemoglobin (Hb) synthesis and structure. These are among the most common single-gene disorders worldwide, affecting millions and contributing significantly to global health burdens.[1] Approximately 7% of the global population are carriers of clinically significant mutations, predominantly leading to thalassemias and hemoglobin variants.[2] The prevalence of clinically significant hemoglobinopathies is estimated at 1.5 per 1,000 live births. Traditionally concentrated in subtropical regions—including the Mediterranean, Middle East, and Southeast Asia—population migration has broadened their prevalence beyond these geographical confines, necessitating heightened awareness and healthcare preparedness globally.[3]

NORMAL HEMOGLOBIN STRUCTURE AND PHYSIOLOGY

Hemoglobin is a tetrameric protein composed of iron-containing heme groups and four globin polypeptide chains: two α-like and two β-like chains. Adult hemoglobin (HbA) predominantly consists of two α and two β chains ($\alpha 2\beta 2$), accounting for approximately 95–98% of total Hb in healthy adults. Minor components include HbA2 ($\alpha 2\delta 2$, ~2-3%) and fetal hemoglobin HbF ($\alpha 2\gamma 2$), which predominates in fetal life and usually constitutes <1% postnatally as it declines after birth.

The globin chains are encoded by gene clusters located on chromosomes 16p (α-globin genes: HBA1 and HBA2) and 11p (β-globin gene: HBB and related genes). The delicate balance in the synthesis of α- and β-chains is crucial for RBC integrity. Disruptions result in imbalanced globin chain production, precipitation, and ineffective erythropoiesis.

CLASSIFICATION OF HEMOGLOBINOPATHIES

1. **Thalassemias:** Quantitative defects characterized by reduced or absent synthesis of one globin chain type, classified primarily as alpha (α), beta (β), or delta-beta (δβ) thalassemia based on chains affected.
2. **Structural/Variant Hemoglobins:** Qualitative abnormalities leading to altered globin chain structure resulting in abnormal hemoglobin function, e.g., Hb S (sickle), Hb E, Hb C, Hb D-Punjab, Hb O-Arab.

   These defects can coexist, compounding clinical severity and heterogeneity.

Molecular Basis

Alpha-globin Gene Cluster

- Encodes α-chains (141 amino acids).
- Two nearly identical genes *HBA1* and *HBA2* reside on chromosome 16p.
- α-thalassemia is commonly caused by deletions involving one or both α-globin genes (α0 or α+).

Beta-globin Gene Cluster

- Single gene *HBB* encodes β chains (146 amino acids), located on chromosome 11p.
- β-thalassemia mutations generally involve single nucleotide substitutions, small insertions, or deletions affecting β-globin synthesis (β0 - absence; β+ - partial reduction).
- Mutations disrupting gene expression or mRNA processing lead to diminished β-chain production and consequent imbalance with α-chains.

PATHOPHYSIOLOGY

- In thalassemias, excess unmatched globin chains precipitate within erythroid precursors causing oxidative membrane damage, ineffective erythropoiesis, hemolysis, and anemia.
- In β-thalassemia, increased HbF and HbA2 partially compensate for deficient HbA but do not fully correct anemia.
- Variant Hbs (e.g., HbS) cause qualitative RBC deformities; HbS polymerizes on deoxygenation, causing sickling, hemolysis, vaso-occlusion, multiorgan complications.

CLINICAL SPECTRUM (TABLE 1)

Diagnostic Evaluation

Routine Testing

- **Complete Blood Count (CBC):** Microcytic hypochromic anemia typical; red cell indices guide differential diagnosis **(Table 2)**.
- **Peripheral Smear:** Shows target cells, nucleated RBCs, and anisocytosis.

Screening Tests

- **NESTROFT:** Simple and cost-effective for β-thalassemia carrier detection.
- **DCIP Test:** For HbE carriers.
- **Solubility Test:** For HbS detection.

Definitive Testing

- **High-Performance Liquid Chromatography (HPLC):** Quantifies Hb fractions (HbA2, HbF, and variants) aiding carrier detection and differentiation.
- **Capillary Electrophoresis:** Similar utility to HPLC.

TABLE 1: Clinical spectrum according to genotype.

Genotype	*Phenotype*	*Clinical features*
Homozygous β-thalassemia major	Severe transfusion-dependent	Severe anemia early infancy, growth retardation, hepatosplenomegaly
Compound heterozygous β-thalassemia intermedia	Variable severity	Moderate anemia; may require intermittent transfusions
Heterozygous β-thalassemia trait	Carrier state	Usually asymptomatic with mild anemia or microcytosis
α-thalassemia silent carriers	Asymptomatic	Normal or mild hematological changes
HbH disease (3 α-gene deletion)	Moderate hemolytic anemia	Hemolysis, pallor, and splenomegaly
Hb Bart's hydrops fetalis (4 α-gene deletion)	Incompatible with life	Severe intrauterine anemia, hydrops fetalis, and stillbirth
Hb S disease (Sickle Cell)	Chronic hemolytic anemia	Pain crises, acute chest syndrome, infections, and organ damage

TABLE 2: Hematologic parameters in differential diagnosis of microcytic anemia.

Parameter	*Normal range*	*α-/β-Thalassemia carriers*	*HbE, HbS, HPFH carriers*	*Iron deficiency Anemia*
Mean Corpuscular Volume (MCV)	80–100 fl	Reduced	Normal	Reduced
Mean Corpuscular Hemoglobin (MCH)	27–32 pg	Reduced	Normal	Reduced
RBC Count	Varies	Normal or Increased	Normal	Reduced
Red Cell Distribution Width (RDW)	Varies	Normal	Normal	Increased
Serum Ferritin	Varies	Normal or Elevated	Normal or Elevated	Reduced

Molecular Testing

- **α-thalassemia:** Large gene deletions analyzed by multiplex ligation-dependent probe amplification (MLPA) or gap-PCR.
- **β-thalassemia:** Mutations detected by ARMS-PCR, reverse dot-blot, or Sanger sequencing.
- **Next-Generation Sequencing (NGS):** For rare or novel mutations.

PREVENTION STRATEGIES

- **Carrier Screening:** Early identification of at-risk couples using CBC and Hb analysis in high-prevalence areas or target populations.
- **Genetic Counseling:** Educating carriers about transmission risk (25% for affected child if both parents are carriers) and reproductive options.
- **Prenatal Diagnosis:** Chorionic villus sampling (10–12 weeks) or amniocentesis (after 16 weeks) with molecular confirmation.

- **Preimplantation Genetic Diagnosis (PGD):** For couples opting for IVF with genetic screening.
- **Cascade Screening:** Testing extended family members of affected individuals to identify additional carriers **(Algorithm 1)**.

Algorithm 1: Screening and Diagnostic Workflow for β-Thalassemia Carriers

Step 1: Clinical suspicion based on anemia or family history
↓
Step 2: CBC shows microcytic hypochromic anemia
↓
Step 3: NESTROFT/DCIP/solubility tests as convenient screening
↓
Step 4: Confirmatory HPLC or capillary electrophoresis
↓
Step 5: Molecular genetic testing for mutation characterization
↓
Step 6: Genetic counseling for at-risk couples
↓
Step 7: Prenatal diagnosis or preimplantation genetic diagnosis offered if both partners carriers

MANAGEMENT HIGHLIGHTS[4]

- **Thalassemia Major:** Regular blood transfusions, iron chelation therapy, folic acid supplementation, and supportive care.
- **Sickle Cell Disease:** Pain crisis management, hydroxyurea, infection prophylaxis, transfusions, and emerging curative options (bone marrow transplantation).
- **HbE Disease and Mild Forms:** Supportive management; may require transfusion during crises or pregnancy.[5]

CHALLENGES AND ETHICAL CONSIDERATIONS

- **Screening Barriers:** Sociocultural stigma, cost, and logistics limit universal carrier screening.
- **Counseling:** Sensitive communication about reproductive choices and options is needed to respect autonomy and cultural beliefs.
- **Prenatal Diagnosis:** Legal and ethical frameworks vary by country regarding pregnancy termination. PGD presents a promising alternative when accepted.

CONCLUSION

Hemoglobinopathies represent a complex group of inherited disorders necessitating a multidisciplinary approach involving molecular diagnostics, genetic counseling, and preventive strategies. With advancing diagnostic technologies and screening programs, early detection and prevention remain the cornerstones of reduced disease burden.[6]

REFERENCES

1. Colah R, Gorakshakar A, Nadkarni A. Global burden, distribution and prevention of β-thalassemias and hemoglobin E disorders. Expert Rev Hematol. 2010;3(1):103-17.
2. Christianson A, Howson CP, Modell B. March of Dimes global repcrt on birth Defects: the hidden toll of dying and disabled children. White Plains, New York: March of Dimes Birth Defects Foundation; 2006.
3. Williams TN, Weatherall DJ. World distribution, population genetics, and health burden of the hemoglobinopathies. Cold Spring Harb Perspect Med. 2012;2(9):a011692.
4. World Health Organization. Management of Hemoglobin Disorders: Report of Joint WHO-TIF Meeting, Nicosia, Cyprus. Geneva, Switzerland: World Health Organization; 2007.
5. Brendel C, Williams DA. Current and future gene therapies for hemoglobinopathies. Curr Opin Hematol. 2020 May;27(3):149-154.
6. Weatherall DJ. The inherited diseases of hemoglobin are an emerging global health burden. Blood. 2010;115(22):4331-6.

CHAPTER 38

Gestational Diabetes Mellitus

Ruchika Garg

INTRODUCTION

Pregnancy is a diabetogenic state driven by insulin resistance and hyperglycemia, exacerbated by placental hormones. Hyperglycemia in pregnancy (HIP), encompassing preexisting type 1 diabetes mellitus (T1DM), type 2 diabetes mellitus (T2DM), and gestational diabetes mellitus (GDM), is a leading cause of maternal, perinatal, and neonatal morbidity and mortality, with long-term implications for both mother and offspring.[1] GDM, defined as impaired glucose tolerance first recognized during pregnancy, constitutes ~90% of HIP cases globally, with a prevalence of ~10%.[1] In India, GDM incidence is notably higher (10–14%) compared to Western populations, earning it the title of a "GDM hub".[1]

PATHOPHYSIOLOGY AND CLASSIFICATION

- **Pathophysiology (Fig. 1):**
  - **Insulin Resistance:** Placental hormones (human placental lactogen, cortisol, and progesterone) and cytokines (TNF-α) increase insulin resistance, peaking in the second and third trimesters.[1]
  - **β-Cell Dysfunction:** Inadequate pancreatic β-cell compensation leads to hyperglycemia, particularly in genetically predisposed individuals.[1]
  - **Fetal Impact:** Maternal hyperglycemia causes fetal hyperinsulinemia, driving macrosomia, organomegaly, and metabolic complications.[1]
- **Classification (Table 1):**[1]
  - **Preexisting Diabetes:** T1DM or T2DM diagnosed before pregnancy.

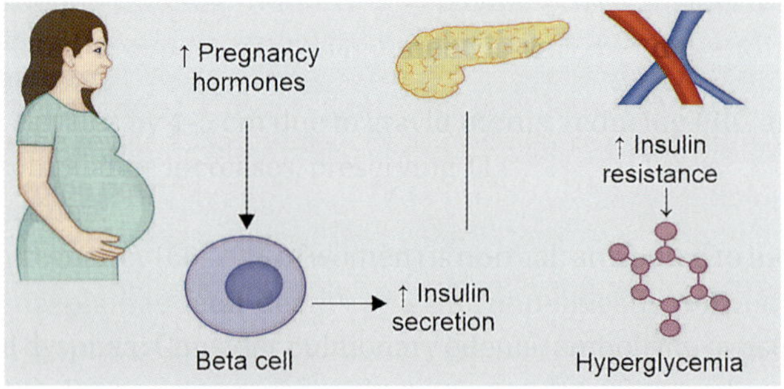

Fig. 1: Pathophysiology of diabetes in pregnancy.
Source: American Diabetes Association.

TABLE 1: Classification of hyperglycemia in pregnancy.

Type	*Definition*	*Key features*
Preexisting T1DM	Autoimmune β-cell destruction	Requires insulin, high congenital anomaly risk
Preexisting T2DM	Insulin resistance, β-cell dysfunction	Often on OADs prepregnancy, obesity common
GDM	Impaired glucose tolerance in pregnancy	90% of HIP, 10–14% prevalence in India
Overt Diabetes	T2DM diagnosed in pregnancy	A1c ≥6.5%, fasting ≥126 mg/dL

Source: Seshiah V, et al. MoHFW Diagnosis and Management of Gestational Diabetes Mellitus: Technical and Operational Guidelines. New Delhi: MoHFW; 2018.[1]

- **GDM:** Impaired glucose tolerance with onset or first recognition during pregnancy.
- **Overt Diabetes:** Newly diagnosed T2DM during pregnancy (e.g., A1c ≥6.5% or fasting glucose ≥126 mg/dL).

Risk Factors[1]

- Personal history of impaired glucose tolerance (A1c ≥5.7%, impaired fasting glucose, prior GDM with 40% recurrence risk).
- Family history of diabetes.
- Prepregnancy BMI >30 kg/m^2 or excessive gestational weight gain.
- Advanced maternal age (>40 years).
- High-risk ethnic groups (South/East Asian, Hispanic, African American, Native American, Pacific Islander).
- Polycystic ovary syndrome (PCOS) or previous macrosomic infant (≥4,000 g).

SCREENING AND DIAGNOSIS

Universal Screening[1]

- **When:** At first antenatal visit for all pregnant women (except known diabetics), regardless of gestational age.
- **Method: DIPSI Test** (Diabetes in Pregnancy Study Group India):
  - 75 g glucose in 300 mL water, consumed within 10 minutes, irrespective of meals.
  - Measure capillary blood glucose using a plasma-calibrated glucometer after 2 hours.
  - **Criteria:**
    - <140 mg/dL: Normoglycemia
    - ≥140 mg/dL: GDM
- **Retest:** Between 24 and 28 weeks (minimum 4-week interval from first test) if initial result is normal.
- **Alternative:** Two-step approach (ACOG):[2]
  - Step 1: 50 g glucose challenge test (GCT), 1-hour glucose ≥135–140 mg/dL.
  - Step 2: 100 g oral glucose tolerance test (OGTT), diagnostic if ≥2 values meet thresholds (fasting ≥95, 1-hour ≥180, 2-hour ≥155, and 3-hour ≥140 mg/dL).

TABLE 2: Diagnostic criteria for GDM.

Test	*Threshold*	*Notes*
DIPSI (2-hour, 75 g)	≥140 mg/dL	Single-step, India-specific
ACOG 2-Step (100 g OGTT)	≥2 abnormal values: Fasting ≥ 95, 1-h ≥ 180, 2-h ≥ 155, and 3-h ≥ 140 mg/dL	Used in Western settings
Overt Diabetes	Fasting ≥ 126 mg/dL, A1c ≥ 6.5%	Diagnosed anytime

Source: MoHFW. Diagnosis and Management of Gestational Diabetes: Technical and Operational Guidelines. New Delhi: MoHFW; 2018; ACOG Practice Bulletin No. 190: Gestational Diabetes Mellitus. Obstet Gynecol. 2018;131(2):e49-e64.[1,2]

TABLE 3: Complications of uncontrolled diabetes in pregnancy.

Category	*Complications*
Maternal	Preeclampsia, polyhydramnios, infections (UTI and pyelonephritis), preterm delivery, obstructed/prolonged labor, postpartum hemorrhage, operative delivery (cesarean and instrumental), and obesity
Fetal	Macrosomia, shoulder dystocia, congenital anomalies (cardiac, CNS, and sacral agenesis), spontaneous abortion, and stillbirth
Neonatal	Hypoglycemia, hypocalcemia, hyperbilirubinemia, polycythemia, respiratory distress syndrome, sepsis, and seizures
Long-term (Mother)	T2DM (10% annual risk, highest in first 5 years), obesity, and cardiovascular disease
Long-term (Offspring)	Early-onset T2DM, obesity, cardiometabolic risk, impaired motor function, and inattention/hyperactivity

Source: MoHFW. Diagnosis and Management of Gestational Diabetes: Technical and Operational Guidelines. New Delhi: MoHFW; 2018.[1]

Diagnosis of Overt Diabetes (Table 2)[2]

- Fasting plasma glucose ≥ 126 mg/dL.
- A1c ≥ 6.5%.
- Random glucose ≥ 200 mg/dL with symptoms.

COMPLICATIONS

Uncontrolled hyperglycemia leads to significant maternal, fetal, and neonatal complications, with long-term risks **(Table 3)**.

Specific Notes:

- **Infections:** Glucosuria exacerbates UTI risk (asymptomatic bacteriuria and pyelonephritis); 10% develop polyhydramnios, increasing abruption and preterm labor risks.[1]
- **Congenital Anomalies:** Preexisting diabetes increases risk (e.g., tetralogy of Fallot, spina bifida, and sacral agenesis); not elevated in GDM.[1]
- **Macrosomia:** Evident at 26–28 weeks, leading to fetopelvic disproportion, shoulder dystocia, and operative delivery.[1]
- **Stillbirth:** Associated with poor glycemic control, particularly in preexisting diabetes.[1]

TABLE 4: Target glucose levels in pregnancy.

Time	*Glucose (mg/dL)*
Fasting	69–90
Premeal (lunch/supper/snack)	60–105
1-hour Postprandial	<120
Overnight (2–6 am)	>60
Optimal (Preexisting Diabetes)	Premeal/overnight: 60–99; Postprandial: 100–129; A1c < 6.0%

Source: MoHFW. Diagnosis and Management of Gestational Diabetes: Technical and Operational Guidelines. New Delhi: MoHFW; 2018; American Diabetes Association. 14. Management of Diabetes in Pregnancy: Standards of Medical Care in Diabetes-2020. Diabetes Care. 2020;43(Suppl 1):S183-S192.[1,3]

TABLE 5: Energy requirements by activity level.

Activity Level	*Energy (kcal/day)*
Sedentary	2,250 (1,900 + 350)
Moderate	2,580 (2,230 + 350)
Heavy	3,200 (2,850 + 350)

Source: ICMR, MoHFW. Diagnosis and Management of Gestational Diabetes: Technical and Operational Guidelines. New Delhi: MoHFW; 2018.[1]

MANAGEMENT

Goals: Achieve euglycemia **(Table 4)** to minimize complications, ensure fetal well-being, and plan timely delivery.[2]

Algorithm 1: Management of GDM

- **Step 1: Diagnosis**: Confirm GDM (DIPSI ≥ 140 mg/dL).
- **Step 2: Medical Nutrition Therapy (MNT)**:
  - Initiate for 2 weeks.
  - Monitor fasting (<95 mg/dL) and 1-hour postprandial (<120 mg/dL) venous blood sugar.
  - If targets met: Continue MNT, monitor fortnightly until 37 weeks, then weekly.
  - If targets unmet: Initiate pharmacotherapy.

- **Step 3: Pharmacotherapy**: Insulin or oral antidiabetic drugs (OADs).
- **Step 4: Obstetric Monitoring**: Fetal and maternal surveillance.
- **Step 5: Delivery Planning**: Based on control and complications.
- **Step 6: Postpartum Care**: Glucose monitoring and follow-up.

Medical Nutrition Therapy

- **Caloric Needs:**[1]
  - Nonobese: 30 kcal/kg/day (prepregnancy weight).
  - Obese (BMI >30): 30–33% calorie reduction, monitor ketonuria weekly.
  - **ICMR Formula:** Energy = BMR × PAL **(Table 5)**
    - BMR (18–30 years): 14 × weight (kg) + 471.

TABLE 6: Guidelines for initiating insulin therapy in gestational diabetes.

Organization	*Recommendation*
International Federation of Gynecology and Obstetrics (FIGO), 2015	• Oral therapy failure **or** the presence of any of the following risk factors: – Diabetes diagnosed before 20 weeks of gestation – Oral therapy used for >30 weeks – Fasting plasma glucose > 110 mg/dL – 1-hour postprandial glucose > 140 mg/dL – Weight gain > 12 kg during pregnancy
Canadian Diabetes Association (CDA), 2018	If glycemic control is not achieved within 2 weeks after starting medical and nutritional interventions
American Diabetes Association (ADA), 2018	First-line therapy if glycemic control is not achieved after diet intervention
American College of Obstetricians and Gynecologists (ACOG), 2018	First-line therapy if glycemic control is not achieved after diet intervention

- BMR (30–60 years): 8.3 × weight (kg) + 788.
- Add 350 kcal/day in second/third trimesters for 10–12 kg weight gain.

- **Diet Structure:**
  - Three small meals, 2–3 snacks daily.
  - Complex carbohydrates (whole grains, oats, bajra, jowar, ragi, vegetables, and fruits with skin) preferred.
  - Carbohydrate serves: 2–3 (15 g each) at meals, 1–2 at snacks.[1]

Pharmacotherapy

- **Insulin:**[3]
  - **Indications:** Fasting >110 mg/dL, 1-hour postprandial >140 mg/dL, diagnosis <20 weeks, or failure of MNT.[2]

  Insulin has always been incorporated in standard care of diabetes in pregnancy but in recent past use of oral antidiabetic medications such as metformin and glyburide for treatment of GDM has also gained importance.

Insulin

Most professional societies recommend insulin as first-line treatment of gestational diabetes after failure of lifestyle modification **(Table 6)**. Insulin does not cross the placenta because of its small molecular size and has an established safety profile in pregnancy.

Mechanism of Action

Insulin initiates its action by binding to a glycoprotein receptor on the surface of the cell. This receptor consists of an α-subunit, which binds the hormone, and a β-subunit, which is an insulin-stimulated, tyrosine-specific protein kinase. These specific receptors are located on practically all cells, but liver and fat cells have these receptors in abundance.

Insulin stimulates glucose transport across cell membrane by ATP-dependent translocation of glucose transporters, GLUT 4 and GLUT 1, to the plasma membrane and achieves hypogycemia. Exogenous insulin improves insulin availability and acts similar to endogenous insulin. Main actions are illustrated in **Figure 3**.

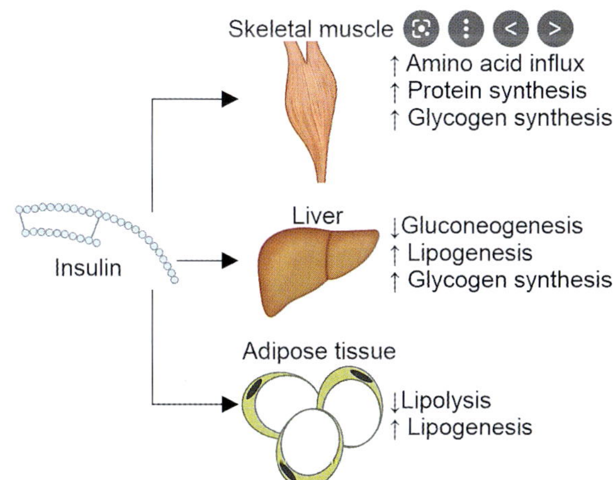

Fig. 3: Mechanism of action of insulin.
Courtesy: Clinical Diabetes and Endocrinology (BioMed Central), 2016.

Flowchart 1: Classification of insulin

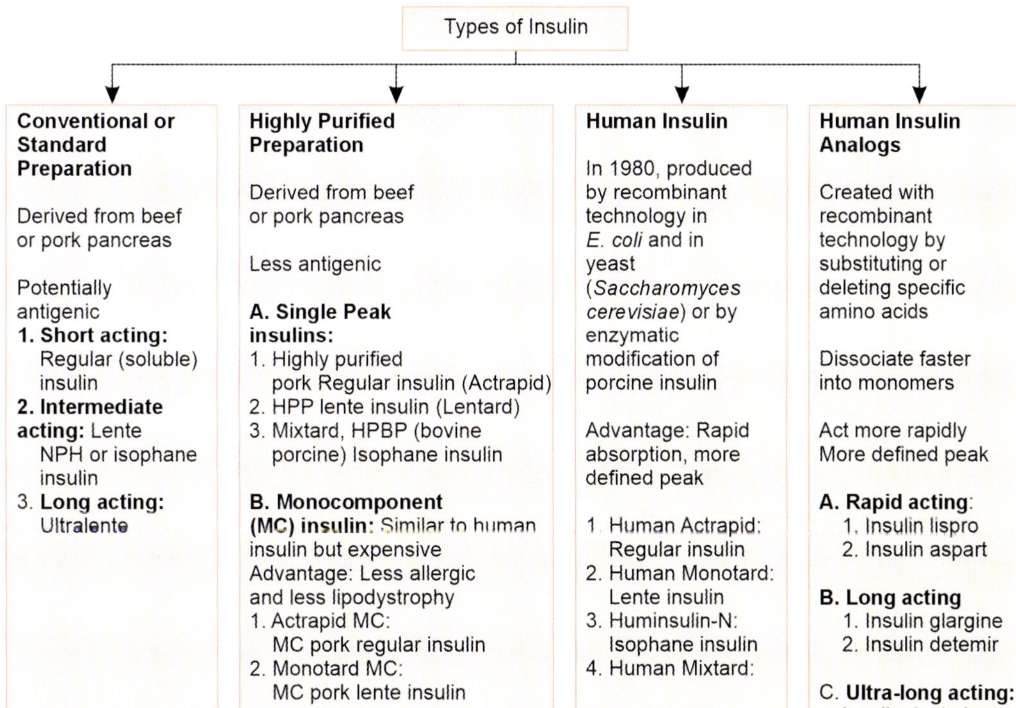

TABLE 7: Types of Insulin.

Types of insulin	*Onset of action*	*Peak of action (hours)*	*Duration of action (hours)*	*Remarks*	*Fda category*
Insulin lispro	1–15 minutes (rapid acting)	1–2	4–5	Decreased risk of severe maternal hypoglycemia compared with regular insulin	Category B
Insulin aspart	1–15 minutes (rapid acting)	1–2	4–5	Impart better glycemic control higher satisfaction of patients than regular insulin	Category B
Regular insulin	30–60 minutes (short acting)	2–4	6–8	Covers insulin needs for meals eaten within 30–60 minutes	Category B
NPH	1–3 hours (intermediate acting)	5–7	13–18	Covers insulin needs for about half the day or overnight	Category B
Insulin glargine	1–2 hours (long acting)	No peak	24	Insulin is delivered at a steady level	Category C
Insulin detemir	1–3 hours	Minimal peak at 8–10	18–26	Less incidence of hypoglycemia compared to NPH	Category B
Premixed 30/70 50/50	 30 minutes 30 minutes	 2–4 hours 2–5 hour	 14–24 hours 18–24 hours	These are usually taken two or three times a day before mealtime	Safe

Table 7 is showing different types of insulin. Thorough knowledge of insulin is mandatory to understand its usage.

Pharmacokinetics: It is shown in **Box 1**.

Pharmacokinetics of most commonly used insulin preparations **(Box 1)**

Salient points about commonly used insulin:

A. Rapidly acting insulin
   1. Insulin aspart (NovoLog):
      Onset: Approximately 15 minutes
      Timing: At the start of a meal (contrast to the timing of regular insulin)
   2. Insulin lispro (Humalog):
      Very similar to aspart.
      Timing: At the start of a meal given

B. Short-acting insulin:
   Regular insulin:
   - *Timing:* At least 10–15 and up to 30 minutes before a meal.
   - Available in U-100 and U-500 strength, U-500 useful in patients with insulin requirement >200 units per day

BOX 1: Insulin pharmacokinetics.

Insulin Regimens

- **Split Mix Regimen or Premix Regimen**
  - Two injections (intermediate +soluble) or premix per day
  - Before breakfast and before bedtime
  - Calculate total insulin requirement as per given formula
    - 2/3 of the total dose given in morning 1/3 in evening

  If NPH (neutral protamine Hagedorn) and regular insulin or rapid-acting insulin is being given.

  ↓

  Morning dose: 2/3 NPH (before breakfast) + 1/3 regular insulin or insulin lispro or aspart (with breakfast)

  Evening dose: ½ NPH (bedtime) + ½ regular insulin or insulin lispro or aspart (with dinner)
- **MDI or Basal Bolus Regimen**
  - Most physiologic and most flexible regimen.
  - Multiple daily injection regimens (4–7 injections before meals and before bedtime)
  - Insulin glargine/detemir and rapidly acting insulin is being given.
  - Divide total required dose into:

    ↓
  - *Half dose (basal insulin):* Insulin glargine (OD, evening) or insulin detemir (BD)
  - *Rest half dose:* Lispro or aspart divided into three equal doses with meals.
- **Continuous Subcutaneous Insulin Infusion**

  If adequate glycemic control is not achieved by MDI regimen.
- **Special Situations**
  - Only fasting glucose levels are high—basal insulin only
  - Only postprandial glucose levels are high—mealtime insulin only

    ↓
  - When regimens one and two are compared, maternal and fetal outcomes, total insulin doses, and overall glycemic control, both found to be equivalent.
  - Adjustments
  - It is necessary

C. Intermediate-acting insulin: NPH insulin (Novolin N and Humulin N)

- D*ose:* 2–3 times daily.
- *Disadvantage:* Increased risk of nighttime hypoglycemia (contrast to longer-acting insulins)

D. Long-acting insulins:

1. Insulin glargine (Lantus):

   Dose: A single daily dose.

   Evidence: Although glargine is comparable to NPH and is associated with fewer hypoglycemic events, there are no data on long-term risks of glargine in pregnancy
2. Insulin detemir (Levemir):

   Dosing for insulin detemir should be every 12 hours.

Special mention:

1. Insulin glulisine:

   Onset: 10–15 minutes

   Peak: 55 minutes

Duration of action: 4–5 hours
Category C drug in pregnancy

2. Nasal insulin:
   Onset: 15 minutes
   Peak: 50 minutes
   Duration of action: 2 hours
   Equivalent to lispro
   Disadvantage: Bronchospasm
   Category C drug in pregnancy
   - Insulin degludec
     Onset: 1 hour
     Long duration of action
     No peak
     Dose: Once daily

   Category C drug in pregnancy
   Insulin regimens: The insulin regimen should be based on the blood glucose profile
   Commonly used insulin regimens are as follows:
   1. Split mix regimen or premix regimen
   2. Multiple daily injections (MDIs) or basal-bolus regimen
   3. Continuous subcutaneous infusion

Different insulin regimens are given in **Box 1**.

Fetomaternal outcomes, total insulin doses, and overall glycemic control, both found to be equivalent in regimen 1 and 2.

Adjustments:

- It is necessary to titrate and individualize the regimen.
- It is utmost important to rapidly adjust dose to achieve glycemic control for better fetal and maternal outcome.
- Target capillary blood glucose levels

As per FIGO (2015), ADA (2018), ACOG (2018) and Government of India guidelines (2018) target capillary blood glucose levels are as follows:

- Capillary preprandial glucose <95 mg/dL (5.3 mmol/L)
- Capillary 1-hour postprandial glucose <140 mg/dL (7.8 mmol/L)
- Capillary 2-hour postprandial glucose <120 mg/dL (6.7 mmol/L)

There is insufficient evidence to suggest the optimal frequency of blood glucose testing in women with GDM. Based on the data available, recommendation is for daily glucose monitoring four times a day, once after fasting and again after each meal.

Route: Subcutaneous for all preparations.

Only regular insulin can be Injected IV (in intensive care settings)

Insulin delivery device

1. Vials and syringes
2. Pen
3. Insulin pump

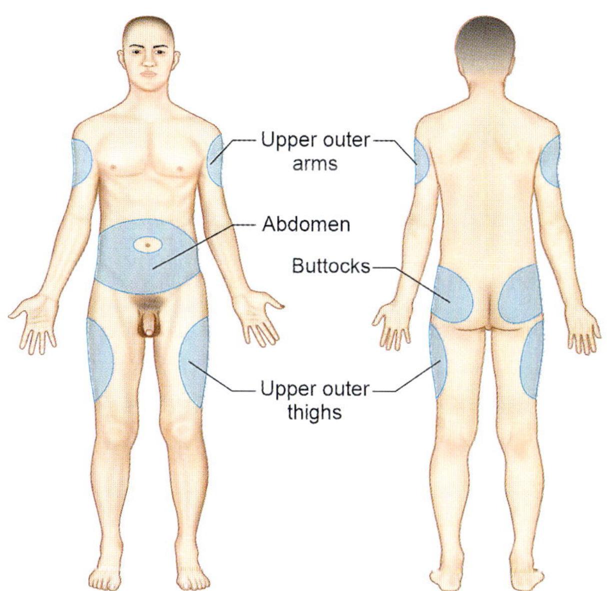

Fig. 4: Insulin injection sites. Source: MoHFW Guidelines 2018.

(especially useful with unstable diabetes without increasing rates of DKA or serious hypoglycemic events)

Injections sites (**Fig. 4**)

1. Abdomen (most common)
2. Upper outer thighs
3. Side of upper arm
4. Buttocks

Storage of insulin

- In refrigerator at 40–80°C (in the door of the refrigerator) and battery backup in areas with an erratic supply of electricity is must.
- Vial should never be kept in freezer compartment of refrigerator.
- If by mistake, vials are stored in freezer and frozen, they should not be used at all and discarded.
- Insulin vials should not be exposed to direct heat/sunlight and are stable up to 250–300°C.
- Open insulin vials (in current use) should be stored in refrigerator or in dark and cool place.
- Insulin vial once opened, it should be used within a month.
- If not used within a month, it should be discarded.
- Date of opening of vial to be written on the vial.
- Syringes can be stored at room temperature without direct exposure to sunlight or heat.
- Unopened insulin pens should be kept in refrigerator, once opened they can be kept at room temperature out of direct sunlight.

Adverse effects

- Hypoglycemia: Most frequent and potentially the most serious reaction.

Causes

1. Inadvertent injection of large doses of insulin
2. Missing a meal
3. Vigorous exercise

Diagnosis of hypoglycemia

Symptoms

- Sweating, anxiety, palpitation, tremor (because of counter regulatory sympathetic stimulation)
- Dizziness, headache, behavioral changes, visual disturbances, hunger, fatigue, weakness, muscular incoordination, sometimes fall (neuroglucopenic symptoms)
- Mental confusion, seizures, and coma (blood glucose levels than 40 mg/dL)

Treatment

- Glucose must be given orally or IV (for severe cases). It reverses the symptoms rapidly.

Pregnant women on insulin therapy should be instructed to keep sugar/jaggery/glucose powder handy at home to treat hypoglycemia if it occurs.

- Local reactions
    - Swelling, erythema, and stinging
    - Lipodystrophy—not seen with newer preparations
- *Allergy:* Very rare with human insulin
- *Edema:* In some patients develop short-lived dependent edema.

Drug Interactions

- β-adrenergic blockers prolong hypoglycemia
- Thiazides, furosemide, corticosteroids, oral contraceptives, salbutamol, and nifedipine tend to raise blood sugar and reduce effectiveness of insulin
- Acute ingestion of alcohol can precipitate hypoglycemia
- Salicylates, lithium, and theophylline may also accentuate hypoglycemia.

Barriers to insulin use:

- Compliance of patients
- Fear of many injections in a day and scarring
- Difficulty in administration and pain
- Risk of hypoglycemia

Oral Hypoglycemic Agents

Insulin has always been incorporated in standard care of diabetes in pregnancy but in recent past use of oral antidiabetic medications such as metformin and glyburide for treatment of GDM has also gained importance. **Table 8** shows comparison of oral hypoglycemic agents and insulin.

Metformin

Recently Society for Maternal-Fetal Medicine (SMFM) endorsed metformin as a safe first-line alternative to insulin.

TABLE 8: Comparison of oral hypoglycemic agents and insulin.

Study	*Details*	*Findings*
Nicholson et al.—4 RCTs (n = 1,229) + 5 observational studies (n = 831)	• 1 RCT of metformin vs. insulin • 3 RCTs of glibenclamide vs. insulin • 1 RCT of acarbose vs. insulin • 5 observational studies	• No difference in maternal and neonatal outcomes • Higher neonatal hypoglycemia in insulin group (8.1%) compared to OHA (3.3%), $p = 0.008$ • Overall no difference in maternal and neonatal outcomes
Dhulkotia et al.—6 RCTs (n = 1,388)	• 2 RCTs of metformin vs. insulin • 4 RCTs of glyburide vs. insulin	• No difference in glycemic control • OR of maternal hypoglycemia = 0.34 (95% CI: 0.02–5.82) with OHA • Higher hypertensive disorders in insulin group • No differences in CS rate, preterm birth, neonatal hypoglycemia, BW, LGA, NICU admission, RDS, SGA, IUFD
Nicholson et al.—8 RCTs	• 2 RCTs of metformin vs. insulin	• No difference in any outcome, trends of increased maternal hypoglycemia in insulin arm

In **Table 9**, Role of metformin as per different guidelines is beautifully depicted.

Mechanism of Action

Metformin is a biguanide analog that functions by:

- Inhibiting hepatic gluconeogenesis
- Stimulating glucose uptake in peripheral tissues
- Decreasing gastrointestinal glucose absorption

Although metformin requires the presence of insulin to potentiate its effect, it does not stimulate insulin secretion and therefore is not associated with hypoglycemia.

Dose

- Starting dose—500 mg in night for the first week, followed by an increase to 500 mg twice daily.
- The maximum daily dose: 2,500–3,500 mg divided into 2–3 doses.
- The half-life of metformin is 2–5 hours.
- Peak plasma concentrations—4 hours extended-release metformin
- Half-life: 7–8 hours
- Maximum limit: 2,000 mg daily.

Advantages:

- Lower gastrointestinal adverse effects
- Easier dosing that can be once daily instead of in divided dose
- Side Effects
- Common side effect (2.5–45.7% of patients):
    - Diarrhea
    - Nausea
    - Stomach pain

TABLE 9: Role of metformin as per different guidelines.

Guide	*Country*	*Year*	*Requirements/Recommendations*
American Diabetes Association (ADA)	American	2020	Insulin is the first-line treatment for GDM in the US. Although trials show metformin and glyburide can reduce glucose levels, they are **not recommended as first-line** due to placental transfer and limited safety data. Metformin may be considered to treat polycystic ovary syndrome and induce ovulation but should be discontinued by the end of the first trimester
American Congress of Obstetricians and Gynecologists (ACOG)	American	2018	For women who decline insulin, metformin is a reasonable second-line option. Patients must be informed about risks such as prematurity, placental drug transfer, and lack of long-term safety data regarding fetal growth
International Federation of Gynecology and Obstetrics (FIGO)	–	2015	Insulin, glyburide, and metformin are safe and effective options for second- and third-trimester treatment of GDM if glycemic targets are not met with lifestyle modification alone
National Institute for Health and Care Excellence (NICE)	UK	2015	Metformin is used if blood sugar targets are not met within 1–2 weeks of lifestyle changes. If metformin is contraindicated or insufficient, insulin is used
International Diabetes Federation (IDF)	–	2009	If blood sugar targets are unmet after 1–2 weeks of lifestyle changes, medication should begin. Insulin is preferred, but metformin and glyburide may be considered when insulin is unsuitable. Combination therapy lacks sufficient evidence
Australasian Diabetes in Pregnancy Society (ADIPS) and Australian Electronic Treatment Guidelines (eTG)	Australian	2015	Insulin is recommended as first line. Metformin may be used only if patients refuse injections

  - Heartburn
- Serious side effects:
  - Lactic acidosis
  - Low blood sugar

Limitations: Crosses the placenta with concentrations reaching similar levels as in the maternal circulation.

Its indication and contraindications are given in **Table 10**

Pros and cons of metformin in GDM is given in **Table 11**.

Glyburide (also known as glibenclamide) is a second-generation sulfonylurea.

Mechanism of action (Table 12)

It binds to pancreatic β-cell adenosine triphosphate–calcium-channel receptors

TABLE 10: Relative indications and contraindications of metformin.

Relative indications	*Contraindications*
As monotherapy:	**Medical status:**
• GDM not responding to medical nutrition therapy and exercise, if FPG < 110 mg/dL	• Diagnosis in early gestation • Elevated BMI with significant hyperglycemia
• Poor compliance or refusal to use insulin	
• Lack of skills and/or resources for self-management of diabetes with insulin	• Gastrointestinal intolerance • Previous adverse reaction or allergy to metformin • Renal or hepatic dysfunction
Add-on to insulin therapy:	**Metabolic status:**
• High insulin dose requirements	• Significant hyperglycemia (FPG ≥ 110 mg/dL)
• Excess maternal weight gain	• Ketosis or ketonuria
	Obstetric status:
	• History of major congenital anomaly in previous pregnancy
	• Presence of hydramnios
	• Maternal distress
	• Fetal distress

- Acts to increase insulin secretion
- Increase sensitivity in peripheral tissues

Dose

- 2.5–20 mg daily, given in a single morning dose or divided into two daily doses.
- Should be taken 30 minutes to 1 hour before meals because peak in 2–3 hours.
- Insulin secretion is directly proportional to glyburide concentration.
- Drug concentrations return to baseline in 8 hours
- Suggesting that three times daily dosing may be more optimal.
- A daily dose >20 mg may increase the risk of hypoglycemic events as well as neonatal hypoglycemia and is therefore not recommended.
- Limitation: Glyburide does appear to cross the placenta, levels are low enough to be considered safe.

Special obstetric care for pregnant women with GDM

Antenatal care

Only salient points pertaining to GDM in pregnancy will be discussed in this section.

- Most of the guidelines worldwide like The American and Canadian guidelines recommend universal screening by two-step approach but In India recently Government of India endorsed the "Single Step Procedure" for screening and diagnosis of GDM by 2-hour 75 g post-blood sugar ≥ 140 mg/dL **(Flowchart 2)**.
- Evidences from India show that women in our country are at much higher risk of developing glucose intolerance during pregnancy as compared to white women and compliance is real problem.

TABLE 11: Pros and cons of metformin in GDM.

Category	*Pros*	*Cons*
Mechanism of action	• Reduces insulin resistance, the main pathophysiology in GDM	May fail to achieve adequate glycemic control in presence of insulinopenia
Pharmacokinetics	• Oral route of administration • Easy dose titration	• Increased renal clearance → need for higher doses • Significant placental transfer → exposure of fetus • Gastrointestinal intolerance
Efficacy	• Glycemic control comparable to insulin or glyburide • Low risk of maternal hypoglycemia	• Failure rate in 14–46% of women, requiring supplemental insulin • Slow onset of action → time lag in presence of significant hyperglycemia
Social and other considerations	• Better patient acceptability • Less cost • Less need for self-monitoring of blood glucose	• Not approved for use in pregnancy (Category B), use is off-label • Discordant views among leading guidelines
Maternal outcomes	• No adverse maternal outcomes • Less risk of hypoglycemia • Lower maternal weight gain • Less risk of pregnancy-induced hypertension	Slightly lower gestational age at delivery
Short-term fetal outcomes	• No increased risk of teratogenicity in fetuses exposed in first trimester • No increased risk of perinatal complications • Reduced neonatal hypoglycemia • Reduced NICU admissions • Lower birth weight; reduced risk of LGA and macrosomia	Increased risk of preterm birth (inconsistent results)
Long-term effects of exposure of fetus	• No evidence of growth or motor-social developmental abnormalities • May result in more favorable adipose tissue distribution	Insufficient data on long-term effects of in utero exposure

Maternal Risk FetaRisk

Once a diagnosis of GDM has been confirmed, initial management involves medical nutrition therapy (MNT) and physical exercise for 2 weeks. After 2 weeks on MNT and physical exercise, 2 hours PPBS (post-meal) should be done. If it is not controlled with MNT (lifestyle changes), metformin or insulin therapy is added.

If 2-hour PPBS is >200 mg/dL at diagnosis, insulin has to be started straightaway.

The dose to be adjusted on follow-up and at the same time MNT and physical exercise has to be followed **(Flowchart 3)**.

- In cases diagnosed before 20 weeks of pregnancy, a fetal anatomical survey by USG should be performed at 18–20 weeks.

TABLE 12: Comparison of insulin, metformin, and glyburide.

Features	*Insulin*	*Metformin*	*Glyburide*
History	Standard of care First-line therapy by most guidelines	Approved recently as alternative to insulin	As second choice after metformin
Placental transfer	Not known to cross the placenta	Crosses placenta	Crosses placenta
Fetomaternal outcome	Safe	Similar to insulin, superior to glyburide	Relatively safe in pregnancy but with more long-term data required
Advantages	Long-term safety data	Satisfaction of patient Less cost Reduce several common short-term adverse outcomes related to GDM	Convenient, cheaper, and easier to administer and store than insulin
Drawbacks	Decreased compliance, Costly Substantial education of patient	No long-term safety data Potential detrimental effect of metformin on fat mass, fetal programming	Meta-analyses suggest that glyburide may increase the risk for LGA infants and neonatal hypoglycemia

Flowchart 2: Universal Screening GDM.

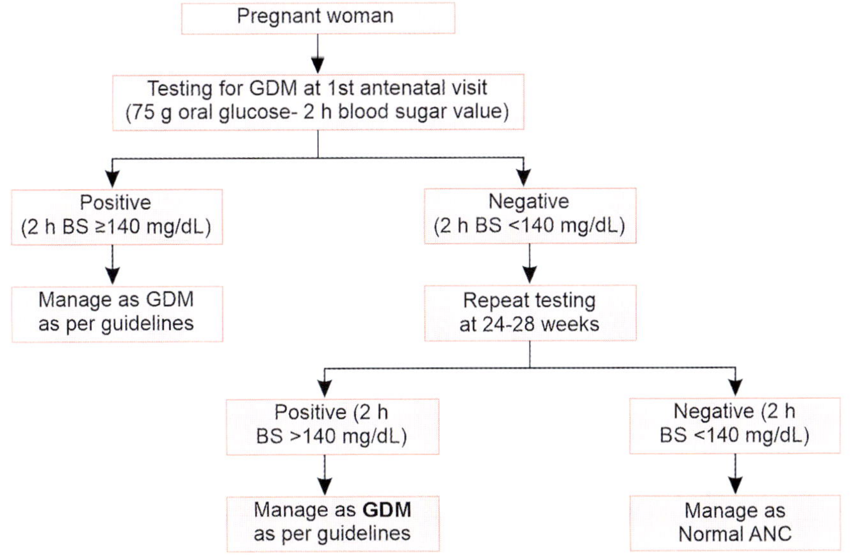

Source: MoHFW. Diagnosis and Management of Gestational Diabetes: Technical and Operational Guidelines. New Delhi: MoHFW; 2018.

Flowchart 3: Management of GDM in pregnancy.

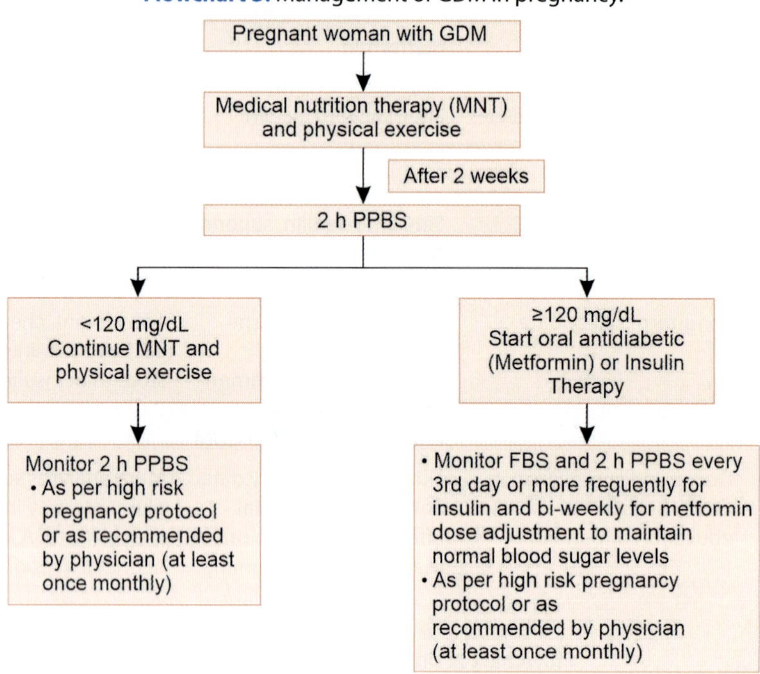

Source: MoHFW. Diagnosis and Management of Gestational Diabetes: Technical and Operational Guidelines. New Delhi: MoHFW; 2018.

- For all pregnancies with GDM, a fetal growth scan should be performed at 28–30 weeks gestation and repeated at 34–36 weeks gestation.
- Pregnant women should be explained about daily fetal activity assessment.
- Pregnant women with GDM in whom blood sugar level is well controlled and there are no complications, should continue with antenatal visits as per high-risk pregnancy protocol.
- Monitor for abnormal fetal growth (macrosomia/growth restriction) and polyhydramnios at each ANC visit.
- Pregnant women with GDM to be diligently monitored for hypertension in pregnancy, proteinuria, and other obstetric complications.
- In pregnant women with GDM between 24 and 34 weeks of gestation and requiring early delivery, antenatal steroids should be given as per GOI guidelines, i.e., injection dexamethasone 6 mg IM 12 hourly for 2 days. More vigilant monitoring of blood sugar levels should be done for next 72 hours following injection. In case of raised blood sugar levels during this period, adjustment of insulin dose should be made accordingly **(Flowchart 4)**.

Labor and Delivery

- If a pregnant women with GDM with well-controlled blood sugar has not already delivered spontaneously, induction of labor should be scheduled at or after 39 weeks pregnancy.
- In pregnant women with GDM with poor blood sugar control, those with risk factors like hypertensive disorder of pregnancy, previous stillbirth and other complications should

Flowchart 4: Insulin therapy in GDM.

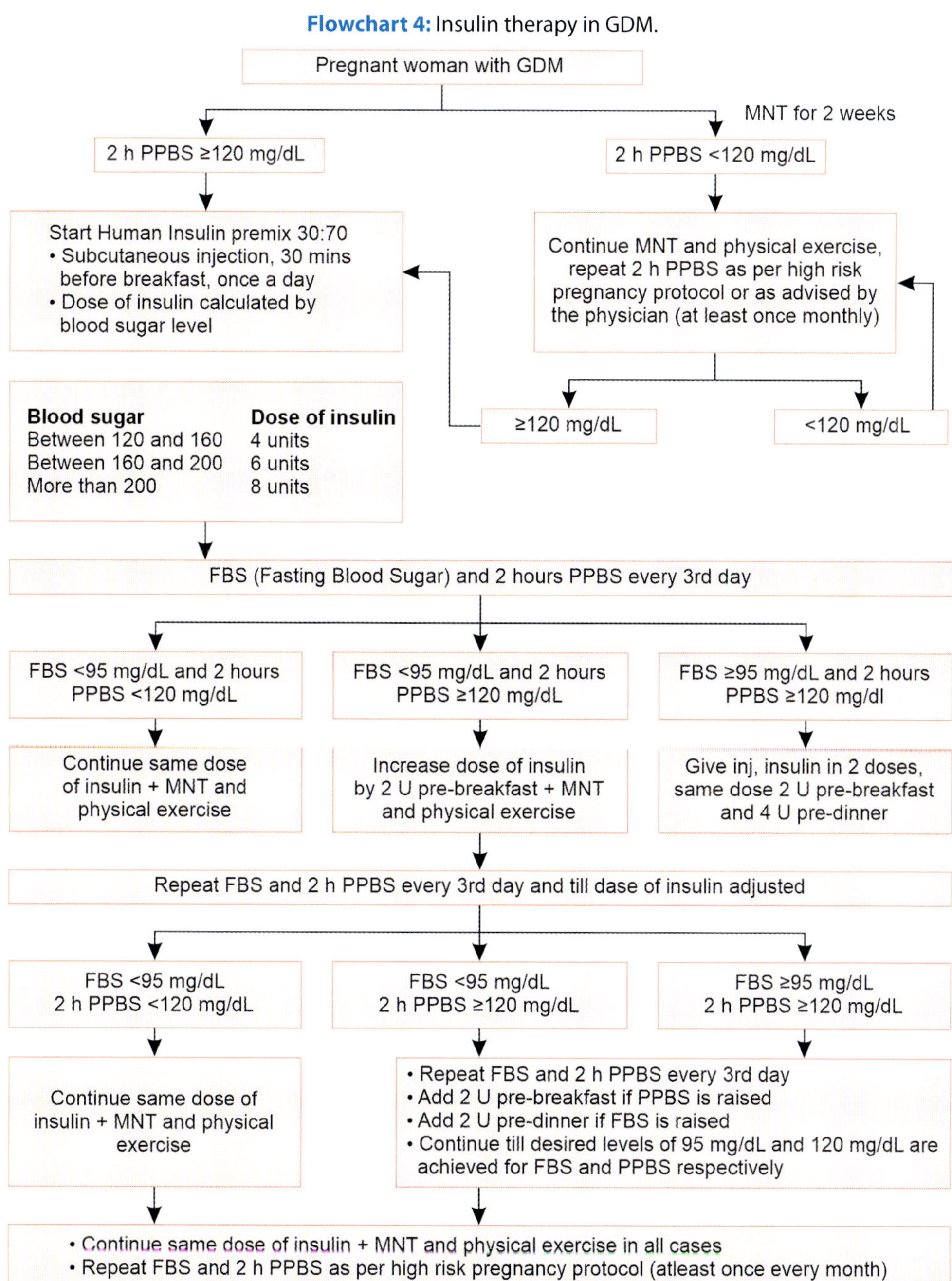

Source: MoHFW. Diagnosis and Management of Gestational Diabetes: Technical and Operational Guidelines. New Delhi: MoHFW; 2018.

TABLE 13: Insulin on sliding scale.

Blood sugar level	*Amount of insulin added in 500 mL NS*	*Rate of NS infusion*
90–120 mg/dL	0	100 mL/hour (16 drops/min)
120–140 mg/dL	4 U	100 mL/hour (16 drops/min)
140–180 mg/dL	6 U	100 mL/hour (16 drops/min)
>180 mg/dL	8 U	100 mL/hour (16 drops/min)

be delivered earlier. The timing of delivery should be individualized by the obstetrician accordingly.
- Vaginal delivery should be preferred and LSCS should be done for obstetric indications only.
- In case of fetal macrosomia (estimated fetal weight > 4 kg), consideration should be given for a primary cesarean section at 39 weeks to avoid shoulder dystocia.
- GDM pregnancies are associated with delay in lung maturity of the fetus; so routine delivery prior to 39 weeks is not recommended.

Special precaution during labor
- Pregnant women with GDM on medical management (metformin or insulin) require blood sugar monitoring during labor by a glucometer.
- The morning dose of insulin/metformin is withheld on the day of induction/labor and the pregnant women should be started on 2 hourly monitoring of blood sugar.
- IV infusion with normal saline (NS) to be started and regular insulin to be added according to blood sugar levels as per the **Table 13**.

Summary of delivery protocol in GDM is given in **Box 2**.

Step 1:
Immediate neonatal care for baby of mother with GDM
- All neonates should receive immediately essential newborn care with emphasis on early breastfeeding to prevent hypoglycemia.
- If required, the sick neonates should be immediately resuscitated as per GOI guidelines.
- Newborn should be monitored for hypoglycemia. Monitoring should be started at 1 hour of In all babies born to diabetic mother, BS should be checked by glucometer between 1 and 2 hours after birth
- Postdelivery follow-up of pregnant women with GDM:
  - Immediate postpartum care of women with GDM is not different from women without GDM but these women are at high risk to develop type 2 diabetes mellitus in future.
  - Maternal glucose levels usually return to normal after delivery.
  - Subsequently, must perform 75 g OGTT (fasting and 2 hours PP) at 6 weeks postpartum to evaluate glycemic status of woman

Flowchart 5 is showing this algorithm.

Preconception care and counseling

BOX 2: Summary of delivery protocol in GDM.

Intradelivery protocol and method of delivery

Elective Cesarean Section

- Women with type 1 diabetes should be placed first on the operating list and admitted either the previous day or early on the morning of surgery
- Long-acting insulin is taken as normal before a light supper
- The mother should fast from 22:00 hour the evening before surgery and should be first on the operating list the next day; rapid-acting insulin should be withheld
- 1–2 hours before surgery, hourly monitoring of blood glucose begins; and a glucose–insulin infusion is commenced, if necessary, to maintain blood glucose between 4 and 7 mmol/L.
- The insulin dose and/or rate are adjusted in response to maternal/capillary glucose

Induction of Labor

- Women should continue their current insulin regimen until labor is confirmed
- Often, an early morning breakfast is consumed with their normal morning insulin dose
- Once labor is confirmed and the mother is fasting, a glucose–insulin infusion is commenced as per protocol, unless delivery is imminent
- Maternal blood glucose levels should be monitored hourly
- Blood glucose levels should be maintained between 4 and 7 mmol/L
- The insulin dose and/or rate is adjusted in response to maternal blood glucose

Spontaneous Labor

- Following admission in spontaneous labor, the patient is fasted
- A blood glucose level should be taken on admission and hourly thereafter
- Once labor is confirmed, a glucose–insulin infusion is commenced as per protocol
- Capillary glucose levels should be maintained between 4 and 7 mmol/L
- The insulin dose and/or rate is adjusted according to the local protocol in response to maternal blood glucose

Source: MoHFW. Diagnosis and Management of Gestational Diabetes: Technical and Operational Guidelines. New Delhi: MoHFW; 2018.

Flowchart 5: Follow-up algorithm.

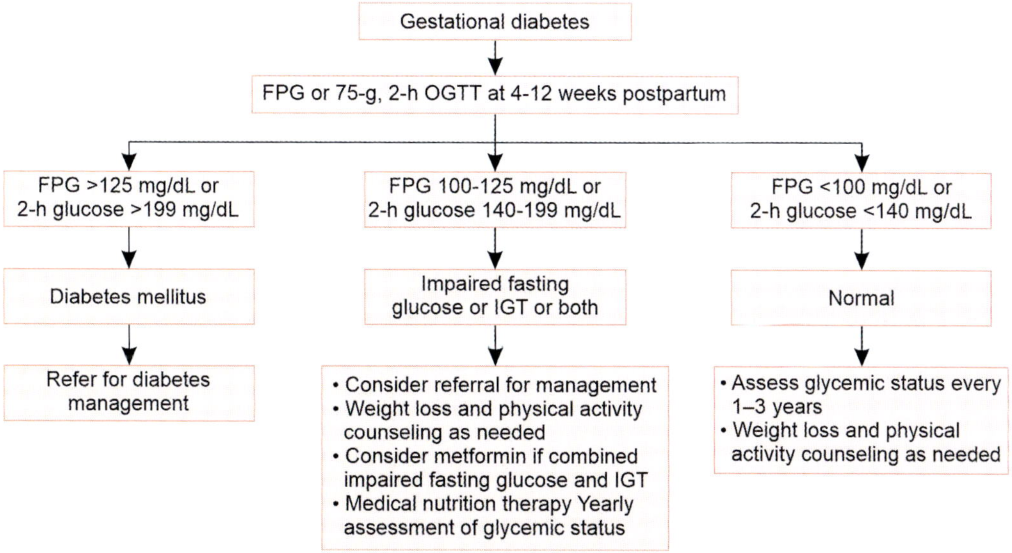

Gestational diabetes
↓
FPG or 75-g, 2-h OGTT at 4-12 weeks postpartum

FPG >125 mg/dL or 2-h glucose >199 mg/dL	FPG 100-125 mg/dL or 2-h glucose 140-199 mg/dL	FPG <100 mg/dL or 2-h glucose <140 mg/dL
Diabetes mellitus	Impaired fasting glucose or IGT or both	Normal
Refer for diabetes management	• Consider referral for management • Weight loss and physical activity counseling as needed • Consider metformin if combined impaired fasting glucose and IGT • Medical nutrition therapy Yearly assessment of glycemic status	• Assess glycemic status every 1–3 years • Weight loss and physical activity counseling as needed

Woman with history of GDM to be counseled about BMI and blood sugar estimation before next pregnancy

Desired blood sugar levels:

- 1 FBS: <100 mg/dL
- 1.2-hour PPBS: <140 mg/dL
- Counseled to consult gynecologist as soon as she misses her period
- **Insulin Pumps:** Reduce HbA1c, hypoglycemia, and dawn phenomenon; disadvantages include cost, education needs, and ketoacidosis risk if malfunctioning.[3]
- **Oral Antidiabetic Drugs (OADs):**[2]
    - **Metformin:** Safe, preferred by patients, equivalent perinatal outcomes to insulin (MiG trial).[1]
    - **Glyburide:** Alternative, safe in breastfeeding.[3]
    - **Evidence:** MiG trial showed no increased perinatal complications with metformin; women preferred it over insulin.[1]

Obstetric Care

- **Preconception (Preexisting Diabetes):**[3]
    - Optimize glycemic control (A1c < 6.5%).
    - Evaluate complications: Funduscopic examination, serum creatinine, eGFR, LFTs, TSH, urine albumin-to-creatinine ratio, and 24-hour proteinuria.
- **Antenatal Monitoring:**[2]
    - Fetal anatomical survey (18–20 weeks if diagnosed early).
    - Growth scans (28–30 weeks and 34–36 weeks).
    - Daily fetal movement count.
    - Insulin/OAD patients: Monthly ultrasounds, twice-weekly NSTs, or weekly BPP/AFI.
    - Monitor hypertension, proteinuria, and polyhydramnios.
    - Antenatal steroids for delivery between 24 and 34 weeks.
- **Delivery Timing (Table 14):**[2]
    - Well-controlled GDM/MNT: 39 0/7–40 6/7 weeks.
    - Well-controlled GDM/medication or preexisting diabetes: 39 0/7–39 6/7 weeks.
    - Poorly controlled: 36 0/7–38 6/7 weeks (preexisting) or individualized (GDM).

TABLE 14: Delivery timing (ACOG).

Condition	*Timing (Weeks)*
Pregestational, well-controlled	39 0/7–39 6/7
Pregestational, poorly controlled	36 0/7–38 6/7
GDM, MNT, well-controlled	39 0/7–40 6/7
GDM, medication, well-controlled	39 0/7–39 6/7
GDM, poorly controlled	Individualized

Source: ACOG Practice Bulletin No. 190: Gestational Diabetes Mellitus. Obstet Gynecol. 2018;131(2):e49-e64.[2]

TABLE 15: Postpartum glucose testing.

Timing	*Test*	*Action*
Day 1	Blood glucose	Confirm normoglycemia
6 weeks	75-g 2-hour OGTT	<140 mg/dL: Annual screening; ≥140 mg/dL: Treat as T2DM
6–13 weeks (NICE)	Fasting glucose	If unavailable, use HbA1c

Source: MoHFW. Diagnosis and Management of Gestational Diabetes: Technical and Operational Guidelines. New Delhi: MoHFW; 2018; NICE, 2015.[1,3]

Intrapartum Management

- **Glycemic Control:**
  - Normal saline infusion typically sufficient; insulin rarely needed.[2]
  - Monitor glucose hourly if on insulin (target 70–110 mg/dL).
- **Anesthesia:** No contraindications for epidural, spinal, or general anesthesia.[2]

POSTPARTUM CARE (TABLE 15)

- **Immediate Postpartum:**
  - Monitor glucose day after delivery to confirm normoglycemia.[3]
  - GDM: 95% return to normal glucose; insulin rarely needed.[3]
- **Glucose Tolerance Testing:**[1]
  - 75-g 2-hour OGTT at 6 weeks:
    - <140 mg/dL: Annual postprandial screening.
    - ≥140 mg/dL: Manage as overt diabetes.
  - **NICE Guidelines:** Fasting plasma glucose at 6–13 weeks; HbA1c if fasting unavailable; avoid routine OGTT.[3]
- **Breastfeeding:**[3]
  - Reduces maternal T2DM, childhood obesity, and T1DM risk.
  - Safe with insulin, metformin, glyburide (no neonatal hypoglycemia).
  - Initiate within 30 minutes post-birth, every 2–3 hours, maintaining neonatal glucose ≥ 2.0 mmol/L.
- **Long-Term Follow-up:** DPPOS Study: GDM increases T2DM risk by 48% over 10 years; intensive lifestyle and metformin reduce progression by 35% and 40%, respectively.[3]

CASE STUDY: PRIMIGRAVIDA AT 32 WEEKS WITH GDM

Scenario: A 28-year-old primigravida at 32 weeks, diagnosed with GDM due to irregular antenatal checkups.

Management[1,2]

- **Diagnosis:** Confirm with DIPSI test (2-hour glucose ≥140 mg/dL).
- **History:** Assess risk factors (BMI, family history, and ethnicity), symptoms, and obstetric history.

- **MNT:**
  - Calculate energy: 30 kcal/kg prepregnancy weight + 350 kcal/day.
  - 3 meals, 2–3 snacks with complex carbohydrates (2–3 serves/meal, 1–2/snack).
  - Monitor fasting (<95 mg/dL) and 1-hour postprandial (<120 mg/dL) for 2 weeks.
- **Pharmacotherapy:** If targets unmet, initiate insulin (0.9 units/kg/day) or metformin (fasting >110 mg/dL, postprandial > 140 mg/dL).
- **Obstetric Care:**
  - Growth scan at 34–36 weeks to assess macrosomia/polyhydramnios.
  - Daily fetal movement count.
  - Twice-weekly NSTs or weekly BPP/AFI.
  - Screen for hypertension, proteinuria, and infections.
- **Delivery:** Plan for 39 0/7–39 6/7 weeks if well-controlled; earlier if poorly controlled or complications (e.g., macrosomia and preeclampsia).
- **Postpartum:**
  - Monitor glucose day 1.
  - 75-g OGTT at 6 weeks; annual screening if normal.
  - Encourage breastfeeding and lifestyle modification.

ADVANCED TOPICS FOR PGs

- **Genetics and Epigenetics:**
  - GDM risk is linked to *TCF7L2, GCK*, and *KCNJ11* gene variants.[1]
  - Fetal exposure to hyperglycemia alters epigenetic markers, increasing T2DM and obesity risk.[1]
- **Emerging Therapies:**
  - **SGLT2 Inhibitors/GLP-1 Agonists:** Not recommended in pregnancy due to limited safety data.[3]
  - **Continuous Glucose Monitoring (CGM):** Improves glycemic control in T1DM and high-risk GDM, reducing neonatal hypoglycemia.[3]
- **Controversies:**
  - **One-Step versus Two-Step Screening:** DIPSI (one-step) is cost-effective in India but may overdiagnose; ACOG's two-step approach is more specific but resource-intensive.[2]
  - **Induction versus Expectant Management:** No clear superiority in GDM; RCTs show similar cesarean and neonatal outcomes.[2]

TABLE 16: Global GDM diagnostic criteria.

Guideline	*Fasting (mg/dL)*	*1-hour (mg/dL)*	*2-hour (mg/dL)*
DIPSI	–	–	≥140
WHO	≥92	≥180	≥153
IADPSG	≥92	≥180	≥153
ACOG (100 g)	≥95	≥180	≥155

Source: MoHFW 2018; ACOG 2018.[1,2]

- **Global Guidelines Comparison:**
  - **WHO:** 75-g OGTT, diagnostic if fasting ≥ 92, 1-hour ≥ 180, or 2-hour ≥ 153 mg/dL.[1]
  - **IADPSG:** Lower thresholds (fasting ≥ 92, 1-hour ≥ 180, and 2-hour ≥ 153 mg/dL) to reduce complications but increase GDM prevalence **(Table 16)**.[1]

REFERENCES

1. Ministry of Health and Family Welfare. Diagnosis and Management of Gestational Diabetes Mellitus: Technical and Operational Guidelines. New Delhi: MoHFW; 2018.
2. ACOG Practice Bulletin No. 190: Gestational Diabetes Mellitus. Obstet Gynecol. 2018;131(2):e49-e64.
3. American Diabetes Association. 14. Management of Diabetes in Pregnancy: Standards of Care in Diabetes—2024. Diabetes Care. 2024;47(Suppl 1):S282-S293. doi:10.2337/dc24-S014.

Hypertensive Disorders in Pregnancy

Ruchika Garg

EPIDEMIOLOGY AND GLOBAL BURDEN

- Hypertensive disorders in pregnancy (HDP) accounts for >90% of maternal deaths in under-resourced countries.
- Approximately 76,000 maternal deaths and 500,000 fetal deaths occur annually due to HDP globally (~14% of maternal and 10–25% of perinatal deaths).
- Incidence of preeclampsia in the USA is rising, affecting 3–5% of pregnancies and contributes to about 32% of maternal deaths during delivery.
- MBRRACE-UK data: Maternal mortality rate 13.56/100,000; 16.2/100,000 directly due to HDP.[1]
- Preterm birth and neonatal morbidity strongly linked to preeclampsia-related NICU admissions.
- Incidence varies by region and ethnicity, e.g., in England, black women have a higher risk compared to white women.

CLASSIFICATION (ISSHP GUIDELINES)

- Chronic hypertension—hypertension present before 20 weeks or before pregnancy
- Gestational hypertension—new-onset hypertension after 20 weeks without proteinuria
- Preeclampsia—hypertension after 20 weeks with proteinuria or end-organ dysfunction.[2]
- Eclampsia—seizures in preeclamptic patients
- Superimposed preeclampsia—chronic hypertension with superimposed preeclampsia **(Tables 1 to 3)**.

TABLE 1: Diagnostic criteria for HDP.

Parameter	*Diagnostic standard*
Blood Pressure (BP)[3]	≥140/90 mm Hg (Korotkoff V for diastolic)
Measurement Technique	Seated position, feet flat, and validated device
Confirmation	Average of two readings, repeat for confirmation
Severe Hypertension	≥160/110 mm Hg, repeat within 15 minutes
Proteinuria	≥300 mg/24 h; or protein: creatinine ratio ≥30 mg/mmol; or dipstick ≥2+ (less reliable)
Urine Analysis	Microscopy for casts, RBCs, WBCs, and bacteriuria screening

TABLE 2: Clinical features and severity markers.

Feature	*Mild HDP*	*Severe HDP*
Systolic BP	<160 mm Hg	≥160 mm Hg
Diastolic BP	<110 mm Hg	≥110 mm Hg
Proteinuria	Absent or positive	Same as mild
Headache	Absent	Present
Visual disturbances	Absent	Present
Epigastric/upper abdominal pain	Absent	Present
Oliguria	Absent	Present
Convulsions (eclampsia)	Absent	Present
Platelets (<100,000/mm^3)	Absent	Present
Elevated liver enzymes	Minimal	Marked
Fetal growth Restriction	Absent	Present
Pulmonary edema	Absent	Present

Mild versus Severe HDP

TABLE 3: Risk factors for preeclampsia (NICE Guidelines).

Major risk factors	*Moderate risk factors*
Previous HDP	Nulliparity
Chronic kidney disease	Age ≥40 years
Autoimmune disease (SLE and APS)	Pregnancy interval >10 years
Type 1 or 2 diabetes	BMI ≥35 at first visit
Chronic hypertension	Family history of preeclampsia
Multiple pregnancy	

DIAGNOSTIC ADVANCES

- Ratio of sFlt-1/PlGF (soluble fms-like tyrosine kinase-1/placental growth factor) predicts early onset preeclampsia.
- Elevated sFlt-1 (antiangiogenic) reduces PlGF/VEGF leading to endothelial dysfunction.
- PlGF testing reduces outpatient visits and ultrasound frequency; cost-effective short-term diagnostic tool.

ETIOPATHOGENESIS

- Abnormal trophoblastic invasion → defective spiral artery remodeling → placental ischemia and hypoxia → systemic inflammation and endothelial dysfunction.
- Immunological Dysregulation: Altered maternal-fetal immune tolerance, HLA incompatibility, and oxidative stress contributing to endothelial injury.
- Genetic Predisposition: Polymorphisms in genes regulating endothelial function, coagulation, and immune response implicated.

- Endothelial Cell Injury: Circulating endothelial cells/microparticles elevated in preeclampsia, contributing to coagulopathy and increased vasopressor sensitivity.
- Imbalance in Prostaglandins: Reduced vasodilator prostacyclin and increased vasoconstrictor thromboxane A2 promote hypertension.
- Nitric oxide deficiency → impaired vasodilation.
- Excess antiangiogenic factors (sFlt-1 and sEng) cause vascular damage and organ ischemia.

Flowchart 1: Clinical Algorithm: Diagnosis and Management of HDP[4,5]

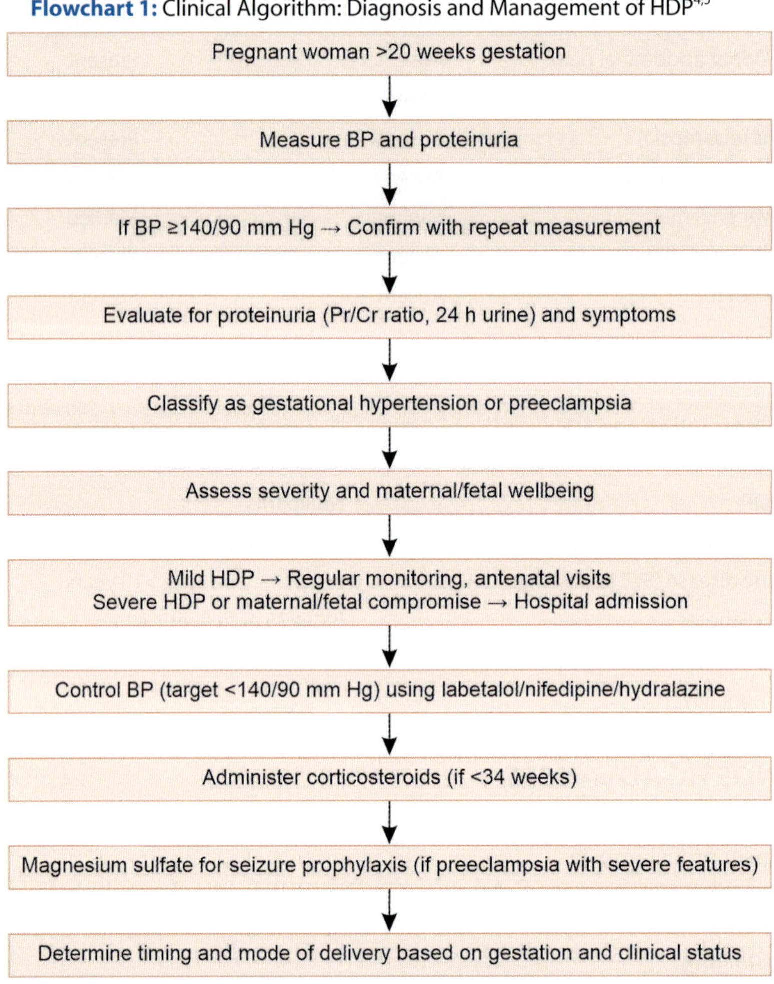

ANTENATAL AND INTRAPARTUM MANAGEMENT SUMMARY

- Blood pressure control essential; reduce severe maternal and fetal complications.
- Aspirin prophylaxis (50–150 mg/day) from 12 to 16 weeks reduces preterm preeclampsia risk (ASPRE trial).
- Regular fetal growth assessment through ultrasound and Doppler.
- Hospitalize in severe cases; magnesium sulfate for eclampsia prevention.

- Timely delivery planned per gestational age and maternal-fetal condition (generally ≥34 weeks or earlier if complications arise).

POSTPARTUM FOLLOW-UP

- BP peaks between days 3 and 7 postpartum; close monitoring recommended (self-monitoring encouraged).
- Continue antihypertensives as needed; calcium channel blockers and ACE inhibitors are breastfeeding safe.
- Counsel on long-term cardiovascular risks; HDP increases lifetime cardiovascular disease, chronic kidney disease, and diabetes risk.
- Annual cardiovascular risk assessments advised for 5–10 years postpartum.
- Lifestyle modifications (weight control, smoking cessation, and healthy diet/exercise) crucial.
- Monitor future pregnancies closely; recurrence risk of HDP is high.

LONG-TERM COMPLICATIONS

- HDP significantly increases risk of cardiovascular disease including coronary artery disease, heart failure, hypertension, and stroke with two-to-fourfold increased risks.
- Pathophysiology includes vascular remodeling abnormalities, persistent endothelial dysfunction, left ventricular hypertrophy, and metabolic syndrome.[6]
- Offspring of HDP pregnancies may also have increased cardiovascular and renal risks.

EMERGING THERAPIES

- Metformin prolongs gestation in early preeclampsia (<32 weeks) (PL2 trial).
- Nitric oxide donors, melatonin, and plasmapheresis show promise though evidence is evolving.
- siRNA targeting *sFlt-1* gene expression is a novel investigational strategy.

Eclampsia

Generalized tonic-clonic, absence, or focal seizures in a pregnant/postpartum woman with preeclampsia that cannot be attributed to another cause.

Epidemiology

- Incidence: 2–8 per 10,000 deliveries in developed countries 20–80 per 10,000 in low-resource settings.
- 1–2% of women with preeclampsia progress to eclampsia
- Antepartum (50%), intrapartum (30%), and postpartum (20%)
- Postpartum eclampsia: 60–80% within 48 hours, but up to 7–10 days possible

Risk Factors (same as severe preeclampsia)

- Nulliparity, extremes of age, and multiple gestation

- Previous preeclampsia, chronic hypertension, renal disease, and APS
- Lack of prenatal care and nonuse of aspirin prophylaxis

Prodromal Symptoms (often present 1–2 h before seizure)

- Persistent severe headache (frontal/occipital)
- Visual disturbances (scotomata, blurred vision, and cortical blindness)
- Severe epigastric/RUQ pain
- Hyperreflexia + clonus (>3 beats)
- Altered sensorium/agitation

Clinical Types

- Antepartum (most common and worst prognosis)
- Intrapartum
- Postpartum (late postpartum >48 h now recognized; up to 4 weeks)

Complications of Eclamptic Convulsion

- Maternal: Aspiration pneumonitis, pulmonary edema, cerebral hemorrhage (10%), AKI, DIC, HELLP, abruption, CVA, and death (1–2% in tertiary centers)
- Fetal: Acute hypoxia → fetal bradycardia/CTG abnormalities, preterm delivery, IUGR, and stillbirth (especially antepartum)

Immediate Management During Seizure (ABC Approach)

- Call for help, left lateral position, and airway protection (no tongue blade)
- High-flow oxygen and suction
- Protect from injury and avoid restraints
- Single seizure usually self-limiting (<90 seconds)

Definitive Treatment

- Delivery is the only cure (timing depends on gestational age, maternal condition, and fetal status)
- ≥34 weeks or maternal/fetal compromise → expedite delivery
- <34 weeks → corticosteroids + delivery within 24–48 hours if stable

Antihypertensive Therapy (same as severe preeclampsia)

Target BP <160/110 mm Hg

- First line: IV labetalol, IV hydralazine, and oral nifedipine
- Avoid nitroprusside and ACE inhibitors

Post-Seizure Care

- Continuous fetal monitoring
- Fluid restriction (80–100 mL/h) to prevent pulmonary edema

- Monitor for recurrent seizures (10–15% risk)
- Neuroimaging (noncontrast CT/MRI) if: Focal signs, prolonged coma (>4 h), and atypical presentation

Postpartum Eclampsia

- Up to 30–40% of all eclampsia
- Most common 2–7 days postpartum
- Often in women with no antepartum preeclampsia diagnosis
- Same management principles; higher index of suspicion needed

Key Points for Examination

- Eclampsia can occur with mild or even normal BP in 20–30%.
- Postpartum eclampsia is real and must be recognized.
- Recurrent seizures: 10–15% (second agent like phenytoin/levetiracetam if >2 seizures despite standard therapy).
- Maternal mortality in eclampsia: 1–2% (developed) versus 5–15% (developing countries).[1]
- Leading causes of death: Intracranial hemorrhage, pulmonary edema, and renal failure.

Prevention = Early recognition of severe preeclampsia + timely delivery + aspirin prophylaxis in high-risk women.

SHORT NOTE: HELLP SYNDROME AND MAGNESIUM SULFATE THERAPY

HELLP Syndrome

- **Full form:** Hemolysis, elevated liver enzymes, and low platelets
- Severe variant of preeclampsia (occurs in 0.5–0.9% of pregnancies; 10–20% of women with severe preeclampsia/eclampsia)
- Usually presents in 27–37 weeks gestation, but 15–30% postpartum (mostly within 48 h)

Classical Diagnostic Criteria (Tennessee or Mississippi classification)

Any three of the following:

1. **Hemolysis:** Abnormal peripheral smear (schistocytes), ↑ bilirubin (>1.2 mg/dL), and ↑ LDH (>600 U/L)
2. **Elevated liver enzymes:** AST ≥70 U/L (or ≥2 × upper limit), ALT elevated
3. **Low platelets:** <100,000/mm^3
    - Class I: platelets <50,000
    - Class II: 50,000–100,000
    - Class III: 100,000–150,000 (newer criteria)

Clinical Features

- Right upper quadrant/epigastric pain (65–90%)
- Nausea/vomiting, headache, and visual changes
- Hypertension (>140/90) in ~85%; may be absent in 15–20%.

- Can rapidly progress to DIC, liver rupture, acute kidney injury, pulmonary edema, and stroke

Management of HELLP

1. **Definitive Treatment:** Delivery (regardless of gestational age if ≥34 weeks or maternal/fetal deterioration).
2. <34 weeks → Corticosteroids for fetal lung maturity (betamethasone 12 mg IM q24h × 2 doses) + expedited delivery within 24–48 hours
3. Blood pressure control (goal <160/110): Labetalol, hydralazine, and nifedipine
4. Platelet transfusion if <20,000–25,000 prior to cesarean (or <50,000 if bleeding)

Magnesium Sulfate Therapy in HELLP

- **Primary Indication:** Seizure prophylaxis (same as in severe preeclampsia/eclampsia)
- HELLP alone is *not* an absolute indication if no preeclampsia features, but most patients have overlapping severe features → Magnesium sulfate ($MgSO_4$) is usually given.
- Standard regimen (Zuspan or Pritchard):

Regimen	*Loading dose*	*Maintenance*	*Duration*
Zuspan (IV)	4–6 g IV over 15–20 minutes	1–2 g/h IV continuous	24 h postpartum (or 24 h after last seizure)
Pritchard (IM)	4 g IV + 10 g IM (5 g each buttock)	5 g IM q4h	Same as above

Monitoring on Magnesium Sulfate

- Patellar reflexes (lost at 8–10 mEq/L)
- Respiratory rate (>12/min)
- Urine output (>100 mL/4 h or >25 mL/h)
- Serum magnesium level if renal impairment (therapeutic 4.8–8.4 mg/dL or 4–7 mEq/L)

Toxicity and Antidote

- 10 mEq/L → Loss of reflexes
- 12–15 mEq/L → Respiratory depression
- 15–20 mEq/L → Cardiac arrest
- Antidote: Calcium gluconate 1 g IV (10 mL of 10%) over 3–5 minutes

Key Points

- $MgSO_4$ does *not* treat hemolysis or thrombocytopenia; only prevents seizures
- Continue 24-hour postpartum (highest risk period)
- In true postpartum HELLP with no antepartum preeclampsia, some centers omit $MgSO_4$ if neurologically stable—controversial

Summary: Deliver promptly + BP control + $MgSO_4$ for seizure prophylaxis (24-h postpartum) is the cornerstone in most cases.

HYPERTENSIVE DISORDERS IN PREGNANCY OVERVIEW AND MANAGEMENT[5,7]

- Classification: Chronic HTN, gestational HTN, preeclampsia, and eclampsia
- Risk Factors: Major and moderate (NICE guidelines)
- Pathogenesis: Abnormal placentation → Endothelial dysfunction → Vasospasm and Oxidative stress
- Clinical Features: BP, proteinuria, and severe features
- Diagnostics: BP measurement, proteinuria assessment, and angiogenic markers (sFlt-1/PlGF)
- Management: BP control, aspirin prophylaxis, $MgSO_4$, and timing of delivery
- Postpartum care: Monitoring, BP control, and cardiovascular risk counseling
- Long-term complications: CVD, renal disease
- Emerging treatments: Metformin, siRNA, and others

REFERENCES

1. Vousden N, Bunch K, Kenyon S, et al. Impact of maternal risk factors on ethnic disparities in maternal mortality: a national population-based cohort study. Lancet Reg Health Eur. 2024;40:100893.
2. Paraskevas T, Gakis G, Papapanou M, et al. Statins for preventing preeclampsia. Cochrane Database Syst Rev. 2025 Mar 18;3(3):CD016133.
3. Tucker KL, Mort S, Yu LM, et al. Effect of Self-monitoring of Blood Pressure on Diagnosis of Hypertension During Higher-Risk Pregnancy: The BUMP 1 Randomized Clinical Trial. JAMA. 2022;327(17):1656-65. Erratum in: JAMA. 2022;328(2):217.
4. Ford ND, Cox S, Ko JY, et al. Hypertensive Disorders in Pregnancy and Mortality at Delivery Hospitalization - United States, 2017-2019. MMWR Morb Mortal Wkly Rep. 2022;71(17):585-91.
5. Traub A, Sharma A, Gongora MC. Hypertensive Disorders of Pregnancy: Pathophysiology and Management. US Cardiology Rev. 2024;18:e03.
6. Rana S, Lemoine E, Granger JP, et al. Preeclampsia: pathophysiology, challenges, and perspectives. Circ Res. 2019;124(7):1094-112.
7. Knight M. Saving Lives, Improving Mothers' Care. UK confidential enquiry. 2015–17.

Epilepsy and Antiepileptic Drugs in Pregnancy

Ruchika Garg

INTRODUCTION

Epilepsy is a prevalent neurological condition in pregnancy, affecting 0.5–1% of pregnant women globally, with a 10-fold increased maternal mortality risk compared to nonepileptic women.[1] Managing epilepsy during pregnancy balances seizure control with minimizing fetal risks from antiepileptic drugs (AEDs).

CLASSIFICATION OF EPILEPSY

Epilepsy is classified based on seizure type and EEG features as per the International League Against Epilepsy (ILAE) 2017 criteria:[2]

- **Primary Generalized Seizures (85% of Cases):**
  - Involve both hemispheres, often hereditary.
  - **Tonic-Clonic (Grand Mal):** Loss of consciousness, tonic muscle contraction, clonic jerks; risk of status epilepticus.
  - **Absence (Petit Mal):** Brief (5–10 seconds) loss of consciousness, no motor disturbance, rapid recovery, 3 Hz spike-and-wave EEG pattern, triggered by hyperventilation.
  - **Myoclonic:** Sudden, brief muscle jerks.
- **Partial (Focal) Seizures (15% of cases):**
  - Originate in one brain region, often secondary to trauma, tumors, or perinatal factors.
  - **Simple Partial:** Preserved consciousness, may involve motor, sensory, autonomic, or psychological symptoms; rapid recovery.
  - **Complex Partial (Temporal Lobe):** Impaired consciousness, aura, duration >1 minute, postictal confusion.

Conditions Mimicking Seizures

- **Pseudoseizures (Nonepileptic Attack Disorders):** Prolonged/repeated episodes without cyanosis, resistance to eye-opening, down-going plantar reflexes, and preserved conjunctival reflex.[3]
- **Syncope:** May include jerking movements; includes cardiac arrhythmia-related, vasovagal, or aortic stenosis-induced episodes.[4]

TABLE 1: Causes of secondary epilepsy.[6]

Cause	*Examples*
Structural	Previous cerebral surgery, intracranial mass (cavernomas, meningiomas, and AVMs)
Vascular	Stroke and subarachnoid hemorrhage
Metabolic	Hypoglycemia (diabetes and hypoadrenalism) and hypocalcemia (hypoparathyroidism)
Infectious	Tuberculoma and toxoplasmosis
Obstetric	Eclampsia, posterior reversible leukoencephalopathy, and gestational epilepsy
Other	Antiphospholipid syndrome, TTP, drug/alcohol withdrawal, and postdural puncture

TABLE 2: Causes of increased seizure frequency in pregnancy.[8]

Factor	*Mechanism*
Physiological	Nausea/vomiting, decreased GI motility, antacid use, hypervolemia, and increased GFR
Pharmacokinetic	Induction of hepatic/placental enzymes, and increased drug metabolism
Behavioral	Medication noncompliance, sleep deprivation, hyperventilation, and labor pain

PATHOGENESIS

- **Primary Epilepsy:** Idiopathic, with 30% familial prevalence; no identifiable cause.[5]
- **Secondary Epilepsy:** Associated with underlying pathologies **(Table 1)**.[6]

CONCERNS DURING PREGNANCY

- **Increased Seizure Frequency:**
  - Occurs in 20–30% of pregnant women with epilepsy due to subtherapeutic AED levels and lower seizure threshold.[7]
  - Causes include altered pharmacokinetics and physiological changes **(Table 2)**.[8]
- **Fetal Risks:**
  - Untreated epilepsy does not increase malformation risk, but AEDs elevate congenital malformation rates (4–8% vs. 2–3% in general population).[9]
  - Risks include pregnancy loss, intrauterine growth restriction (IUGR), developmental delay, behavioral issues, and fetal anticonvulsant syndrome.
  - Recurrence risk of major congenital malformations is 16.8% if a previous child was affected.[10]
  - Teratogenic mechanisms **(Table 3):**
    - **Oxidative Metabolites:** AEDs (e.g., phenytoin and valproate) form embryotoxic oxide radicals, disrupting DNA/RNA synthesis.[11]
    - **Folate Deficiency:** AEDs reduce serum folate by up to 90%, impairing neural tube closure.[12]
    - **Genetic Predisposition:** Reduced epoxide hydrolase activity increases teratogen accumulation.[13]

TABLE 3: Teratogenic effects of common AEDs.[9,14]

Drug	*Abnormalities*	*Risk*	*Pregnancy category*
Valproate	Neural tube defects, skeletal anomalies, and developmental delay	1–2% (monotherapy) and 9–12% (polytherapy)	D
Phenytoin	Fetal hydantoin syndrome, craniofacial defects, and cardiac defects	5–11%	D
Carbamazepine	Spina bifida and fetal hydantoin syndrome	1–2%	D
Phenobarbital	Clefts, cardiac anomalies, and urinary tract defects	10–20%	D
Lamotrigine	Oral clefts (fourfold increase)	~2%	C
Topiramate	Oral clefts	~2%	C
Levetiracetam	Skeletal anomalies (animal studies)	Insufficient data	C

TABLE 4: Common AED side effects.[14,21]

Drug	*Maternal effects*	*Fetal effects*
Phenytoin	Nystagmus, ataxia, hirsutism, and gingival hyperplasia	Teratogenesis, coagulopathy, and hypocalcemia
Carbamazepine	Drowsiness, leukopenia, and hepatotoxicity	Craniofacial defects and spina bifida
Valproate	Ataxia, alopecia, and hepatotoxicity	Neural tube defects and skeletal defects
Lamotrigine	Rash, headache, and diplopia	Oral clefts

Pharmacokinetics of Antiepileptic Drugs in Pregnancy

Pregnancy alters AED pharmacokinetics due to increased plasma volume, hepatic metabolism, and renal clearance.[15]

- **Carbamazepine:**
  - 70–80% protein-bound, hepatic metabolism.
  - Increased metabolism and epoxide metabolite accumulation lower bioavailability.[16]
- **Phenytoin:** 90–93% protein-bound, hepatic 8-hydroxylation increases clearance, reducing serum levels.[17]
- **Phenobarbital:** 50% protein-bound, induces hepatic enzymes, long half-life, causes sedation.[18]
- **Valproate:** 88–92% protein-bound, concentration-dependent binding, requires dose adjustments.[19]
- **Newer AEDs (e.g., Lamotrigine, Levetiracetam, and Topiramate) (Table 4):** Primarily renally cleared, minimal hepatic metabolism, no antifolate effects, and safer in pregnancy.[20]

MANAGEMENT OF EPILEPSY IN PREGNANCY

Management aims to prevent seizures, minimize teratogenic risks, and ensure maternal-fetal safety, guided by RCOG Green-top Guideline No. 68 (2023) and NICE NG217 (2022).[22,23]

Preconception Counseling

- **Objectives:** Optimize AED regimen, reduce teratogenic risk, and ensure folate supplementation **(Table 5)**.[24]
- **Key Actions:**
  - Initiate folic acid 5 mg/day 3 months preconception, continue through pregnancy to reduce neural tube defect risk.[25]
  - Review AEDs: Avoid valproate if possible; consider lamotrigine/levetiracetam (lower teratogenicity).[26]
  - Reduce valproate dose (<600 mg/day) or switch to safer AEDs before conception (neural tube closure occurs by day 26).[27]
  - Counsel on seizure recurrence risk post-AED withdrawal: 25% within 1 year, 40% by 2 years, and >50% with structural lesions or abnormal EEG.[28]
  - Advise smoking/alcohol cessation, genetic counseling, and medication compliance.[29]
  - Discontinue AEDs only in women seizure-free >2 years, after neurologist consultation (not suitable for juvenile myoclonic epilepsy).[30]

Antenatal Care

- **AED Management:**
  - Continue carbamazepine, lamotrigine, or levetiracetam if well-controlled; avoid abrupt cessation.[31]
  - Valproate: Reduce to <600 mg/day, use divided doses or modified-release forms to minimize peak levels.[32]
  - Monitor free drug levels monthly in women with frequent seizures; adjust doses based on seizure frequency/severity.[33]
  - Lamotrigine may require two-to-threefold dose increase due to increased clearance; phenytoin/carbamazepine may also need adjustments.[34]
- **General Measures:**
  - Advise shallow baths/showers, recovery position training for family to prevent aspiration.[35]

TABLE 5: Preconception counseling for women with epilepsy.[24]

Action	*Details*
Folic Acid	5 mg/day from 3 months preconception to end of first trimester
AED Review	Avoid valproate; prefer lamotrigine/levetiracetam; reduce doses
Lifestyle	Adequate sleep, no smoking/alcohol, and maintain nutrition
Counseling	Seizure risks, teratogenicity, genetic predisposition, and compliance
Withdrawal	Consider if seizure-free >2 years; avoid in high-risk cases

- Offer prenatal screening: Nuchal translucency (11–13 weeks), detailed anomaly scan (18–20 weeks), and fetal cardiology assessment.[36]
- Serial growth scans for IUGR detection; no routine cardiotocography unless indicated.[37]
- Avoid high-dose corticosteroids for lung maturation in women on enzyme-inducing AEDs (e.g., carbamazepine and phenytoin) due to increased metabolism.[38]

- **Complications:** Increased risks of preeclampsia, postpartum hemorrhage, cesarean section, labor induction, nonproteinuric hypertension, postpartum depression, and offspring seizure disorders.[39]

Intrapartum Management

- **Seizure Risk:** 1–2% risk during labor and 24 hours postpartum.[40]
- **AED Continuation:** Administer regular AEDs; use parenteral forms if oral intake is not feasible.[41]
- **Pain Management:** Early epidural to reduce seizure triggers (pain and anxiety); avoid pethidine (seizure risk); use diamorphine or TENS/Entonox.[42]
- **Seizure Management:** For non-self-limiting seizures, administer IV lorazepam (4 mg over 2 minutes) or diazepam (10–20 mg IV/rectal).[43]
- **Delivery:** Vaginal delivery preferred; cesarean section for recurrent seizures in late pregnancy. Continuous fetal monitoring for high-risk cases.[44]

Postnatal Management

- **Neonatal Care:**
  - Administer 1 mg IM vitamin K to newborns of mothers on enzyme-inducing AEDs (e.g., carbamazepine and phenytoin) to prevent hemorrhagic disease.[45]
  - Monitor for withdrawal symptoms in neonates exposed to phenobarbital (rare with newer AEDs).[46]
- **Breastfeeding:**
  - Encouraged for all women; AEDs in breast milk are minimal (3–5% of therapeutic dose), except lamotrigine/phenobarbital (30–50%).[47]
  - Avoid initiating lamotrigine in breastfeeding mothers due to neonatal accumulation (immature glucuronidation).[48]
  - Feed before AED dose to minimize peak milk levels.[49]
- **AED Adjustment:** Gradually reduce doses increased during pregnancy (e.g., lamotrigine and phenytoin) over weeks postpartum, as clearance normalizes.[50]
- **Safety:** Advise changing diapers on the floor, shallow bathing with supervision to prevent injury during seizures.[51]
- **Mental Health:** Screen for postpartum depression; provide support contacts.[52]

Management of Newly Diagnosed Epilepsy

- **Incidence:** 20–30 per 100,000 women of childbearing age annually.[53]
- **Approach:**
  - Exclude secondary causes (e.g., eclampsia, stroke, and hypoglycemia).[54]
  - Single seizure: Treatment not mandatory; counsel on risks.

TABLE 6: Contraceptive advice for women on AEDs.[56]

Method	*Effectiveness with enzyme-inducing AEDs*	*Recommendation*
Combined Oral Contraceptives (COCs)	Reduced efficacy	Use 50 µg ethinyl estradiol or double 30 µg COCs
Progestin-Only Pills (POPs)	Reduced efficacy	Double dose
Emergency Contraception	Reduced efficacy	Double levonorgestrel/ulipristal dose
Implants/Rings/Patches	Reduced efficacy	Use alternative method
Medroxyprogesterone Injection	Effective	Standard dose
Levonorgestrel IUD (Mirena)	Effective	Preferred

- Treatment: Lamotrigine/carbamazepine for focal seizures; levetiracetam for generalized seizures; avoid valproate.[55]

Contraception

- **Enzyme-inducing AEDs** (phenytoin, carbamazepine, phenobarbital, and primidone):
  - Reduce efficacy of hormonal contraceptives; require higher estrogen doses or nonhormonal methods **(Table 6)**.[56]
- **Nonenzyme-inducing AEDs** (valproate, levetiracetam, and gabapentin): Compatible with all contraceptives.[57]
- **Lamotrigine:** Estrogen-containing contraceptives lower levels, risking seizures; nonhormonal methods preferred.[58]

RCOG AND NICE GUIDELINES

- **RCOG Green-top Guideline No. 68 (2023):**
  - Recommends preconception counseling, folate 5 mg/day, and avoiding valproate unless no alternative.
  - Advocates lamotrigine/levetiracetam as first line; monitor AED levels in women with frequent seizures.
  - Supports breastfeeding and neonatal vitamin K administration.[22]
- **NICE NG217 (2022):**
  - Emphasizes multidisciplinary care (obstetrician, neurologist, and midwife).
  - Advises against routine AED level monitoring in seizure-free women; adjust doses based on clinical need.
  - Highlights contraception counseling for enzyme-inducing AEDs.[23]

KEY POINTS

- Epilepsy affects 0.5–1% of pregnant women, with a 10-fold increased mortality risk.
- Seizure frequency increases in 20–30% of pregnancies due to altered AED pharmacokinetics and physiological changes.

- AEDs elevate congenital malformation risk (4–8%); valproate is most teratogenic (9–12% with polytherapy).
- Preconception: Use folate 5 mg/day, prefer lamotrigine/levetiracetam, avoid valproate, and counsel on seizure recurrence.
- Antenatal: Continue AEDs, monitor levels in frequent seizures, offer anomaly scans, and avoid high-dose corticosteroids.
- Intrapartum: Use epidural, benzodiazepines for seizures, vaginal delivery preferred, and continuous fetal monitoring if high risk.
- Postnatal: Administer neonatal vitamin K, encourage breastfeeding, screen for depression, and adjust AED doses.
- Contraception: Enzyme-inducing AEDs require higher-dose hormonal methods or IUDs; nonenzyme-inducing AEDs are compatible with all methods.
- RCOG/NICE advocate safer AEDs, multidisciplinary care, and patient education.

REFERENCES

1. Harden CL, Meador KJ. Epilepsy in pregnancy: Risks and management. Lancet Neurol. 2015;14(5):448-54.
2. Fisher RS, Cross JH. ILAE 2017 classification of seizures. Epilepsia. 2017;58(4):522-30.
3. Reuber M, Elger CE. Psychogenic non-epileptic seizures. Lancet Neurol. 2017;16(6):464-73.
4. Manolis TA, Manolis AS. Syncope and seizures. Curr Neurol Neurosci Rep. 2016;16(5):47.
5. Perucca P, Gilliam FG. Idiopathic generalized epilepsy. Neurol Clin. 2015;33(1):149-63.
6. Stephen LJ, Brodie MJ. Secondary epilepsy causes. Epilepsy Res. 2018;147:63-71.
7. Pennell PB. Seizure frequency in pregnancy. Epilepsia. 2016;57(Suppl 1):46-50.
8. Tomson T, Battino D. Pharmacokinetics of AEDs in pregnancy. Clin Pharmacokinet. 2019;58(6):697-709.
9. Meador KJ, Loring DW. AED teratogenicity. Neurology. 2016;86(14):1301-9.
10. Campbell E, Kennedy F. Malformation recurrence in epilepsy. BJOG. 2017;124(5):769-76.
11. Pennell PB, Hovinga CA. AED oxidative metabolites. Epilepsia. 2015;56(8):1170-9.
12. Asadi-Pooya AA. AED-induced folate deficiency. Seizure. 2017;50:128-34.
13. Finnell RH, Buehler BA. Genetic predisposition in teratogenicity. Teratology. 2018;97(3):201-10.
14. Tomson T, Battino D. Teratogenic effects of AEDs. Lancet Neurol. 2019;18(2):174-86.
15. Reimers A, Brodtkorb E. AED pharmacokinetics in pregnancy. Expert Opin Drug Metab Toxicol. 2016;12(3):281-92.
16. Johannessen SI, Landmark CJ. Carbamazepine pharmacokinetics. CNS Drugs. 2018;32(7):627-36.
17. Patsalos PN, Perucca E. Phenytoin in pregnancy. Clin Pharmacokinet. 2017;56(9):1007-16.
18. Patsalos PN. Phenobarbital pharmacokinetics. Epilepsy Res. 2015;110:183-90.
19. Bialer M, Midha KK. Valproate pharmacokinetics. CNS Drugs. 2018;32(2):109-27.
20. Perucca E, Tomson T. Newer AEDs in pregnancy. Epilepsia. 2019;60(Suppl 1):6-17.
21. Patsalos PN, Spencer EP. AED side effects. Ther Adv Neurol Disord. 2018;11:1756286418757830.
22. Royal College of Obstetricians and Gynaecologists (RCOG). (2016). Epilepsy in pregnancy. Green-top Guideline No. 68. [online] Available from https://www.rcog.org.uk/guidance/browse-all-guidance/green-top-guidelines/epilepsy-in-pregnancy-green-top-guideline-no-68/ [Last accessed December, 2025].
23. NICE. (2022). Epilepsies in children, young people and adults. NICE guideline: NG217. [online] Available from https://www.nice.org.uk/guidance/ng217 [Last accessed December, 2025].
24. Harden CL, Pennell PB. Preconception counseling in epilepsy. Epilepsy Behav. 2017;74:91-8.

25. Wilson RD, O'Connor DL. Folic acid in epilepsy. J Obstet Gynaecol Can. 2019;41(5):697-705.
26. Herzog AG, Mandle HB. AED optimization in pregnancy. Neurology. 2018;91(15):e1395-404.
27. Tomson T, Marson A. Valproate in pregnancy. Lancet Neurol. 2016;15(2):210-8.
28. Specchio LM, Beghi E. AED withdrawal risks. Epilepsia. 2015;56(10):1515-22.
29. Johnson EL, Burke AE. Lifestyle counseling in epilepsy. Seizure. 2019;64:1-8.
30. Lossius MI, Tauboll E. AED discontinuation in pregnancy. Acta Neurol Scand. 2017;136(Suppl 200):7-13.
31. Pennell PB. AED management in pregnancy. Continuum. 2016;22(1):159-79.
32. Bromley R, Weston J. Valproate dose reduction. Cochrane Database Syst Rev. 2018;10:CD012554.
33. Voinescu PE, Pennell PB. AED level monitoring. Epilepsia. 2017;58(Suppl 1):51-9.
34. Sabers A, Tomson T. Lamotrigine dose adjustments. Seizure. 2016;37:87-92.
35. Sveberg L, Svalheim S. Safety measures in epilepsy. Epilepsy Behav. 2018;80:9-15.
36. Mawhinney E, Campbell J. Prenatal screening in epilepsy. Ultrasound Obstet Gynecol. 2017;50(4):418-24.
37. Battino D, Tomson T. Fetal growth in epilepsy. Epilepsia. 2016;57(Suppl 1):60-6.
38. Westin AA, Reimers A. Corticosteroids and AEDs. Epilepsy Res. 2018;140:171-8.
39. Viale L, Allotey J. Pregnancy complications in epilepsy. BJOG. 2015;122(10):1367-74.
40. Edey S, Moran N. Intrapartum seizures. Seizure. 2016;36:1-6.
41. Reisinger TL, Newman M. AED administration in labor. Epilepsy Behav. 2019;94:172-8.
42. Walker JJ, Kaplan PW. Pain management in epilepsy. Obstet Gynecol Clin North Am. 2019;46(2):265-78.
43. Rajiv KR, Radhakrishnan A. Seizure management in labor. Epilepsia. 2017;58(Suppl 1):66-71.
44. Alsaadi T, El-Hammer Z. Delivery in epilepsy. Int J Gynaecol Obstet. 2018;143(3):297-303.
45. Harden CL, Sethi NK. Neonatal vitamin K in epilepsy. Neurology. 2015;85(1):82-8.
46. Veiby G, Bjørk M. Neonatal withdrawal from AEDs. Epilepsia. 2016;57(2):195-202.
47. Meador KJ, Baker GA. Breastfeeding and AEDs. Neurology. 2019;92(5):e451-9.
48. Nordmo E, Aronsen L. Lamotrigine in breast milk. Ther Drug Monit. 2018;40(3):377-82.
49. Tomson T, Battino D. AEDs in breast milk. Epilepsia. 2017;58(Suppl 1):80-6.
50. Reimers A, Helde G. Postpartum AED adjustments. Seizure. 2017;45:115-21.
51. Thomas SV, Jose M. Safety strategies in epilepsy. Epilepsy Behav. 2019;91:36-41.
52. Bjørk MH, Veiby G. Postpartum depression in epilepsy. Acta Neurol Scand. 2018;137(6):556-61.
53. Manford M. Incidence of epilepsy in women. J Neurol. 2017;264(9):1865-73.
54. Beghi E, Giussani G. Secondary seizures in pregnancy. Epilepsia. 2019;60(Suppl 1):18-24.
55. Weston J, Bromley R. Treatment of new-onset epilepsy. Cochrane Database Syst Rev. 2017;2:CD010914.
56. Reimers A, Brodtkorb E. Contraception and AEDs. Seizure. 2015;24:78-85.
57. Dutton C, Foldvary-Schaefer N. Contraception in epilepsy. Neurology. 2016;87(19):e229-36.
58. Herzog AG. Lamotrigine and contraception. Epilepsia. 2017;58(4):575-83.

Anemia in Pregnancy

Kalpana Kumari, Vandana Verma

INTRODUCTION

Anemia is qualitative or quantitative reduction in the oxygen carrying capacity of blood usually resulting from reduced hemoglobin that leads to reduced oxygen supply to peripheral tissues. The World Health Organization (WHO), the American College of Obstetrician and Gynecologist, and The Center for Disease Control and Prevention (CDC) have defined anemia in pregnant women as hemoglobin (Hb) concentration of less than 11g% and hematocrit (HCT) of less than 33% in first and third trimesters and 10.5g% and HCT of less than 32% during second trimester.

Anemia is the most common medical disorder during pregnancy, resulting in increased maternal morbidity and mortality. According to WHO, about 32.4 million pregnant women suffer from anemia disease. The prevalence percentage of anemia in pregnant women in India using the NFHS-4 survey remained 50.2%.

According to the WHO and the Indian Council of Medical Research (ICMR), anemia in pregnancy is classified based on severity into categories such as mild, moderate, and severe. The classification is summarized in **Table 1**.

TABLE 1: Grading of anemia.

Severity	*WHO Criteria (g/dL)*	*ICMR Criteria (g/dL)*
Mild	10.0–10.9	10.0–10.9
Moderate	7.0–9.9	7.0–10.0
Severe	<7.0	7.0–4.0
Very Severe	—	<4.0

There are various causes of anemia during pregnancy that are listed in **Table 2**.

TABLE 2: Various causes of anemia.

Acquired causes	*Inherited causes*
• Physiological anemia • Deficiency anemia • Anemia of chronic disease • Hemolytic anemia • Aplastic anemia	• Thalassemia • Sickle cell anemia • Inherited hemolytic anemia • Hemoglobinopathies other than sickle cell anemia

EFFECTS OF ANEMIA ON PREGNANCY

Anemia during pregnancy is associated with a spectrum of adverse maternal and fetal outcomes. In the maternal context, antepartum complications include preterm birth, preterm premature rupture of membranes (PPROM), antepartum hemorrhage (APH), congestive heart failure, prolonged labor, and placental abruption. Postpartum complications may manifest as postpartum hemorrhage (PPH), puerperal sepsis, lactation failure, thromboembolism, subinvolution of the uterus, and postpartum depression. For the fetus, anemia in the mother can lead to low birth weight, prematurity, neonatal anemia, increased susceptibility to infections, poor mental and psychomotor development, and perinatal mortality.

CLINICAL PRESENTATION

The clinical presentation of anemia varies based on its severity. In mild anemia, individuals are often asymptomatic. Moderate anemia may manifest as general weakness, fatigue, tiredness, reduced appetite, indigestion, dizziness, and breathlessness on exertion. In severe cases, symptoms become more pronounced, including palpitations, rapid heartbeat (tachycardia), significant breathlessness, and generalized swelling (edema). General physical signs may be absent in mild anemia but become evident as the condition progresses. These include pallor of the skin and mucous membranes, nail abnormalities such as depressed nails or koilonychia (spoon-shaped nails), angular cheilitis, glossitis (smooth tongue), stomatitis, and signs of hyperdynamic circulation like a soft systolic murmur. In decompensated states, signs of heart failure such as basal lung crepitations and peripheral edema may be present.

Physiological anemia: During pregnancy, the bone marrow undergoes erythroid hyperplasia, leading to a 15–25% rise in red blood cell (RBC) mass in women carrying a single fetus.

However, the plasma volume expands disproportionately—by about 40–50%—which causes hemodilution (also known as hydremia of pregnancy) and increases the body's demand for iron. As a result, a physiological anemia develops, with the HCT falling from around 38–45% in healthy, nonpregnant women to approximately 34% by the end of a singleton pregnancy, and to about 30% in multiple pregnancies. Despite this dilutional change, the overall oxygen-carrying capacity of the blood remains adequate throughout gestation. After childbirth, the HCT level typically rises again because blood from the placental circulation is transferred back into the maternal bloodstream.

DEFICIENCY ANEMIAS

Iron Deficiency Anemia

Iron deficiency anemia (IDA) is the most prevalent form of anemia during pregnancy. A woman's nutritional status largely reflects her long-term iron balance, which is supported by sufficient dietary intake of iron and the use of iron supplements.[1]

Iron deficiency anemia develops in progressive stages. The initial stage involves **depletion of iron stores**, where the body's reserve iron is reduced or absent, though serum iron levels, transferrin saturation, and hemoglobin levels in the blood remain within normal limits. In the next stage, known as **iron-deficient erythropoiesis**, iron stores are still lacking or significantly reduced, serum iron and transferrin saturation are typically low, but anemia has not yet developed. The final and most severe stage—**iron deficiency anemia**—is marked by absent or markedly reduced iron stores, low serum iron levels, decreased transferrin saturation, and a drop in hemoglobin concentration, resulting in clinical anemia.

Causes: Iron deficiency anemia in pregnancy arises from several contributing factors. One of the primary reasons is the increased physiological demand for iron during pregnancy, with an estimated additional requirement of about 900 mg to support fetal growth, placental development, and the expansion of maternal red cell mass. Inadequate dietary intake remains the most common cause in India, where iron-rich foods are often limited in the daily diet.

Impaired absorption of iron, due to gastrointestinal conditions or poor bioavailability of dietary iron, also plays a role. Additionally, increased blood loss—whether from chronic hookworm infestation or frequent, closely spaced pregnancies—can further deplete iron reserves. These factors together contribute to the high prevalence of iron deficiency anemia among pregnant women

Diagnosis: The diagnosis of iron deficiency anemia in pregnancy involves a thorough evaluation using both general and specific laboratory investigations. A complete blood count (CBC) provides vital information including hemoglobin levels, red blood cell indices (MCV, MCH, and MCHC), reticulocyte count, total leukocyte count, and platelet count. A peripheral blood smear further helps by revealing characteristic microcytic, hypochromic red cells typical of iron deficiency. To identify possible sources of blood loss or infection, urine microscopy and culture, as well as stool examination for occult blood and parasitic ova or cysts, are essential. The NESTROFT test is a simple screening tool used to differentiate thalassemia trait from iron deficiency anemia. Iron studies—including serum iron, ferritin, total iron-binding capacity (TIBC), and transferrin saturation—are definitive for confirming iron deficiency. Additional tests such as liver function tests (LFTs), vitamin B12 and folate levels, renal function tests, or hemoglobin electrophoresis may be required to rule out other causes or coexisting types of anemia.[2]

Prevention: The prevention of iron deficiency anemia is a lifelong process that ideally begins in childhood and continues through adolescence and reproductive years. Early prevention strategies include dietary modifications such as regular consumption of iron-rich foods (green leafy vegetables, legumes, jaggery, and meat), cooking in iron utensils to enhance iron content, and avoiding practices that reduce iron absorption like excessive intake of tea or coffee and overcooking food. Food fortification is another key preventive measure—iron is added to commonly consumed staples such as wheat flour, salt, and rice. Among iron compounds used for fortification, sodium iron EDTA (NaFeEDTA) is preferred for its superior bioavailability, while micronized ferric pyrophosphate is used for fortifying color-sensitive foods like salt and rice. Preventive strategies also include regular screening of adolescent girls for anemia and providing iron supplementation where necessary, chemoprophylaxis for malaria in endemic regions, and promoting adequate birth spacing (a minimum of two years) to allow for maternal recovery of iron stores. Regular deworming with antihelminthic agents such as albendazole (400 mg single dose) is recommended, especially for adolescent girls and pregnant women after the first trimester, as per WHO and Government of India guidelines.[3,4]

TABLE 3: Summary of recommendations by WHO and MoHFW.

	During pregnancy		
	Prophylaxis	*Treatment*	*Postpartum*
WHO	Daily 60 mg iron + 400 µg folic acid till term	Daily 120 mg iron + 400 µg folic acid till term	Daily 60 mg iron and 400 µg folic acid—3 months
MoHFW	Daily 60 mg iron + 500 µg folic acid—for 100 days starting after the first trimester, at 14–16 weeks of gestation	Mild anemia—2 IFA tablets/day—100 days Moderate anemia—IM iron therapy + oral folic acid	Daily 60 mg iron + 500 µg folic acid—6 months

Treatment

The primary goal in treating iron deficiency anemia during pregnancy is to raise hemoglobin levels to near-normal and replenish iron stores before the onset of labor. The choice of treatment—particularly the route of iron administration—depends on the severity of anemia, gestational age, and the presence of any complicating factors.

Oral iron therapy (Table 3) is the first-line approach for most cases. Government of India, Ministry of Health, recommends 200 mg elemental iron with 1 mg folic acid per day for treatment until Hb levels come back to normal followed by 100 mg per day as maintenance therapy until 6 months after delivery to replenish the stores. Iron is best absorbed on an empty stomach; however, this often leads to gastrointestinal side effects, so it may alternatively be taken before meals or one hour after eating. To enhance absorption, vitamin C is recommended, while substances such as tea, coffee, milk, and calcium supplements should be avoided as they inhibit iron uptake.

Compliance with therapy can be indirectly assessed by asking about black-colored stools, a common side effect of iron intake. A follow-up hemoglobin test is usually advised after 3–4 weeks of therapy to evaluate response. Once hemoglobin levels normalize, daily prophylactic iron should be continued throughout the pregnancy and for at least 6 months postpartum. A positive clinical response to oral iron therapy includes improved well-being, reduced fatigue and palpitations, better sleep, and increased exercise tolerance.

Parenteral Iron Therapy offers a reliable and effective alternative to oral iron, especially in cases where rapid correction of anemia is needed or when oral iron is not tolerated.

Although the rise in hemoglobin levels is approximately 0.7–1.0 g/dL per week, which is comparable to oral therapy, the key benefit of parenteral administration is its assured bioavailability and patient compliance, particularly in late pregnancy. Indications for parenteral iron include intolerance to oral iron (due to side effects), impaired absorption, chronic blood loss, and gastrointestinal conditions that worsen with oral iron such as peptic ulcers or ulcerative colitis. After 32 weeks of gestation, parenteral therapy is often preferred due to better compliance and quicker results. It is also used in conjunction with erythropoietin to enhance erythropoiesis in anemia with renal disease. However, parenteral iron is contraindicated in cases with a history of anaphylaxis, during the first trimester, in patients with chronic liver disease, or in those with ongoing infections. Oral iron should be discontinued at least 24 hours before starting parenteral therapy to reduce the risk of toxicity.

The required dose of iron can be calculated using the **Ganzoni formula:**

Required iron dose (mg) = 2.4 × (Target Hb – Actual Hb) × Body weight in kg + 1,000 mg (for iron store replenishment).

A common regimen includes 200 mg of iron sucrose diluted in 200 mL of normal saline, administered intravenously over 20 minutes on alternate days, typically three times a week until the total calculated dose is delivered.

Ferric carboxymaltose (FCM) is an intravenous iron formulation used for parenteral therapy. It allows administration of large single doses of up to 1,000 mg elemental iron in one sitting, can be infused over a short period of about 15–30 minutes, carries a lower risk of anaphylaxis compared to other iron formulations, and does not require a test dose before administration.

ROLE OF BLOOD TRANSFUSION

Blood transfusion during pregnancy is reserved for specific indications where the severity of anemia poses a threat to maternal or fetal health, or when conservative treatment fails.

Indications of Blood Transfusion in Pregnancy

Antepartum Period

1. Pregnancy <34 weeks:
    - Hb <5 g/dL with or without signs of cardiac failure or hypoxia
    - Hb 5–7 g/dL in presence of impending heart failure
2. Pregnancy >34 weeks
    - Hb <7 g/dL without signs of cardiac failure or hypoxia
    - Severe anemia with decompensation

Intrapartum Period

- Hb <7 g/dL (in labor)
- Decision of blood transfusion depends on medical history or symptoms

Postpartum Period

- Anemia with signs of shock/acute hemorrhage with signs of hemodynamic instability.
- Hb <7 g% (postpartum): Decision of blood transfusion depends on medical history or symptoms

MANAGEMENT OF ANEMIA IN LABOR

Ideally, hemoglobin levels at the time of delivery should be at least 7 g/dL. If levels are lower, blood transfusion with one or more units of packed red cells is necessary, administered slowly over 4–6 hours.

- During the first stage of labor, patients should be counseled and informed consent obtained.
- Oxygen may be administered if required.
- The number of vaginal examinations should be minimized to reduce infection risk.
- Continuous monitoring for signs of cardiac failure—including pulse, blood pressure, and chest auscultation—is essential.

- Fluids must be restricted, and blood transfusions should be given under diuretic cover (e.g., frusemide) to prevent fluid overload.
- Prophylactic antibiotics are recommended to reduce infection risk.
- In the second stage, labor may be shortened by using ventouse or forceps to limit maternal exertion.
- Strict aseptic precautions must be followed.
- If oxytocin is used, it should be given in a concentrated form to avoid excess fluid administration.
- Intravenous fluids should remain restricted.
- During the **third stage**, active management is crucial to prevent postpartum hemorrhage.
- Intravenous frusemide may be administered postdelivery to reduce cardiac strain.
- In the **puerperium**, close observation for at least 6 hours postpartum is vital to detect signs of heart failure.
- Early ambulation is encouraged to reduce the risk of thromboembolism.

FOLATE AND VITAMIN B12 DEFICIENCY ANEMIA

It is characterized by megaloblasts on peripheral blood smear. Megaloblastic anemia in pregnancy may present with a variety of symptoms such as anorexia, vomiting, diarrhea, constitutional complaints, and in vitamin B12 deficiency, neurological manifestations like numbness, paraesthesia, weakness, ataxia, and subacute combined degeneration of the spinal cord. On examination, pallor, atrophic glossitis, and hepatosplenomegaly may be observed. Laboratory findings typically reveal macrocytosis with RBC indices showing MCV >100 fL, MCH > 33 pg, normal MCHC, and pancytopenia on CBC. Peripheral smear demonstrates megaloblastic changes, reticulocyte count is low due to ineffective erythropoiesis, and lactate dehydrogenase (LDH) is elevated. Diagnosis of vitamin B12 deficiency is confirmed when cobalamin levels are <150 ng/L, while folic acid deficiency is indicated by folate levels <2.5 ng/mL or RBC folate <150 ng/mL.

Treatment depends on the underlying cause. For folate deficiency, folic acid 5 mg/day is administered, continued until 4 weeks postdelivery, along with iron and vitamin B12 supplementation. Response to therapy includes an increased sense of well-being and improvement in symptoms, reduction in LDH levels within 3–4 days, an increase in reticulocyte count within 5–7 days, and hemoglobin improvement within 2–3 weeks (approximately 0.8 g/dL per week). Peripheral smear findings normalize by 6–8 weeks, while neurological deficits may take 6 weeks to 3 months to recover.

DIMORPHIC ANEMIA

Dimorphic anemia in pregnancy is characterized by the simultaneous presence of **microcytic (small-cell)** and **macrocytic (large-cell)** red blood cells. This dual pattern indicates a combined deficiency of **iron and vitamin B12 and/or folate**. It is a significant type of anemia during pregnancy and often results from inadequate dietary intake or poor absorption of these essential nutrients. Management includes **supplementation with iron, folate, and vitamin B12**, along with **dietary modifications** to correct the nutritional deficiencies. Early identification and timely intervention are vital to ensure optimal **maternal and fetal health outcomes**.

HEMOGLOBINOPATHIES

Hemoglobinopathies are a group of **inherited single-gene disorders** affecting the **structure or production** of the hemoglobin (Hb) molecule. These disorders can be broadly classified into **qualitative** and **quantitative** defects.

- **Qualitative defects** result from genetic mutations that alter the structure of the globin protein chains, leading to amino acid deletions or substitutions and giving rise to abnormal hemoglobin variants such as **HbS, HbD, and HbE**.
- **Quantitative defects** lead to reduced synthesis of structurally normal globin chains.

A classic example is **thalassemia**, a genetically heterogeneous **autosomal recessive** disorder caused by germline mutations that lead to partial or complete reduction in the synthesis of **alpha or beta globin chains**. This imbalance in globin production causes **anemia, tissue hypoxia, and hemolysis** of red blood cells.[5]

- **Alpha-thalassemia** is characterized by defective synthesis of alpha chains.
- **Beta-thalassemia** results from deficient synthesis of beta chains.

In normal adult hemoglobin (HbA), **alpha chains** are encoded by a pair of identical genes on **chromosome 16**, while the **beta chains** are encoded by a single gene on **chromosome 11**.

Globally, over **270 million people** are estimated to carry hereditary hemoglobin disorders, with about **300,000 newborns** affected annually as homozygotes or compound heterozygotes. This highlights the importance of **screening and clinical management policies during pregnancy** to reduce complications.

The geographical distribution shows that **alpha-thalassemia** is more common in **Southeast Asia, the Eastern Mediterranean, and the Middle East**, whereas **beta-thalassemia** is prevalent in the **Mediterranean region, Africa, the Middle East, India, Pakistan, and Southeast Asia**.

SICKLE CELL DISEASE

Sickle cell disease (SCD) encompasses a spectrum of disorders caused by the presence of abnormal hemoglobin S (HbS). It includes **homozygous sickle cell anemia (SS)** and various **compound heterozygous** forms such as:

- Sickle hemoglobin C disease (SC)
- Sickle beta-plus thalassemia ($S\beta^{+}$Thal)
- Sickle beta-zero thalassemia ($S\beta^{0}$Thal)
- Sickle cell anemia with alpha thalassemia (SS αThal)
- Sickle cell anemia with elevated fetal hemoglobin (SS+F)

The most severe form, **sickle cell anemia (SCA)**, results from a **homozygous HbS mutation**. It is characterized by **chronic anemia** and recurrent **painful crises** due to microvascular occlusion caused by sickling of red blood cells.[6]

Pregnancy in women with SCD carries an increased risk of **obstetric complications**, including **preeclampsia, eclampsia, gestational diabetes**, and **spontaneous abortions or**

stillbirths, largely due to **microvascular damage** and **reduced uteroplacental perfusion**. Maternal malnutrition, poor general health, and substance abuse further worsen outcomes.

Pregnancy tends to **worsen anemia** in SCD patients, increasing the need for **blood transfusions**. While the rate of **cesarean delivery** is higher, SCD itself is **not an indication for cesarean section**. Additionally, complications such as **vaso-occlusive crises (VOCs)** and **acute chest syndrome (ACS)** are more common during pregnancy. The combined effect of **auto-splenectomy** and **pregnancy-induced immunosuppression** increases susceptibility to infections such as **pneumonia, urinary tract infections, and postpartum sepsis**. The hypercoagulable state of pregnancy also predisposes to **thromboembolic events** such as **deep vein thrombosis** and **cerebral venous thrombosis**.

Maternal **hypoxia and anemia** contribute to **intrauterine growth restriction (IUGR)** due to impaired placental perfusion and oxygen delivery to the fetus.[6]

MAJOR ADVERSE EVENTS AND MANAGEMENT STRATEGIES

1. **Painful Crisis (Vaso-occlusive Crisis):** Hospitalization is recommended. Ensure bed rest, adequate hydration, and pain relief with **paracetamol or NSAIDs**; **opioids** may be used if required. **Meperidine** should be avoided due to toxicity and seizure risk.
2. **Acute Chest Syndrome (ACS):** Suspect in cases of cough and chest pain. Evaluate with chest X-ray, leukocyte count, and cultures. Management includes **oxygen therapy, antibiotics, hydration, analgesia,** and **blood transfusion** if needed.
3. **Pulmonary Embolism:** Consider in women with chest pain and dyspnea but normal chest X-ray. Begin **LMWH** treatment pending confirmation, as **D-dimer** may be elevated in other conditions like ACS.
4. **Stroke:** Any acute neurological deficit should raise suspicion for infractive or hemorrhagic stroke. **Emergency exchange transfusion** is the treatment of choice, as **thrombolysis** is ineffective in SCD-related strokes.
5. **Hematological Complications:** Anemia may worsen due to blood loss, bone marrow suppression, or nutritional deficiencies. Some centers advocate **prophylactic transfusion**, but **RCOG guidelines** recommend transfusion only if **Hb <7 g/dL** to ensure adequate fetal oxygenation. **HELLP syndrome** may develop in up to 10% of cases with preeclampsia and requires individualized management based on gestational age.
6. **Infections:** Common infections include **UTIs and respiratory tract infections**. Less frequently, **endometritis, hepatitis, osteomyelitis,** and **HIV** may occur. Fever and acidosis exacerbate sickling. Early initiation of **appropriate antibiotics** is essential. **Acute cholecystitis** may mimic hepatic complications; diagnosis relies on **LFTs and ultrasound**, and treatment includes antibiotics and postpartum **elective cholecystectomy**.

THALASSEMIA

Thalassemias are a group of hereditary blood disorders characterized by the reduced or suppressed production of synthesis of the globin chains of hemoglobin. They are classified according to the impaired globin chains, resulting in variable phenotypes ranging from severe anemia to clinically asymptomatic individuals.

Deletion of three α-globin genes results in hemoglobin H (Hb H) disease. In addition to deletional forms, there are at least 70 forms of nondeletional hemoglobin H disease, which may require occasional or frequent transfusions. A clear phenotype-genotype correlation is found in terms of hemoglobin and reticulocyte values, MCV, bilirubin in children, LDH and splenomegaly. Hb H disease needs regular monitoring for early detection and treatment of possible complications, such as worsening anemia that may require red cell transfusion, cholelithiasis, and iron overload.

Patients with beta-thalassemia intermedia present after the first 2 years of life with moderate anemia and do not require regular transfusions. The main clinical features in these patients are hypertrophy of erythroid marrow with medullary and extramedullary hematopoiesis and its complications (osteoporosis, masses of erythropoietic tissue that primarily affect the spleen, liver, lymph nodes, chest and spine, and bone deformities and typical facial changes), gallstones, painful leg ulcers and an increased predisposition to thrombosis.[1]

Individuals with beta-thalassemia major usually present within the first 2 years of life with severe anemia, requiring regular red blood cell transfusions for survival.

Prenatal Testing

For beta-thalassemia status, blood typing of the partner must be known. Couples at risk of having children with beta-thalassemia should be informed of the risk (25%) of having a thalassemia major fetus. Diagnosis can be made either earlier during the first trimester (11th week) by chorionic villus sampling or after the 16th week by amniocentesis. The risk of miscarriage does not differ between these invasive procedures and is estimated to be less than 1%.

Pregnancy has been reported safe in most women with thalassemia intermedia under multidisciplinary management. Most successful pregnancies are conceived without assisted reproductive technologies.

Management of Thalassemia in Pregnancy

Thalassemia Minor (Trait)

Usually heterozygous and clinically mild.

Preconception and Antenatal Counseling

- Genetic counseling: Essential to assess risk of fetal thalassemia major if partner is also a carrier.
- Partner screening: CBC and Hb electrophoresis.
- Prenatal diagnosis: If both partners are carriers → offer chorionic villus sampling (CVS) at 10–12 weeks or amniocentesis at 16–18 weeks for genetic testing of the fetus.

Maternal Management

- Usually no need for transfusion.
- Folic acid 5 mg/day throughout pregnancy.
- Iron supplementation only if iron deficiency is documented (serum ferritin <30 ng/mL).
- Monitor Hb each trimester (target >10 g/dL).

Obstetric Care

- Routine antenatal care.
- Monitor for mild anemia and IUGR.
- No special delivery precautions unless obstetric indication.

Fetal Considerations

- If partner noncarrier → normal fetus.
- If both carriers → 25% chance of thalassemia major → prenatal diagnosis and counseling essential.

Thalassemia Major (Homozygous β-thalassemia)

Patients are usually transfusion-dependent and have multiple complications due to iron overload.

Preconception Counseling

- Multidisciplinary approach: Hematologist, obstetrician, cardiologist, and endocrinologist.
- Assess organ function before conception:
  - Cardiac: ECG and echocardiogram (iron cardiomyopathy risk).
  - Liver: LFTs, iron studies, and ferritin.
  - Endocrine: Screen for diabetes, thyroid dysfunction, and hypogonadism.
- Chelation therapy (e.g. deferoxamine) ideally optimized before conception, then stopped once pregnancy confirmed (due to teratogenicity).

During Pregnancy

1. **Anemia Management:**
   - Maintain Hb ≥ 10 g/dL via regular blood transfusions every 2–4 weeks.
   - Use leukoreduced, matched blood to minimize alloimmunization.
   - Monitor for iron overload, though chelation is usually withheld (can restart deferoxamine in second to third trimester if severe overload).
2. **Iron Chelation:**
   - First trimester: Avoid all chelators.
   - Second/third trimester: Deferoxamine may be cautiously used if maternal cardiac function compromised.
3. **Give Folic acid: 5 mg/day.**
4. **Avoid iron supplementation unless proven deficiency.**
5. **Endocrine and Cardiac Monitoring**
   - Check thyroid, blood sugar, and cardiac function each trimester.
   - Monitor for heart failure, arrhythmia, and gestational diabetes.
6. **Anticoagulation:**
   - Thalassemia major → hypercoagulable; if splenectomized or immobilized, use LMWH prophylaxis.
7. **Fetal Monitoring**
   - Serial growth scans (risk of IUGR).
   - Fetal echocardiography if maternal cardiac compromise.

8. **Delivery**
    - Mode: Usually vaginal unless obstetric indication.
    - Anesthesia: Cardiac and hepatic status should guide choice.
    - Active management of third stage (risk of PPH).
9. **Postpartum**
    - Resume iron chelation after delivery.
    - Contraception: Nonhormonal or progesterone-only methods preferred if thrombophilic.
    - Breastfeeding: Deferoxamine is poorly excreted in breast milk → can be used.

CONCLUSION

Anemia in pregnancy remains one of the most common and preventable medical disorders worldwide. It significantly contributes to maternal morbidity, mortality, and adverse perinatal outcomes. Iron deficiency continues to be the leading cause, though other etiologies must be identified and treated appropriately. Early screening and regular antenatal monitoring are essential for timely diagnosis. Adequate iron, folic acid, and balanced nutrition play a vital role in prevention. Rational use of iron therapy and blood transfusions improves maternal and fetal outcomes. Health education and community-based interventions are key to reduce prevalence.

Addressing anemia strengthens overall maternal health and pregnancy safety. A multidisciplinary approach ensures comprehensive management and follow-up. Ultimately, prevention and early correction of anemia are the cornerstones of safe motherhood.

REFERENCES

1. World Health Organization. Iron Deficiency Anemia: Assessment, Prevention and Control: A Guide for Programme Managers, Geneva, Switzerland: World Health Organization; 2001.
2. WHO. Hemoglobin concentrations for the diagnosis of anemia and assessment of severity. Vitamin and Mineral Nutrition Information System. Geneva, Switzerland: World Health Organization; 2011.
3. Centres for Disease Control and Prevention. Recommendations to prevent and control iron deficiency in the United States. Centers for Disease Control and Prevention. MMWR Recomm Rep. 1998;47 (RR-3):1-29.
4. Ministry of Health and Family Welfare, Govt of India. NFHS IV, 2015-16: India. New Delhi: MOFHW, 2017.
5. Origa R, Comitini F. Pregnancy in Thalassemia. Mediterr J Hematol Infect Dis. 2019;11(1):e2019019.
6. Jain D, Atmapoojya P, Colah R, et al. Sickle Cell Disease and Pregnancy. Mediterr J Hematol Infect Dis. 2019;11(1):e2019040.

Cardiac Disease in Pregnancy

Ruchika Garg

1. Physiological Changes in Cardiac and Circulatory System

Ans.

Pregnancy induces significant hemodynamic adaptations to meet maternal and fetal demands. These changes begin early in gestation and peak in the third trimester, with further alterations during parturition. A detailed overview is given in **Table 1**.

Changes During Parturition:

- **Labor Stages**:
  - **First Stage**: CO increases by 25% due to uterine contractions and pain-induced tachycardia.

TABLE 1: Physiological cardiac and circulatory changes in pregnancy.

Parameter	*Change*	*Mechanism/Impact*
Cardiac output (CO)	Increases by 40–50% by 32 weeks	Driven by increased plasma volume (40%) initially, later by heart rate (HR) rise (10–15 bpm)
Heart rate (HR)	Increases by 10–15 bpm from 20–32 weeks, plateaus until postpartum	Compensates for increased metabolic demand; normalizes by 6 weeks postpartum
Blood pressure (BP)	Diastolic BP decreases by ~10 mm Hg in 1st–2nd trimesters, normalizes in 3rd	Vasodilation due to prostacyclin and nitric oxide; rises in late pregnancy
Plasma volume	Increases by 40–50%	Supports increased CO; peaks at 32 weeks
Systemic vascular resistance	Decreases by 20–30%	Facilitates increased CO; mediated by vasodilatory hormones
Heart sounds	Exaggerated S1 splitting, audible S3, and Grade I–II systolic murmurs	Due to hyperdynamic circulation and increased blood flow
Cardiac size	Cardiomegaly with 10–20% increase in left ventricular mass	Accommodates increased preload; leftward rotation due to gravid uterus
ECG changes	Left axis deviation (15–20°), inverted T waves, attenuated Q waves	Reflects cardiac displacement and increased workload
Multiple gestation	Amplified CO and cardiomegaly	Greater hemodynamic stress due to increased fetal demand

- **Second Stage**: CO rises by 50% due to increased preload from autotransfusion and straining.
- **Immediate Postpartum**: CO peaks by 80% due to autotransfusion from uterine involution and venous return from lower limbs.

- **Blood Pressure**: Systolic and diastolic BP increase by 15–20% during contractions.
- **Supine Hypotension**: Supine position may compress the inferior vena cava, reducing preload and fetal perfusion; left lateral position is preferred.
- **Postpartum Recovery**: Hemodynamic parameters normalize by 6 weeks postpartum.

Epidemiology of Cardiac Disorders in Pregnancy

Cardiac diseases complicate 1–4% of pregnancies globally, with higher prevalence in developing countries like India due to rheumatic heart disease (RHD). Key disorders include:

- **Rheumatic Heart Disease**: Predominant in India, affecting 60–70% of cardiac cases in pregnancy.[1] Mitral stenosis is the most common lesion.
- **Hypertensive Disorders**: Preeclampsia and gestational hypertension affect 5–10% of pregnancies, contributing to cardiac strain.[2]
- **Congenital Heart Disease (CHD)**: Increasing due to improved surgical corrections in childhood; affects ~0.8% of pregnancies[3]
- **Cardiomyopathies**: Peripartum cardiomyopathy (PPCM) has an incidence of 1:1,000–4,000 pregnancies, higher in African populations.[4]
- **Ischemic Heart Disease**: Rare, with an incidence of 1:10,000–15,000; more common with advanced maternal age.[5]

2. Risk Stratification of Cardiac Diseases in Pregnancy and NYHA Classification

Ans.

Risk Stratification

The modified World Health Organization (mWHO) classification is used to stratify maternal cardiac risk in pregnancy, integrating comorbidities and contraindications **(Table 2)**.[6]

TABLE 2: WHO risk classification for cardiac diseases in pregnancy.

Class	*Risk level*	*Examples*	*Follow-up*
I	No increased mortality, minimal morbidity	Mild PS, PDA, MVP, repaired ASD/VSD, and ectopic beats	1–2 cardiac consultations
II	Small increased mortality, moderate morbidity	Unoperated ASD/VSD, repaired tetralogy of Fallot, and arrhythmias	Each trimester
II–III	Significant mortality/ morbidity risk	Mild LV dysfunction, hypertrophic cardiomyopathy, and Marfan's (aorta <45 mm)	Bimonthly
III	High mortality/morbidity risk	Mechanical valves, Fontan circulation, and moderate LV dysfunction	Monthly
IV	Pregnancy contraindicated	Severe MS/AS, pulmonary hypertension, and severe LV dysfunction (LVEF <30%)	Monthly/fortnightly

TABLE 3: NYHA classification.

Class	*Symptoms*	*Activity limitation*
I	No symptoms during ordinary activity	None
II	Mild symptoms and slight limitation	Comfortable at rest, limited by ordinary activity
III	Marked limitation with less than ordinary activity	Comfortable only at rest
IV	Symptoms at rest and severe limitation	Unable to perform any physical activity

NYHA Classification for Heart Failure Symptoms

The New York Heart Association (NYHA) classification assesses functional limitations due to heart failure **(Table 3)**.[7]

3. Mitral Valve Disorders in Pregnancy and Management of Mitral Stenosis (MS) in Rheumatic Heart Disease (RHD)

Ans.

Mitral Valve Disorders in Pregnancy

- Mitral Stenosis
- Mitral Regurgitation (MR)
- Mitral Valve Prolapse (MVP)
- Prosthetic Mitral Valves

Management of Mitral Stenosis in Pregnancy and Parturition

Pathophysiology of MS in RHD:

- **Cause**: Primarily RHD in India, leading to mitral valve narrowing
- **Severity Grading (Table 4)**[8]
- **Hemodynamic Impact**: Increased plasma volume (40%) and tachycardia reduce diastolic filling, elevating left atrial pressure, leading to pulmonary edema, atrial fibrillation (AF), and thromboembolism
- **Maternal Risks**: Heart failure (NYHA III–IV), pulmonary edema, and arrhythmias
- **Fetal Risks**: Intrauterine growth restriction (IUGR) and preterm delivery

Management:[9,10]

- **Medical**:
  - **Beta-Blockers** (e.g., metoprolol): Control HR to improve diastolic filling.
  - **Diuretics** (e.g., furosemide): Reduce preload, manage pulmonary edema.

TABLE 4: Grading of mitral stenosis.

Severity	*Valve area (cm^2)*	*Mean gradient (mm Hg)*	*Complications*
Mild	>1.5	<5	Minimal symptoms
Moderate	1–1.5	5–10	Dyspnea and pulmonary edema
Severe	<1	>10	Pulmonary hypertension and heart failure

- **Anticoagulation**: Heparin for AF or thromboembolism risk; warfarin avoided in 1st trimester due to teratogenicity.
- **Penicillin Prophylaxis**: Prevents RHD progression and endocarditis

- **Surgical**:
  - **Percutaneous Balloon Mitral Valvuloplasty (BMV)**: Preferred after 20 weeks for severe MS (valve area <1 cm^2, NYHA III–IV)
  - **Mitral Valve Replacement**: For nonpliable valves or restenosis; high fetal mortality risk
- **Labor and Delivery**:
  - **Vaginal Delivery**: Preferred with epidural analgesia to minimize tachycardia
  - **Instrumental Delivery**: Shortens 2nd stage to avoid Valsalva
  - **Cesarean Section**: Reserved for obstetric indications or severe MS (NYHA III–IV)
  - **Fluid Management**: Restrict fluids (<75 mL/h) to prevent overload; monitor for autotransfusion postdelivery.
  - **Antibiotics**: Broad-spectrum to prevent endocarditis

Postpartum:

- Monitor for heart failure due to autotransfusion; use diuretics and invasive monitoring if needed.

4. Cardiomyopathies in Pregnancy and Peripartum Cardiomyopathy (PPCM)

Ans.

Cardiomyopathies in Pregnancy

- **Dilated Cardiomyopathy (DCM)**: Ventricular dilation and systolic dysfunction; includes PPCM
- **Hypertrophic Cardiomyopathy (HCM)**: Left ventricular hypertrophy, risk of arrhythmias
- **Restrictive Cardiomyopathy**: Rare, with impaired ventricular filling
- **Secondary Cardiomyopathies**: Due to systemic diseases (e.g., diabetes and thyroid disorders).

Peripartum Cardiomyopathy[11,12]

- **Definition**: Heart failure with left ventricular systolic dysfunction (LVEF <45%) in the last month of pregnancy or within 5 months postpartum, without other identifiable causes.
- **Incidence**: 1:1,000–4,000 pregnancies; higher in African descent, multiparity, and preeclampsia[4]
- **Risk Factors**:
  - Multiparity
  - Advanced maternal age
  - Preeclampsia
  - African ethnicity
  - Diabetes mellitus
- **Pathophysiology**:[13]
  - Oxidative stress and prolactin cleavage into antiangiogenic fragments (e.g., 16-kDa prolactin).
  - Increased sFlt-1 (anti-angiogenic factor) impairs myocardial vascularity.

- Two-hit hypothesis: Genetic predisposition + environmental triggers (e.g., preeclampsia).

- **Presentation**:
  - Dyspnea, orthopnea, fatigue, and edema
  - Echocardiogram: Global LV hypokinesia and reduced LVEF (<45%)
- **Management (BOARD Protocol):**[14]
  - **Bromocriptine**: Inhibits prolactin to reduce myocardial damage; dose 2.5 mg twice daily for 2 weeks
  - **Oral Heart Failure Drugs**:
    - Hydralazine and nitrates (antenatal)
    - ACE inhibitors (e.g., captopril) postdelivery or during breastfeeding
    - Beta-blockers (e.g., metoprolol) for HR control
  - **Anticoagulation**: Heparin/warfarin for LVEF <35% to prevent thromboembolism
  - **Relaxants**: Vasodilators to reduce afterload
  - **Diuretics**: Furosemide to manage pulmonary edema; use cautiously antenatally to avoid fetal hypoperfusion.
  - **Advanced Therapies**: Intra-aortic balloon pump, ventricular assist devices, or cardiac transplant for refractory cases
- **Delivery**:
  - **Vaginal**: Preferred for stable patients with epidural analgesia
  - **Cesarean**: For hemodynamic instability or obstetric indications
- **Prognosis**:
  - Recovery in 50–60% within 6 months; persistent LV dysfunction contraindicates future pregnancies
  - Relapse risk in subsequent pregnancies, even with recovered LVEF.

SMALL QUESTIONS AND ANSWERS

1. Prosthetic Heart Valves in Pregnancy

Ans.

- **Types**:[15]
  - **Mechanical Valves**: Durable (20–30 years), require lifelong anticoagulation (e.g., warfarin, heparin)
  - **Bioprosthetic Valves**: Less durable (10–15 years), lower thrombogenic risk, and no anticoagulation needed
- **Challenges in Pregnancy**:
  - Mechanical valves: High risk of valve thrombosis due to hypercoagulable state; warfarin embryopathy risk (1st trimester)
  - Bioprosthetic valves: Accelerated deterioration due to hyperdynamic circulation.
- **Management**:
  - **Anticoagulation**: Heparin (UFH/LMWH) in 1st trimester and peripartum; warfarin in 2nd–3rd trimesters (INR 2–3)

- **Monitoring**: Regular echocardiography; Wilkins' score (>8) indicates poor BMV candidacy, favoring valve replacement
- **Delivery**: Vaginal preferred; cesarean for obstetric indications or severe symptoms

- **Complications**: Heart failure, thromboembolism, fetal loss, and IUGR

2. Role of Anticoagulation in Pregnancy for Cardiac Indications

Ans.

- **Indications**:[16]
  - Mechanical prosthetic valves
  - Atrial fibrillation with thromboembolism risk (e.g., MS with left atrial thrombus)
  - PPCM with LVEF <35%
- **Anticoagulants**:
  - **Warfarin**: Effective but teratogenic (1st trimester); dose >5 mg increases embryopathy risk (9%).[17]
  - **Unfractionated Heparin (UFH)**: Does not cross placenta; risk of HIT, and osteoporosis.
  - **Low Molecular Weight Heparin (LMWH)**: Preferred; lower HIT risk, monitored via anti-Xa levels (0.8–1.2 U/mL)
- **Regimen**:
  - Preconception: Switch to LMWH/UFH.
  - 2nd–3rd Trimester: Warfarin (INR 2–3) or continue LMWH.
  - Peripartum: Switch to UFH (aPTT 2x control) to minimize bleeding risk.
  - Postpartum: Resume warfarin with heparin bridging until INR is therapeutic.
- **Reversal**:
  - Warfarin: Vitamin K, fresh frozen plasma
  - UFH: Protamine sulfate

3. Aortic Stenosis (AS) and Its Management in Pregnancy

Ans.

- **Definition and Grading (Table 5)**:[18]
- **Etiology**: RHD (India), congenital bicuspid aortic valve (Western countries)
- **Pathophysiology**:
  - Fixed cardiac output due to narrowed valve; preload reduction (e.g., blood loss, epidural) worsens output.
  - Concentric LV hypertrophy, reduced LVEF.
- **Management**:[19]
  - **Preconception**: Severe AS (mWHO IV) contraindicates pregnancy; consider valvuloplasty or transcatheter aortic valve replacement (TAVR) post-20 weeks.

TABLE 5: Grading of aortic stenosis.

Severity	*Valve area (cm^2)*	*Mean gradient (mm Hg)*	*Symptoms*
Mild	>1.5	<25	Asymptomatic
Moderate	1–1.5	25–40	Dyspnea and chest pain
Severe	<1	>40	Syncope, heart failure, and sudden death

- **Medical**: Beta-blockers for arrhythmias; cautious diuresis for pulmonary edema
- **Delivery**:
  - Vaginal: Preferred for mild/moderate AS with epidural analgesia.
  - Cesarean: For severe AS to avoid preload reduction; general anesthesia preferred.
  - Fluid Management: Maintain preload (125 mL/h); avoid supine position.
- **Monitoring**: Echocardiography, central venous pressure for severe cases.
- **Complications**: Aortic dissection (bicuspid valve), heart failure, and fetal loss.

REFERENCES

1. Soma-Pillay P, Nelson-Piercy C, Tolppanen H, et al. Physiological changes in pregnancy. Cardiovasc J Afr. 2016;27(2):89-94.
2. Regitz-Zagrosek V, Roos-Hesselink JW, Bauersachs J, et al. 2018 ESC Guidelines for the management of cardiovascular diseases during pregnancy. Eur Heart J. 2018;39(34):3165-241.
3. van Oppen SA, et al. Congenital heart disease and pregnancy: A review. Neth Heart J. 2015;23(10):480-8.
4. Bauersachs J, et al. Peripartum cardiomyopathy: Current management and future perspectives. Eur Heart J. 2016;37(40):3267-78.
5. Elkayam U, Goland S, Pieper PG, et al. High-risk cardiac disease in pregnancy: Part I. J Am Coll Cardiol. 2016;68(4):396-410.
6. Thorne S, et al. Pregnancy and heart disease: Risk stratification and management. Heart. 2018;104(12):1017-24.
7. Nishimura RA, Otto CM, Bonow RO, et al. 2017 AHA/ACC focused update of valvular heart disease guidelines. Circulation. 2017;135(25):e1159-95.
8. Chandrashekhar Y, et al. Mitral stenosis: Diagnosis and management. Lancet. 2018;391(10124):1045-55.
9. Siu SC, et al. Pregnancy outcomes in women with heart disease: The CARPREG II study. J Am Coll Cardiol. 2017;69(20):2511-20.
10. van Hagen IM, et al. Global cardiac risk assessment in pregnancy: The ROPAC registry. Eur Heart J. 2015;36(21):1307-16.
11. Arany Z, Elkayam U. Peripartum cardiomyopathy. Circulation. 2016;133(14):1397-409.
12. Hilfiker-Kleiner D, et al. Peripartum cardiomyopathy: From pathogenesis to treatment. Nat Rev Cardiol. 2017;14(10):589-604.
13. Patten IS, et al. Prolactin and anti-angiogenic pathways in peripartum cardiomyopathy. J Clin Invest. 2015;125(8):3038-51.
14. Bauersachs J, et al. Bromocriptine for peripartum cardiomyopathy: A randomized trial. Eur Heart J. 2019;40(35):2947-55.
15. Vahanian A, et al. 2021 ESC/EACTS Guidelines for the management of valvular heart disease. Eur Heart J. 2021;42(35):3561-629.
16. D'Souza R, et al. Anticoagulation for pregnant women with mechanical heart valves. Obstet Gynecol. 2017;130(5):1124-36.
17. Steinberg ZL, et al. Maternal and fetal outcomes with anticoagulation in pregnancy. J Am Coll Cardiol. 2017;69(6):777-86.
18. Writing Committee Members; Otto CM, Nishimura RA, Bonow RO, et al. 2020 ACC/AHA Guideline for the management of patients with valvular heart disease. J Am Coll Cardiol. 2021;77(4):e25-197.
19. Orwat S, et al. Aortic stenosis in pregnancy: A case series. Int J Cardiol. 2016;223:1018-23.

Liver Disorders in Pregnancy

Ruchika Garg

CAUSES OF JAUNDICE IN PREGNANCY

Jaundice in pregnancy, occurring in approximately 1 in 1,000 pregnancies, is defined by serum bilirubin levels exceeding 2 mg/dL, leading to yellowish discoloration of tissues.[1] Causes are classified based on their relation to pregnancy **(Table 1)**.

NORMAL LIVER CHANGES IN PREGNANCY

- **Skin Findings:** Palmar erythema and spider angiomata, often indicative of liver dysfunction, are normal in pregnancy due to hyperestrogenism.
- **Laboratory Findings:**
  - Serum bilirubin, alanine transaminase (ALT), and aspartate transaminase (AST) levels remain unchanged
  - Serum alkaline phosphatase may increase up to 4 times normal in the third trimester due to placental production.
  - Serum albumin decreases due to hemodilution.[3]

1. **Causes, Etiopathogenesis, Investigations, and Management of Intrahepatic Cholestasis of Pregnancy (ICP)**

INTRAHEPATIC CHOLESTASIS OF PREGNANCY

Introduction

Intrahepatic cholestasis of pregnancy, also known as obstetric cholestasis, is a pregnancy-specific liver disorder characterized by elevated serum bile acids and pruritus, with or without

TABLE 1: Causes of jaundice in pregnancy.[2]

Jaundice peculiar to pregnancy	*Jaundice unrelated to pregnancy*
Intrahepatic cholestasis of pregnancy (ICP)	Viral hepatitis (A, B, C, D, and E)
Acute fatty liver of pregnancy (AFLP)	Gallstone (obstructive jaundice)
Severe preeclampsia/HELLP syndrome	Drug-induced (e.g., isoniazid and phenothiazines)
Severe hyperemesis gravidarum	Hemolytic jaundice
Endotoxic shock	Chronic hepatitis
	Liver cirrhosis
	Hepatic tumors

jaundice. It typically presents in the third trimester and resolves postpartum. The global prevalence ranges from 0.3 to 15%, with 1.2–1.5% in Indian Asian populations.[4]

Etiopathogenesis

Intrahepatic cholestasis of pregnancy has a multifactorial etiology involving genetic, hormonal, and environmental factors:

- **Genetic Factors:**
  - Sex-linked dominant inheritance, with familial clustering reported in 20–30% of cases[5]
  - Mutations in **ABCB4** (encodes MDR3 and canalicular phospholipid transporter) account for 15% of cases, and **ABCB11** (encodes bile salt export pump, BSEP) mutations contribute to 5%.[6]
- **Hormonal Influence:** Increased sensitivity of bile ducts and hepatocytes to estrogen and progesterone disrupts bile acid transport, leading to accumulation in maternal and fetal circulation.
- **Pathophysiology:** Impaired bile acid clearance from the fetus to the mother results in elevated bile acids in fetal blood, umbilical cord, and amniotic fluid. High bile acid levels cause vasoconstriction of chorionic veins, reducing fetal oxygenated blood flow and leading to hypoxia.[7]
- **Environmental Factors:** Seasonal variation (higher in winter) and dietary factors (e.g., selenium deficiency) may contribute.[8]

Fetal Effects*:*

- Preterm delivery (30–40% of cases)
- Fetal distress due to asphyxia
- Meconium-stained amniotic fluid
- Sudden intrauterine fetal demise (IUFD, risk increases with bile acids >100 μmol/L)
- Respiratory distress syndrome
- Increased perinatal mortality (1–2%)[9]

Maternal Effects*:*

- Increased risk of gallstones and gallbladder disease long term
- No evidence of permanent liver damage.[10]

Clinical Presentation

- **Pruritus:** Generalized, worse at night, starting on palms and soles, progressing to limbs, trunk, and face. It causes sleep deprivation and emotional distress.
- **Jaundice:** Develops 2–4 weeks after pruritus in 20–25% of cases, resolving rapidly postpartum.
- **Other Symptoms:** Fat malabsorption (diarrhea), nausea, vomiting, and abdominal discomfort[11]

Investigations

Intrahepatic cholestasis of pregnancy is a diagnosis of exclusion, confirmed by symptom resolution and normalized liver function tests (LFTs) postpartum. Key investigations include **(Table 2)**:

- **Serum Bile Acids:** Diagnostic if >10 μmol/L. Severity classification:

TABLE 2: Laboratory features of ICP.[12]

Parameter	*Finding*	*Comments*
Serum bile acids	>10 μmol/L (diagnostic)	>100 μmol/L increases stillbirth risk
Direct bilirubin	<5 mg/dL	Mild elevation
AST/ALT	2–4-fold increase	Rarely >400 IU/L
Alkaline phosphatase	1–2-fold increase	Placental contribution
Cholesterol/triglycerides	Elevated	Nonspecific
Viral hepatitis serology	Negative	Rule out viral causes
Ultrasound	Normal	Excludes gallstones

TABLE 3: Management of ICP.[15,17]

Intervention	*Details*	*Notes*
UDCA	10–15 mg/kg/day (300 mg TID or 500 mg BID)	First-line, improves pruritus and fetal outcomes
Vitamin K	5–10 mg/day orally	For coagulopathy
Antihistamines	Chlorpheniramine 4 mg every 6 hours	Relieves pruritus
Delivery	36–37 weeks gestation	Reduces IUFD risk
Fetal monitoring	Ultrasound, NST, and maternal fetal movement tracking	Continuous intrapartum monitoring
Postpartum	LFTs at 4–6 weeks	Rule out other liver disorders

    - **Mild:** 19–39 μmol/L
    - **Moderate:** 40–99 μmol/L
    - **Severe:** >100 μmol/L (increased stillbirth risk)[12]
- **Liver Function Tests:**
    - Elevated direct bilirubin (<5 mg/dL)
    - AST/ALT increased 2–4-fold (100–400 IU/L)
    - Alkaline phosphatase elevated 1–2-fold (placental contribution)
- **Other Markers:** Elevated serum cholesterol and triglycerides
- **Screening:** Rule out viral hepatitis (A, B, C, D, and E) with serology.
- **Imaging:** Upper abdominal ultrasound to exclude cholelithiasis or other causes of cholestasis.[13]
- **Histology:** Liver biopsy (rarely performed) shows centrilobular cholestasis without inflammation.[14]

Management

Management focuses on symptom relief, maternal/fetal monitoring, and timely delivery to minimize complications. It aligns with RCOG Green-top Guideline No. 43 (2022) and NICE NG194 (2023; **Table 3**).[15,16]

- **Symptom Relief:**
    - **Ursodeoxycholic Acid (UDCA):** First-line treatment (10–15 mg/kg/day, typically 300 mg 2–3 times daily or 500 mg twice daily). UDCA reduces bile acid toxicity, improves

pruritus within 1–2 weeks, and enhances fetal bile acid clearance. Up to 25% of patients may experience mild nausea/dizziness.[17]
    - **Antihistamines:** Chlorpheniramine (4 mg every 6 hours) for pruritus relief
    - **Topical Emollients:** Lactocalamine for temporary relief
    - **Adjuncts:** S-adenosyl methionine or rifampicin may enhance UDCA effects in refractory cases.[18]
    - **Vitamin K:** 5–10 mg/day orally for prolonged prothrombin time to prevent bleeding.[19]
- **Maternal Monitoring:**
    - Weekly LFTs and bile acid levels for mild/moderate ICP
    - Monitor for coagulopathy (PT/INR).
- **Fetal Monitoring:**
    - Routine ultrasound and nonstress test (NST) to assess fetal well-being
    - Patient education on monitoring fetal movements; immediate reporting of reduced movements is critical.
    - No evidence that NST or biophysical profile prevents stillbirth.[20]
- **Delivery:**
    - **Timing:** ACOG and RCOG recommend delivery at 36 0/7–37 0/7 weeks to reduce IUFD risk, particularly if bile acids >100 μmol/L.[15,21]
    - **Mode:** Vaginal delivery preferred with continuous intrapartum fetal monitoring. Cesarean section for obstetric indications only.
    - **Intrapartum Care:** Continuous cardiotocography to detect fetal distress.
- **Postpartum Care:**
    - Repeat LFTs and bile acid levels 4–6 weeks postpartum. Persistent abnormalities warrant investigation for other hepatobiliary disorders (e.g., primary biliary cholangitis).
    - **Contraception:** Avoid estrogen-containing oral contraceptives due to cholestasis risk. Progesterone-only pills or nonhormonal methods (e.g., IUDs) recommended.[15]
- **Future Risk:**
    - **Recurrence risk in subsequent pregnancies:** 45–90%.[22]
    - Familial ICP increases risk of chronic liver disease (e.g., gallstones and cholangitis).

RCOG and NICE Guidelines

- **RCOG Green-top Guideline No. 43 (2022):** It recommends UDCA as first-line therapy, delivery at 36–37 weeks, and continuous fetal monitoring. Avoid estrogen-based contraceptives postpartum.[15]
- **NICE NG194 (2023):** It emphasizes early diagnosis with bile acid levels, multidisciplinary care, and patient education on fetal movement monitoring.[16]

Key Points

- Intrahepatic cholestasis of pregnancy is a pregnancy-specific liver disorder with a prevalence of 0.3–15%, characterized by pruritus and elevated bile acids.
- Etiology involves genetic (ABCB4/ABCB11 mutations), hormonal, and environmental factors, leading to bile acid accumulation and fetal hypoxia.
- Diagnosis is confirmed by bile acids >10 μmol/L and resolution postpartum.
- UDCA is the cornerstone of treatment, with delivery at 36–37 weeks to prevent IUFD.
- Recurrence risk is high (45–90%), and familial cases increase chronic liver disease risk.

ACUTE FATTY LIVER OF PREGNANCY

INTRODUCTION

Acute fatty liver of pregnancy (AFLP), also known as acute yellow atrophy of the liver, is a rare but life-threatening obstetric emergency characterized by acute liver failure due to microvesicular steatosis. It occurs primarily in the third trimester with a prevalence of 1 in 7,000–16,000 deliveries.[23] AFLP is associated with significant maternal and fetal morbidity and mortality if not managed promptly.

ETIOPATHOGENESIS

Acute fatty liver of pregnancy results from mitochondrial dysfunction leading to impaired fatty acid metabolism. The key mechanisms include:

- **Fetal Genetic Defect:** Deficiency of long-chain 3-hydroxyacyl-CoA dehydrogenase (LCHAD), an enzyme critical for fatty acid β-oxidation, leads to accumulation of medium- and long-chain fatty acids in the fetus. These metabolites are transferred to the maternal circulation via the placenta, causing maternal hepatotoxicity.[24]
- **Genetic Basis:** AFLP is linked to autosomal recessive mutations, with the E474Q mutation in the G1528C gene being the most common, accounting for a significant proportion of cases.[25] Mothers and fetuses heterozygous for this mutation are particularly susceptible.
- **Pathophysiology:** Accumulated fatty acids cause mitochondrial oxidative stress, apoptosis, and microvesicular steatosis in hepatocytes, leading to acute liver failure. This is exacerbated by increased metabolic demands of pregnancy.
- **Risk Factors:** Primiparity, multiple gestation, male fetus, and preeclampsia are associated with higher risk.[26]

LABORATORY FEATURES

Diagnosis of AFLP relies on clinical suspicion supported by laboratory and imaging findings. Key laboratory features include:

- **Hyperbilirubinemia:** Serum bilirubin levels often exceed 5–10 mg/dL, reflecting severe cholestasis.[27]
- **Elevated Transaminases:** Aspartate aminotransferase (AST) and alanine aminotransferase (ALT) levels are elevated 3–10 times the upper limit of normal (300–500 IU/L), though less than in viral hepatitis.[28]
- **Coagulopathy:** Prolonged prothrombin time (PT) and activated partial thromboplastin time (aPTT) due to impaired hepatic synthesis of clotting factors
- **Hypoglycemia:** Blood glucose <72 mg/dL due to impaired gluconeogenesis
- **Elevated Ammonia:** Serum ammonia levels >66 µmol/L, indicating hepatic dysfunction.
- **Renal Impairment:** Elevated serum creatinine (>1.7 mg/dL) and urea (>950 mg/dL)
- **Other Findings:** Neutrophilic leukocytosis, elevated uric acid, and thrombocytopenia are common
- **Imaging:** Ultrasound may show a “bright liver” due to fatty infiltration, though findings can be normal in early stages. Liver biopsy, rarely performed due to bleeding risk, confirms micro vesicular steatosis with oil-red-O staining.[29]

TABLE 1: Swansea criteria for diagnosis of AFLP.[30]

Criterion	*Description*
Vomiting	Persistent nausea and vomiting
Abdominal pain	Right upper quadrant or epigastric pain
Polydipsia/polyuria	Excessive thirst or urination
Encephalopathy	Altered mental status or coma
WBC count	$>11 \times 10^9$/L
Bilirubin	>0.8 mg/dL
ALT	>42 IU/L
Ammonia	>66 μmol/L
Prothrombin time	>14 s or coagulopathy
Ascites	Detected on imaging
Urea	>950 mg/dL
Creatinine	>1.7 mg/dL (acute kidney injury)
Hypoglycemia	<72 mg/dL
Micro vesicular steatosis	Confirmed on liver biopsy
Bright liver	Seen on ultrasound

The **Swansea criteria (Table 1)** are used for diagnosis, requiring 6 out of 15 criteria for confirmation, with 100% sensitivity and 57% specificity.[30]

MANAGEMENT

Acute fatty liver of pregnancy requires urgent, multidisciplinary management in a high-dependency unit involving obstetricians, hepatologists, intensivists, and hematologists. The primary goals are maternal stabilization, supportive care, and prompt delivery.

Monitoring

- **Maternal Monitoring:**
  - Hourly vital signs (pulse, blood pressure, and respiratory rate)
  - Input/output charting to assess fluid balance
  - Central venous pressure monitoring via central line
  - Blood glucose every 2 hours to detect hypoglycemia
  - Coagulation studies (PT and aPTT) every 6 hours
- **Fetal Monitoring:**
  - Continuous cardiotocography to assess fetal well-being
  - Regular ultrasound to monitor fetal growth and amniotic fluid

Supportive Care

- **Intravenous Fluids:** Glucose-containing fluids (e.g., 10% dextrose) to correct hypoglycemia and maintain hydration
- **Blood Products:** Fresh-frozen plasma, cryoprecipitate, or platelets to correct coagulopathy and thrombocytopenia.

- **Antibiotics:** Prophylactic antibiotics to prevent sepsis in critically ill patients.
- **Management of Complications:**
    - Treat hepatic encephalopathy with lactulose and supportive care.
    - Manage acute kidney injury with careful fluid management and, if necessary, dialysis.

Delivery

- **Timing:** Immediate delivery is critical after maternal stabilization, regardless of gestational age, to halt disease progression. The Royal College of Obstetricians and Gynaecologists (RCOG) recommends delivery as soon as possible in confirmed AFLP cases.[31]
- **Mode:** Vaginal delivery is preferred unless obstetric indications (e.g., fetal distress and maternal instability) necessitate cesarean section.
- **Intrapartum Care:** Continuous fetal monitoring is mandatory due to the high risk of fetal distress.

Specific Treatments

- **N-Acetylcysteine:** Emerging evidence suggests that it may reduce oxidative stress and improve liver function, though not yet standard in RCOG/NICE guidelines.[32]
- **Liver Transplantation:** Rarely required in cases of fulminant liver failure with severe disseminated intravascular coagulation (DIC) or encephalopathy

Postpartum Care

- **Monitoring:** Repeat liver function tests (LFTs) 4–6 weeks postpartum. Normalization typically occurs within 1–2 weeks.
- **Complications:** Monitor for diabetes insipidus (due to elevated vasopressin) and persistent liver dysfunction, which warrants further investigation for alternative diagnoses.
- **Neonatal Screening:** Test newborns for LCHAD deficiency, as they may carry the genetic mutation.

Recurrence Risk

The risk of recurrence in subsequent pregnancies is 15–25%.[33] Genetic counseling is recommended for mothers with confirmed LCHAD mutations.

Maternal and Fetal Outcomes

- **Maternal Outcomes:**
    - **Liver Failure:** AFLP can progress to fulminant hepatic failure, with risks of coagulopathy, DIC, and hepatic encephalopathy.
    - **Multiorgan Dysfunction:** Renal failure, respiratory distress, and cardiovascular instability may occur.
    - **Mortality:** Maternal mortality has decreased from 85% to 10–18% with early recognition and management.[34]
- **Fetal Outcomes:**
    - **Preterm Delivery:** Common due to early delivery to protect maternal health

TABLE 2: Differential diagnosis of AFLP.[35]

Condition	*Key features*	*Differentiating factors*
HELLP syndrome	Hemolysis, elevated liver enzymes, and low platelets	Associated with preeclampsia, severe hypertension, and hemolysis prominent
Intrahepatic cholestasis of pregnancy (ICP)	Pruritus, elevated bile acids	Pruritus is hallmark, bile acids >10 µmol/L, and less severe liver dysfunction
Viral hepatitis	High transaminases (500–3000 IU/L), positive serology	Viral markers (e.g., anti-HAV IgM and HBsAg) positive, no microvesicular steatosis

- **Fetal Distress:** Caused by placental insufficiency and maternal hypoxia
- **Stillbirth:** Risk is high (up to 10%) without timely intervention
- **Neonatal Complications:** Prematurity-related issues, such as respiratory distress syndrome, are common.

DIFFERENTIAL DIAGNOSIS

Acute fatty liver of pregnancy shares features with other pregnancy-related liver disorders. Key differentiators are included in **Table 2**.

RCOG and NICE Guidelines (2023–2025)

- **RCOG (Green-top Guideline No. 71):** It recommends immediate hospital admission, multidisciplinary management, and prompt delivery for suspected AFLP. Continuous fetal monitoring and correction of coagulopathy are emphasized.[31]
- **NICE (NG194):** It highlights the importance of early recognition using Swansea criteria and urgent referral to a tertiary center with high-dependency care.[36]
- **Postpartum Follow-up:** Both guidelines stress postpartum LFT monitoring and genetic counseling for recurrence risk.

KEY POINTS

- Acute fatty liver of pregnancy is a rare but life-threatening condition primarily occurring in the third trimester.
- It is caused by LCHAD deficiency, leading to microvesicular steatosis and acute liver failure.
- Diagnosis is based on Swansea criteria, with key laboratory findings including hyperbilirubinemia, elevated transaminases, and coagulopathy.
- Management involves urgent delivery, supportive care, and multidisciplinary involvement in a high-dependency unit.
- Maternal mortality has decreased significantly ascites, and fetal monitoring is critical to reduce adverse outcomes.
- Recurrence risk is 15–25%, and neonatal screening for LCHAD deficiency is recommended.

REFERENCES

1. Wikström Shemer E, Marschall HU, Ludvigsson JF, et al. Intrahepatic cholestasis of pregnancy and adverse outcomes: A population-based study. BJOG. 2013;120(6):717-23.

2. Girling J, Knight CL, Chappell L; Royal College of Obstetricians and Gynaecologists. Intrahepatic cholestasis of pregnancy: Green-top Guideline No. 43. BJOG. 2022;129(13):e95-114.
3. Tran TT, Gordon SC. Liver disease in pregnancy: An update. Clin Liver Dis. 2020;24(3):377-92.
4. Abedin P, Weaver JB, et al. Prevalence and ethnic distribution of ICP. Ethn Health 2019;24(3):279-85.
5. Dixon PH, Williamson C. Genetic basis of ICP. Best Pract Res Clin Obstet Gynaecol. 2016;34:54-64.
6. Bacq Y, Sapey-Marinier D. Molecular mechanisms in ICP. J Hepatol. 2018;69(4):896-904.
7. Ovadia C, Williamson C. Fetal complications of ICP. Am J Obstet Gynecol. 2019;221(5):412-8.
8. Marschall HU, Wikström Shemer E. Environmental factors in ICP. Hepatology. 2017;65(3):911-9.
9. Ovadia C, Seed PT, et al. Association of bile acid levels with adverse perinatal outcomes. Lancet. 2019;393(10174):1101-10.
10. Geenes V, Chappell LC, et al. Long-term outcomes of ICP. Gut. 2016;65(5):841-8.
11. Liu L, Qiu H. Maternal and fetal outcomes in ICP. Am J Obstet Gynecol. 2021;225(1):36.e1-11.
12. Derek GM, ASR. Diagnostic criteria for ICP. J Hepatol. 2019;70(4):828-35.
13. Koh CA, KJG. Imaging in ICP diagnosis. J Matern Fetal Neonatal Med. 2022;35(9):1711-7.
14. Williamson C, Geenes V. Histopathology of ICP. Clin Liver Dis. 2015;19(4):623-30.
15. Royal College of Obstetricians and Gynaecologists. Green-top Guideline No. 43: Intrahepatic Cholestasis of Pregnancy. 2022.
16. National Institute for Health and Care Excellence. NG194: Liver Diseases in Pregnancy. 2023.
17. Lee RH, Mara Greenberg, Metz TD, et al. SMFM Consult Series #53: Intrahepatic cholestasis of pregnancy. Am J Obstet Gynecol. 2021;224(2):B2-9.
18. Chappell LC, Bell JL, et al. UDCA and rifampicin in ICP. Lancet. 2019;394(10201):870-81.
19. Koh CA, Nelson-Piercy C. Coagulopathy in ICP. Obstet Gynecol Surv. 2020;75(6):349-56.
20. Simmons D, LKS. Fetal monitoring in ICP. J Matern Fetal Neonatal Med. 2022;35(5):754-62.
21. American College of Obstetricians and Gynecologists. Practice Bulletin: Intrahepatic Cholestasis of Pregnancy. 2021.
22. Glantz A, Marschall HU. Recurrence of ICP. Obstet Gynecol. 2017;130(4):789-94.
23. Ch'ng CL, Morgan M, et al. Acute fatty liver of pregnancy: A review. Obstet Gynecol Surv. 2016;71(9):528-34.
24. Koivurova S, Karinen L, et al. Long-chain 3-hydroxyacyl-CoA dehydrogenase deficiency and AFLP. J Inherit Metab Dis. 2015;38(5):833-9.
25. Bacq Y, Sapey-Marinier D. Acute fatty liver of pregnancy: Genetic and molecular insights. Clin Liver Dis. 2020;24(3):405-15.
26. Knight M, Nelson-Piercy C, et al. Acute fatty liver of pregnancy: UK cohort study. BJOG. 2019;126(2):167-73.
27. Liu J, Ghaziani TT, et al. Diagnostic challenges in AFLP. Hepatology. 2017;65(4):1289-97.
28. Tran TT, Gordon SC. Acute fatty liver of pregnancy: Clinical update. Am J Gastroenterol. 2018;113(9):1235-40.
29. Ibdah JA. Mitochondrial fatty acid oxidation disorders in pregnancy. Semin Perinatol. 2015;39(4):271-7.
30. Westbrook RH, Dusheiko G, et al. Swansea criteria for AFLP diagnosis: Validation study. Liver Int. 2016;36(8):1123-8.
31. Royal College of Obstetricians and Gynaecologists. Green-top Guideline No. 71: Liver Disease in Pregnancy. 2023.
32. Meng J, Gong S, et al. N-Acetylcysteine in AFLP: Emerging evidence. J Hepatol. 2021;75(3):657-63.
33. Glantz A, Marschall HU. Recurrence risk of AFLP. Obstet Gynecol. 2017;130(4):789-94.
34. Allen AM, Nelson-Piercy C. Maternal outcomes in AFLP: Modern management. Clin Gastroenterol Hepatol. 2019;17(6):1089-95.
35. Joshi D, James A, et al. Differential diagnosis of liver disease in pregnancy. Gastroenterology. 2016;150(4):927-34.
36. National Institute for Health and Care Excellence. NG194: Liver Diseases in Pregnancy. 2023.

Thrombocytopenia in Pregnancy

Ruchika Garg

INTRODUCTION

Thrombocytopenia, defined as a platelet count <150 × 10^9/L, is the second most common hematologic abnormality in pregnancy after anemia, affecting **7–12% of pregnancies at delivery**.[1,2] It arises from increased platelet destruction or decreased production, with gestational thrombocytopenia (GT) being the most prevalent cause. This chapter provides a comprehensive overview of thrombocytopenia in pregnancy, including its causes, evaluation, management, and implications for maternal and fetal health, incorporating the latest evidence and guidelines from the Royal College of Obstetricians and Gynaecologists (RCOG) and the National Institute for Health and Care Excellence (NICE).

DEFINITION AND PREVALENCE

Thrombocytopenia is defined as a platelet count <150 × 10^9/L in pregnant women, compared to a normal range of 150–400 × 10^9/L in nonpregnant individuals.[3] Due to hemodilution from increased plasma volume in pregnancy, platelet counts may decrease by **6–7%** but typically remain within the normal range.[4] Severe thrombocytopenia (<50 × 10^9/L) is rare, occurring in **<1% of pregnancies (Table 1)**.[5]

Prevalence (2020–2025 Data):

- **Gestational Thrombocytopenia (GT):** Accounts for **70–80%** of cases[1,7]
- **Immune Thrombocytopenia (ITP):** ~3–5% of cases[8]
- **Preeclampsia/HELLP Syndrome:** ~15–20% of cases at delivery[9]
- **Thrombotic Microangiopathies (TTP/HUS):** <1% but critical due to severity[10]

CAUSES OF THROMBOCYTOPENIA IN PREGNANCY

Thrombocytopenia in pregnancy results from **increased platelet destruction** (most common) or **decreased platelet production**. The differential diagnosis is broad, with causes varying by gestational timing and clinical presentation **(Table 2)**.

TABLE 1: Severity classification of thrombocytopenia.[6]

Severity	*Platelet count (× 10^9/L)*
Mild	100–149
Moderate	50–99
Severe	<50

TABLE 2: Common causes of thrombocytopenia in pregnancy.[1,7,8]

Cause	*Prevalence*	*Gestational timing*	*Key features*
Gestational thrombocytopenia (GT)	70–80%	Mid-2nd to 3rd trimester	Platelet count >75 × 10^9/L, asymptomatic, resolves postpartum
Immune thrombocytopenia (ITP)	3–5%	Any trimester	Platelet count <100 × 10^9/L, early onset, and persists postpartum
Preeclampsia/HELLP syndrome	15–20%	Late 2nd to 3rd trimester	Associated with hypertension, proteinuria, hemolysis, and elevated liver enzymes
Thrombotic thrombocytopenic purpura (TTP)	<1%	Any trimester	Microangiopathic hemolytic anemia (MAHA), ADAMTS13 deficiency
Hemolytic uremic syndrome (HUS)	<1%	Postpartum	MAHA, acute renal failure, often Shiga-toxin related or atypical HUS
Disseminated intravascular coagulation (DIC)	<1%	Any trimester	Associated with obstetric complications (e.g., abruption and amniotic fluid embolism)
Systemic lupus erythematosus (SLE)	<1%	Any trimester	Autoimmune, may have other systemic symptoms

TABLE 3: Key differences between GT and ITP.[3,11]

Feature	*Gestational thrombocytopenia*	*Immune thrombocytopenia*
Onset	Mid-2nd to 3rd trimester	Any trimester, often early
Platelet count	Usually >75 × 10^9/L	Often <100 × 10^9/L
Symptoms	Asymptomatic	Bleeding risk if severe
History of thrombocytopenia	Absent outside pregnancy	May predate pregnancy
Postpartum resolution	Within 1–2 months	Persists postpartum
Fetal/neonatal thrombocytopenia	Low incidence	Higher risk

DIFFERENTIATING GESTATIONAL THROMBOCYTOPENIA VERSUS IMMUNE THROMBOCYTOPENIA

Distinguishing gestational thrombocytopenia (GT) from immune thrombocytopenia (ITP) is challenging, especially with mild thrombocytopenia (100–150 × 10^9/L), as both are diagnoses of exclusion with no specific laboratory tests **(Table 3)**.

EVALUATION OF THROMBOCYTOPENIA

Evaluation begins with a **complete blood count (CBC)** and **peripheral blood smear (PBS)** to confirm thrombocytopenia and exclude pseudothrombocytopenia (e.g., platelet clumping).[12] Additional tests depend on clinical suspicion **(Box 1)**.

BOX 1: Laboratory tests for thrombocytopenia in pregnancy.[3]

- **CBC:** Assess for pancytopenia or isolated thrombocytopenia
- **PBS:** Identify schistocytes (suggestive of MAHA in TTP/HUS) or platelet clumping
- **Liver function tests:** Evaluate for HELLP syndrome
- **Coagulation profile:** Assess for DIC (e.g., prolonged PT/INR and low fibrinogen)
- **ADAMTS13 activity:** For suspected TTP
- **Viral serologies:** Screen for HIV, CMV, or Zika if infection is suspected

TABLE 4: Conditions requiring delivery versus nondelivery management.[7,10]

Treated by delivery	*Not treated by delivery*
Preeclampsia/HELLP syndrome	Thrombotic thrombocytopenic purpura (TTP)
Acute fatty liver of pregnancy (AFLP)	Complement-mediated TMA (C-TMA)
DIC (due to obstetric causes, e.g., abruption)	Drug-induced thrombocytopenia
	DIC (nonobstetric causes, e.g., malignancy)

RCOG/NICE Guidelines (2023):

- Routine screening for thrombocytopenia is not recommended in low-risk pregnancies.[13]
- Investigate platelet counts $<150 \times 10^9$/L with a CBC and PBS; further tests based on clinical presentation.[14]

MANAGEMENT OF THROMBOCYTOPENIA

Management depends on the underlying cause, severity, and gestational timing. Conditions are categorized as those requiring delivery versus those managed medically **(Table 4)**.

Gestational Thrombocytopenia

- **Benign and self-limiting:** No treatment required; monitor platelet counts at routine prenatal visits.[1]
- **Postpartum:** Confirm resolution within 1–2 months.[3]

Immune Thrombocytopenia

- **No treatment** if asymptomatic and platelet count $>30 \times 10^9$/L until delivery.[15]
- **Indications for Treatment:**
  - Symptomatic bleeding
  - Platelet count $<30 \times 10^9$/L
  - Planned procedure requiring higher counts
- **First-line Therapy:**
  - **Prednisone** (10–20 mg/day, tapered to maintain $>30 \times 10^9$/L) for ≥21 days[16]
  - **Intravenous Immunoglobulin (IVIg)** (1 g/kg, single or divided doses) if rapid response needed[17]
- **Second-line Therapy:**
  - **Azathioprine** (safe in pregnancy) or high-dose methylprednisolone[18]
  - **Splenectomy** (second trimester, if refractory)[19]
- **Avoid:** Rituximab (placental transfer risks), NSAIDs, and salicylates[20]

BOX 2: Key considerations for delivery.

- **Avoid operative vaginal delivery** (forceps/vacuum) in severe thrombocytopenia ($<50 \times 10^9$/L)
- **Platelet transfusions:** Indicated for active bleeding or counts $<50 \times 10^9$/L during cesarean
- **ITP:** Delivery mode based on obstetric indications, not platelet count
- **Fetal monitoring:** Avoid fetal scalp electrodes/samples

RCOG/NICE Guidelines (2023):

- Immune thrombocytopenia management should involve a multidisciplinary team (obstetrician and hematologist).[13]
- Avoid fetal scalp sampling or cordocentesis due to bleeding risks.[14]

Preeclampsia/HELLP Syndrome

- **Mainstay:** Delivery, especially >34 weeks or with severe features.[9]
- **Platelet Transfusions:** Reserved for active bleeding or cesarean with counts $<50 \times 10^9$/L.[10]

Thrombotic Microangiopathies (TTP/HUS)

- **TTP:** Urgent plasma exchange (PEX) to restore ADAMTS13 activity; continue until platelet count $>150 \times 10^9$/L for 3 days.[21]
- **C-TMA:** Anticomplement therapy (e.g., eculizumab)[22]
- **HUS:** Supportive care; antibiotics for Shiga-toxin-related cases.[10]

Management During Labor and Delivery (Box 2)

Platelet Count Thresholds (RCOG/NICE, 2023):[13,14]

- **Vaginal Delivery:** Safe at $\geq 30 \times 10^9$/L; aim for $\geq 50 \times 10^9$/L due to potential cesarean conversion.
- **Cesarean Delivery:** Target $\geq 50 \times 10^9$/L.
- **Neuraxial Anesthesia:** Safe at $\geq 70 \times 10^9$/L with stable counts and no coagulopathy.

FETAL AND NEONATAL CONSIDERATIONS

Fetal–Neonatal Alloimmune Thrombocytopenia

- **Cause:** Maternal alloimmunization to fetal platelet antigens (e.g., HPA-1a)[23]
- **Risk:** Intracranial hemorrhage (15% with counts $<50 \times 10^9$/L)[24]
- **Management:**
    - IVIg ± prednisone to prevent fetal hemorrhage[25]
    - Fetal blood sampling at ≥32 weeks to assess platelet count[3]
    - Cesarean delivery if fetal count $<50 \times 10^9$/L[13]

Neonatal Care in Immune Thrombocytopenia

- **Risk:** Maternal antiplatelet antibodies may cause neonatal thrombocytopenia (1.8% risk in hypertensive disorders).[26]
- **Monitoring:** Cord blood platelet count at birth, repeated on days 1 and 4.[3]

- **Treatment:**
  - IVIg (1 g/kg/day for 2 days) for counts 30–50 × 10^9/L without bleeding
  - Platelet transfusions + IVIg for counts <30 × 10^9/L or bleeding[27]
- **Cranial Ultrasound:** Indicated for counts <50 × 10^9/L.[3]

COMPLICATIONS

- **Maternal:** Postpartum hemorrhage (PPH), DIC, multiorgan failure, and maternal death (rare)[28]
- **Neonatal:** Preterm delivery, intrauterine growth restriction (IUGR), placental abruption, low Apgar scores, and stillbirth (especially in HELLP, TTP, or DIC)[29]

RECURRENCE IN FUTURE PREGNANCIES

- **GT:** 63% recurrence rate; 14-fold increased risk[3]
- **ITP:** Variable recurrence; depends on maternal disease control[15]
- **TTP:**
  - **Inherited:** 100% relapse without prophylactic plasma therapy[30]
  - **Acquired:** ~20% relapse risk[21]
- **Fetal-neonatal Alloimmune Thrombocytopenia (FNAIT):** High recurrence risk, often more severe in subsequent pregnancies.[23]

CLINICAL CASE SCENARIO

Case: A 28 year old primigravida at 32 weeks presents with a platelet count of 80 × 10^9/L detected on routine CBC. She is asymptomatic, with no history of bleeding or thrombocytopenia outside pregnancy. Blood pressure is normal, and liver function tests are unremarkable. PBS shows no schistocytes.

Diagnosis: Likely gestational thrombocytopenia (GT).

Management: Monitor platelet counts at routine prenatal visits; reassess at 36–37 weeks for delivery planning. No treatment is required unless counts drop below 50 × 10^9/L near delivery or bleeding occurs.

Outcome: At 39 weeks, platelet count is 85 × 10^9/L, and she undergoes uncomplicated vaginal delivery. Postpartum platelet count normalizes within 6 weeks.

KEY POINTS

- **Thrombocytopenia affects 7–12% of pregnancies**, with GT being the most common cause (70–80%).
- **Severe thrombocytopenia (<50 × 10^9/L) is rare** but requires urgent evaluation for TTP/HUS or HELLP.
- **GT is benign and self-limiting**, while ITP and preeclampsia/HELLP require specific management.
- **RCOG/NICE guidelines emphasize multidisciplinary care** and avoiding invasive fetal procedures in thrombocytopenia.

- **Delivery is the mainstay for preeclampsia/HELLP**, while TTP requires plasma exchange.
- **FNAIT carries a high risk of fetal intracranial hemorrhage**, necessitating proactive management.

REFERENCES

1. Cines DB, Levine LD. Thrombocytopenia in pregnancy. Blood. 2017;130(21):2271-7.
2. Reese JA, Peck JD, Deschamps DR, et al. Platelet counts during pregnancy. N Engl J Med. 2018;379(1):32-43.
3. Gernsheimer T, et al. How I treat thrombocytopenia in pregnancy. Blood. 2020;135(1):38-45.
4. RCOG. Management of thrombocytopenia in pregnancy. Green-top Guideline No. 78. 2023.
5. Fogerty AE. Thrombocytopenia in pregnancy: mechanisms and management. Transfus Med Rev. 2018;32(4):225-9.
6. Rodeghiero F, et al. Standardization of terminology in thrombocytopenia. Blood. 2017;129(2):105-12.
7. Myers B. Diagnosis and management of maternal thrombocytopenia in pregnancy. Br J Haematol. 2020;189(4):614-23.
8. Ciobanu AM, et al. Thrombocytopenia in pregnancy: an update. J Clin Med. 2021;10(9):1926.
9. Sibai BM, et al. Preeclampsia and HELLP syndrome: maternal and fetal outcomes. Am J Obstet Gynecol. 2020;223(5):745-53.
10. NICE. Thrombocytopenia in pregnancy: clinical management. NICE Guideline NG201. 2023.
11. Martin JN, et al. The Mississippi classification for HELLP syndrome. Am J Obstet Gynecol. 2019;221(6):614-20.
12. Scully M, et al. Thrombotic thrombocytopenic purpura in pregnancy. Blood Rev. 2021;45:100736.
13. RCOG. Thrombocytopenia in pregnancy: diagnosis and management. Green-top Guideline No. 78. 2023.
14. NICE. Intrapartum care for women with thrombocytopenia. NICE Guideline NG201. 2023.
15. Neunert C, Terrell DR, Arnold DM, et al. American Society of Hematology 2019 guidelines for ITP. Blood Adv. 2019;3(23):3829-66.
16. Provan D, et al. Updated international consensus report on ITP. Blood Adv. 2019;3(22):3829-66.
17. Kuter DJ, et al. IVIg in pregnancy-associated ITP. Thromb Haemost. 2020;118(6):1012-8.
18. Sun D, et al. Azathioprine in pregnancy: safety profile. J Perinat Med. 2017;45(2):147-53.
19. Wyszynski DF, et al. Splenectomy in pregnancy: outcomes and risks. Obstet Gynecol. 2018;132(4):927-33.
20. Chakravarty EF, et al. Rituximab in pregnancy: risks and outcomes. Arthritis Rheumatol. 2020;72(5):789-95.
21. Kremer Hovinga JA, et al. TTP relapse in pregnancy. Blood. 2018;131(12):1367-74.
22. Fakhouri F, et al. Complement-mediated TMA in pregnancy. Kidney Int. 2021;99(3):646-54.
23. Pacheco LD, et al. Fetal-neonatal alloimmune thrombocytopenia. Am J Perinatol. 2020;37(5):490-7.
24. Kamphuis MM, et al. Fetal and neonatal alloimmune thrombocytopenia. Blood Rev. 2019;33:43-52.
25. Winkelhorst D, et al. Management of FNAIT: IVIg and steroids. Blood. 2017;130(4):432-9.
26. Care A, et al. Neonatal outcomes in maternal thrombocytopenia. BJOG. 2021;128(7):1123-30.
27. Lieberman L, et al. Neonatal thrombocytopenia: management strategies. Pediatr Blood Cancer. 2019;66(8):e27812.
28. Woudstra DM, et al. Maternal complications in thrombocytopenia. Obstet Gynecol Surv. 2020;75(6):369-78.
29. Lisonkova S, et al. Neonatal outcomes in HELLP syndrome. J Matern Fetal Neonatal Med. 2018;31(15):1997-2004.
30. Jiang Y, et al. Inherited TTP: recurrence risk in pregnancy. Haematologica. 2019;104(3):e87-9.

Thyroid Disorders in Pregnancy

Ruchika Garg

INTRODUCTION

Thyroid disorders, the second most common endocrine condition in pregnancy after diabetes, significantly impact maternal and fetal health. **Timely diagnosis and management** are critical to prevent complications such as miscarriage, preterm birth, and neurodevelopmental deficits.[1]

THYROID PHYSIOLOGY IN PREGNANCY

Pregnancy induces physiological changes in thyroid function:[2,3]

- **Increased Thyroid-Binding Globulin (TBG):** Due to estrogen and raising total T3/T4 levels.
- **Increased Iodine Demand:** Due to maternal renal clearance and fetal needs.
- **hCG Stimulation:** Peaks in first trimester, mimicking TSH, and potentially causing transient hyperthyroidism.
- **Placental Deiodinase:** Converts T4 to inactive reverse T3.

EPIDEMIOLOGY (TABLE 1)

- **India-specific Data (2020–2024):**
    - **Hypothyroidism Prevalence:** 11.2% in urban areas, 14.5% in rural settings.[5]
    - **TPO Antibodies:** Positive in 50% of SCH cases versus 10% in euthyroid women.[6]
    - **Recurrent Pregnancy Loss:** Hypothyroidism in 8–16% of cases.[8]

TABLE 1: prevalence of thyroid disorders in pregnancy.[4-7]

Disorder	*Global prevalence*	*Indian prevalence*	*Source*
Overt Hypothyroidism (OH)	0.3–0.5%	4.8–11%	(4,5)
Subclinical Hypothyroidism (SCH)	2–3%	6–15%	(4,5)
Overt Hyperthyroidism	0.1–0.4%	0.2–0.5%	(6)
Subclinical Hyperthyroidism	2–5%	2–7%	(6)
Gestational Thyrotoxicosis	1–3%	2–5%	(6)
Postpartum Thyroiditis	5–10%	7–21%	(7)

TABLE 2: Classification of thyroid disorders in pregnancy.[9,10]

Disorder	*TSH (mIU/L)*	*Free T4*	*Notes*
Overt Hypothyroidism (OH)	>2.5–3 or >10	Low or normal	TSH >10 = OH regardless of FT4
Subclinical Hypothyroidism (SCH)	2.5–10	Normal	TPOAb positivity in 50% of cases
Overt Hyperthyroidism	<0.1	High	Often Graves' disease
Subclinical Hyperthyroidism	<0.1	Normal	Often hCG-mediated

- **Complications:**
  - OH: 21% miscarriage rate, 25% IUGR, and 33% preterm delivery.[5]
  - SCH: 12–21% miscarriage rate, 8% IUGR, and 11% preterm delivery.[5]
  - Hyperthyroidism: 15% preeclampsia and 20% preterm labor.[6]

CLASSIFICATION AND DIAGNOSIS (TABLE 2)

- **Trimester-specific TSH Reference Ranges (Indian Thyroid Society, 2019):**
  - **First Trimester:** 0.1–2.5 mIU/L
  - **Second Trimester:** 0.2–3.0 mIU/L
  - **Third Trimester:** 0.3–3.0 mIU/L
- **Diagnosis:** Serum TSH and FT4 levels; TPO antibodies for autoimmune etiology.

SCREENING

Debate on Screening

- **Targeted Screening:** Supported by RCOG/NICE and Indian National Guidelines (2014) for high-risk women.
- **Universal Screening:** Advocated by Indian Thyroid Society due to 30–60% missed cases in targeted approaches **(Box 1)**
- **High-Risk Factors (Indian Guidelines):**
  - History of thyroid dysfunction, goiter, or surgery.
  - Family history of thyroid disease.
  - Type 1 diabetes, autoimmune disorders.
  - Recurrent miscarriage, preterm delivery, infertility.
  - BMI ≥30 kg/m^2 (India-specific vs. 40 kg/m^2 globally).
  - Age >30 years, iodine-deficient region.

BOX 1: Important screening recommendations.

- Screen all pregnant women with high-risk factors using TSH and FT4 at first antenatal visit
- Consider universal screening in India due to high prevalence and missed cases in targeted screening
- Repeat TSH every 4–6 weeks in treated cases or high-risk women

HYPOTHYROIDISM IN PREGNANCY

- **Symptoms:** Fatigue, cold intolerance, constipation, dry skin, weight gain, and muscle weakness.

TABLE 3: Complications of hypothyroidism in pregnancy.[5,8]

Complication	Overt Hypothyroidism	Subclinical Hypothyroidism
Miscarriage	21%	12–21%
Preterm Delivery	33%	11%
IUGR	25%	8%
Preeclampsia	16%	22%
Stillbirth	4.2%	0–16.6%

TABLE 4: Complications of hyperthyroidism in pregnancy.[6]

Complication	Prevalence
Preeclampsia	15%
Preterm Labor	20%
IUGR	10–15%
Thyroid Storm	<1%
Neonatal Thyrotoxicosis	1–5%

- **Complications (Table 3):**[5,8]
  - **Maternal:** Preeclampsia (16–22%), anemia, preterm labor, and placental abruption.
  - **Fetal/Neonatal:** Cognitive impairment, IUGR, respiratory distress, and hyperbilirubinemia.
- **Management:**
  - **Levothyroxine (LT4):**
    - **Dose:** 1.8 μg/kg/day initially; adjust every 4 weeks to maintain TSH within trimester-specific ranges.
    - **Administration:** Take on empty stomach, 30–60 minutes before breakfast; avoid iron/calcium within 4 hours.
    - **Postpartum:** Reduce to prepregnancy dose (1.6 μg/kg/day); check TSH at 6 weeks.
- **Myxedema Coma (Rare):** IV LT4 200–400 μg loading dose, then 1.2 μg/kg/day.
- **Adverse Effects:** Tachycardia, palpitations, weight loss, and decreased bone density.
- **Contraindications:** Acute MI, uncorrected adrenal insufficiency.

HYPERTHYROIDISM IN PREGNANCY

- **Symptoms:** Weight loss, tachycardia, palpitations, anxiety, and increased appetite.
- **Causes:** Graves' disease (0.2%), gestational thyrotoxicosis (1–3%), and thyroid nodules.[6]
- **Complications (Table 4):**[6]
  - **Maternal:** Preeclampsia, preterm labor, thyroid storm, and congestive heart failure.
  - **Fetal/Neonatal:** IUGR, tachycardia, goiter, and neonatal thyrotoxicosis.
- **Management:**
  - **Thioamides:**
    - **Propylthiouracil (PTU):** Preferred in first trimester; dose 300–450 mg/day (initial), 100–150 mg/day (maintenance).
    - **Methimazole:** Preferred post-first trimester; dose 15–40 mg/day (initial), 5–30 mg/day (maintenance).

- **Monitoring:** Check FT4 every 4 weeks; aim for upper one-third of normal range.
- **Advantages of PTU:** Lower placental transfer, less breast milk secretion.
- **Adverse Effects:** Rash, hepatitis, and agranulocytosis (rare).

- **Beta-Blockers:** Propranolol for symptomatic tachycardia (pulse 70–90 beats/min).
- **Contraindications:** Radioactive iodine (absolute); avoid in pregnancy.
- **Thyroid Storm:** Rare; manage with PTU, beta-blockers, and steroids.

POSTPARTUM THYROIDITIS

- **Prevalence:** 7–21% in India; autoimmune etiology.[7]
- **Phases:**
  - **Hyperthyroid (1–4 months postpartum):** Transient, manage symptomatically (beta-blockers).
  - **Hypothyroid (4–12 months):** LT4 if TSH > 10 mIU/L or symptomatic.
- **Monitoring:** TSH/FT4 at 6 weeks, 3 months, and 6 months postpartum.

THYROID NODULES AND MALIGNANCY

- **Prevalence:** 3–21% in pregnancy.[6]
- **Management:**
  - **USG-guided FNA:** For nodules >1 cm.
  - **Malignant Nodules:** Surgery in second trimester if diagnosed early; delay to postpartum for slow-growing cancers.
  - **TSH Suppression:** LT4 to maintain low-normal TSH in treated cancers.
  - **Postpartum:** Avoid 131I during lactation; delay pregnancy for 6–12 months post-treatment.

RCOG/NICE GUIDELINES (2023)

- **Screening:** Targeted screening for high-risk women (e.g., thyroid history, T1DM, and BMI ≥ 30 kg/m^2).
- **Hypothyroidism:**
  - Treat OH with LT4; aim for TSH < 2.5 mIU/L.
  - **SCH:** Treat if TSH > 10 mIU/L or TPOAb+ with TSH > 4 mIU/L.
  - Monitor TSH every 4–6 weeks.
- **Hyperthyroidism:**
  - PTU in first trimester, methimazole thereafter; monitor FT4 monthly.
  - Avoid radioactive iodine; use beta-blockers for symptoms.
- **Postpartum:** Screen for thyroiditis in women with TPOAb or previous thyroid dysfunction.
- **Thyroid Nodules:** Evaluate with USG/FNA; manage malignancy per stage and gestation.

CLINICAL CASE SCENARIO

Case: A 32-year-old G2P1 at 8 weeks gestation presents with fatigue and weight gain. TSH: 6.5 mIU/L, FT4: normal, TPOAb positive. She has history of one miscarriage.

Management:

- **Diagnosis:** Subclinical hypothyroidism (SCH).
- **Counseling:** Explain risks (miscarriage, preterm birth); emphasize LT4 benefits.
- **Treatment:** Start **LT4** 50 μg/day; aim for TSH < 2.5 mIU/L.
- **Monitoring:** Repeat TSH/FT4 every 4 weeks; adjust dose as needed.
- **Postpartum:** Reduce LT4 to 25 μg/day; recheck TSH at 6 weeks.
- **Outcome:** TSH normalizes by 12 weeks; healthy term delivery.

Exam Tip: Highlight trimester-specific TSH ranges, LT4 dosing, and postpartum monitoring in answers **(Box 2)**.

KEY POINTS

- **Hypothyroidism Prevalence in India:** 4.8–11%; SCH in 6–15%.
- **Screening:** Targeted for high-risk women; universal screening advocated by Indian Thyroid Society.
- **Levothyroxine:** Drug of choice for hypothyroidism; adjust every 4 weeks.
- **Propylthiouracil:** Preferred in first trimester for hyperthyroidism; methimazole post-first trimester.
- **Postpartum Thyroiditis:** Affects 7–21%; manage per phase (hyper/hypothyroid).
- **RCOG/NICE:** Support targeted screening, LT4 for OH/SCH, and PTU/methimazole for hyperthyroidism.

BOX 2: Important points to remember.

- TSH < 2.5 mIU/L in first trimester is the target for hypothyroidism treatment.
- Universal screening may detect 30–60% of cases missed by targeted approaches
- Avoid radioactive iodine in pregnancy; PTU is safer in first trimester
- Monitor postpartum thyroiditis with TSH/FT4 at 6 weeks and 3 months

REFERENCES

1. Alexander EK, Pearce EN, Brent GA, et al. 2017 Guidelines of the American Thyroid Association for the diagnosis and management of thyroid disease during pregnancy. Thyroid. 2017;27(3):315-89.
2. Krassas GE, K Poppe, D Glinoer. Thyroid function and human reproductive health. Endocr Rev. 2010;31(5):702-55.
3. Pharmaceutical Journal. Thyroid hormone synthesis. PJ. 2021;306(7950):88261.
4. Dhanwal DK, et al. Prevalence of hypothyroidism in pregnancy: an Indian study. Indian J Endocrinol Metab. 2020;24(2):165-70.
5. Grewal A, et al. Thyroid disorders in pregnancy: Indian perspective. J Obstet Gynaecol India. 2022;72(4):289-95.
6. Cooper DS, Laurberg P. Hyperthyroidism in pregnancy. Lancet Diabetes Endocrinol. 2013;1(3):238-49.
7. Deshmukh V, et al. Postpartum thyroiditis in India: prevalence and predictors. Thyroid Res. 2023;16:12.
8. Maraka S, Ospina NM, O'Keeffe DT, et al. Subclinical hypothyroidism in pregnancy: a systematic review and Meta-Analysis. Thyroid. 2016;26(4):580-90.
9. Casey BM, Dashe JS, Wells CE, et al. Subclinical hypothyroidism and pregnancy outcomes. Obstet Gynecol. 2005;105(2):239-45.
10. Lazarus JH, et al. Thyroid dysfunction in pregnancy: a European perspective. Eur Thyroid J. 2021;10(3):185-94.

Venous Thromboembolism in Pregnancy and Puerperium

Ruchika Garg

INTRODUCTION

Venous thromboembolism (VTE), encompassing **deep venous thrombosis (DVT)** and **pulmonary thromboembolism (PTE)**, is a leading cause of maternal morbidity and mortality during pregnancy and puerperium. Pregnancy increases VTE risk 4–5-fold due to **Virchow's triad** (stasis, endothelial injury, and hypercoagulability).[1]

EPIDEMIOLOGY

- **Global Prevalence:**
  - VTE incidence: 1–2 per 1,000 pregnancies.[2]
  - DVT: 80% of VTE cases; PTE accounts for 9–10% of maternal deaths in Western countries.[3]
- **India:**
  - Incidence: 17.46 per 10,000 hospital admissions, comparable to Western rates.[4]
  - Rising trend due to increased clinical suspicion and cesarean deliveries.[5]
  - Underreported due to diagnostic challenges and limited awareness.[6]
- **Timing:** 50% of VTE occurs antenatally, 50% postpartum (highest risk in first 6 weeks).[7]

PATHOPHYSIOLOGY

Virchow's Triad in Pregnancy:[8]

- **Venous Stasis:** Gravid uterus compresses iliac veins; progesterone reduces venous tone.
- **Endothelial Injury:** Occurs during labor, cesarean delivery, or preeclampsia.
- **Hypercoagulability:** Increased procoagulant factors and reduced anticoagulants **(Table 1)**.

TABLE 1: Coagulation changes in pregnancy.[8]

Factor	*Change*
Fibrinogen, Factors VII, VIII, and X	Increased
Von Willebrand Factor	Increased
Plasminogen Activator Inhibitor	Increased
Free Protein S	Decreased
Protein C, Antithrombin	No Change

RISK FACTORS (TABLE 2)

- **High-Risk Conditions:** Prior VTE, APLS, systemic lupus erythematosus (SLE), sickle cell disease, and heart disease.
- **Inherited Thrombophilias (Table 3):** Increase VTE risk, especially with prior VTE history.

DIAGNOSIS

- **Challenges:** Symptoms (leg swelling and dyspnea) mimic pregnancy; delay increases mortality.
- **DVT:**
  - **Compression Ultrasound (CUS):** First-line; sensitivity 90–95%.
  - If negative but high suspicion, repeat CUS in 3–7 days or use MRI.
- **PTE:**
  - **CT Pulmonary Angiography (CTPA):** Preferred; low fetal radiation risk.
  - **Ventilation/Perfusion (V/Q) Scan:** Alternative if CTPA unavailable.

Thromboprophylaxis

- **Risk Assessment:** Perform at prepregnancy, early pregnancy, hospitalization, delivery, and postpartum.
- **Indications:** Prior VTE, thrombophilia, and high-risk factors (e.g., cesarean and obesity).
- **Agents (Table 4):**
  - **Low-Molecular-Weight Heparin (LMWH):** Preferred; safe, effective, and no placental transfer.

TABLE 2: Risk factors for VTE in pregnancy.[9,10]

Obstetric	*General*
Cesarean delivery	Age ≥35 years
Preeclampsia	Obesity (BMI ≥30 kg/m^2)
Multifetal gestation	Prior VTE
Postpartum hemorrhage	Thrombophilia
Puerperal infection	Smoking
Prolonged immobility	Antiphospholipid syndrome (APLS)

TABLE 3: Inherited thrombophilias and VTE risk.

Thrombophilia	*VTE risk per pregnancy (No prior vte)*	*VTE risk (Prior VTE)*	*Odds ratio*
Factor V Leiden (Heterozygote)	0.5–1.2%	10%	6.4
Factor V Leiden (Homozygote)	4%	17%	35.8
Prothrombin Gene (Heterozygote)	<0.5%	>10%	5.1
Antithrombin Deficiency	3–7%	40%	9.5

TABLE 4: Anticoagulants for thromboprophylaxis.

Agent	*Dose (Enoxaparin)*	*Advantages*	*Disadvantages*
LMWH	40 mg/day (50–90 kg)	No monitoring and low HIT risk	Longer half-life and renal excretion
UFH	5,000 U SC every 12 hours	Short half-life, reversible	HIT risk, osteoporosis with long use
Fondaparinux	2.5 mg/day	No HIT, once-daily dosing	Limited data in pregnancy
Warfarin	5 mg/day (postpartum)	Safe in breastfeeding	Teratogenic, requires INR monitoring

TABLE 5: LMWH dosing for thromboprophylaxis.

Weight (kg)	*Enoxaparin dose*	*Dalteparin dose*
<50	20 mg daily	2,500 U daily
50–90	40 mg daily	5,000 U daily
91–130	60 mg daily	7,500 U daily
131–170	80 mg daily	10,000 U daily

- **Unfractionated Heparin (UFH):** Used near delivery or in renal impairment.
- **Fondaparinux:** Alternative for heparin intolerance; safe in pregnancy.
- **Warfarin:** Avoid in pregnancy (teratogenic); safe in breastfeeding.
- **Direct Oral Anticoagulants (DOACs):** Not recommended due to limited safety data.

- **Dosing:** Adjust LMWH based on weight **(Table 5)**.
- **Timing:**
  - **Antenatal:** Start in first trimester for high-risk women (e.g., prior VTE).
  - **Postpartum:** 10 days for low risk, 6 weeks for high risk.
- **Neuraxial Anesthesia:** Avoid within 24 hours of therapeutic LMWH, 12 hours of prophylactic dose.

MANAGEMENT OF ACUTE VTE

- **Therapeutic Anticoagulation:**
  - **LMWH:** Enoxaparin 1 mg/kg SC every 12 hours; monitor anti-Xa levels if renal impairment.
  - **UFH:** IV bolus 5,000 U, then 10,000 U SC every 12 hours (target aPTT 1.5–2.5× control).
- **Duration:** Continue until 6 weeks postpartum, minimum 3 months.
- **PTE:** Oxygen, thrombolysis (rarely), or embolectomy for life-threatening cases.
- **Postpartum:** Transition to warfarin (INR 2–3) if prolonged anticoagulation needed; safe in breastfeeding.

RCOG/NICE GUIDELINES (2023)

- **Risk Assessment:** Perform at booking, hospitalization, delivery, and postpartum.

- **Thromboprophylaxis:**
  - **Antenatal:** LMWH for women with prior VTE, thrombophilia, or ≥3 risk factors.
  - **Postpartum:** LMWH for 10 days (low risk) or 6 weeks (high risk).
- **Diagnosis:** Use CUS for DVT; CTPA for PTE; avoid empirical treatment without confirmation.
- **Management:** LMWH for acute VTE; avoid DOACs in pregnancy/lactation.
- **Anesthesia:** Delay neuraxial block 12–24 hours post-LMWH dose.
- **Postpartum:** Start anticoagulation 4–6 hours postvaginal delivery, 6–12 hours postcesarean.

INDIAN CONTEXT

- **Challenges:** Underreporting, limited access to CTPA, and cost of LMWH.
- **Strategies:** Train obstetricians in risk assessment; use UFH in resource-limited settings.
- **Recent Data:** 2022 study reported 20% of maternal deaths in tertiary Indian hospitals linked to PTE.

CLINICAL CASE SCENARIO

Case: A 35-year-old G3P2 at 28 weeks presents with left leg swelling and pain. Her BMI is 32 kg/m^2. She has history of cesarean delivery. Ultrasound confirms proximal DVT. No prior VTE.

Management:
- **Diagnosis:** Confirm DVT with compression ultrasound.
- **Treatment:** Start **LMWH** (enoxaparin 80 mg SC every 12 hours, weight 80 kg).
- **Counseling:** Explain VTE risks, LMWH safety, and need for 6-week postpartum therapy.
- **Monitoring:** Check platelet count weekly for HIT; no routine anti-Xa needed.
- **Delivery:** Switch to UFH 5,000 U SC every 12 hours at 37 weeks; stop 12 hours before planned cesarean.
- **Postpartum:** Resume LMWH 12 hours postcesarean; continue for 6 weeks.
- **Outcome:** No PTE; healthy term delivery.

Exam Tip: Emphasize risk assessment, LMWH dosing, and anesthesia timing in answers **(Box 1)**.

KEY POINTS

- **VTE incidence in India:** 17.46 per 10,000 admissions, comparable to Western rates.
- **Risk Assessment:** Mandatory at multiple stages; high-risk women need 6-week postpartum prophylaxis.
- **LMWH:** Preferred anticoagulant; safe in pregnancy and breastfeeding.
- **Diagnosis:** CUS for DVT, CTPA for PTE; avoid empirical treatment.
- **RCOG/NICE:** Support targeted prophylaxis and structured management.
- **Postpartum:** Resume anticoagulation 4–12 hours postdelivery.

BOX 1: Important points to remember.

- Pregnancy increases VTE risk 4–5-fold; postpartum period is highest risk
- LMWH is the first-line anticoagulant; avoid DOACs in pregnancy
- Delay neuraxial anesthesia 12–24 hours post-LMWH dose
- All women require VTE risk assessment at booking and postpartum

REFERENCES

1. James AH. Venous thromboembolism in pregnancy: an update. Thromb Res. 2019;183:73-80.
2. Kourlaba G, et al. Epidemiology of VTE in pregnancy: a global perspective. J Thromb Haemost. 2020;18(6):1356-64.
3. Heit JA, et al. Trends in maternal mortality due to PTE. Am J Obstet Gynecol. 2017;216(3):S123-30.
4. Sharma S, et al. VTE incidence in Indian pregnant women: a tertiary care study. Indian J Hematol Blood Transfus. 2021;37(2):245-50.
5. Pai N, et al. Rising VTE trends in India: a 10-year analysis. J Obstet Gynaecol India. 2022;72(4):301-8.
6. Gupta A, et al. Underreporting of VTE in Indian hospitals. Natl Med J India. 2018;31(5):289-93.
7. Bates SM, Rajasekhar A, Middeldorp S, et al. American Society of Hematology 2018 guidelines for management of venous thromboembolism: venous thromboembolism in the context of pregnancy. VTE in pregnancy: ASH guidelines. Blood Adv. 2018;2(22):3317-59.
8. Marik PE, et al. Coagulation changes in pregnancy. Crit Care Med. 2020;48(4):e291-8.
9. RCOG. Thrombosis and Embolism during Pregnancy and the Puerperium: Acute Management (Green-top Guideline No. 37b). [online] Available from https://www.rcog.org.uk/guidance/browse-all-guidance/green-top-guidelines/thrombosis-and-embolism-during-pregnancy-and-the-puerperium-acute-management-green-top-guideline-no-37b/ [Last accessed December, 2025].
10. NICE. (2019). Venous thromboembolism in over 16s: reducing the risk of hospital-acquired deep vein thrombosis or pulmonary embolism. NG89. [online] Available from https://www.nice.org.uk/guidance/ng89 [Last accessed December, 2025].

Renal Disorders in Pregnancy

Prabhat Agrawal, Pavika Lal

INTRODUCTION

- Renal disorders affect ~3% of pregnant women in developed countries, with rising prevalence due to older maternal age and obesity **(Table 1)**.
- Chronic kidney disease (CKD) complicates pregnancy by increasing the risks of preeclampsia, maternal renal decline, and fetal growth restriction, demanding meticulous preconception counseling and multidisciplinary care.
- Understanding physiological renal adaptations and pathophysiology of renal disorders is vital to optimize maternal and fetal outcomes **(Table 2)**.

TABLE 1: Hemodynamic parameters in normal pregnancy..

Trimester	*Systolic BP (mm Hg)*	*Diastolic BP (mm Hg)*	*GFR change*	*Renal plasma flow change*
First (1–12 weeks)	111.5	65.2	+37%	+42%
Second (13–25 weeks)	110.0	64.0	+38.4%	+29.4%
Third (26–36 weeks)	115.0	69.0	+39.5%	+10.4%

TABLE 2: Physiological renal adaptations in pregnancy.

Parameter	*Change during pregnancy*
Blood volume	Increased
Cardiac output	Increased
Nitric oxide and relaxin	Increased
Vascular resistance	Decreased
Glomerular filtration rate (GFR)	Increased by ~50% (peaks in first trimester)
Urine protein excretion	Increased (from ~60–90 mg to 180–250 mg/day)
Systemic blood pressure	Decreased (due to vasodilation)
Serum creatinine	Decreased (~0.4–0.6 mg/dL)
Th2 immune phenotype	Increased (enhanced fetal tolerance)
Regulatory T cells (Tregs)	Increased (support placental development)

TABLE 3: Antihypertensive treatment guidelines.

Guideline	*Treatment threshold (BP mm Hg)*	*Delivery recommendation*
American (ACOG)	≥160/110	Delivery at ≥37 weeks
UK (NICE)	≥150/100	No specific recommendation
Canadian	≥140/90	No specific recommendation

TABLE 4: Risk factors and symptoms of preeclampsia.

Category	*Details*
Risk Factors	Age >40 years, obesity, previous/family preeclampsia, primiparity, multiple gestations, CKD, diabetes, and connective tissue disorders
Symptoms	Headache, visual changes, epigastric pain, nausea, vomiting, and severe edema
Signs	Hypertension, proteinuria, epigastric tenderness, papilledema, clonus, convulsions, and abnormal labs (LFT, platelets, and creatinine)

PREGNANCY-RELATED RENAL DISORDERS

Hypertensive Disorders of Pregnancy (HDP)[1]

- Affect 6–8% of pregnancies, including chronic hypertension, gestational hypertension, and preeclampsia.
- Gestational hypertension prevalence: 6–7%.
- A 10 mm Hg drop in mean arterial pressure correlates with a 176 g reduction in birth weight, highlighting the importance of blood pressure control **(Table 3)**.

PREECLAMPSIA DIAGNOSIS AND RISK FACTORS

- Diagnosis: BP ≥140/90 mm Hg after 20 weeks + proteinuria ≥300 mg/24 h or protein:creatinine ratio ≥0.3
- Severe features include neurological symptoms, elevated liver enzymes, thrombocytopenia, and fetal growth restriction.
- Endothelial dysfunction and angiogenic imbalance (elevated sFlt-1/reduced PlGF) underlie severe early-onset (<34 weeks) preeclampsia[2] **(Table 4)**.

ACUTE KIDNEY INJURY IN PREGNANCY[3]

- Defined by a rapid rise in serum creatinine (>0.3 mg/dL), 50% rise from baseline, or oliguria (<0.5 mL/kg/h >6 hours).
- Major causes: Preeclampsia, sepsis, hemorrhage, and septic abortion.
- Acute kidney injury (AKI) has declined in developed settings due to better prenatal care; dialysis needed in ~1/10,000 pregnancies **(Tables 5 and 6)**.

URINARY TRACT INFECTIONS IN PREGNANCY

- Anatomical changes increase risk of urinary tract infections (UTIs) during pregnancy.

TABLE 5: AKI causes in pregnancy.

AKI category	*Features*
Prerenal AKI	Ischemia-induced reversible injury due to hypoperfusion
Acute Tubular Necrosis	Prolonged ischemia causing tubular damage, usually reversible
Acute Cortical Necrosis	Severe ischemia causing irreversible cortical necrosis; obstetric causes mainly placental abruption

TABLE 6: Causes of AKI in pregnancy with examples.

Category	*Examples*
Hypertensive disorders	Preeclampsia, HELLP syndrome
Hemorrhage	Placental abruption, uterine atony
Sepsis	Septic abortion, chorioamnionitis
Volume depletion	Hyperemesis, pyelonephritis
Obstruction	Gravid uterus, hydramnios
Others	Acute fatty liver, amniotic fluid embolism

- Asymptomatic bacteriuria in 2–10%, screening recommended with urine culture early in pregnancy (ACOG)
- Acute cystitis diagnosed by symptoms + urine culture (≥100,000 CFU/mL).
- Treatment with targeted antibiotics for 5–7 days, avoiding amoxicillin/ampicillin due to resistance.
- Pyelonephritis requires hospital admission and 14-day antibiotic course.
- Recurrent UTI managed with postcoital or continuous prophylaxis.

CHRONIC KIDNEY DISEASE IN PREGNANCY[4]

- Major causes: Diabetic nephropathy, lupus nephritis, and glomerulonephritis.
- Chronic kidney disease (CKD) severity based on serum creatinine: Mild (≤1.4 mg/dL), moderate (1.5–2.5 mg/dL), and severe (≥2.5 mg/dL).
- Moderate/severe CKD increases risks of preeclampsia (40%), anemia (48%), and hypertension (56%).
- Early detection essential; postpartum renal monitoring to reduce progression.

MANAGEMENT OVERVIEW

Antenatal Care

- Multidisciplinary; assess CKD stage, blood pressure, renal function, medication side effects, and UTIs.
- Monitor renal function biweekly until 32 weeks, then weekly in moderate/severe CKD.
- Fetal monitoring 4–6 weekly in mild CKD, 2–4 weekly in advanced CKD.

Intrapartum Care

- Prefer vaginal delivery unless obstetric contraindications.
- Continuous fetal monitoring is recommended.
- Maintain fluid balance; avoid dehydration and pulmonary edema.
- Avoid ergometrine and syntometrine in hypertensive patients.
- Use magnesium sulfate in severe preeclampsia for seizure prophylaxis and fetal neuroprotection.[5]

Dialysis in Pregnancy

- Dialysis indicated if creatinine ≥3.5 mg/dL, GFR < 20 mL/min, volume overload, hyperkalemia, or uremic symptoms.
- Target urea <56 mg/dL.
- Avoid hypotension with frequent, gentle fluid removal.

CONCLUSION

- Pregnancy with renal disease warrants early identification, close monitoring, and multidisciplinary management.
- Careful blood pressure control, fetal surveillance, infection prevention, and renal function monitoring are essential.
- Awareness of physiological changes prevents misinterpretation of renal laboratory tests during pregnancy.
- Optimizing maternal and perinatal outcomes depends on individualized care plans.[6]

REFERENCES

1. Magee LA, Pels A, Helewa M, et al.; Canadian Hypertensive Disorders of Pregnancy Partnership. Diagnosis, evaluation, and management of the hypertensive disorders of pregnancy. Pregnancy Hypertens. 2023;29:205-23.
2. Al Turkistani AH, et al. The role of angiogenic biomarkers in predicting preeclampsia: an updated systematic review. J Obstet Gynaecol Res. 2024;50(4):982-93.
3. Tomlinson J, Macedo E, Heerspink HJL, et al. Advances and future challenges in gestational kidney disease: a Global Kidney Health Atlas Report. Kidney Int Suppl (2011). 2025;15(1):1-9.
4. Levin A, Bellamy C, Jiang H, et al. Chronic kidney disease and pregnancy outcomes: a systematic review and meta-analysis. Kidney Int Rep. 2024;9(1):33-47.
5. Nair MF, Puthumana J, Balachandran V, et al. Effectiveness of aspirin prophylaxis in hypertensive disorders of pregnancy: updated meta-analysis and clinical guidelines. Hypertens Pregnancy. 2024;43(3):237-46.
6. Syed A, Maxwell C, Coppell KJ, et al. Pregnancy outcomes in women with pre-existing chronic kidney disease: a multicentre prospective cohort study. BJOG. 2024;131(4):522-30.

Psychiatric Disorders in Pregnancy and Postpartum

Ruchika Garg

INTRODUCTION

Psychiatric disorders during **pregnancy** and the **postpartum period** are common, affecting maternal and fetal outcomes if untreated. These include **depression**, **anxiety**, **bipolar disorder**, and **postpartum psychosis**, with prevalence rates of 10–20% for depression and anxiety, and 1–2% for severe disorders such as psychosis.[1]

EPIDEMIOLOGY

- **Global Prevalence:**
  - Depression: 10–15% in pregnancy, 10–20% postpartum[2]
  - Anxiety: 15–20% in pregnancy, 10–15% postpartum[3]
  - Bipolar disorder: 1–2% of women; relapse risk 50–70% postpartum[4]
  - Postpartum psychosis: 1–2 per 1,000 births[5]
- **India:**
  - Depression: 20–30% in urban areas, higher in rural settings due to socioeconomic stressors[6]
  - Anxiety: 15–25%, often underreported[7]
  - Postpartum psychosis: ~1 per 1,000; higher in women with bipolar history[8]
- **Risk Factors:** Previous psychiatric history, domestic violence, unplanned pregnancy, low socioeconomic status, and lack of social support.[9]

COMMON PSYCHIATRIC DISORDERS

See **Table 1**.

SCREENING AND DIAGNOSIS

- **Screening Tools**
  - **Edinburgh Postnatal Depression Scale (EPDS):** 10-item questionnaire; score ≥10 indicates possible depression.
  - **Generalized Anxiety Disorder-7 (GAD-7):** For anxiety, score ≥8 suggests further evaluation.
  - **Mood Disorder Questionnaire (MDQ):** Screens for bipolar disorder.

TABLE 1: Psychiatric disorders in pregnancy and postpartum.[10]

Disorder	*Symptoms*	*Onset*	*Risks*
Antenatal depression	Sadness, anhedonia, fatigue, sleep/appetite changes, and suicidal ideation	Pregnancy	Preterm birth, low birth weight, and bonding issues
Postpartum depression	Similar to antenatal; guilt, inability to care for infant	Within 4–6 weeks postpartum	Infant developmental delays and maternal suicide
Anxiety disorders	Excessive worry, panic attacks, OCD symptoms (e.g., intrusive thoughts)	Pregnancy/postpartum	Fetal distress and parenting difficulties
Bipolar disorder	Mania/hypomania (euphoria and irritability) and depression; high relapse risk	Pregnancy/postpartum	Psychosis and infanticide risk
Postpartum psychosis	Delusions, hallucinations, confusion, and mood swings	Within 2 weeks postpartum	Suicide, infanticide, hospitalization.

- **Timing:**
  - Antenatal: At booking visit and third trimester
  - Postpartum: 6–8 weeks postdelivery
- **Challenges in India:** Stigma, lack of trained staff, and low awareness; integration into ANC visits essential.

MANAGEMENT

Management involves a multidisciplinary approach with **nonpharmacological** and **pharmacological** interventions, tailored to severity and pregnancy stage.

Nonpharmacological Interventions

- **Counseling/Psychotherapy:**
  - **Cognitive Behavioral Therapy (CBT):** First line for mild-moderate depression/anxiety; effective in 60–70% of cases
  - **Interpersonal Therapy (IPT):** Focuses on relationship issues; useful postpartum
- **Support Groups:** Peer support reduces isolation, especially in rural India.
- **Lifestyle:** Exercise, sleep hygiene, and nutrition (e.g., omega-3 supplementation)
- **Psychoeducation:** Educate family to reduce stigma and enhance support.

Pharmacological Interventions (Table 2)

- **Principles:**
  - Use lowest effective dose; avoid first trimester if possible.
  - Monitor fetal growth and neonatal outcomes.
  - Breastfeeding: Sertraline, paroxetine preferred due to low milk transfer.
- **Contraindications:**
  - Avoid paroxetine (cardiac defects risk).
  - Valproate contraindicated (teratogenic: neural tube defects).

TABLE 2: Pharmacological management of psychiatric disorders.

Drug class	*Examples*	*FDA category*	*Use in pregnancy/postpartum*	*Risks*
SSRIs	Sertraline and escitalopram	C	First line for depression/anxiety; sertraline preferred	Neonatal adaptation syndrome (5–10%)
SNRIs	Venlafaxine and duloxetine	C	Second line for resistant cases	Similar to SSRIs; hypertension risk
Mood Stabilizers	Lithium	D	Bipolar disorder; use if benefits outweigh risks	Ebstein's anomaly (0.1%); monitor levels
Antipsychotics	Olanzapine and quetiapine	C	Psychosis and bipolar mania; low-dose use	Sedation and gestational diabetes risk
Benzodiazepines	Lorazepam (short term)	D	Severe anxiety; avoid long-term use	Floppy infant syndrome and withdrawal

Postpartum Psychosis

- **Emergency:** Requires hospitalization due to suicide/infanticide risk
- **Treatment:**
  - Antipsychotics (e.g., olanzapine 5–10 mg/day)
  - Mood stabilizers (e.g., lithium, monitor levels 0.6–1.2 mmol/L)
  - Benzodiazepines for acute agitation
- **Electroconvulsive Therapy (ECT):** Effective for severe cases unresponsive to drugs; safe in pregnancy/postpartum.

RCOG/NICE Guidelines (2023)

- **Screening:** Use EPDS at antenatal visits and 6–8 weeks postpartum; GAD-7 for anxiety.
- **Mild-Moderate Depression/Anxiety:** Offer CBT/IPT; consider SSRIs (sertraline) if no response.
- **Severe Depression/Bipolar/Psychosis:** Refer to perinatal mental health team; start SSRIs, antipsychotics, or lithium as needed.
- **Postpartum Psychosis:** Urgent psychiatric admission; antipsychotics + mood stabilizers.
- **Breastfeeding:** Prefer sertraline, quetiapine; avoid high-dose benzodiazepines.
- **Monitoring:** Regular follow-up; assess mother-infant bonding and infant development.

SPECIAL CONSIDERATIONS FOR INDIA

- **Cultural Stigma:** Address myths (e.g., mental illness as weakness) through community education.
- **Resource Constraints:** Train ASHA workers for screening; integrate mental health into ANC.
- **Postpartum Practices:** Confinement traditions may exacerbate isolation; involve family in care plans.

CLINICAL CASE SCENARIO (DNB/MS EXAM-RELEVANT)

Case: A 28-year-old primigravida at 32 weeks presents with low mood, anhedonia, and suicidal thoughts for 3 weeks. EPDS score: 14. History of depression 5 years ago, untreated. No substance use.

Management

- **Screening:** Confirm depression with EPDS; rule out bipolar disorder (MDQ negative).
- **Counseling:** Refer for CBT; educate husband on support role.
- **Pharmacotherapy:** Start **sertraline** 50 mg/day (titrate to 100 mg if needed); discuss neonatal adaptation risk.
- **Monitoring:** Follow up in 2 weeks; repeat EPDS; fetal growth ultrasound at 36 weeks.
- **Postpartum:** Continue sertraline if breastfeeding; screen for postpartum depression at 6 weeks.
- **Outcome:** Symptoms improve by 36 weeks; normal delivery. Postpartum EPDS score: 6 at 6 weeks.

KEY POINTS FOR MS/DNB EXAMINATION

- **Prevalence:** Depression/anxiety affect 20–30% of Indian pregnant/postpartum women; psychosis is rare (1–2/1,000).
- **Screening:** EPDS (≥10) for depression; GAD-7 for anxiety; mandatory at ANC and postpartum visits.
- **Management:** CBT for mild cases; sertraline for moderate-severe depression; antipsychotics for psychosis.
- **Postpartum Psychosis:** Psychiatric emergency; hospitalize, use olanzapine/lithium.
- **Guidelines:** Follow RCOG/NICE for evidence-based care; integrate mental health into ANC in India.
- **Fetal Risks:** Untreated disorders increase preterm birth, low birth weight; SSRIs safe with monitoring.

REFERENCES

1. Howard LM, et al. Perinatal mental health: a review. Lancet. 2016;387(10018):1779-88.
2. Gelaye B, et al. Epidemiology of maternal depression in low-income settings. BMC Pregnancy Childbirth. 2019;19:210.
3. Dennis CL, et al. Prevalence of antenatal anxiety: a meta-analysis. Br J Psychiatry. 2017;211(6):315-23.
4. Wesseloo R, et al. Bipolar disorder relapse in the perinatal period. Am J Psychiatry. 2018;175(2):141-9.
5. Jones I, et al. Postpartum psychosis: an update. Lancet Psychiatry. 2019;6(2):166-76.
6. Upadhyay RP, et al. Postpartum depression in India: a systematic review. Indian J Med Res. 2017;145(5):632-45.
7. George C, et al. Anxiety disorders in pregnancy: Indian perspective. J Obstet Gynaecol India. 2018;68(4):245-50.
8. Sharma V, et al. Postpartum psychosis in India: a cohort study. Asian J Psychiatr. 2019;40:33-9.
9. Fisher J, et al. Risk factors for perinatal mental disorders in low-resource settings. Bull World Health Organ. 2016;94(8):577-84.
10. NICE. Antenatal and postnatal mental health [CG192]. London: National Institute for Health and Care Excellence; 2020.

Placenta Accreta Spectrum

Ruchika Garg

DEFINITION AND CLASSIFICATION (FIGO 2019/ISUOG 2023)

Placenta Accreta Spectrum (PAS) refers to abnormal adherence/invasion of placental trophoblast into/through the myometrium due to defective decidua basalis (Nitabuch layer).

Grade (Histological)	*Depth of invasion*	*Prevalence*	*Clinical implication*
Grade 1—Accreta	Villi adhere to myometrium (no decidua)	60–65%	Severe PPH on attempted removal
Grade 2—Increta	Villi invade into myometrium	15–20%	Hysterectomy almost always required
Grade 3—Percreta	Villi penetrate through serosa ± adjacent organs (bladder most common)	15–20%	Highest morbidity (bladder/bowel injury)

EPIDEMIOLOGY

- Global incidence: 1 in 300–500 deliveries (10-fold increase since 1980s)
- India (2023-2025 multicenter data): 1 in 800–1,100 deliveries
- Accounts for 7–10% of all peripartum hysterectomies and 30–50% of emergency hysterectomies
- Maternal mortality: 0.05% (high-resource) to 7% (low-resource)
- Neonatal prematurity rate: 70–80% (planned delivery <37 weeks)

RISK STRATIFICATION

Number of prior CS + current placenta previa	*Risk of PAS (%)*
0 prior CS	<1
1 prior CS	3–5
2 prior CS	11–25
3 prior CS	40–60
≥4 prior CS	61–67
≥5 prior CS	>80

Other significant risks: Previous myomectomy entering cavity, Asherman surgery, endometrial ablation, ART, and age ≥35 years.

PATHOPHYSIOLOGY

1. Uterine scar → defective decidualization
2. Absent/reduced Nitabuch fibrinoid layer
3. Unregulated extravillous trophoblast invasion
4. Abnormal deep placentation with dilated spiral arteries → lacunae and hypervascularity
5. Loss of normal cleavage plane → catastrophic hemorrhage on separation attempt

ANTENATAL DIAGNOSIS (ISUOG/FIGO 2023 CONSENSUS)

First-line: 2D + Color Doppler Ultrasound (18–20 weeks and 32–34 weeks)—Highly suggestive signs (≥2 required for diagnosis):

Ultrasound sign	*Sensitivity*	*Specificity*	*PPV*
Loss of retroplacental clear zone	80–90%	90–95%	High
Myometrial thinning <1 mm	85%	90%	High
Multiple irregular lacunae (Swiss-cheese)	85–95%	95%	Very High
Bladder wall interruption	80%	98%	Very High
Bridging vessels (uterovesical/ parametrial hypervascularity)	90–95%	98%	Very High
Focal exophytic mass (percreta)	90%	99%	Very High

Placenta Accreta Index (PAI)—Race and Cali 2023 modification Score ≥6 → 75% risk; Score ≥8 → >90% risk of hysterectomy

MRI—Complementary (not superior) Indications: Posterior placenta, obesity, inconclusive USG, suspected percreta with bladder/bowel invasion Key MRI signs: Dark T2 intraplacental bands, uterine bulging, bladder tenting, and focal serosal interruption

MANAGEMENT (2025 FIGO/ACOG/RCOG/SMFM CONSENSUS)

Antenatal Care

- Confirm diagnosis → Refer to Level III/IV PAS Centre of Excellence
- Multidisciplinary team (MDT): MFM, gyne-oncologist, urologist, vascular surgeon, IR, anesthesia, blood bank, and neonatology
- Optimize Hb ≥ 11 g/dL, treat anemia aggressively
- Corticosteroids 34–35^{+6} weeks (or earlier if bleeding)
- Hospital admission if bleeding, contractions, or remote residence

Timing of Delivery (Stable Patient)

- Planned elective CS-hysterectomy at 34^{+0} to 36^{+6} weeks
  - ACOG/SMFM: 34–35^{+6} weeks
  - FIGO/RCOG: 35–36^{+6} weeks
  - ISUOG 2024: Individualize; most centers 35–36 weeks

Definitive Surgical Management (Gold Standard)

1. Classical/high vertical uterine incision (avoid cutting through placenta)

2. Deliver baby → clamp and cut cord close to placenta → leave placenta in situ
3. Immediate total hysterectomy (no attempt at placental removal)
4. Hypogastric/internal iliac artery ligation or preoperative balloon catheters (if available)
5. Partial cystectomy if bladder invasion

BLOOD LOSS MINIMIZATION TECHNIQUES

Technique	*Reduction in EBL*	*Level of evidence*
Tranexamic acid 1 g IV	30–40%	Strong
Preoperative UAE or IIA balloons	40–60%	Moderate
Aortic compression/tourniquet	50–70%	Moderate
Uterine/devascularization steps (Jauniaux 2018)	40–50%	Strong
Cell salvage	Variable	Recommended

CONSERVATIVE/FERTILITY-PRESERVING OPTIONS (SELECTED CASES ONLY)

Indications: Strong desire for fertility, focal accreta, hemodynamically stable, and no percreta

Techniques:

- One-step conservative surgery (resect invaded area + reconstruction)
- Triple-P procedure (perioperative balloon + pelvic devascularization + placental nonseparation)
- Expectant (leave placenta in situ) ± adjuvant MTX (not recommended)
  Success rate: 70–80%; secondary hysterectomy 15–25%; severe sepsis 6–10%

UNEXPECTED PAS (INTRAOPERATIVE DIAGNOSIS)

1. Do NOT attempt placental removal
2. Call senior help immediately
3. Close uterine incision temporarily if needed → proceed to hysterectomy
4. Activate massive transfusion protocol
5. Survival depends on rapid decision-making

COMPLICATIONS

Maternal	*Incidence (%)*
Massive transfusion (≥10 units)	40–60
ICU admission	30–50
Bladder injury	15–25
Ureteric injury	3–7
Relaparotomy	10–15
Maternal mortality	0.05–7
Neonatal (prematurity-related)	RDS 40%, sepsis 15%

PREVENTION

- Judicious primary cesarean rate (<15–19%)
- Proper surgical technique (high uterine incision in second-stage CS)
- Early referral of placenta previa + previous CS for expert sonography

KEY POINTS

- Prior CS + placenta previa = strongest risk
- Ultrasound + Doppler = diagnostic modality of choice
- MRI only complementary
- Planned CS-hysterectomy at 34–36^{+6} weeks in tertiary center = standard of care
- Never attempt manual removal
- Conservative management only in highly selected cases in expert centers
- Tranexamic acid and cell salvage mandatory

SUGGESTED READING

1. American College of Obstetricians and Gynecologists; Society for Maternal-Fetal Medicine. Obstetric care consensus no. 7: Placenta accreta spectrum. Obstet Gynecol. 2018;132(6):e259-75.
2. Bonanni G, Lopez-Giron MC, Allen L, Fox K, Silver RM, Hobson SR, et al. Guidelines on placenta accreta spectrum disorders: a systematic review. JAMA Netw Open. 2025;8(7):e2521909.
3. Jauniaux E, Bhide A, Kennedy A, et al. FIGO consensus guidelines on placenta accreta spectrum disorders: Prenatal diagnosis and screening. Int J Gynecol Obstet. 2018;140(3):274-80.
4. Kayem G, Seco A, Beucher G, et al. Clinical profiles of placenta accreta spectrum: the PACCRETA population-based study. BJOG 2021 Jan 3.
5. Tan GSE, Jobling TW, Wallace EM, et al. Surgical management of placenta accreta: a 10-year experience. Acta Obstet Gynecol Scand. 201;92(4):445-50.

High Risk Obstetrics

50. **Antepartum Hemorrhage**
Ruchika Garg

51. **Oligohydramnios and Polyhydramnios**
Ruchika Garg

52. **Antepartum Fetal Surveillance**
Ruchika Garg

53. **Intrapartum Fetal Heart Rate Monitoring**
Ruchika Garg

54. **Fetal Growth Restriction**
Ruchika Garg

55. **Induction of Labor**
Aditi Vishal Phulpagar, Ankita Mathur

56. **Shock in Obstetrics**
Ruchika Garg, Rekha Rani

57. **Advanced Maternal Age**
Ruchika Garg

58. **Obesity in Pregnancy**
Anurekha

59. **Preterm Premature Rupture of Membranes**
Ruchika Garg

60. **Rh Alloimmunization**
Ruchika Garg

61. **Maternal Near Miss Mortality**
Ruchika Garg

62. **Imaging in Obstetrics Fetal MRI**
Vandana Bansal, Meera Agalawe

63. **Cesarean Myomectomy**
Ruchika Garg

64. **Artificial Intelligence in Obstetrics and Gynecology**
Ruchika Garg

65. **Government Programs**
Ruchika Garg

66. **Vesicovaginal Fistula**
Ruchika Garg, Shaifali Singh

67. **Multifetal Pregnancy**
Ruchika Garg

68. **Monochorionic Twin Pregnancy**
Ruchika Garg

69. **Fetal Monitoring**
Ruchika Garg

70. **Abnormal Puerperium**
Ruchika Garg

71. **Puerperal Sepsis**
Ruchika Garg

72. **Lactation Suppression**
Ruchika Garg

73. **Vaccination in Pregnancy**
Ruchika Garg

74. **Telemedicine in Gynecology**
Ruchika Garg

75. **Magnesium Sulphate in Obstetrics**
Ruchika Garg

76. **Postpartum Hemorrhage**
Ruchika Garg

77. **Cesarean Section: Indications and Techniques**
Ruchika Garg

78. **Strategies to Reduce Cesarean Section Rates**
Ruchika Garg

79. **Pregnancy in Scarred Uterus**
Ruchika Garg

80. **Difficult Situations in Cesarean Delivery**
Ruchika Garg

81. **Amniotic Fluid Embolism**
Ruchika Garg

82. **Intrauterine Fetal Death**
Ruchika Garg

83. **HIV in Pregnancy**
Ruchika Garg

84. **High Dependency Unit in Maternal Health Care**
Ruchika Garg

85. **Enhanced Recovery After Surgery**
Ruchika Garg

86. **Dengue in Pregnancy**
Ruchika Garg

87. **Toxoplasmosis in Pregnancy**
Ruchika Garg

88. **Chickenpox in Pregnancy**
Ruchika Garg

89. **Malaria in Pregnancy**
Ruchika Garg

90. **Cervical Cancer in Pregnancy**
Ruchika Garg

91. **Ethics in Obstetrics and Gynecology**
Ruchika Garg

92. **Pre-conception and Pre-natal Diagnostic Techniques Act**
Ruchika Garg

93. **Breaking Bad News in Obstetrics**
Savita Somalwar

Antepartum Hemorrhage

Ruchika Garg

DEFINITION

Bleeding from or into the genital tract from period of viability (24 + 0 weeks) of pregnancy until delivery.

CAUSES AND INCIDENCE

Cause	*Incidence (%)*
Placenta previa[1]	31
Placental abruption[2]	22
Marginal/unclassified	28
Cervicitis	4.0
Trauma[3]	3.0
Uterine rupture	5.0
Coagulopathies	3.0
Domestic violence	2.0
Vasa previa[4]	0.5
Vulvovaginal varicosities	0.5

RISK FACTORS FOR ANTEPARTUM HEMORRHAGE[5]

- Advanced maternal age
- Multiparity
- Hypertension
- Trauma (accidents and domestic violence)
- Prior uterine surgery or C-section
- Smoking and cocaine abuse
- Multiple gestation
- Polyhydramnios
- Premature rupture of membranes (PROM and PPROM)

Abruptio Placentae

Definition

Premature separation of a normally implanted placenta before delivery causing bleeding.

Etiology

- Rupture/shearing of maternal blood vessels at decidua basalis
- Mechanical trauma (accident, fall, and uterine decompression)
- Chronic vascular pathology: decidual necrosis, infarction, and inflammation

Incidence

- Occurs in about 1 in 100 pregnancies
- Contributes to 1/3 of APH cases
- 2/3 occur in third trimester

Risk Factors

- Advanced maternal age
- Multiparity
- Maternal smoking (2× risk)
- Cocaine abuse
- Trauma
- Hypertension, hypothyroidism, and bronchial asthma
- PROM/PPROM
- Polyhydramnios
- Multiple gestations
- Placental bed leiomyomas
- History of prior abruption[6]

Classification (Sher's Classification)

Grade	*Description*	*Notes*
Grade 1	Mild, retroplacental clot at delivery	Minimal symptoms
Grade 2	Tense, tender abdomen, and live fetus	Moderate severity
Grade 3a	Fetal demise without coagulopathy	Severe
Grade 3b	Fetal demise with coagulopathy (DIC)	Most severe, DIC risk

Clinical Features[7]

Symptoms	*Signs*
Abdominal pain (common)	Vaginal bleeding (may be concealed)
Vaginal bleeding (variable)	Tachycardia and hypotension (shock signs)
Uterine tenderness	Increased uterine tone and size
Uterine contractions (high frequency and low amplitude)	Fetal heart rate abnormal or absent

Investigations

- Laboratory
  - Hypofibrinogenemia
  - Elevated maternal alpha-fetoprotein
  - Pregnancy-associated plasma protein A (PAPP-A)
- Imaging
  - Ultrasound shows retroplacental or subchorionic hemorrhage.
  - Retroplacental hemorrhage worse prognosis than subchorionic

Histopathology

- Retroplacental clots and surface depression
- Chronic decidualitis, necrosis, hemorrhage, vasculitis, infarction, and hemosiderosis

Management Algorithm for Abruption Placentae[8,9]

1. Assess maternal hemodynamic status and fetal wellbeing.
2. Secure IV access, resuscitate with fluids and blood products as required.
3. Continuous monitoring of maternal vitals and fetal heart rate
4. Correct coagulopathy if present
5. If ≥34 weeks or fetal/maternal compromise → expedite delivery (usually cesarean)
6. If preterm and stable → conservative management with close monitoring
7. Prevent complications: AKI, DIC, and hemorrhagic shock
8. Postpartum: Watch for PPH, consider uterotonics, and surgical intervention if needed

Complications

Maternal	*Fetal/Neonatal*[10]
Hypovolemic shock	Fetal distress
Postpartum hemorrhage[11]	Intrauterine fetal demise
Acute kidney injury	Stillbirth
Disseminated intravascular coagulation (DIC)	Perinatal morbidity/mortality (20–30%)[12]

Placenta Previa

Definition

Placenta lying over (true) or near (low lying) the internal cervical os.

Types

Type	*Description*
True placenta previa	Placenta covers internal os completely
Low-lying placenta	Placenta edge within 2 cm of internal os

Risk Factors

- Multiparity
- Advanced maternal age
- Previous cesarean or uterine surgery

- Assisted reproductive technologies (ART)
- Multiple gestations
- Maternal smoking

Role of Imaging

- Transvaginal ultrasound (TVS) preferred for sensitivity and safety
- Transabdominal (TAS) and transperineal ultrasound less sensitive
- TVS sensitivity ~100% for placental localization
- TVS also measures cervical length (short cervix increases preterm delivery risk)[13]
- Placental position re-assessed at 32 and 36 weeks for resolution or persistence

Management of Low-lying Placenta with Bleeding at 34 Weeks

- Admission in hospital; continuous monitoring maternal/fetal status
- Assess bleeding severity, hemodynamic stability
- Secure IV access; cross-match blood products[14]
- Administer corticosteroids (if <34 + 6 weeks gestation) to mature fetal lungs[13]
- Tocolytics may be considered if preterm contractions, but discontinue if delivery indicated.
- Continuous fetal heart monitoring
- Plan for cesarean delivery at 36–37 weeks or earlier if bleeding uncontrolled or fetal distress.
- Prepare for potential massive hemorrhage: uterotonics, blood products available, and surgical backup

Feature	*Placenta previa*	*Abruptio placentae*
Bleeding	Painless, bright red vaginal bleeding	Painful abdominal bleeding, dark blood
Uterine tenderness	Usually none	Marked uterine tenderness and rigidity
Onset of labor	Usually premature uterine contractions absent until bleeding	Contractions often occur with bleeding
Fetal heart rate	Usually normal	Often abnormal or absent
Diagnosis[7]	Ultrasound (TVS best)	Clinical + Ultrasound for hematoma
Management	Elective cesarean often required	Depends on severity; often urgent delivery

- Patient counseling on risks and signs of emergency

Differences between Placenta Previa and Abruptio Placentae

Antepartum Hemorrhage Causes and Management

Condition	*Key features*	*Diagnostic method*	*Management summary*
Placenta previa[1]	Painless bright red bleeding, TVS diagnosis	TVS with cervical length	Hospital admission, corticosteroids, and planned cesarean 36–37 weeks
Abruptio placentae	Painful bleeding, uterine tenderness, and fetal distress	Clinical + Ultrasound	Stabilize mother, fetal monitoring, and expedite delivery if needed
Vasa previa[4,15]	Catastrophic fetal bleeding, rupture of exposed vessels	Doppler ultrasound	High-risk monitoring and planned cesarean at 34–36 weeks

REFERENCES

1. Lockwood CJ, Russo-Stieglitz K. Clinical features, diagnosis, and course of placenta previa. UpToDate.
2. Calleja-Agius J, Custo R, Brincat MP, et al. Placental abruption and placenta praevia. European Clinics in Obstetrics and Gynaecology (Vol 2). Springer UK; 2006.
3. Melamed N, Aviram A, Silver M, et al. Pregnancy course and outcome following blunt trauma. J Matern Fetal Neonatal Med. 2012;25(9):1612-7.
4. Gagnon R, Morin L, Bly S, et al. Guidelines for the management of vasa previa. Int J Gynaecol Obstet. 2010;108:85-9.
5. Department of Health. Savings Mothers 2005-2007. Fourth report on confidential enquiries into maternal deaths in South Africa. Pretoria: Department of Health; 2009.
6. Oyelese Y, Ananth C V. Placental Abruption. Obstet Gynecol. 2006;108(4):1005-16.
7. Elsasser DA, Ananth CV, Prasad V, et al. Diagnosis of placental abruption: relationship between clinical and histopathological findings. Eur J Obstet Gynecol Reprod Biol. 2010;148(2):125-30.
8. Neilson JP. Interventions for treating placental abruption. Cochrane Database Syst Rev. 2012;2:CD000117.
9. Jauniaux ERM, Alfirevic Z, et al. Placenta Praevia and Placenta Accreta: Diagnosis and Management. Green-top Guideline No. 27a. BJOG. 2018.
10. Reddy UM, Abuhamad AZ, Levine D, et al. Fetal Imaging. Obstet Gynecol. 2014;123(5):1070-82.
11. WHO. WHO postpartum haemorrhage (PPH) summit. Project Brief. 2022.
12. Pariente G, Wiznitzer A, Sergienko R, et al. Placental abruption: critical analysis of risk factors and perinatal outcomes. J Matern Fetal Neonatal Med. 2011;24(5):698-702.
13. Roberts D, Brown J, Medley N, et al. Antenatal corticosteroids for accelerating fetal lung maturation for women at risk of preterm birth. Cochrane Database Syst Rev. 2017;3(3):CD004454.
14. Kandasamy D, Kumar Selvarajan A, Jeyakumar JD. Outcome of audit and education on blood transfusion practice in obstetrics setting. Hematol Transfus Cell Ther. 2022;44(2).
15. Gagnon R, Morin L, Bly S, et al. SOGC CLINICAL PRACTICE GUIDELINE: management of vasa previa. Int J Gynaecol Obstet. 2010;108(1):85-9.

Oligohydramnios and Polyhydramnios

Ruchika Garg

Amniotic fluid plays a critical role in fetal development by cushioning the fetus, promoting lung maturation, and supporting musculoskeletal growth. Oligohydramnios (reduced amniotic fluid) and polyhydramnios (excess amniotic fluid) represent significant deviations from normal amniotic fluid volume (AFV), affecting approximately 4–8% and 1–2% of pregnancies, respectively. These conditions increase maternal and perinatal morbidity, demanding vigilant antenatal surveillance and multidisciplinary management. This chapter synthesizes current pathophysiology, diagnosis, risks, management algorithms, and evidence-based guidelines from 2024–2025.

PHYSIOLOGY AND REGULATION

- AFV peaks at 800–1000 mL between 28 and 34 weeks, then gradually declines to 600–700 mL by term.
- Production is mainly from fetal urine (after 16 weeks) and lung secretions; removal via fetal swallowing and intramembranous absorption.
- Balance maintained by fetal renal function, placental perfusion, and maternal factors.

EMERGING BIOMARKERS AND RESEARCH

- Novel biochemical markers such as amniotic fluid cytokines, matrix metalloproteinases, and proteomic profiles are under investigation for idiopathic polyhydramnios and oligohydramnios.
- These biomarkers may improve early diagnosis, differentiate between infectious and noninfectious etiologies, and guide personalized management in the future.
- Prophylactic amnioinfusion's role for idiopathic oligohydramnios is being studied in ongoing clinical trials.

DIAGNOSIS AND MONITORING

- Utilize single deepest pocket (SDP) for diagnosing oligohydramnios (preferred over AFI to reduce unnecessary interventions).
- Serial ultrasounds assess fluid volume and fetal growth; use Doppler studies and biophysical profiles (BPP) for surveillance, especially in oligohydramnios.
- Fetal surveillance with NST, Doppler velocimetry, and BPP is crucial to detect fetal compromise early.
- Screening for maternal diabetes and fetal anomalies mandatory in polyhydramnios.

COUNSELING AND MULTIDISCIPLINARY CARE

- Patients should be counseled on risks associated with abnormal AFV including preterm birth, fetal distress, and mode of delivery implications.
- Include neonatologists early in cases of severe oligohydramnios or polyhydramnios.
- A multidisciplinary team—obstetricians, radiologists, maternal-fetal medicine specialists, and neonatologists—ensures optimal management.
- Psychosocial support for parents regarding potential neonatal complications and long-term outcomes is essential.

KEY GUIDELINE SUMMARIES

- ACOG (2024): Recommend SDP <2 cm for oligohydramnios diagnosis; prompt delivery ≥36 weeks if isolated oligohydramnios.[1]
- RCOG (2024): Advise routine diabetes screening in polyhydramnios; amnioreduction limited to symptomatic relief.[2]
- NICE (2024): Emphasizes individualized surveillance plans, avoiding unnecessary interventions in mild cases.[3]

TABLES AND ALGORITHMS

Table 1 summarizes key clinical features in oligohydramnios and polyhydramnios.

Management Algorithm for Oligohydramnios

Suspected reduced fetal movements or routine USG
↓
Confirm with SDP/AFI + detailed anomaly and Doppler scan
↓
Determine etiology: Maternal (BP, meds), Fetal (echocardiography, karyotype <24 weeks)
↓
<24 weeks: Counsel poor prognosis, consider termination
24–36 weeks: Close monitoring with daily NST/BPP from 32 weeks; aspirin if FGR
>37 weeks: Induce labor (per ACOG)
↓
Interventions: Hydration, amnioinfusion (intrapartum), shunts for LUTO;
delivery timing based on fetal status

TABLE 1: Comparison of key clinical features in oligohydramnios and polyhydramnios.

Aspect	*Oligohydramnios*	*Polyhydramnios*
Prevalence	4–8%	1–2%
Diagnostic criteria	SDP <2 cm; AFI <5 cm	SDP ≥8 cm; AFI ≥24 cm
Common risks	FGR, pulmonary hypoplasia, and CS	Preterm labor, PPH, and malpresentation
Management	Hydration, fetal monitoring, and timely delivery	Glycemic control, amnioreduction if symptomatic
Perinatal mortality	Increased 4-fold if early onset	Increased 4-fold if severe cases

Management Algorithm for Polyhydramnios

Detected abdominal distension or USG suggestive
↓
Confirm with ultrasound, OGTT, anomaly scan, and MCA-PSV for anemia
↓
Mild/Idiopathic: Regular surveillance every 2-4 weeks; manage GDM if present
Moderate/Severe: Referral to MFM; initiate NST monitoring
↓
Symptomatic dyspnea or contractions: Amnioreduction (1–2 L) with counseling on PTB risk
>37 weeks: Induce labor to reduce PPH risk
↓
Delivery mode: Vaginal if cephalic; cesarean if malpresentation or placenta issues

KEY TAKE-HOME MESSAGES

- Use SDP over AFI to avoid overdiagnosis and unnecessary intervention in oligohydramnios.
- Prioritize underlying etiology workup before management.
- Timely delivery (≥36 weeks) recommended for isolated oligohydramnios.
- In polyhydramnios, exclude diabetes and anomalies; use amnioreduction cautiously.
- Multidisciplinary antenatal care and thorough counseling improve maternal-fetal outcomes.
- Emerging biomarkers and prophylactic strategies represent future avenues for optimized care.

REFERENCES

1. ACOG Committee. Opinion No. 831: Medically Indicated Late-Preterm and Early-Term Deliveries, 2021; reaffirmed 2024. [online] available from https://www.acog.org/clinical/clinical-guidance/committee-opinion/articles/2021/07/medically-indicated-late-preterm-and-early-term-deliveries. [December, 2025].
2. RCOG. Green-top Guideline No. 51: Management of Multiple Pregnancy; Reviewed 2024.
3. NICE. NG201: Antenatal Care for Uncomplicated Pregnancies, 2021; Updated 2024.

CHAPTER 52

Antepartum Fetal Surveillance

Ruchika Garg

INTRODUCTION

Antepartum fetal surveillance assesses fetal well-being to prevent adverse outcomes in high-risk pregnancies. Techniques include maternal perception of fetal movements, nonstress test (NST), biophysical profile (BPP)/modified BPP, and fetal Doppler velocimetry. Despite high negative predictive value, limitations exist in predicting acute events and fetal compromise.

TECHNIQUES OF ANTEPARTUM FETAL SURVEILLANCE

- **Maternal Perception of Fetal Movements:**[1]
    - Mothers count daily fetal movements (e.g., ≥10 in 2 hours).
    - Cost-free, noninvasive; detects reduced movements signaling distress.
    - Limitations: Subjective, varies by maternal perception; poor positive predictive value.
- **Nonstress Test (Fig. 1)**[2]
    - Monitors fetal heart rate (FHR) response to movements using cardiotocography

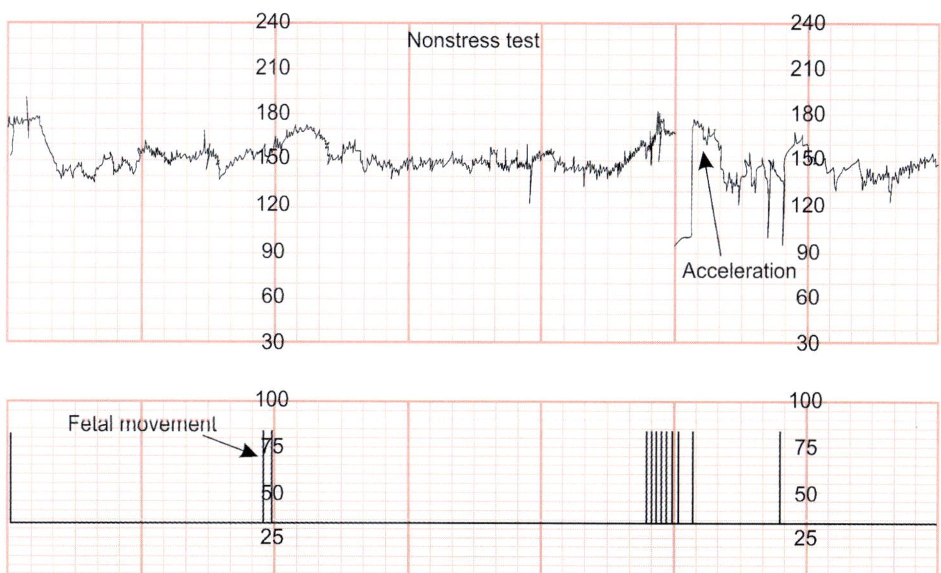

Fig. 1: A reactive nonstress test.

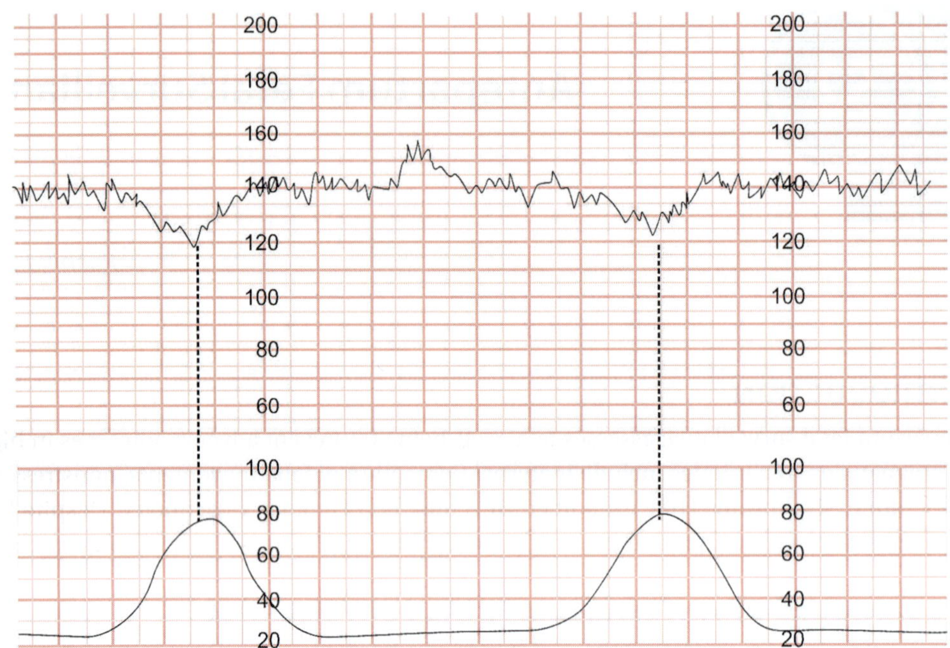

Fig 2: Early deceleration.

- Reactive: ≥2 accelerations (15 bpm × 15 seconds) in 20 minutes
- Noninvasive, outpatient-friendly; no maternal/fetal risk
- Limitations: Nonreactive results may reflect sleep cycles, not compromise.

- **Biophysical Profile (BPP)/Modified BPP (Table 1):**[3]
  - BPP: Ultrasound assesses fetal movement, tone, breathing, amniotic fluid volume (AFV), and plus NST (score 0–10).
  - Modified BPP: NST + AFV [deepest vertical pocket (DVP)]
  - High negative predictive value (~99.9%); predicts acute hypoxia
  - Limitations: Time-consuming, requires expertise; false positives
- **Fetal Doppler Velocimetry:**[4]
  - Measures blood flow in umbilical artery, middle cerebral artery, or ductus venosus
  - Used in fetal growth restriction (FGR); detects placental insufficiency
  - Limitations: Not predictive of acute events; requires specialized equipment

LIMITATIONS OF ANTEPARTUM FETAL SURVEILLANCE

- **Acute Events:** Cannot predict sudden catastrophes (e.g., abruption, cord prolapse) causing rapid fetal deterioration[5]
- **Poor Positive Predictive Value:** Abnormal tests (10–40% PPV) weakly correlate with acidemia severity or long-term outcomes; normal tests have 99.8% NPV.[6]
- **Focus on Wellness:** Tests forecast fetal health rather than illness, limiting specificity for compromise.[7]

TABLE 1: Biophysical Profile (BPP).

Variables	*Normal score = 2*	*Abnormal score = 0*
Fetal breathing movements	≥1 episode in 30 minutes, each lasting ≥30 seconds	Absent OR no episode ≥30 seconds in 30 minutes
Gross body movements	Three or more discrete body or limb movements in 30 minutes (episodes of active continuous movement count as a single movement)	Fewer than 3 episodes of body or limb movements in 30 minutes
Fetal tone	≥1 episode of active extension with return to flexion of fetal limbs or trunk; opening and closing of hand considered normal tone	Slow extension without return to flexion; movement of limb in full extension; fetal movement absent
Reactive fetal heart rate	≥2 episodes of accelerations (≥15 beats/min) in 20 minutes, each lasting ≥15 seconds and associated with fetal movement	≤2 episodes of accelerations OR acceleration <15 beats/min in 20 minutes
Qualitative amniotic fluid volume	>1 pocket of fluid measuring ≥1 cm in 2 perpendicular planes	Pockets absent OR pocket <1 cm in 2 perpendicular planes
Variables	*Score*	*Notes*
Normal	8–10	CNS is functional, and fetus is not hypoxemic
Equivocal	6	—
Abnormal	<4	Often associated with oligohydramnios → labor induction

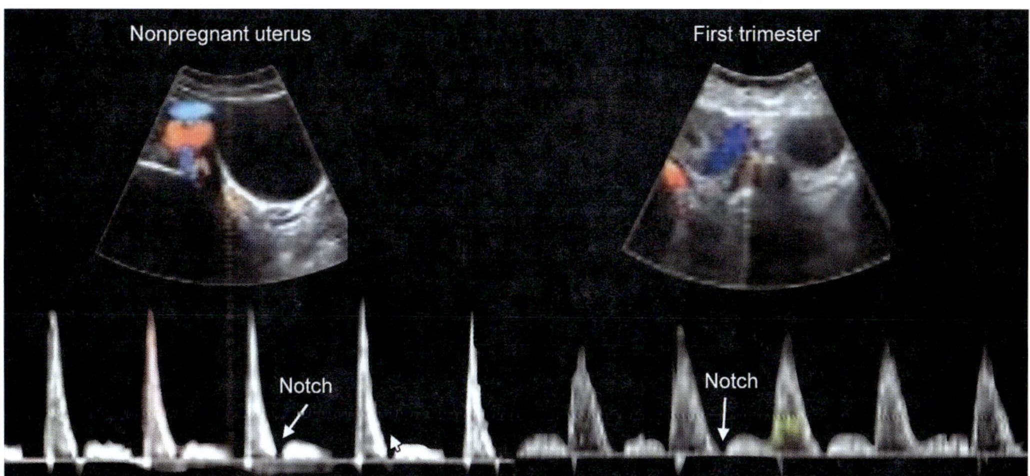

Fig. 3: Diastolic notch in uterine artery is normal.

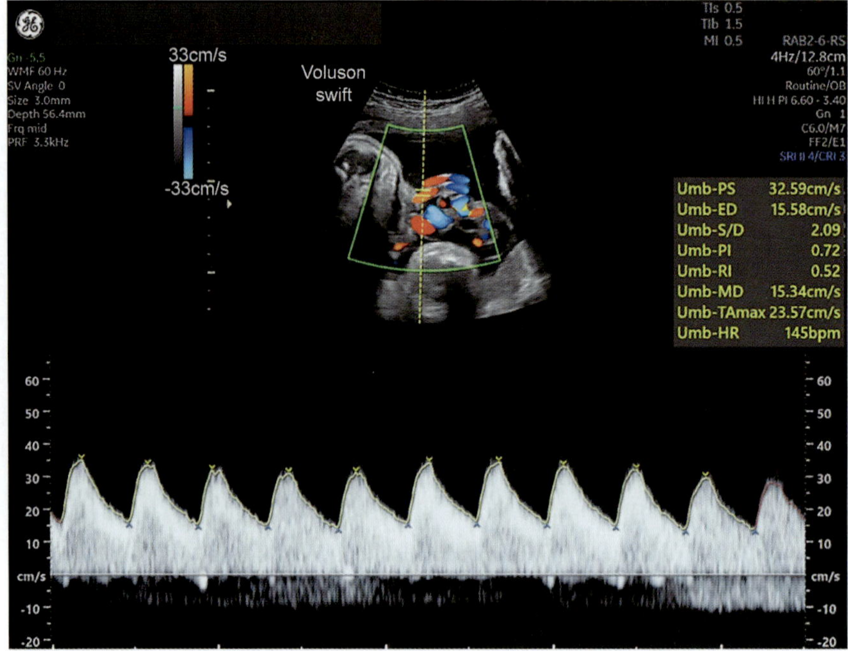

Fig. 4: Normal umbilical artery Doppler.

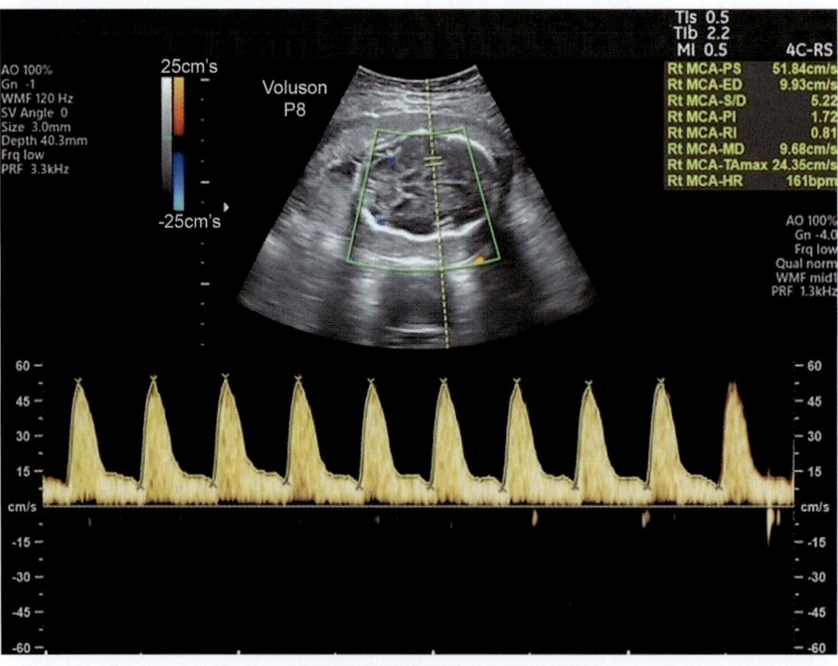

Fig. 5: Middle cerebral artery Doppler.

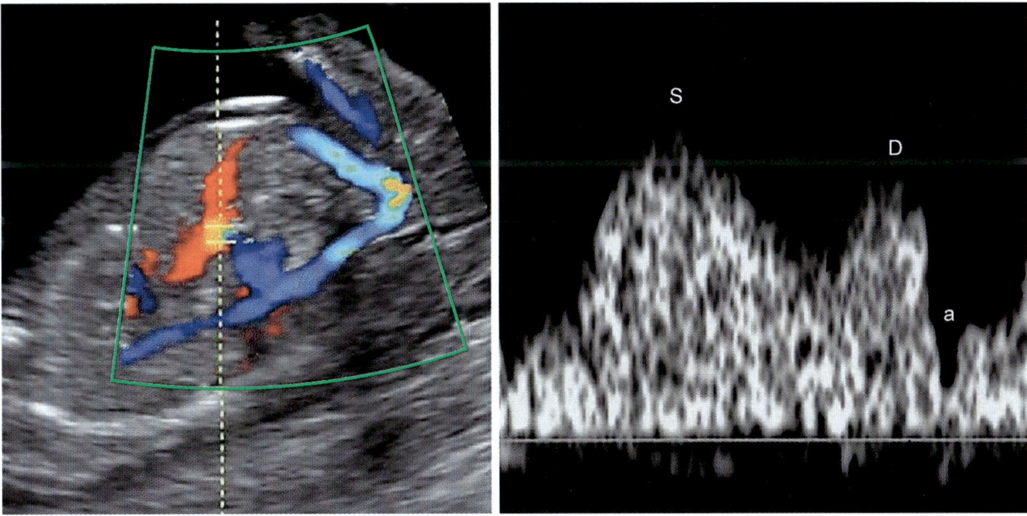

Fig. 6: Ductus venosus color Doppler.

TABLE 2: Antepartum fetal surveillance techniques.[1-4]

Technique	*Components*	*Advantages*	*Limitations*
Fetal movements	Maternal counting	Noninvasive and cost free	Subjective
NST	FHR accelerations	Outpatient, safe	Nonreactive in sleep cycles
BPP/modified BPP	Ultrasound + NST	High NPV	Time consuming
Doppler	Blood flow assessment	Detects FGR	Not for acute events

- **False Positives:** Nonreactive NST or low BPP may reflect benign causes (e.g., fetal sleep), leading to unnecessary interventions.[8]

INDICATIONS

Fetal Factors:[9]

- FGR: Initiate twice-weekly testing at diagnosis.
- Multiple pregnancy: Weekly or twice weekly from 32 weeks

Maternal Factors:[10]

- **Hypertensive Disorders:**
  - Without severe features: Twice weekly from diagnosis
  - Severe features: Daily from 32 weeks
- **Gestational Diabetes:**
  - Controlled: Once/twice weekly from 32 weeks
  - Poorly controlled: Twice weekly
- **Pregestational Diabetes:** Twice weekly from 32 weeks
- **Other Conditions:** Systemic lupus erythematosus (SLE), antiphospholipid syndrome, sickle cell disease, renal disease, and thyroid disorders

- **Obesity:**
  - BMI 35.0–39.9: Weekly from 37 weeks
  - BMI ≥40.0: Weekly from 34 weeks

Obstetric Factors:[11]

- Previous stillbirth: Weekly/twice weekly from 32 weeks or individualized if <32 weeks
- Previous FGR/preeclampsia: Weekly from 32 weeks
- Cholestasis: Once/twice weekly at diagnosis
- Late-term (≥41 weeks): Once/twice weekly
- Abnormal serum markers (e.g., PAPP-A ≤0.4 MoM): Weekly from 36 weeks

Placental/Cord Factors:[12]

- Chronic placental abruption: Once/twice weekly at diagnosis
- Umbilical cord abnormalities (e.g., single umbilical artery): Weekly from diagnosis

Fluid Abnormalities:[13]

- Oligohydramnios (DVP <2 cm): Once/twice weekly at diagnosis
- Polyhydramnios (DVP ≥12 cm or AFI ≥30 cm): Once/twice weekly from 32–34 weeks

TABLE 3: Indications and timing.[9-13]

Category	*Condition*	*Timing/Frequency*
Fetal	FGR	Twice weekly at diagnosis
Maternal	Severe preeclampsia	Daily from 32 weeks
Obstetric	Late term	Once/twice weekly from 41 weeks
Placental	Abruption	Once/twice weekly at diagnosis
Fluid	Oligohydramnios	Once/twice weekly at diagnosis

PHYSIOLOGICAL BASIS OF NONSTRESS TEST

- **FHR Regulation:** FHR is modulated by autonomic nervous system (ANS) inputs from chemoreceptors, baroreceptors, and central nervous system (CNS). Parasympathetic (vagus nerve) slows FHR; sympathetic stimulation increases it.[14]
- **Gestational Age Effects:**
  - Early gestation: High baseline FHR due to sympathetic dominance
  - Third trimester: Parasympathetic maturation lowers baseline; accelerations increase with sympathetic activity.[15]
- **Hypoxemia Response:**
  - **Late Decelerations:** Uterine contractions reduce oxygen, triggering chemoreceptor-mediated sympathetic vasoconstriction, then vagal slowing via baroreceptors.[16]
  - **Variable Decelerations:** Umbilical cord compression causes transient hypovolemia (FHR rise) or arterial compression (FHR slowing).[17]
  - **Prolonged Decelerations:** Result from acute maternal or placental insults (e.g., hypotension and abruption).[18]
  - **Chronic Hypoxia:** Reduces FHR variability, indicating acidosis[19]

TABLE 4: FHR patterns and causes.[16-19]

Pattern	*Cause*	*Implication*
Late deceleration	Uterine contraction hypoxia	Chemoreceptor reflex
Variable deceleration	Cord compression	Transient hypovolemia
Prolonged deceleration	Maternal hypotension and abruption	Acute distress hypoxia
Reduced variability	Chronic hypoxia	Acidosis risk

Flowchart 1: FHR regulation pathway.[14]

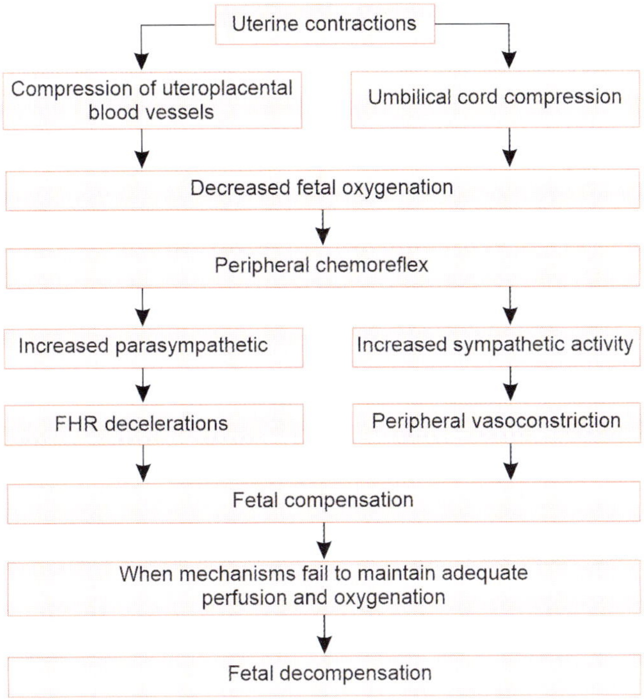

Uterine contractions

Compression of uteroplacental blood vessels → Decreased fetal oxygenation

Umbilical cord compression → Decreased fetal oxygenation

Decreased fetal oxygenation → Peripheral chemoreflex

Peripheral chemoreflex → Increased parasympathetic → FHR decelerations → Fetal compensation

Peripheral chemoreflex → Increased sympathetic activity → Peripheral vasoconstriction → Fetal compensation

Fetal compensation → When mechanisms fail to maintain adequate perfusion and oxygenation → Fetal decompensation

PERFORMANCE AND TIMING

- **Initiation:** Begin at 32–34 weeks for most indications; 26–28 weeks for severe conditions (e.g., severe FGR and uncontrolled diabetes).[20]
- **Frequency:** Weekly (7-day interval) for mild conditions; twice/thrice weekly for severe cases (e.g., severe preeclampsia).[21]
- **Equipment:** Cardiotocogram (CTG) with Doppler transducer for FHR and pressure transducer for contractions/fetal movement; autocorrelation minimizes artifacts.[22]
- **Reactive NST:**
  - ≥2 accelerations (15 bpm × 15 seconds) in 20 minutes (ACOG) post-32 weeks; 10 bpm × 10 seconds pre-36 weeks.[23]
  - Extended to 40–60 minutes if nonreactive initially (accounts for sleep cycles).

- Vibroacoustic stimulation: Shortens NST by ~4 minutes, reduces nonreactive results by 34%; applied 1–3 seconds up to 3 times.[24]

- **Nonreactive NST:**
    - Causes: Fetal sleep (most common), immaturity, maternal smoking, drugs (e.g., narcotics and magnesium sulfate), or fetal anomalies[25]
    - Management: Repeat in 30–60 minutes, perform vibroacoustic stimulation, or escalate to BPP/modified BPP or Doppler.[26]

CLINICAL SIGNIFICANCE

- **Reactive NST:** 99.8% NPV; fetal death within 7 days is rare, confirming normal oxygenation[2]
- **Nonreactive NST:** Mean umbilical vein pH 7.28 ± 0.11; requires further evaluation[27]
- **Decelerations:**
    - Nonrepetitive, brief (<30 seconds): Benign, no intervention needed[28]
    - Repetitive (>3 in 20 minutes): Increased risk of fetal distress, CS[29]
    - Prolonged (>1 minute): Warrants urgent ultrasound, Doppler, or delivery[30]
- **Terminal CTG:** Baseline <5 bpm, absent accelerations, late decelerations; indicates severe compromise, necessitating immediate delivery.[31]
- **2018 Cochrane Review:** No significant maternal/infant outcome improvement with NST alone vs. no testing; combined NST + ultrasound may enhance prediction[32]
- **2023 Study:** Modified BPP (NST + AFV) reduced stillbirth rates in FGR by 30% compared to NST alone, highlighting complementary testing[33]

TABLE 5: NST interpretation and actions.[23-31]

Finding	*Interpretation*	*Action*
Reactive NST	Normal oxygenation	Continue surveillance
Nonreactive NST	Possible sleep cycle	Repeat, vibroacoustic, and BPP
Repetitive decelerations	Fetal distress risk	Ultrasound and Doppler
Terminal CTG	Severe compromise	Immediate delivery

RCOG/NICE GUIDELINES

- **RCOG Green-top Guideline No. 57 (2019):** Recommends NST/BPP for FGR, diabetes, and late-term pregnancies; twice-weekly testing from 32 weeks in high-risk cases.[34]
- **NICE NG201 (2021):** Advises fetal movement monitoring for all pregnancies; NST/modified BPP for diabetes, hypertension, or reduced movements from 32 weeks; Doppler for FGR.[35]

CLINICAL CASE SCENARIO

Case: A 34-year-old G2P1 at 36 weeks with gestational diabetes (well-controlled) presents with reduced fetal movements for 12 hours. BMI is 36 kg/m^2. NST shows no accelerations over 20 minutes, moderate variability, and no decelerations. AFV is normal (DVP 3 cm).

Questions:

1. **What is the next step?**
2. **What are potential causes of the NST result?**

Ans.

1. **Next Step:** Extend NST to 40 minutes or perform vibroacoustic stimulation. If still nonreactive, conduct modified BPP or Doppler to assess FGR/hypoxia (NICE 2021). Counsel on risks and consider delivery if abnormal.
2. **Causes:** Fetal sleep cycle (most likely), maternal obesity affecting perception, or early fetal compromise due to diabetes. Exclude drug effects or anomalies.

   Discussion: Well-controlled diabetes warrants twice-weekly testing from 32 weeks. Reduced movements and nonreactive NST require urgent escalation to rule out hypoxia.

FUTURE RESEARCH

- Optimal frequency and combination of surveillance techniques
- Predictive models integrating NST, BPP, and Doppler for acute events
- Impact of maternal obesity on fetal movement perception accuracy
- Cost-effectiveness of routine Doppler in low-resource settings like India

INDIAN EXAMINATION RELEVANCE

Appeared in NEET-PG (2023), DNB (2020, Paper-2), AIIMS PG (2022). Focus: Indications, NST interpretation, management of nonreactive results. Challenges: Limited Doppler access in rural India (20% availability), reliance on NST, and training gaps in CTG interpretation.

KEY POINTS

- **Techniques:** Fetal movements, NST, BPP, Doppler; high NPV (99.8%) but low PPV (10–40%) **(Table 1)**
- **Indications:** FGR, diabetes, hypertension, late-term, and oligohydramnios **(Table 2)**
- **NST Basis:** FHR reflects ANS maturity; hypoxia causes decelerations/reduced variability **(Table 3)**.
- **Management:** Reactive NST reassures; nonreactive or decelerations prompt BPP/Doppler **(Table 4)**.
- **Guidelines:** RCOG/NICE advocate NST/BPP from 32 weeks in high-risk cases **(Table 5)**
- **India:** Enhance Doppler access, standardize CTG training.

REFERENCES

1. Unterscheider J, et al. Fetal movement counting. BJOG. 2016;123(4):543-9.
2. ACOG. Practice Bulletin No. 145: Antepartum fetal surveillance. Obstet Gynecol. 2020;136(4):e1-14.
3. Manning FA, et al. Biophysical profile updates. Ultrasound Obstet Gynecol. 2018;51(3):298-305.
4. Alfirevic Z, et al. Doppler velocimetry in FGR. Cochrane Database Syst Rev. 2017;6:CD012073.
5. Grivell RM, et al. Limitations of fetal surveillance. Aust N Z J Obstet Gynaecol. 2019;59(2):171-8.
6. Signore C, et al. Predictive value of fetal testing. J Perinatol. 2017;37(5):489-94.
7. O'Neill E, et al. Fetal surveillance accuracy. Eur J Obstet Gynecol Reprod Biol. 2020;245:29-35.

8. Chauhan SP, et al. False positives in NST. Am J Perinatol. 2018;35(7):625-31.
9. SMFM. Indications for fetal surveillance. Am J Obstet Gynecol. 2021;224(5):B2-12.
10. RCOG. Fetal surveillance in high-risk pregnancy. Green-top Guideline No. 57. 2019.
11. Dawes GS, et al. FHR maturation. J Physiol. 2016;594(12):3241-50.
12. Freeman RK, et al. FHR accelerations. Obstet Gynecol. 2019;134(4):683-91.
13. Serra V, et al. Sympathetic maturation in FHR. Ultrasound Obstet Gynecol. 2018;52(2):214-20.
14. Nijhuis JG, et al. FHR autonomic control. Early Hum Dev. 2017;105:1-8.
15. Martin CB, et al. FHR baseline changes. Am J Obstet Gynecol. 2019;220(3):219-27.
16. Parer JT, et al. Late decelerations and hypoxia. Clin Perinatol. 2018;45(2):199-212.
17. Garite TJ, et al. Variable decelerations. Am J Obstet Gynecol. 2020;222(4):321-8.
18. Simpson KR, et al. Prolonged decelerations. MCN Am J Matern Child Nurs. 2017;42(3):136-43.
19. Macones GA, et al. Chronic hypoxia and FHR. Obstet Gynecol. 2019;134(5):879-86.
20. Signore C, et al. Timing of fetal surveillance. J Matern Fetal Neonatal Med. 2020;33(8):1345-52.
21. EFM. Frequency of NST in high-risk pregnancy. J Perinat Med. 2018;46(6):589-95.
22. Devoe LD, et al. CTG equipment advances. Clin Obstet Gynecol. 2017;60(3):554-64.
23. ACOG. NST interpretation guidelines. Obstet Gynecol. 2020;136(4):e15-e24.
24. Smith CV, et al. Vibroacoustic stimulation in NST. Am J Obstet Gynecol. 2019;220(2):159-65.
25. Tan KH, et al. Causes of nonreactive NST. Acta Obstet Gynecol Scand. 2017;96(8):933-40.
26. Brown R, et al. Management of nonreactive NST. J Obstet Gynaecol. 2018;38(5):597-603.
27. Clark SL, et al. Umbilical pH in nonreactive NST. Am J Perinatol. 2021;38(6):543-9.
28. Cahill AG, et al. Benign decelerations in NST. Obstet Gynecol. 2018;132(4):873-80.
29. Sholapurkar SL. This study demonstrates that the "cumulative deceleration area" performs poorly and the study data calls for scientific classification of FHR decelerations. J Matern Fetal Neonatal Med. 2022 Apr;35(8):1583-1584. doi: 10.1080/14767058.2020.1759537. Epub 2020 Apr 29. PMID: 32349569.
30. Gibb D, et al. Prolonged decelerations management. J Perinatol. 2019;39(7):901-8.
31. Grivell RM, et al. Terminal CTG and outcomes. BJOG. 2017;124(9):1352-60.
32. Grivell RM, et al. NST Cochrane review. Cochrane Database Syst Rev. 2018;2:CD006593.
33. Lees C, et al. Modified BPP in FGR. Lancet. 2023;401(10377):683-91.
34. RCOG. Green-top Guideline No. 57: Fetal surveillance. 2019.
35. NICE. NG201: Antenatal care. 2021.

Intrapartum Fetal Heart Rate Monitoring

Ruchika Garg

DEFINITION

Intrapartum fetal heart rate (FHR) monitoring assesses fetal well-being during labor by detecting changes in FHR patterns, reflecting cardiac and central nervous system responses to oxygenation, blood pressure, and acid–base status. It aims to identify hypoxia to guide timely interventions while avoiding unnecessary procedures.[1]

KEY POINTS

- **Objective:** Detect fetal hypoxia to prevent hypoxic-ischemic encephalopathy (HIE), cerebral palsy, or death; avoid unnecessary interventions in well-oxygenated fetuses.[1]
- **Prevalence:** Used in 85–90% of labors in high-resource settings; continuous electronic fetal monitoring (EFM) common in high-risk cases.[2]
- **Methods:** Structured intermittent auscultation (SIA) for low-risk; continuous EFM for high-risk or abnormal SIA findings.[3]
- **Limitations:** High false-positive rates (60–80%); no significant reduction in perinatal mortality or cerebral palsy.[4]
- **Guidelines:** RCOG/NICE advocate SIA for low-risk women, continuous EFM for high-risk.[5,6]

OBJECTIVES OF INTRAPARTUM FETAL HEART RATE MONITORING

- Identify FHR changes indicating inadequate oxygenation for timely intervention to reduce hypoxic injury.[1]
- Accurately confirm well-oxygenated fetuses to prevent unnecessary cesarean or instrumental deliveries.[1]
- Monitor high-risk pregnancies [e.g., preeclampsia, intrauterine growth restriction (IUGR)] to optimize outcomes.[3]

RATIONALE FOR INTRAPARTUM FETAL HEART RATE MONITORING

- **Purpose:** Developed in the 1960s to detect events leading to HIE (1–3/1,000 live births), cerebral palsy (2/1,000), or fetal death (0.5–1/1,000).[2]
- **Physiology:** FHR reflects fetal responses to hypoxia, mediated by baroreceptors (cord compression), and chemoreceptors (hypoxemia).[1]
- **Impact:** Reduced intrapartum stillbirths (50% decline since 1980s) and neonatal seizures (RR: 0.5), but no significant decrease in cerebral palsy or perinatal mortality.[4]

- **Challenges:** High false-positive rates (60–80%) increase cesarean (RR: 1.63) and instrumental delivery rates (RR: 1.15).[4]

PREVALENCE AND TRENDS

- **Global Use:** 85–90% of labors in high-resource settings; 30–50% in low-resource settings.[2]
- **High-risk Cases:** Continuous EFM used in 60–70% of labors with risk factors (e.g., preeclampsia, oxytocin use).[3]
- **Trends:** Increasing EFM use due to rising high-risk pregnancies (e.g., obesity and diabetes).[7]
- **Outcomes:**
    - Metabolic acidosis: 1–2% of deliveries.[2]
    - HIE: 1–3/1,000 live births; 10–20% progress to cerebral palsy.[7]
    - Perinatal mortality: 0.5–1/1,000 in high-resource settings.[2]

METHODS OF FETAL HEART RATE MONITORING

Structured Intermittent Auscultation

- **Technique:** Doppler device at 15–30 minutes intervals in first stage, every 5 minutes in second stage.[3]
- **Indication:** Low-risk pregnancies; equivalent to EFM for perinatal outcomes (RR: 1.0).[4]
- **Advantages:** Noninvasive, promotes mobility, and lower intervention rates.[3]
- **Limitations:** Misses subtle FHR changes; requires skilled staff.[4]

TABLE 1: Prevalence of intrapartum fetal heart rate monitoring and outcomes.[2,7]

Parameter	*Prevalence*	*Notes*
EFM Use	85–90% (high-resource)	60–70% in high-risk cases
Metabolic Acidosis	1–2%	Cord pH < 7.0
HIE	1–3/1,000	10–20% cerebral palsy risk
Perinatal Mortality	0.5–1/1,000	No significant EFM impact

Continuous Electronic Fetal Monitoring

- **Technique:** External (Doppler ultrasound) or internal (fetal scalp electrode) monitoring.[1]
- **Indication:** High-risk pregnancies or abnormal SIA findings.[5]
- **Advantages:** Detects subtle FHR changes; continuous data.[1]
- **Limitations:** High false-positive rate (60–80%), increased cesarean rate (RR: 1.63).[4]

TABLE 2: Comparison of SIA versus continuous EFM.[3,4]

Parameter	*SIA*	*Continuous EFM*
Indication	Low risk	High risk, abnormal SIA
Frequency	15–30 minutes (1st stage), 5 minutes (2nd stage)	Continuous
False-positive Rate	Low	60–80%
Cesarean Risk	RR: 1.0	RR: 1.63

INDICATIONS FOR CONTINUOUS ELECTRONIC FETAL MONITORING

- **Maternal Risk Factors:**
  - Preeclampsia (≥160/110 mm Hg), diabetes, cardiac disease, and anemia.[5]
  - Oxytocin use, chorioamnionitis, prolonged rupture of membranes (>24 h).[6]
  - Previous cesarean, regional analgesia (initial bolus).[5]
- **Fetal Risk Factors:**
  - IUGR, oligohydramnios, meconium-stained liquor, and preterm (<32 weeks).[6]
  - Abnormal Doppler, breech presentation, and multiple pregnancies.[5]

TABLE 3: Indications for continuous EFM.[5,6]

Category	*Risk factor*	*Example*
Maternal	Hypertension	Preeclampsia (≥160/110 mm Hg)
Maternal	Labor factors	Oxytocin use, prolonged rupture
Fetal	Growth issues	IUGR, oligohydramnios
Fetal	Presentation	Breech, multiple pregnancies

TECHNIQUES FOR FETAL HEART RATE MONITORING

- **External Monitoring:**
  - Doppler ultrasound detects cardiac motion; prone to signal loss (20–30% in second stage).[8]
  - Preferred initial method; noninvasive.[1]
- **Internal Monitoring:**
  - Fetal scalp electrode measures R-R intervals; accurate for arrhythmias.[1]
  - Contraindications: Maternal infections (HIV and hepatitis), fetal bleeding disorders, and preterm (<32 weeks).[9]
- **Maternal Position:** Lateral recumbent or half-sitting preferred to avoid aortocaval compression.[10]
- **Paper Scales:** 1–3 cm/min (horizontal), 20–30 bpm/cm (vertical).[1]
- **Uterine Contractions:**
  - Normal: ≤5 in 10 minutes over 30 minutes.[1]
  - Tachysystole: >5 in 10 minutes; increases hypoxia risk.[1]

ANALYSIS OF FETAL HEART RATE TRACINGS

Baseline Fetal Heart Rate

- **Definition:** Mean FHR rounded to 5 bpm over 10 minutes, excluding periodic changes.[1]
- **Normal:** 110–160 bpm.[1]
- **Tachycardia (>160 bpm, >10 minutes):**
  - Causes: Maternal fever (most common), drugs (β-agonists), and fetal arrhythmias.[11]
- **Bradycardia (<110 bpm, >10 minutes):**
  - Causes: Maternal hypothermia, β-blockers, and fetal heart block.[12]

Variability

- **Definition:** Fluctuations in baseline FHR (3–5 cycles/min).[1]
- **Normal:** 6–25 bpm (moderate).[1]
- **Reduced (<5 bpm):** Hypoxia, sedation, and infection.[13]
- **Increased (>25 bpm):** Rapid hypoxia with decelerations (saltatory pattern).[13]

Accelerations

- **Definition:** Abrupt FHR increase (≥15 bpm for ≥15 seconds, <2 minutes).[1]
- **Significance:** Indicates fetal well-being; absent in deep sleep or hypoxia.[14]
- **Preterm:** ≥10 bpm for ≥10 seconds.[1]

Decelerations

- **Early:** Symmetrical, nadir with contraction peak; head compression; benign.[15]
- **Variable:** Abrupt (<30 seconds to nadir), V-shaped; cord compression; hypoxia if prolonged (>3 minutes).[15]
- **Late:** Delayed nadir postcontraction; uteroplacental insufficiency.[15]
- **Prolonged:** ≥2 minutes but <10 minutes; hypoxia if <80 bpm with reduced variability.[15]

Sinusoidal Pattern

- **Definition:** Regular oscillations (3–5 cycles/min, ≥20 minutes), absent variability.[1]
- **Causes:** Severe fetal anemia, acute hypoxia, and infection.[16]

TABLE 4: FHR pattern definitions (ACOG).[1]

Feature	*Definition*	*Significance*
Baseline	110–160 bpm	Normal fetal status
Variability	6–25 bpm	Fetal CNS activity
Acceleration	≥15 bpm, ≥15 s	Fetal well-being
Deceleration	Early, variable, late, prolonged	Varies by type
Sinusoidal	3–5 cycles/min, ≥20 minutes	Severe hypoxia/anemia

Classification of Fetal Heart Rate Tracings

- **NICHD 3-Tier System:**
  - **Category I:** Normal; continue monitoring.[1]
  - **Category II:** Indeterminate; general measures (e.g., maternal repositioning and oxygen).[1]
  - **Category III:** Abnormal; expedite delivery.[1]

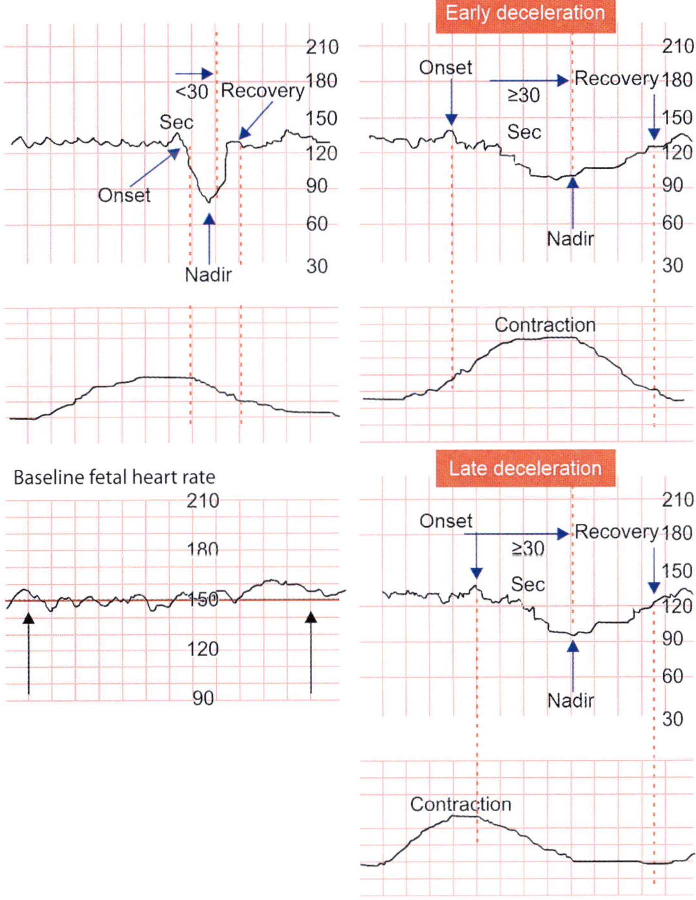

Fig. 1: CTG tracing

TABLE 5: NICHD FHR categories and management.[1,5]

Category	*Features*	*Management*
I	Normal baseline, variability; no late/variable decelerations	Continue SIA/EFM
II	Tachycardia, minimal variability, recurrent decelerations	Reposition, oxygen, amnioinfusion, consider delivery
III	Absent variability with recurrent decelerations, bradycardia, and sinusoidal	Expedite delivery

RCOG/NICE GUIDELINES

- **RCOG (2017):**[5]
  - SIA for low-risk women; continuous EFM for high-risk or abnormal SIA.
  - Use NICHD 3-tier system for CTG interpretation.
  - Avoid fetal scalp blood sampling; consider delivery for category III tracings.

- **NICE (2023):**[6]
  - Offer SIA every 15 minutes (first stage) and 5 minutes (second stage) for low-risk women.
  - Switch to EFM if risk factors (e.g., meconium and oxytocin) or abnormal SIA.
  - Remove EFM if 20 minutes normal tracing after initial concern.
- Do not use fetal ST analysis (STAN) routinely.

ANCILLARY TESTS

- **Fetal Scalp Blood Sampling:** Measures pH/lactate; not recommended due to invasiveness, limited predictive value.[6]
- **Scalp/Vibroacoustic Stimulation:** Elicits accelerations; unreliable for hypoxia.[17]
- **Fetal Pulse Oximetry:** Not recommended; no outcome improvement.[6]
- **ST Analysis (STAN):** Assesses fetal ECG ST-segment changes; no significant benefit (RR: 1.0 for HIE).[18]

TABLE 6: Ancillary tests for fetal assessment.[6,17,18]

Test	*Purpose*	*Status*
Scalp Sampling	pH/lactate	Not recommended
STAN	ECG ST changes	Not routine
Pulse Oximetry	Oxygen saturation	Not recommended

LIMITATIONS OF FETAL HEART RATE MONITORING

- **Inter-/Intraobserver Variability:** 20–30% disagreement in CTG interpretation.[19]
- **Poor Predictive Value:** Category II/III tracings predict acidosis in <50% cases.[4]
- **Increased Interventions:** Continuous EFM raises cesarean (RR: 1.63) and instrumental delivery (RR: 1.15) rates.[4]
- **Underpowered Trials:** No evidence for reducing perinatal mortality or cerebral palsy due to rare outcomes.[4]

RECENT ADVANCES

- **Computerized CTG Analysis:** Reduces observer variability (10–15% improvement); not yet standard.[20]
- **Fetal Oxygen Saturation Monitoring:** Under research; inconclusive benefits.[17]
- **Machine Learning:** Predicts acidosis with 80% accuracy; experimental.[21]

KEY POINTS FOR POSTGRADUATE EDUCATION

- Intrapartum FHR monitoring detects hypoxia to prevent HIE (1–3/1,000) and fetal death (0.5–1/1,000).
- Used in 85–90% of labors in high-resource settings; continuous EFM in 60–70% of high-risk cases.
- SIA recommended for low risk; EFM for high risk (e.g., preeclampsia and IUGR).
- NICHD 3-tier system classifies tracings: Category I (normal), II (indeterminate), III (abnormal).

- High false-positive rates (60–80%) increase cesarean (RR: 1.63) and instrumental delivery (RR: 1.15).
- RCOG/NICE advocate SIA for low risk, EFM for high risk; avoid scalp sampling/STAN.
- Limitations: Observer variability (20–30%), poor acidosis prediction (<50%).
- Advances: Computerized CTG and machine learning improve accuracy (10–15%).

REFERENCES

1. American College of Obstetricians and Gynecologists. Intrapartum fetal heart rate monitoring: Nomenclature, interpretation, and general management principles. Obstet Gynecol. 2017; 130(1):e1-e12.
2. Ayres-de-Campos D. Intrapartum fetal monitoring: Where are we now? Best Pract Res Clin Obstet Gynaecol. 2016;36:3-8.
3. Alfirevic Z, Devane D, Gyte GM, et al. Continuous cardiotocography (CTG) as a form of electronic fetal monitoring (EFM) for fetal assessment during labour. Cochrane Database Syst Rev. 2017;2:CD006066.
4. Al Wattar BH, Honess E, Bunnewell S, et al. Effectiveness of intrapartum fetal surveillance: A systematic review and network meta-analysis. CMAJ. 2021;193(14):E468-E478.
5. Royal College of Obstetricians and Gynaecologists. Intrapartum care: Care of healthy women and their babies during childbirth. RCOG Guideline. 2017.
6. National Institute for Health and Care Excellence. Intrapartum care for women and babies (CG190). London: NICE; 2023.
7. Parer JT, et al. Fetal heart rate monitoring: Past, present, and future. Am J Obstet Gynecol. 2017;217(5):S2-S6.
8. Nurani R, Chandraharan E, Lowe V, et al. Misidentification of maternal heart rate as fetal on cardiotocography during the second stage of labor: the role of the fetal electrocardiograph. Acta Obstet Gynecol Scand. 2012;91(12):1428-32.
9. Maiques V, García-Tejedor A, Perales A, et al. Intrapartum fetal invasive procedures and perinatal transmission of HIV. Eur J Obstet Gynecol Reprod Biol. 1999;87(1):63-7.
10. Carbonne B, Benachi A, Lévèque ML, et al. Maternal position during labor: effects on fetal oxygen saturation measured by pulse oximetry. Obstet Gynecol. 1996;88(5):797-800.
11. Segal S, et al. Maternal fever and epidural analgesia: Effects on FHR. Anesth Analg. 2016;122(5):1467-75.
12. Jadhon ME, Main EK. Fetal bradycardia associated with maternal hypothermia. Obstet Gynecol. 1988;72(3 Pt 2):496-7.
13. Nunes I, et al. Prolonged saltatory FHR pattern and neonatal acidosis. Clin Exp Obstet Gynecol. 2016;43(5):507-11.
14. Suwanrath C, et al. Fetal sleep-wake cycles and FHR patterns. Arch Gynecol Obstet. 2016;294(3):449-54.
15. Holzmann M, et al. CTG patterns and risk of intrapartum fetal acidemia. J Perinat Med. 2017;45(4):411-18.
16. Modanlou HD, et al. Sinusoidal FHR pattern: Clinical significance. J Obstet Gynaecol Res. 2016;42(6):169-80.
17. Sacco A, et al. ST analysis for intrapartum fetal monitoring. Obstet Gynaecol. 2017;19(1):5-12.
18. Blix E, et al. Fetal scalp blood sampling: A systematic review. BJOG. 2016;123(8):1273--81.
19. Blackwell SC, et al. Interobserver reliability of the NICHD 3-tier FHR system. Am J Obstet Gynecol. 2016;215(3):378.e1-e5.
20. Georgieva A, et al. Computerized CTG analysis in intrapartum monitoring. BJOG. 2017;124(7):1121-9.
21. Warrick PA, et al. Machine learning for predicting fetal acidosis in labour. J Matern Fetal Neonatal Med. 2019;32(14):2350-7.

Fetal Growth Restriction

Ruchika Garg

DEFINITION

Fetal growth restriction (FGR) is the failure of a fetus to reach its genetically determined growth potential, typically defined as an estimated fetal weight (EFW) below the 10th or 3rd percentile for gestational age.

PATHOPHYSIOLOGY

Fetal growth restriction arises from impaired nutrient and oxygen delivery to the fetus, categorized into maternal, fetal, and placental factors.

- **Maternal Factors:**
  - Nutritional deficiencies
  - Chronic conditions (e.g., hypertension and diabetes)
  - Infections (e.g., TORCH and varicella)
  - Lifestyle factors (e.g., smoking, alcohol, and drug use)
- **Fetal Factors:**
  - Genetic/chromosomal abnormalities (e.g., trisomy 21, 18, and 13)
  - Congenital infections
  - Structural malformations
- **Placental Factors:**
  - Placental insufficiency
  - Vascular abnormalities (e.g., inadequate spiral artery remodeling)
  - Thrombus/infarcts

DIAGNOSIS

Diagnosis involves clinical assessment, ultrasound, and Doppler studies **(Tables 1 and 2)**.

- **Diagnostic Methods:**
  - **Clinical Assessment:**
    - Maternal history (risk factors and comorbidities)
    - Symphysis-fundal height (SFH) measurement
  - **Ultrasound Measurements:**
    - EFW <3rd percentile
    - Abdominal circumference (AC) <3rd percentile
    - Growth velocity drop (>2 quartiles or >50 percentiles)

TABLE 1: Symmetric versus asymmetric FGR.

Type	*Timing*	*Characteristics*	*Common causes*
Symmetric FGR	Early pregnancy	Proportionate reduction in all biometric parameters	Chromosomal abnormalities, infections, and severe malnutrition
Asymmetric FGR	Late pregnancy	Reduced abdominal circumference and spared head/femur	Placental insufficiency

TABLE 2: Strengths and limitations.

Method	*Strengths*	*Limitations*
Clinical Assessment	Simple, noninvasive, and cost-effective	Less accurate, affected by maternal factors
Ultrasound	Accurate, serial monitoring, and noninvasive	Operator-dependent, less accurate late-term
Doppler Studies	Assesses circulation, fetal well-being	Requires expertise, intraobserver variation
Amniotic Fluid	Quick, complements other tests	Nonspecific, affected by maternal factors
BPP	Comprehensive, multiparameter	Time-consuming, intraobserver variation

- **Doppler Studies:**
  - Umbilical artery (UA): Increased resistance or absent/reversed end-diastolic flow
  - Middle cerebral artery (MCA): Low pulsatility index (PI) indicating cerebral redistribution
  - Ductus venosus (DV): Increased PI or absent/reversed "a" wave. Management—immediate delivery is often indicated, irrespective of the gestation age, due to the high risk of intrauterine death and severe fetal compromise.
- **Amniotic Fluid Assessment:** Oligohydramnios (AFI < 5 cm, SDP < 2 cm)
- **Biophysical Profile (BPP):** Combines fetal movement, tone, breathing, AFI, and nonstress test (NST)

MANAGEMENT AND MONITORING

- **Ultrasound Surveillance:**
  - **Mild-Moderate FGR:** Growth ultrasound every 2–4 weeks, Doppler every 1–2 weeks
  - **Severe FGR:** Growth ultrasound every 2 weeks, Doppler weekly/biweekly, and BPP weekly/twice weekly
  - Tailored based on clinical scenario and Doppler findings **(Table 3)**

CLASSIFICATIONS

- **Timing:**
  - Early-onset (<32 weeks): Severe, often due to placental insufficiency or chromosomal issues
  - Late-onset (>32 weeks): Less severe, milder placental dysfunction

TABLE 3: Therapeutic interventions.

Intervention	*Mechanism*	*Evidence*	*Limitations*
Low-dose Aspirin	Improves placental function	Reduces FGR risk if started <16 weeks	Less effective post-16 weeks. It does not directly improve growth in established FGR but can prevent its onset
Nutritional Supplements	Enhance fetal growth	Modest benefit in deficient populations	Limited impact in well-nourished women
Heparin	Improves placental blood flow	Limited benefit in thrombophilia cases	Risk of bleeding, weak evidence
Bed Rest	Increases uteroplacental flow	No clear benefit, potential harm	Risk of thrombosis, deconditioning
Oxygen Therapy	Improves fetal oxygenation	Transient benefit, no long-term impact	Inconvenient, limited evidence
Sildenafil	Enhances uteroplacental flow	Experimental, mixed results	Needs further research

TABLE 4: Gratacos classification (based on Doppler).

Stage	*UA Doppler*	*DV Doppler*	*Management*
Stage 1	PI >95th, positive EDF	Normal	Regular monitoring, term delivery
Stage 2	PI >99th, absent EDF	Normal	Frequent monitoring, early delivery
Stage 3	PI >99th, reversed EDF	Normal	Intensive surveillance, delivery 30–34 weeks
Stage 4	Abnormal flow	Abnormal (elevated PI, absent/reversed "a" wave)	Immediate delivery

- **Symmetry:**
    - Symmetric: Proportionate growth restriction
    - Asymmetric: Head-sparing, reduced abdominal growth
- **Severity:**
    - Mild: EFW 3rd–10th percentile
    - Severe: EFW <3rd percentile or abnormal Doppler **(Table 4)**

Role of MCA Doppler and BPP

- **MCA Doppler:**
    - Detects cerebral redistribution (low PI) due to hypoxia
    - Monitors disease progression
    - Used with UA Doppler for cerebroplacental ratio (CPR)
- **BPP:**
    - Assesses fetal well-being (movement, tone, breathing, AFI, and NST)
    - Scoring: 8–10 (normal), 6 (equivocal), and <4 (abnormal)
    - Guides intervention timing (normal allows monitoring, abnormal prompts delivery)

OUTCOMES

- **Short-term:** Preterm birth, fetal distress
- **Long-term:** Increased risk of diabetes and cardiovascular disease

MULTIPLE CHOICE QUESTIONS

1. **What is the most common cause of fetal growth restriction (FGR)?**
   a. Maternal hypertension
   b. Fetal genetic disorders
   c. Placental insufficiency
   d. Maternal diabetes

2. **Which maternal factor is least likely to contribute to FGR?**
   a. Smoking
   b. Excessive weight gain
   c. Hypertension
   d. TORCH infections

3. **Which ultrasound parameter is the strongest indicator of FGR?**
   a. Head circumference (HC)
   b. Abdominal circumference (AC)
   c. Femur length (FL)
   d. Biparietal diameter (BPD)

4. **What Doppler finding indicates severe placental insufficiency in FGR?**
   a. Normal umbilical artery (Ua. waveform
   b. Absent end-diastolic flow in UA
   c. Increased MCA peak systolic velocity
   d. Normal ductus venosus (DV) flow

5. **Which intervention is most effective for preventing FGR in high-risk pregnancies?**
   a. Bed rest
   b. Low-dose aspirin
   c. Maternal oxygen therapy
   d. Vitamin C and E supplementation

6. **Which infection is most strongly associated with FGR?**
   a. Herpes simplex virus (HSV)
   b. Cytomegalovirus (CMV)
   c. Rubella
   d. Toxoplasmosis

7. **How does symmetric FGR differ from asymmetric FGR?**
   a. Symmetric FGR spares the head, asymmetric affects all parameters
   b. Symmetric FGR affects all parameters proportionately, asymmetric primarily affects abdomen
   c. Symmetric FGR is late-onset, asymmetric is early-onset.
   d. Symmetric FGR is due to placental issues, asymmetric is due to chromosomal issues.

8. **What is the recommended frequency of Doppler ultrasound in severe FGR?**
   a. Every 4 weeks
   b. Weekly or biweekly
   c. Every 6 weeks
   d. Once per trimester

9. **What does a low MCA pulsatility index (PI) indicate in FGR?**
   a. Improved placental perfusion
   b. Fetal hypoxia and cerebral redistribution
   c. Normal fetal circulation
   d. Reduced risk of fetal distress

10. **What BPP score suggests the need for immediate intervention in FGR?**
   a. 8–10
   b. 6
   c. 4 or less
   d. 7

11. Which Gratacos stage of FGR requires immediate delivery?
a. Stage 1
b. Stage 2
c. Stage 3
d. Stage 4

12. What is a long-term complication of FGR?
a. Reduced risk of diabetes
b. Increased risk of cardiovascular disease
c. Increased risk of asthma
d. Reduced risk of obesity

13. Which finding is typical in asymmetric FGR?
a. Proportionate reduction in all parameters
b. Reduced head circumference
c. Reduced abdominal circumference
d. Increased amniotic fluid volume

14. What is the role of the cerebroplacental ratio (CPR) in FGR?
a. Assesses maternal blood flow
b. Indicates fetal compensation for placental insufficiency
c. Measures amniotic fluid volume
d. Predicts maternal hypertension

Explanations

Ans. 1 c. Placental insufficiency

Placental insufficiency is the leading cause of FGR, as it impairs nutrient and oxygen delivery to the fetus, often due to vascular abnormalities or infarcts. Maternal hypertension and diabetes contribute but are less common, and fetal genetic disorders typically cause symmetric FGR.

Ans. 2 b. Excessive weight gain

Smoking, hypertension, and TORCH infections impair placental function or fetal development, contributing to FGR. Excessive weight gain is not a direct risk factor and may be associated with macrosomia instead.

Ans. 3 b. Abdominal circumference

AC <3rd percentile is a key diagnostic criterion for FGR, reflecting reduced liver size and glycogen stores due to nutrient deprivation, particularly in asymmetric FGR.

Ans. 4 b. Absent end-diastolic flow in UA

Absent or reversed end-diastolic flow in the UA signifies high placental resistance, a hallmark of severe placental insufficiency, requiring urgent intervention.

Ans. 5 b. Low-dose aspirin

Low-dose aspirin (started <16 weeks) reduces preeclampsia and FGR risk by improving placental function. Bed rest, oxygen therapy, and antioxidants lack consistent evidence for efficacy.

Ans. 6 b. Cytomegalovirus (CMV)

CMV is the most common congenital infection linked to FGR, causing symmetric growth restriction via direct fetal infection and placental dysfunction.

Ans. 7 b. Symmetric FGR affects all parameters proportionately, asymmetric primarily affects abdomen

Symmetric FGR involves proportionate reduction in all biometric parameters (early insults like chromosomal issues), while asymmetric FGR shows reduced AC with spared head/femur (late placental insufficiency).

Ans. 8 b. Weekly or biweekly

Severe FGR requires frequent Doppler monitoring (weekly/biweekly) to assess UA, MCA, and DV flows, detecting worsening fetal compromise promptly.

Ans. 9 b. Fetal hypoxia and cerebral redistribution

A low MCA PI reflects increased blood flow to the brain (cerebral redistribution), a compensatory response to hypoxia in FGR due to placental insufficiency.

Ans. 10 c. 4 or less

A BPP score of ≤4 indicates fetal compromise, necessitating urgent intervention (e.g., delivery) to prevent adverse outcomes in FGR.

Ans. 11. d. Stage 4

Stage 4 (abnormal DV Doppler with absent/reversed "a" wave) indicates critical fetal compromise, requiring immediate delivery due to high risk of intrauterine death.

Ans. 12 b. Increased risk of cardiovascular disease

FGR infants face higher risks of metabolic and cardiovascular diseases in adulthood due to fetal programming and altered organ development.

Ans. 13 c. Reduced abdominal circumference

Asymmetric FGR is characterized by reduced AC (due to liver glycogen depletion) with spared head and femur, reflecting head-sparing growth.

Ans. 14 b. Indicates fetal compensation for placental insufficiency

CPR (MCA PI/UA PI) reflects fetal adaptation to placental insufficiency, with a reduced ratio indicating cerebral redistribution due to hypoxia.

Induction of Labor

Aditi Vishal Phulpagar, Ankita Mathur

The artificial initiation of uterine contractions before the onset of spontaneous labor is known as the **induction** of labor. Conversely, **augmentation** refers to the stimulation of existing but insufficient spontaneous contractions to facilitate cervical dilatation and fetal descent.

METHODS OF INDUCTION

1. Pharmacological
2. Nonpharmacological

Pharmacological Methods

A. Prostaglandins
B. Oxytocin
C. Other Methods: Hyaluronidase, corticosteroids, estrogen, relaxin, mifepristone, and nitric oxide donors

Prostaglandins

Prostaglandins, derived from arachidonic acid endogenously, are naturally present in the myometrium, decidua, and fetal membranes during pregnancy. Their production in the cervix increases as pregnancy progresses toward term. Synthetic preparations such as dinoprostone (PGE2) and misoprostol (PGE1) are commonly used for labor induction.

They are available in various formulations, including intravaginal gel, intracervical gel and intravaginal inserts (dinoprostone; **Fig. 1**) and tablets (misoprostol; **Fig. 2**).

Intracervical gel containing 0.5 mg of PGE2 is administered by bringing it to room temperature before insertion into the cervical canal below the internal os. After insertion, the patient should lie supine for 15–30 minutes to prevent leakage. It can be repeated every 6 hours, with

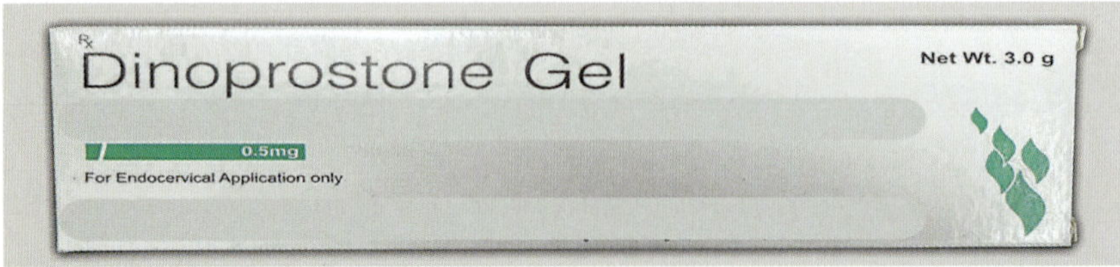

Fig. 1: Dinoprostone Gel: A common prostaglandin preparation used for cervical ripening and labor induction.

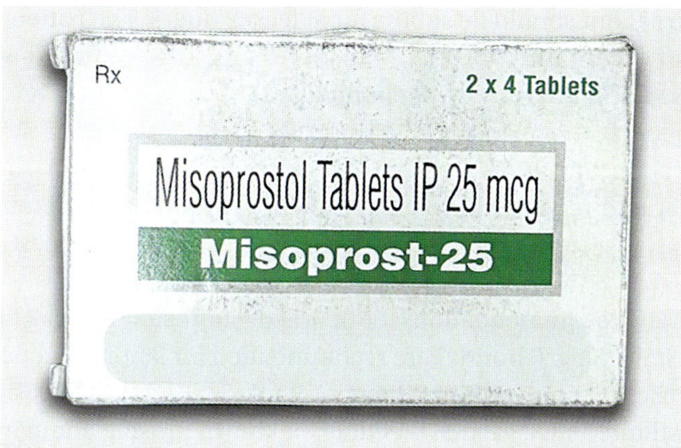

Fig. 2: Tablet misoprostol 25 µg, used for labor induction with advantages of cost effectiveness, ease of administration and stability at room temperature.

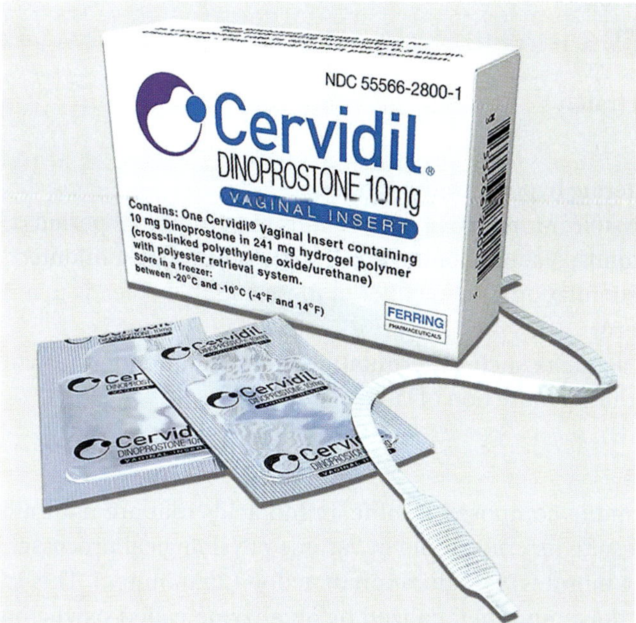

Fig. 3: Cervidil insert: A controlled-release vaginal insert containing 10 mg of dinoprostone, utilized for cervical ripening and labor induction. Placement involves insertion high into the vagina next to the cervix by a healthcare professional, with the patient lying supine for at least 2 hours following insertion.

a maximum dose of 1.5 mg or 3 insertions allowed within 24 hours. If oxytocin is needed, it should only be administered after 6–12 hours from the last gel insertion. Similarly, intravaginal gel preparations (2 mg) can be used following the same guidelines.

The vaginal controlled release insert, Cervidil **(Fig. 3)**, contains a 10 mg insert that releases 0.3 mg of PGE2 per hour. Unlike other preparations, there is no need to prewarm the insert.

After insertion, the patient should lie supine for at least 2 hours. The patient can move around freely while the insert continues to work. The insert should be removed after 12 hours, or if active labor begins, or in the case of hyperstimulation.

In labor induction, the intravaginal route is often considered superior due to its ease of administration and higher effectiveness compared to other routes. Intravaginal insertion is simpler and tends to have fewer side effects such as hyperstimulation. Among intravaginal options, inserts are particularly favored as they have the least chance of causing hyperstimulation.

According to WHO recommendations, both oral misoprostol (25 µg, 2 hourly) and vaginal low-dose misoprostol (25 µg, 6 hourly) are recommended for labor induction.

Prostaglandin use requires caution in patients with conditions such as glaucoma, hepatic or renal disease, asthma, active vaginal bleeding, or known prostaglandin hypersensitivity.

Side effects of prostaglandins:
- Tachysystole with or without fetal heart changes (hyperstimulation)
- Uterine rupture
- Fever and shivering
- Nausea/vomiting
- Diarrhea
- Genital edema (rarely)

Key Notes:
Terminology for uterine hyperactivity includes:
- Uterine tachysystole: More than 4 contractions in a 10-minute period
- Uterine hypertonus: A single contraction lasting longer than 1 minute
- Uterine hyperstimulation: When either of these conditions leads to a nonreassuring fetal heart rate pattern

Beta receptor agonists such as terbutaline are recommended for women with uterine hyperstimulation during induction of labor.

Oxytocin

Oxytocin is a hormone composed of nine amino acids that are naturally produced in the hypothalamus. Despite its crucial role in various physiological processes, it has a relatively short half-life (3–4 minutes) and duration of action (20 minutes). This is because oxytocin is quickly broken down and metabolized by an enzyme called oxytocinase. As a result, its effects are relatively short-lived, requiring careful administration and monitoring when used therapeutically.

MECHANISM OF ACTION

Myometrial oxytocin receptor concentration increases significantly during labor (100–200 times) from 20 weeks of gestation and the response to oxytocin is facilitated by activating the phospholipase C-inositol pathway, leading to increased calcium levels in the myometrium. It also enhances uterine contractions by increasing prostaglandin levels.

Routes of administration of oxytocin:
1. Intravenous
2. Intranasal
3. Buccal

Oral administration is not recommended as oxytocin is destroyed in the gastrointestinal tract by peptidases.

1. How do we titrate oxytocin while labor induction or augmentation?

Ans. Titration of oxytocin

Titration of oxytocin is a critical aspect of managing labor induction to ensure optimal uterine contractions while minimizing the risk of complications.

Typically, two titration approaches are employed: low dose and high dose.

Low-dose titration initiates oxytocin infusion at a rate of 1–2 mIU/min, gradually increasing contractions while reducing the likelihood of tachysystole, or excessively frequent contractions. This dosage is adjusted every 30–45 minutes to carefully control uterine activity and avoid adverse effects.

Conversely, high-dose titration begins at 4–6 mIU/min, leading to more intense uterine contractions and a higher risk of tachysystole. Due to this increased risk, high-dose oxytocin requires more frequent adjustments, typically every 15–30 minutes, to maintain safe and effective contractions **(Table 1)**.

To achieve a concentration of 1 mIU/mL **(Table 1)**, administer 1 mL of the solution per minute, equivalent to 16 drops per minute using an adult drip set or 60 drops per minute using a micro drip set **(Fig. 4)**. Alternatively, the infusion can be set directly in an infusion pump for precise control.

Oxytocin is commonly supplied in 5 IU/mL ampoules **(Fig. 5)**, which are diluted for administration. Dilution involves mixing 1 mL of oxytocin solution with 4 mL of normal saline, resulting in a solution containing 1 IU (1,000 mIU) per milliliter. To achieve a 1 mIU/mL concentration suitable for infusion, 0.5 mL (500 mIU) of this diluted solution is added to 500 mL of either normal saline or Ringer's lactate (1 mL/min = 1 mIU/min).

To simplify, titration aims for three contractions every 10 minutes, each lasting over 45 seconds, with a uterine pressure of 50–60 mm Hg or 150 MVU. We adjust the oxytocin concentration accordingly to maintain this pattern, ensuring an easier and more controlled induction process, known as optimum response. An infusion pump can be utilized to deliver oxytocin precisely during labor induction, ensuring accurate dosing and optimal control over uterine contractions **(Fig. 6)**.

TABLE 1: Oxytocin infusion reference.

Adult Drip Set (drops/min)	8	16	24	32	40	48	56	64	–
Dial Flow (mL/hour) (micro-drop/min)	30	60	90	120	150	180	210	240	–
Dose (mIU/min)	0.5	1	1.5	2	2.5	3	3.5	4	Maximum 10 mIU/min

Note: 1 mL/min = 1 mIU/min = 16 drops/min with adult drip set = 60 drops/min with dial flow/ micro-drip set.

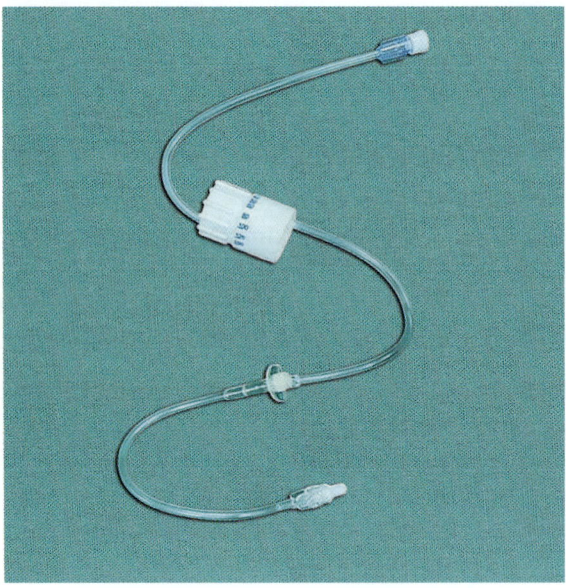

Fig. 4: A micro drip set with dial flow, used commonly for oxytocin titration.

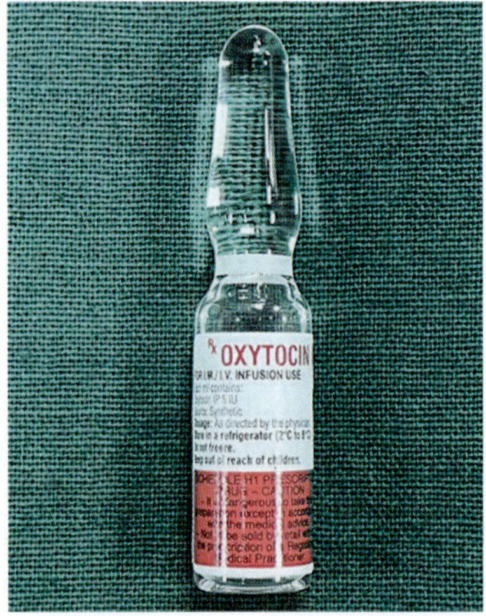

Fig. 5: Commonly available oxytocin ampoule containing 5 IU (international units) in 1 mL, used for labor induction and augmentation.

Key Notes:

- Oxytocin should not be initiated until 6 hours after the administration of vaginal prostaglandins.
- The minimum effective dose of oxytocin should be used and titrated against uterine contractions.

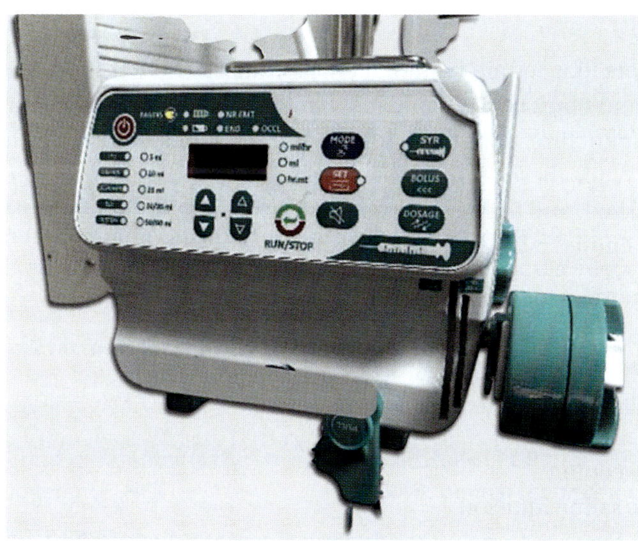

Fig. 6: An infusion set.

- The maximum licensed dose is 20 milliunits per minute and should not exceed 32 milliunits per minute.

2. What are the side effects of oxytocin?

Ans.

- Uterine hyperstimulation
- Uterine rupture
- Water intoxication, especially with high doses (>40 milliunits/min), due to its antidiuretic function
- Hypotension if given as an intravenous bolus
- Hyponatremia if administered with large amounts of sodium-poor fluids
- Antidiuresis
- Fetal distress, fetal hypoxia, or fetal death may occur due to uterine hyperstimulation.

Key Notes:

Certain methods for inducing labor lack sufficient evidence to support their effectiveness according to RCOG. These include oral and intravenous forms of dinoprostone, extra-amniotic dinoprostone or PGF2, intracervical dinoprostone, vaginal PGF2, intravenous oxytocin alone, hyaluronidase, corticosteroids, estrogen, relaxin, mifepristone (except in specific cases such as intrauterine fetal death), and vaginal nitric oxide donors.

3. What are nonpharmacological methods of induction?

Ans.

Nonpharmacological Methods

A. Natural Methods
B. Mechanical Methods
C. Surgical Methods

A. Natural Methods:

It is important to note that certain natural methods, such as herbal supplements (like evening primrose oil, blue and black cohosh, and raspberry leaves), breast stimulation, castor oil, hot baths, enemas, acupuncture, and sexual intercourse, are not supported by available evidence for inducing labor. While these methods have been traditionally used, their efficacy and safety are not well established, and they are not commonly recommended in clinical practice due to potential risks and limited evidence of effectiveness.

4. Describe Mechanical Methods of Labor induction.

Ans.

Mechanical Methods:

I. Hygroscopic dilators
II. Balloon devices
III. Mechanical sweeping
IV. Extra amniotic saline infusion

I. *Hygroscopic dilators:* These include both *natural* osmotic dilators like Laminaria japonicum and Laminaria digitata, as well as *synthetic* osmotic dilators such as Lamicel, Dilapan, and Gelatin.

   They work by absorbing endocervical and local tissue fluids, causing the device to expand 4–5 times within the endocervix leading to mechanical dilatation and release of prostaglandins.

   Hygroscopic dilators, such as laminaria tents, offer several advantages for cervical dilation, including their relatively low cost and ease of use. Compared to other methods, they are less likely to cause hyperstimulation of the uterus, which can be a concern with some pharmacological methods of cervical ripening. However, one significant disadvantage is their higher risk of infection, particularly when used in cases of ruptured membranes. Therefore, they are contraindicated in such situations to avoid the risk of introducing infection into the uterus.

   However, the Royal College of Obstetricians and Gynaecologists (RCOG) advises against their routine use.

II. *Balloon Devices:* Balloon catheters, both single and double, are safe and cost-effective methods for labor induction, especially when uterine hyperstimulation needs to be avoided or prostaglandins are contraindicated. Balloon stimulates the release of prostaglandins by separating the fetal membranes from the lower uterine segment.

   - Single Balloon Device:

     A Foley's catheter **(Fig. 7)** or specially designed device with a fluid-filled balloon can be inserted into the cervix for mechanical cervical ripening.

     During the procedure, the catheter is carefully placed in the endocervix and inflated with normal saline (~30–50 mL, maximum 80 mL). It is retracted by applying constant pressure near the internal os using a fluid-filled bag (1 L) attached to the catheter or intermittent pressure by pulling.

     The catheter remains in place until the membranes rupture or are spontaneously expelled, indicating cervical dilation and labor progression.

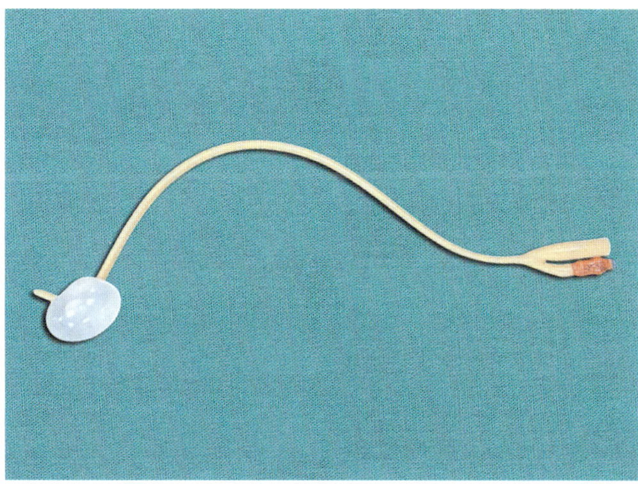

Fig. 7: Foley's catheter can be used as single balloon device for labor induction.

- *Double Balloon Device:*
  It involves the insertion of two balloons (one intrauterine and other extra-amniotic) into the cervix with controlled saline infusion into the extra-amniotic space. This creates separation between the fetal membranes and the uterine wall, promoting cervical ripening and the release of endogenous prostaglandins.
  Both types of balloon devices offer advantages such as low cost, stability at room temperature, and reduced risk of uterine hyperstimulation.
  It is recommended to use balloon catheter with oxytocin if prostaglandins are contraindicated (previous caesarean) or not available for induction of labor.

III. *Membrane Stripping/Sweeping (or)*

Describe the role of membrane sweeping in labor induction and effectiveness.

(MUHS 2018)

Membrane stripping is a safe and cost-effective method for labor induction. During the examination, the healthcare provider will gently sweep his fingers around the cervix's circumference to separate the membranes from the lower part of the uterus. This action stimulates the release of prostaglandins, which can help trigger labor naturally.

At antenatal visits after 39 weeks, membrane sweeping can be discussed with women and verbal consent should be obtained before the procedure. Additional sweeps may be required if labor does not start spontaneously.

However, it is crucial to acknowledge the potential risks associated with this method, including pelvic discomfort, risk of infection, bleeding, and premature rupture of membranes (PROM).

IV. Extra Amniotic Saline Infusion: Sterile saline is infused at the rate of 30–40 mL/h into extra amniotic space using infusion set. It is also a low cost and safe procedure for induction of labor.

5. What is amniotomy? How is it performed? What are the indications and contraindication of amniotomy?

Ans.

Surgical Methods

Amniotomy: It refers to the artificial rupture of the fetal membranes (amniotic sac) during labor to accelerate the progress of labor.

Indications:

- To expedite labor progress
- Examination of amniotic fluid for signs of fetal distress, such as meconium or blood staining, indicating possible fetal compromise or placental abruption
- Facilitate internal fetal monitoring and scalp blood sampling for continuous assessment of fetal well-being during labor.

Contraindications:

- Intrauterine fetal death
- Maternal AIDS
- Active genital herpes infection
- Free floating head or ill-applied cervix
- Cord presentation
- Uncertain fetal presentation and unstable lie
- Suspected vasa previa

6. How to perform artificial rupture of membranes (ARM)?

Ans.

Method of Amniotomy (ARM)

During amniotomy, the patient is positioned in dorsal lithotomy position, ensuring a sterile environment. A vaginal examination is conducted. Using a tool like an amniotic hook or Kocher's forceps **(Fig. 8)**, guided by two fingers to prevent injury, it is advanced to reach the

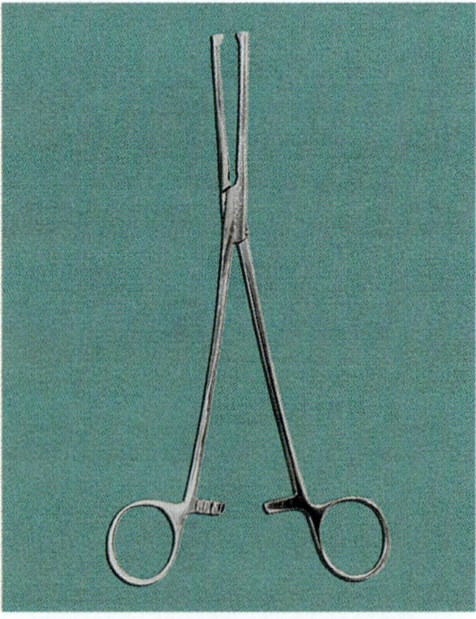

Fig. 8: A pair of Kocher's forceps can be used for ARM.

amniotic sac, piercing the membranes to create a hole and allowing the amniotic fluid to drain. Care is taken to monitor for any signs of umbilical cord prolapse. After the procedure, the fluid's color and fetal heart rate are observed. If necessary, external pressure may be applied to facilitate engagement of the baby. In cases where the presenting part is not well engaged, a speculum is inserted, and a spinal needle is used to slowly release the amniotic fluid, allowing the baby to move into the proper position within the pelvis.

7. What are risks associated with amniotomy?

Ans.

Risks of Amniotomy:
- Cord prolapse
- Fetal heart rate deceleration
- Bleeding through vasa previa
- Fetal injury
- Maternal and fetal infection

Key Notes:

Immediate beneficial effects of amniotomy:
- Lowers blood pressure in hypertensive women
- Reliefs maternal distress in polyhydramnios
- Controls bleeding in abruption and relieves tension

According to WHO, amniotomy alone is not a method of induction of labor. It should be combined with simultaneous or delayed oxytocin infusion.

8. Discuss preinduction cervical assessment.

Ans.

Preinduction Cervical Assessment

Assessment before induction

Maternal:
- Confirm indication and review contraindications.
- Confirm absence of significant uterine contractions.
- Perform clinical pelvimetry.
- Assess cervical condition and assign Modified Bishop score.
- Review risks, benefits, and alternatives of induction of labor with the patient

Fetal:
- Confirm gestational age and wellbeing.
- Assess and document fetal lung maturity status.
- Estimate fetal weight, lie and fetal presentation (either by clinical examination or ultrasound).

9. What are indications and contraindications of induction of labor? (DNB 2021)

Ans.

Indications

In general, obstetric indications to induce labor are based on conditions whereby allowing pregnancy to advance could pose maternal or fetal/neonatal complications.

Obstetric indications	*Fetal indications*	*Others*
• Post-term pregnancy (>41 weeks) • Prelabor rupture of membranes • Hypertensive disorders of pregnancy • Chorioamnionitis • Placental abruption • Intrahepatic cholestasis of pregnancy	• Growth restriction • Rh Isoimmunization • Oligohydramnios • Fetal malformations incompatible with life	• Maternal medical conditions: Diabetes, renal disease, and chronic pulmonary disease • Previous stillbirth with unknown cause • Elective labor induction

Key Notes:

The American College of Obstetricians and Gynecologists (ACOG) recently updated its guidelines on elective induction of labor at term based on findings from the ARRIVE trial. While previously, elective induction was not recommended for convenience, ACOG now suggests offering it to low-risk, first-time mothers at 39 weeks of pregnancy.

However, before proceeding with elective induction, care providers should consider three key factors: the pregnant woman's preferences, the availability of staffing and facility resources to support longer labors, and the protocol for managing a "failed" induction. In the absence of complications, early labor can last for 24 hours or more, and oxytocin can be administered for 12–18 hours after the rupture of membranes before considering the induction unsuccessful.

Contradictions

When vaginal delivery is contraindicated

- Major degree of Placenta previa or Vasa previa
- Previous classical uterine incision or incision due to metroplasty or extensive myomectomy when the uterine cavity is opened
- History of uterine rupture in past
- Fetopelvic disproportion
- Active genital herpes infection
- Invasive cervical carcinoma
- Transverse and oblique lie

Emergency Conditions:

- Cord presentation or prolapse
- Fetal distress

Known hypersensitivity to cervical ripening agents

10. What are risks associated with induction of labor? (or)

What are the complications of labor induction? How can they be managed? (DNB 2017)

Ans.

Risks associated with Induction of Labor

Maternal risks	*Fetal risks*
Failure of induction Uterine hyperstimulation and rupture Chorioamnionitis Amniotic fluid embolism Dysfunctional labor or precipitate labor Placental abruption Increased risk of operative vaginal delivery or cesarean section Increased risk of postpartum hemorrhage (PPH)	Fetal distress Cord prolapse Increased risk of birth trauma Neonatal jaundice Increased NICU admission Fetal death

11. What are the conditions requiring special caution with induction of labor?

Ans.

- Multiple Pregnancy: Due to increased risk of complications such as uterine hyperstimulation, cord prolapse, and operative delivery and higher chance of malpresentation.
- Polyhydramnios: Due to risk of umbilical cord prolapse, uterine hyperstimulation and uterine rupture.
- Grand Multiparity: Due to increased risk of uterine atony and prolonged labor. These patients also have higher risk of uterine rupture on induction.
- Maternal Heart Disease: Hemodynamic changes during induction may exacerbate preexisting cardiac conditions. Induction can precipitate heart failure and arrhythmias.
- Collaboration with a multidisciplinary team is essential for safe induction.
- Severe Hypertension: These patients are at risk of hypertensive crises and placental abruption.
  Due to compromised uteroplacental perfusion, there remains an increased risk of fetal distress and sudden fetal death.
- Breech Presentation:
  Increased labor complications like cord prolapse and fetopelvic disproportion.
  Expert obstetric management and monitoring during induction are essential.
- One Previous Cesarean Section (FNB 2018):
  Careful assessment of the uterine scar and consideration of the type of previous uterine incision prior to trial of labor is essential because there is increased risk of uterine rupture.

12. Where should induction of labor be performed and ideally when?

Ans.

Setting for induction of Labor

- Time of Induction:
  It is preferred to induce early morning, allowing for optimal staffing and resources availability, as well as maximizing daytime hours for monitoring and intervention.
- Place of Induction:
  Induction should occur in a setting where facilities for intervention and continuous fetal monitoring are readily available. This typically includes hospitals or birth centers equipped with obstetricians, midwives, anesthetists, and neonatal specialists, ensuring comprehensive care and timely response to any emergent situations. Outpatient induction is not recommended

13. Describe methods to predict the success of induction of labor. What is a bishop's score? How does it differ from modified bishop's score? (MUHS 2020)

Ans.

Bishop's Score and Ultrasound Examination before labor induction

The success of labor induction relies heavily on the readiness of cervix, assessed using the Bishop's Score **(Table 2)**, a tool developed by Bishop in 1964. This scoring system evaluates various cervical parameters to predict induction outcomes. It was later refined by Burnett, who modified it to enhance accuracy by considering cervical length in place of effacement **(Table 3)**.

TABLE 2: Bishop's Score.

Score	*Dilatation (cm)*	*Cervical length (in cm)*	*Station (–3 to +2)*	*Consistency*	*Position*
0	Closed	>2	–3	Firm	Posterior
1	1–2	2-1	2	Medium	Mid position
2	3–4	1-0.5	1, 0	Soft	Anterior
3	5–6	0.5	+1, +2	—	

TABLE 3: Modified Bishop's Score.

Additional 1 point: Previous vaginal birth
Subtraction of 1 point: Primigravida, postdated pregnancy, and PPROM

Interpretation:
- Score <6: Unfavorable Cervix—cervical ripening agent can be used (prostaglandins or mechanical methods)
- Score ≥6: Favorable Cervix—amniotomy and/or oxytocin infusion can be started
- Score <3: High chances of failure of induction
- Score >8: High chances of spontaneous labor

Additionally, ultrasound imaging can be used as an adjunct in assessing cervical ripeness. Parameters such as cervical length, internal cervical os, shape, and the angle between the cervical axis and the uterine segment wall can be measured using transvaginal ultrasound. While modified Bishop's Score remains a cornerstone in cervical assessment, ultrasound provides a more objective evaluation and complements the clinical assessment.

Score	*Dilatation (cm)*	*Effacement (%)*	*Station (–3 to +2)*	*Consistency*	*Position*
0	Closed	0–30	–3	Firm	Posterior
1	1–2	40–50	–2	Medium	Mid position
2	3–4	60–70	–1, 0	Soft	Anterior
3	5–6	80	+1, +2	-	

14. What is failure of Induction? What is its management? (2019)

Ans.

Failure of Induction

In labor and delivery, failure of induction (FOI) occurs when attempts to medically induce labor do not result in a vaginal delivery within a reasonable timeframe. This can happen if contractions are not effective in dilating or thinning the cervix, or if induction takes longer than expected, typically exceeding 24 hours. Fetal distress during the process may also prompt a cesarean delivery to ensure the baby's safety. Factors contributing to FOI include an unfavorable cervix, fetal positioning issues, and underlying maternal health conditions.

The main outcome of FOI is often a cesarean delivery, which prioritizes the well-being of both mother and baby. Prolonged induction can also increase the risk of complications such as infections and postpartum hemorrhage.

In general, 2 cycles of prostaglandin gel or tablets and 1 cycle of insert use is considered as failure of induction.

15. Describe recommendations of induction in following specific conditions:
- Postdated pregnancy
- PROM and pPROM
- Previous C section
- IUFD: Intrauterine fetal death
- FGR: Fetal growth restriction
- Diabetes in pregnancy
- Hypertension in pregnancy
- Breech presentation
- ICP: Intrahepatic cholestasis of pregnancy
- Abruption of placenta

Ans.

Induction of labor (IOL) recommendations in specific conditions:
- Postdated Pregnancy:
  - Induction of labor is typically recommended for women who have reached 41 + 0 weeks of gestation to reduce the risk of complications.
  - Inducing labor at term can lower the chances of perinatal mortality and meconium aspiration syndrome, neonatal morbidity, and stillbirth or neonatal deaths.
  - For women who decline induction, it is crucial to increase antenatal monitoring, which may include regular cardiotocography (CTG) and ultrasound checks to assess the amniotic fluid index (AFI) twice a week.
- Premature Rupture of Membranes (PROM) and Preterm PROM:
  - In cases of preterm prelabor rupture of membranes (PPROM) before 34 + 0 weeks of gestation, induction of labor is generally avoided unless there are additional obstetric concerns such as infection or fetal compromise.
  - Expectant management is usually offered until 37 + 0 weeks.
  - For women experiencing PPROM after 34 + 0 weeks but before 37 + 0 weeks, the options of expectant management until 37 + 0 weeks or induction of labor are discussed, considering factors such as risks to the woman and baby, availability of neonatal intensive care facilities, and the woman's preferences.
  - If a woman with PPROM after 34 + 0 weeks has a positive Group B streptococcus test during the current pregnancy, immediate induction of labor or cesarean birth is typically offered to reduce the risk of complications related to infection.
  - In cases of prelabor rupture of membranes at term (at or after 37 + 0 weeks), women are offered a choice between expectant management for up to 24 hours or induction of labor as soon as possible.
  - For women who opt for expectant management at term, induction of labor is offered if labor has not commenced naturally after approximately 24 hours.
  - Watch for signs of chorioamnionitis if patient is managed expectantly (maternal fever, uterine tenderness, foul-smelling vaginal discharge, elevated maternal C-reactive protein (CRP) levels, and increased white blood cell count)
  - Induction can be planned as early as 34 + 0 weeks of gestation, if needed.

- Previous Cesarean Section (CS):
  When discussing induction options with a woman who had a previous caesarean, it is crucial to consider:
  - Induction increases emergency cesarean risk (1.5 times).
  - Risk of uterine rupture increases 2–3 times.
  - Mechanical methods like Foley's catheter might be safer.
  - Avoid dinoprostone and misoprostol due to risk of uterine rupture.
  - Offer choice between induction and planned cesarean.
  - Induction can be done by mechanical methods like foley's catheter. Oxytocin can be used.
- Intrauterine Fetal Death (IUFD):
  - Expectant management can be offered to women with intact membranes and no evidence of internal bleeding or other complication.
  - For women with a nonscarred uterus and intrauterine fetal death, induction of labor may involve oral mifepristone 200 mg followed by vaginal dinoprostone or oral/vaginal misoprostol. A mechanical method of induction can be considered.
  - If a woman has a previous caesarean birth, mechanical induction should be done.
  - For pregnancies between 27 and 28 weeks, the recommended dosage of misoprostol is 100 micrograms administered via the intravaginal, sublingual, or buccal route every 4 hours. For pregnancies beyond 28 weeks, the dosage is reduced to 25 micrograms administered intravaginally every 6 hours, following FIGO guidelines.
  - Amniotomy is not done as increases the risk of infections.
- Fetal Growth Restriction:
  - In cases of early intrauterine growth restriction (IUGR) or decreased end-diastolic flow, induction of labor is typically delayed until 37 weeks of gestation or later.
  - If there is absent or reversed flow, delivery may be indicated as early as 32 weeks.
  - Administration of betamethasone to enhance fetal lung maturity is crucial in these situations.
  - However, if there is confirmed fetal compromise, induction of labor should not be offered, and alternative management strategies should be considered.
- Diabetes Mellitus:
  - Women with uncomplicated gestational diabetes should be advised to give birth no later than 40 + 6 weeks.
  - Induction should be planned at 38–39 weeks in women with pregestational diabetes.
  - Earlier induction can be considered in overt diabetes with complications.
- Hypertensive Disorders of Pregnancy:
  - Gestational hypertension and mild preeclampsia: Delivery is recommended at 37 weeks of gestation or later.
  - Severe preeclampsia or HELLP syndrome: Earlier delivery is necessary, typically beyond 34 weeks, and induction of labor may be required.
  - Eclampsia: The decision regarding induction or cesarean delivery should be individualized

- Breech presentation:
  Induction of labor is not typically advised for breech-positioned babies. However, it may be considered if:
  - There is a need to expedite birth.
  - External cephalic version is not successful, declined, or not recommended.
  - The woman prefers not to have a planned cesarean birth. Discuss the pros and cons of induction with the woman to make an informed decision.
- Intrahepatic Cholestasis of Pregnancy:
  - Mild increases in bile acids (19–39 micromole/L): Delivery is recommended at 40 weeks of gestation.
  - Moderate increase in bile acids (40–99 micromole/L): Delivery is recommended between 38 and 39 weeks of gestation.
  - Severe increase in bile acids (>100 micromole/L): Delivery is recommended between 35 and 36 weeks of gestation.
- Abruption
  Minor degree of abruption without fetal distress can be induced by amniotomy and oxytocin infusion.

In conclusion, during induction of labor, the benefits should be weighed against the risks, alternatives should be considered, and the necessity of intervention should be adjudged. However, indiscriminate use of labor-inducing agents should be avoided.

Key Notes:
- Induction should only be considered, if necessary, with the benefits outweighing the risks.
- Take into account the woman's condition and preferences when deciding on induction.
- Exercise caution due to potential risks such as hyperstimulation and fetal distress.
- Ensure facilities are available for monitoring and performing a cesarean section if needed.
- A failed induction does not necessarily mean a cesarean section is required.

REFERENCES

1. World Health Organization. (2011). WHO recommendations for induction of labour. [online] Available from https://www.who.int/publications/i/item/9789241501156 [Last accessed December, 2025].
2. World Health Organization. (2022). WHO recommendations on mechanical methods for induction of labour. [online] Available from https://www.who.int/publications/i/item/9789240055780 [Last accessed December, 2025].
3. World Health Organization. WHO recommendations: Induction of labour at or beyond term. [online] Available from https://www.who.int/publications/i/item/9789240052796 [Last accessed December, 2025].
4. FOGSI- ICOG. Good Clinical Practice Recommendations. 2018.
5. FIGO good practice recommendations for induced or spontaneous labor at term: Prep-for-Labor triage to minimize risks and maximize favorable outcomes. Int J Gynecol Obstet. 2023;163(Suppl. 2):51-6.
6. Institute for Health and Care Excellence. (2021). Inducing labour: NICE guideline. 2021.
7. NICE. (2023). Hypertension in pregnancy: diagnosis and management. NICE Guideline. [online] Available from http://nice.org.uk/guidance/ng133 [Last accessed December, 2025].

8. Sanchez-Ramos L, Levine LD, Sciscione AC, et al. (2024). Methods for the induction of labor: efficacy and safety. Am J Obstet Gynecol. 2024;230(3S):S669-695.
9. FIGO. (2017). Misoprostol-only recommended regimens. [online] Available from chrome-extension://efaidnbmnnnibpcajpcglclefindmkaj/https://www.figo.org/sites/default/files/2020-06/FIGO%20Dosage%20Chart%20%20-%20ENGLISH.pdf [Last accessed December, 2025].
10. NICE. (2020). Diabetes in Pregnancy: Management from preconception to the postnatal period. NICE guideline [NG3]. [online] Available from https://www.nice.org.uk/guidance/ng3 [Last accessed December, 2025].
11. Girling J, Knight CL, Chappell L. (2022). Intrahepatic Cholestasis of Pregnancy (Green-top Guideline No. 43). [online] Available from https://www.rcog.org.uk/guidance/browse-all-guidance/green-top-guidelines/intrahepatic-cholestasis-of-pregnancy-green-top-guideline-no-43/ [Last accessed December, 2025].

CHAPTER 56

Shock in Obstetrics

Ruchika Garg, Rekha Rani

"As life takes root within, the physiological transformations in pregnancy create a critical symphony, harmonizing the vibrant promise of new life with the sobering truth of maternal vulnerability."

—Dr Michael A Belfort

INTRODUCTION

Obstetric shock strikes with little warning, transforming moments of hope into crises. It is a reminder that even in the modern era, where medical advancements reign supreme, nature holds the power to challenge us with its most severe twists.

Shock is defined as "The failure of circulatory system to maintain adequate blood flow to organs and tissues, leading to cellular dysfunction and potential organ failure." Cardiovascular collapse syndrome which is life threatening and associated with obstetric causes is known as Obstetric Shock.[1] It can result from various obstetric emergencies, including severe hemorrhage, sepsis, and complications of preeclampsia or embolic events. Early recognition and management are the key to improve maternal and fetal outcomes.[2,3]

The term "Obstetric Shock" often refers to events directly related to perinatal period and resulting from altered response as a result of pregnancy, whereas "Shock in Obstetrics" loosely refers to indirect nonobstetric causes present during pregnancy/puerperium (polytrauma, anesthetic incidents, cardiovascular, or cerebrovascular incidents).[1]

Exact prevalence of shock in obstetrics/obstetric shock is not known because of difficulties in evaluation in a situation of crisis. It is also known that commonly used index Shock index threshold varies in different maternal conditions. Few studies propose an SI cut-off of 0.9 for referral and a cut-off of 1.1 for intervention in a tertiary care hospital. It was also observed that patients with PIH/eclampsia tend to have lower mean SI values compared to the rest of the study population.[4]

EVOLUTION OF UNDERSTANDING: FROM MYSTICISM TO MODERN MEDICINE

- **Ancient and Medieval Times:** In these times, obstetric shock was not understood as a clinical condition, and maternal mortality from hemorrhage was commonly attributed to divine intervention or fate.[5]

- **18th and 19th Centuries:** Figures such as William Smellie made strides in recognizing the role of blood loss in maternal deaths. His observations helped shift the view of maternal hemorrhage from an inescapable event to a clinical condition that could be managed.[6]
- **Early 20th Century:** With advances in medicine, blood transfusions and surgical interventions became more common, and the understanding of circulatory collapse during childbirth evolved into the formalized concept of "shock."[7]
- **Mid-20th Century to Present:** By the early 20th century, the term "shock" began to take on its modern meaning, not just in obstetrics but in all branches of medicine. The realization that shock could be caused by not only blood loss but also infection and organ failure led to a revolution in medical care. Blood transfusions—once considered impossible—became a lifeline. Antibiotics introduced in the mid-20th century gave obstetricians a weapon against septic shock, which had previously claimed the lives of countless new mothers.[8]

WHY IS OBSTETRIC SHOCK DIFFERENT?

Obstetric shock is unlike any other form of shock seen in medical practice. The intricacies of pregnancy transform a woman's body, reshaping how it responds to life-threatening conditions. Here is why obstetric shock is both unique and especially challenging for clinicians.

The Maternal Body's Unique Adaptations

Pregnancy finely tunes the woman's body, ready to support two lives at once. To meet the demands of both the mother and fetus, the body makes significant physiological changes, especially in the cardiovascular and hematological systems:

- **Supercharged Blood Volume:** By the time a woman reaches her third trimester, her blood volume has surged by 30–50%. This expansion is nature's way of safeguarding against blood loss during childbirth, but it can also make early signs of shock harder to detect. This protective buffer masks symptoms until a large amount of blood has already been lost.[9]
- **Dilutional Anemia:** The blood's plasma volume grows faster than the red blood cell count, creating a state of "physiological anemia." This dilution helps keep the blood flowing smoothly to the placenta, but it also delays the usual signs of hypovolemic shock.[10]
- **Hypercoagulability:** Pregnancy prepares the body for childbirth by enhancing its ability to clot, but this heightened state of coagulation also increases the risk of blood clots (thrombosis), which can complicate the management of shock, especially in cases like sepsis where clotting can spiral into coagulopathy.[11]

These changes protect the pregnant body under normal conditions but may blur the clinical presentation of shock, creating a dangerous delay in diagnosis and treatment.

Obstetric Shock is Triggered by Unique Causes

Pregnancy introduces specific challenges that can push the body into shock, challenges you will not find outside the maternal context:

- **Postpartum Hemorrhage (PPH):** One of the most dramatic examples, PPH, can cause a woman to lose a life-threatening amount of blood in mere minutes after childbirth. While hemorrhagic shock is seen in many settings, its rapid onset and scale in obstetrics—often without prior warning—set it apart.[12]

- **Amniotic Fluid Embolism** (AFE)**:** This rare but devastating complication is unique to pregnancy. Amniotic fluid enters the maternal bloodstream, causing a sudden, severe allergic-like reaction that can lead to cardiovascular collapse and coagulopathy. It is a catastrophic event found only in the obstetric world (Williams, 2022).[13]
- **Hypertensive Disorders (Eclampsia, HELLP Syndrome):** Pregnancy-induced hypertension can escalate into life-threatening conditions. In cases like eclampsia or HELLP syndrome, the shock is driven by systemic damage, affecting the liver, kidneys, and cardiovascular system, all tied to pregnancy-specific complications.[14]

These are no ordinary causes of shock—they are uniquely obstetric in nature, highlighting the need for specialized knowledge and rapid interventions.

Dual Concern: The Mother and the Baby

In obstetric shock, there is not just one life at risk, but two vulnerable individuals. The challenge of managing shock in pregnancy is that the clinician must constantly weigh the needs of both mother and fetus:

- *Placental Perfusion:* During shock, blood flow to the placenta—the lifeline between mother and baby—drops dangerously, cutting off oxygen and nutrients. Fetal distress can set in rapidly, meaning clinicians are fighting not just to stabilize the mother, but also to protect the fetus from hypoxia.[15]
- *The Balancing Act:* Tocolysis versus Delivery: One of the hardest decisions during obstetric shock is whether to deliver the baby to save the mother or to delay delivery in the hope of improving fetal survival. Every minute counts, and the decision-making process is unlike anything seen in nonpregnant patients.[16]

Speed and Severity of Onset

Obstetric shock does not just creep in—it crashes through the door. The rapid progression of conditions like hemorrhage or sepsis in pregnancy leaves little room for delay. In the case of postpartum hemorrhage, for instance, a woman can lose over 1,500 mL of blood in a matter of minutes (Williams, 2022). This speed requires immediate action, with clinicians often needing to initiate resuscitation measures within seconds of recognition.[17]

Altered Clinical Presentation

Pregnancy masks the typical symptoms of shock, making it harder to detect until it is almost too late:

- *Hidden Tachycardia:* A pregnant woman's heart rate is already elevated, making it harder to notice when tachycardia—one of the earliest warning signs of shock—begins. The baseline "normal" in pregnancy may already be at 100 beats/min, meaning that a rise to 120 beats/min might not immediately trigger alarm.
- *Normotensive Shock:* Pregnant women can maintain normal blood pressure longer in shock due to the expanded blood volume and vascular changes. This "silent" shock delays the onset of hypotension, which is often a key indicator in nonpregnant patients.[18]

PHYSIOLOGICAL CHANGES IN PREGNANCY: HEMATOLOGICAL AND CARDIOVASCULAR ADAPTATIONS

Pregnancy is a period of profound physiological transformation, where the maternal body adapts remarkably to meet the demands of the growing fetus. These adaptations are particularly evident in the hematological and cardiovascular systems, ensuring that the mother can withstand the physiological stresses of pregnancy and labor, including the possibility of hemorrhage and shock **(Fig. 1)**. The body's ability to modify its baseline functions creates a buffer against such emergencies, safeguarding both maternal and fetal health.

Hematological Changes

One of the most striking changes during pregnancy is the increase in blood volume—a phenomenon known as **pregnancy-induced hypervolemia**. This expansion begins early in the first trimester and continues until around the 34th week of gestation. By full term, maternal blood volume has increased by 40–50% above nonpregnant levels. This increase is essential for several reasons:

- **Facilitating Placental Circulation:** The increased blood volume ensures adequate perfusion to the placenta, the vital organ that supplies the growing fetus with oxygen and nutrients.
- **Buffer Against Blood Loss:** As childbirth is accompanied by inevitable blood loss, this expanded volume acts as a protective reservoir, allowing the mother to tolerate hemorrhage without immediate hemodynamic collapse.
- **Metabolic Demands:** The augmented intravascular volume supports the heightened metabolic needs of the enlarged uterus and the growing fetus.[19]

During this period, **plasma volume increases disproportionately** more than red cell mass, leading to a state of **dilutional anemia**. This is characterized by a drop in hemoglobin concentration and hematocrit, which are generally lowest in the second trimester. Hemoglobin concentrations typically average 12.5 g/dL by term, with some women falling <11.0 g/dL, a condition considered abnormal only if it arises from iron deficiency rather than the expected hypervolemia of pregnancy.[15]

To meet the increased erythropoietic demand, moderate **erythroid hyperplasia** occurs, and reticulocyte counts are elevated, driven by heightened erythropoietin production. However, the maternal iron requirement also surges, peaking in the third trimester, when the

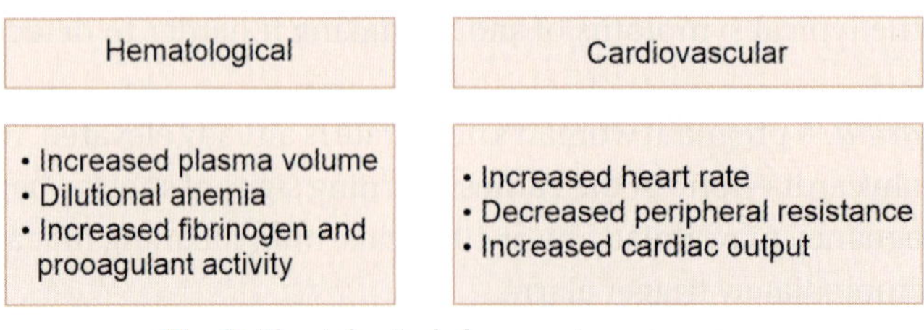

Fig. 1: Physiological changes in pregnancy.

body demands additional iron for both the mother and fetus. This state necessitates careful monitoring of iron levels to avoid deficiency, which could compromise both maternal well-being and fetal development.[20]

Coagulation and Fibrinolysis

Pregnancy brings a shift toward a **hypercoagulable state**, a natural adaptation to prevent hemorrhage during delivery. Both **coagulation** and **fibrinolysis** are finely balanced, though coagulation dominates slightly to prepare the body for the blood loss anticipated during labor.[21]

- **Fibrinogen Levels:** Fibrinogen levels rise significantly in pregnancy, sometimes by as much as 50% by term, reaching 450 mg/dL or more. This increase contributes to a heightened erythrocyte sedimentation rate and aids in clot formation, reducing the risk of excessive bleeding postpartum.[22]
- **Procoagulant Activity:** There is also an increase in clotting factors, particularly factors XI and XIII, which play critical roles in stabilizing clots.[23] These changes ensure that the body can respond swiftly to vascular injury during childbirth.

However, this hypercoagulable state comes with risks, including an increased propensity for **thromboembolic events**, such as deep vein thrombosis and pulmonary embolism (PE). Careful monitoring is required, especially in women with other risk factors for clot formation.[24]

Cardiovascular Changes

Pregnancy also imposes substantial cardiovascular demands. As early as the first trimester, the **cardiac output** begins to rise, driven by both an increased heart rate and stroke volume. By mid-pregnancy, cardiac output may increase by 30–50%, reflecting the need to support the expanded circulatory system.[3] These changes ensure the body is well-prepared to handle the challenges of labor and delivery, where blood loss and fluid shifts are inevitable.

- **Heart Rate:** The maternal heart rate increases by about 10–15 beats/min during pregnancy. This elevation helps maintain the increased cardiac output necessary to perfuse both the maternal organs and the placenta.
- **Vascular Resistance:** Systemic vascular resistance decreases due to the effects of **progesterone**, which causes smooth muscle relaxation in the vessel walls, contributing to the body's ability to accommodate increased blood volume without a corresponding rise in blood pressure.[25] This lowered resistance is crucial for maintaining placental perfusion and preventing hypertensive disorders.

Despite these adaptations, the cardiovascular system remains vulnerable. For example, in cases of **obstetric shock**, the loss of blood volume (due to hemorrhage) or systemic inflammation (as seen in sepsis) can overwhelm the body's compensatory mechanisms, leading to rapid deterioration. However, because the cardiovascular system has been primed by pregnancy-induced hypervolemia and vasodilation, the early signs of shock, such as tachycardia or hypotension, may be masked or delayed.[24]

CLASSIFICATION

TABLE 1: Classification of shock—obstetric causes vs. nonobstetric causes[1]

Pathophysiology/ shock classification	*Obstetrics shock*	*Shock in obstetrics*
Hypovolemic Shock		
1. Hemorrhagic shock	• Hemoperitoneum with/or massive vaginal bleeding • Ruptured ectopic pregnancy • Antenatal, peripartum and postpartum hemorrhage • terine rupture • Placenta previa • Morbid invasive malplacentation • Placental abruption • Obstetric coagulopathy	• Intra-abdominal nontraumatic and traumatic hemorrhage • Ruptured vessels and organs (liver, spleen), ruptured aortic aneurysm • Non-traumatic or traumatic hemothorax • Ruptured aortic aneurysm, pulmonary and cardiac penetration injuries • Limb injuries (traumatic amputation, vessel lesion) • Pre-existent coagulopathy
2. Nonhemorrhagic shock	• Gestational hyperemesis, rapid loss of amniotic fluid	• Severe diarrhea, severe burns, excessive gastric suction, ileus, peritonitis, persistent febrility with dehydration
Septic Shock (endotoxic, bacteremic, viremic shock)	• Obstetric sepsis • Pan metritis (amnio-infection syndrome) • *Puerperal sepsis* • Toxic shock syndrome • Postoperative obstetrics septic complications (e.g., post-cesarean peritonitis, uterine dehiscence)	• No obstetric severe infection (e.g., meningitis, pneumonia, peritonitis, pyothorax) • Postoperative non-obstetric septic complications (peritonitis)
Cardiac and Cardiogenic Shock	Peripartum dilatative decompensated cardiomyopathy	• Traumatic cardiogenic shock with hemopericardia and cardiac tamponade • Acute myocardial infarction
Traumatic Shock	• Uterine rupture • Uterine avulsion	• Severe truncal and limb injuries, polytrauma
Anaphylactic and Anaphylactoid Shock	Amniotic fluid embolism (fetal debris trophoblast)	Severe allergic reaction—anaphylactic shock
Neurogenic Shock	Uterine inversion, uterine rupture, uterine avulsion, severe pain	Spinal shock, spinal cord injuries
Metabolic and Endocrinologic Shock	Unregulated gestational diabetes or diabetes in pregnancy (ketoacidosis coma, hypoglycemic coma, hyperosmolar coma)	Acute adrenal crisis, severe hypoglycemia, hyperthyroid/ hypothyroid coma, uremia

Few common varieties of shock encountered in obstetrics are:

- **Hypovolemic Shock:**
  - **Hemorrhagic Shock:** Caused by significant blood loss (e.g., uterine rupture, placenta previa, or retained placenta).
  - **Nonhemorrhagic Shock:** Caused by fluid loss (e.g., severe dehydration, third-spacing of fluids).
- **Cardiogenic Shock:** Caused by the heart's inability to pump effectively (e.g., myocardial infarction and peripartum cardiomyopathy).
- **Obstructive Shock:** Due to physical obstruction to blood flow (e.g., pulmonary embolism and aortic dissection).
- **Distributive Shock:**
  - **Septic Shock:** Resulting from severe infection leading to systemic vasodilation and hypoperfusion.
  - **Anaphylactic Shock:** Caused by a severe allergic reaction leading to vasodilation and increased vascular permeability.

EXPLORATION: CAUSES AND ETIOPATHOGENESIS OF OBSTETRIC SHOCK (MANAGEMENT)

Few salient features to be remembered and common to management of critical obstetric patient are:

- Resuscitation protocol in pregnant/parturient is almost similar to that of nonpregnant critical patient.
- Physiological changes to be kept in mind while assessment and resuscitation.
- Scoring systems such as Early Warning System (EWS) and Shock Index (OSI) should be used for initial triage, resource allocation, and timely shifting of patient. Thereafter system specific scoring system may be used for outcome prediction and prognostication.
- If spontaneous return of circulation is not expected soon and period of gestation is beyond 24 week, then perimortem cesarean must be initiated within 4 minutes of maternal collapse.

Hemorrhagic (Hypovolemic) Shock

Hemorrhagic shock remains the most common cause of maternal mortality globally, often due to complications such as postpartum hemorrhage (PPH), placenta previa, placental abruption, and ruptured ectopic pregnancy. Understanding the intricate mechanisms behind each cause helps illustrate the severity of this condition in obstetrics.

Postpartum Hemorrhage (PPH)

Causes:

- Incidence of PPH reported around 12% in India
- *Uterine Atony:* The leading cause of PPH, uterine atony refers to the failure of the uterus to contract after childbirth. Without contraction, blood vessels that supplied the placenta remain open, leading to massive blood loss. This is commonly associated with prolonged labor, overdistended uterus (as in multiple gestations or polyhydramnios), or a history of uterine surgery.[14]

- *Trauma:* Trauma to the birth canal, such as lacerations of the cervix, vagina, or perineum, may also lead to hemorrhage. Episiotomies, especially extensive or improperly repaired ones, can be significant sources of blood loss.[17]
- Retained Placental Fragments: Retention of placental tissue prevents complete uterine contraction and predisposes the mother to heavy bleeding.

Etiopathogenesis:

- *Inadequate Myometrial Contraction:* Following delivery, the uterus is expected to contract, compressing the blood vessels at the placental site. In uterine atony, this process fails, resulting in unrelenting blood loss.
- *Coagulation Disorders:* In severe hemorrhagic cases, particularly in the context of prolonged labor or abruptio placentae, disseminated intravascular coagulation (DIC) may develop. This condition depletes the body's clotting factors, exacerbating blood loss.[14]
- Volume Depletion and Hypoperfusion: As blood volume rapidly diminishes, the heart is unable to maintain adequate perfusion to vital organs. The body's initial compensatory mechanisms—vasoconstriction and tachycardia—are overwhelmed, leading to cellular hypoxia, anaerobic metabolism, and lactic acidosis.

Placental Abruption

Causes:

- Reported to affect about 2.5–3.8% pregnancies in India
- *Trauma:* Abdominal trauma, often from accidents or domestic violence, can cause the placenta to prematurely separate from the uterine wall.
- *Hypertension:* Chronic hypertension or preeclampsia significantly increases the risk of placental abruption due to weakened placental attachment.
- *Cocaine Use:* Illicit drug use, particularly cocaine, is associated with placental abruption due to its vasoconstrictive effects.[17]

Etiopathogenesis:

- *Vascular Compromise:* Placental abruption is initiated by bleeding into the decidua basalis, the part of the uterine lining that attaches to the placenta. This leads to placental separation and progressive accumulation of blood between the placenta and uterine wall, impairing fetal oxygenation and causing maternal hemorrhage.
- *Hypovolemic Shock:* The maternal body compensates initially with increased heart rate and peripheral vasoconstriction. As blood loss progresses, perfusion to organs like the kidneys and brain becomes critically compromised.
- *Coagulopathy:* Placental abruption is often complicated by DIC, where excessive clotting factors are consumed, leading to uncontrollable bleeding.[14]

Ruptured Ectopic Pregnancy

Causes:

- Reported incidence of about 0.91–2.8%
- Pertinent to have high index of suspicion in all reproductive age women

- *Delayed Diagnosis:* An undiagnosed ectopic pregnancy that continues to develop may rupture, causing life-threatening internal bleeding. This is common in fallopian tube pregnancies.
- *Previous Tubal Surgery or Infection:* Scar tissue from prior pelvic inflammatory disease (PID) or surgery increases the risk of ectopic pregnancy.

Etiopathogenesis:

- *Tubal Rupture and Hemorrhage:* As the ectopic pregnancy grows within the fallopian tube, the tube stretches until it ruptures, causing hemorrhage into the peritoneal cavity. This can result in rapid hemodynamic collapse.
- *Massive Intraperitoneal Hemorrhage:* With tubal rupture, blood pools into the abdominal cavity, causing acute hypovolemia and shock. The maternal cardiovascular system responds with peripheral vasoconstriction and increased heart rate, but this is often insufficient without immediate surgical intervention.[17]

Management: Hemorrhagic shock is primarily due to massive blood loss, common in conditions like postpartum hemorrhage (PPH), placental abruption, and ruptured ectopic pregnancy. The primary focus is on volume resuscitation, controlling the bleeding, and preventing coagulopathy.

Algorithm for PPH Management:

- Initial Assessment and Resuscitation:
  - Ensure patent airway, breathing, and circulation (ABC)
  - Insert two large-bore IV lines and administer crystalloids
  - Immediate administration of oxytocin or carbetocin
- First-line Management:
  - Administer uterotonics:
  - Oxytocin (10–40 units IV/IM for uterine atony)
  - Second-line agents include ergometrine, misoprostol, or carboprost tromethamine
  - Manual uterine massage
  - If bleeding persists, consider TXA administration

  Investigations:
  - **Hemoglobin and Hematocrit**: To assess the degree of blood loss
  - **Coagulation Profile**: Including platelet count prothrombin time (PT) activated partial thromboplastin time (aPTT), and fibrinogen
  - **Ultrasound**: To assess for retained placental fragments or ongoing bleeding.
- Second-line Management:
  - Balloon tamponade (Bakri balloon insertion).
  - Uterine compression sutures (B-Lynch sutures).
- Third-line Management:
  - Perform uterine artery embolization
  - Surgical intervention: hysterectomy if unresponsive

- *Immediate Resuscitation (ABC Approach):*
  - Airway and Breathing: Ensure a patent airway and provide supplemental oxygen (10–15 L/min) to maintain oxygen saturation above 94%

- *Circulation:* Initiate two large-bore intravenous (IV) lines. Rapid infusion of isotonic crystalloids (e.g., Ringer's lactate or normal saline) is recommended, followed by blood transfusion.

- *Transfusion Protocols:*
  - Massive Transfusion Protocol: In cases where blood loss exceeds 1,500 mL or is rapid, initiate massive transfusion protocols (1:1:1 ratio of packed red blood cells, fresh frozen plasma, and platelets) to prevent dilutional coagulopathy. Platelet transfusions should be guided by laboratory values.

Recent advances:
- Early use of tranexamic acid (TXA), within 3 hours of PPH onset, reduces maternal mortality from hemorrhage.[26]
- Recombinant activated factor VII (rFVIIa) may be considered for intractable bleeding, but only after coagulation abnormalities are corrected.

Uterotonics:
- *Carbetocin:* A long-acting oxytocin analogue has emerged as a first-line treatment for PPH prevention in cesarean deliveries. It has a longer duration of action, reducing the need for additional uterotonic drugs.
- *Misoprostol:* Though traditionally used for cervical ripening and labor induction, misoprostol has become a vital adjunct in the management of PPH, especially in low-resource settings.
- *Nonpneumatic Anti-shock Garment (NASG):*
  - *Application:* Particularly useful in resource-limited settings, the NASG is designed to stabilize women experiencing hypovolemic shock due to PPH. This device wraps around the lower limbs and abdomen, redistributing blood flow to vital organs (heart and brain).
  - *Impact:* NASGs are found to reduce maternal mortality significantly by slowing bleeding and enhancing survival until definitive care is available.
- The E-MOTIVE TRIAL (Early Detection and Treatment of Postpartum Hemorrhage) is a groundbreaking clinical study aimed at improving maternal outcomes by optimizing the management of postpartum hemorrhage (PPH). The trial tested the efficacy of a standardized intervention bundle, which includes early detection through clinical tools and immediate treatment protocols. By focusing on the early identification of blood loss and systematic management, the E-MOTIVE trial demonstrated significant reductions in severe PPH cases and associated maternal morbidity[27] **(Fig. 2)**.

Nonhemorrhagic Hypovolemic Shock

Nonhemorrhagic hypovolemic shock in obstetrics is less frequent but can occur due to significant fluid losses.

Causes
- *Severe Hyperemesis Gravidarum:* Hyperemesis gravidarum, a complication in early pregnancy characterized by intractable vomiting, results in severe dehydration and electrolyte imbalance.[2]

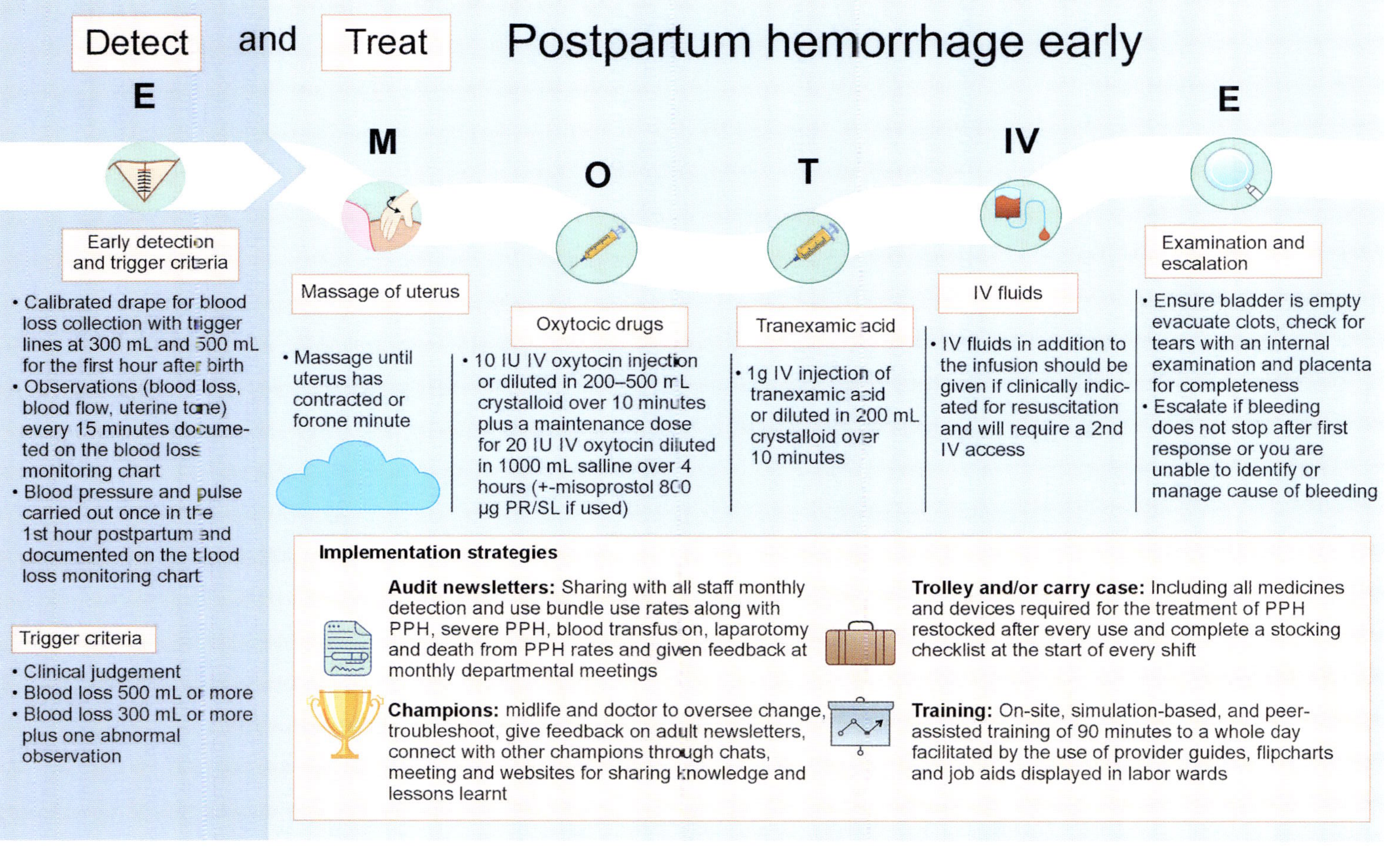

Fig. 2: Early detection and treatment of postpartum hemorrhage.

Source: Gallos I, Devall A, Martin J, et al. Randomized Trial of Early Detection and Treatment of Postpartum Hemorrhage I. New Engl J Med. 2023;389(1):11-21.

- *Amniotic Fluid Leakage:* Amniotic fluid loss, especially in cases of preterm premature rupture of membranes (PPROM), may result in severe dehydration if not managed.

Etiopathogenesis:

- *Fluid Depletion:* In nonhemorrhagic causes, fluid loss through excessive vomiting or amniotic fluid leakage reduces circulating plasma volume. Dehydration diminishes venous return to the heart, resulting in decreased preload and, consequently, lower cardiac output.
- *Hormonal Compensation:* The body compensates through the activation of the renin-angiotensin-aldosterone system (RAAS), which causes vasoconstriction and fluid retention. However, prolonged fluid loss overwhelms these compensatory mechanisms, leading to inadequate tissue perfusion and hypovolemic shock.[14]

Management:

Rapid restoration of fluid balance is key in managing nonhemorrhagic hypovolemic shock, often triggered by severe dehydration from hyperemesis or amniotic fluid leakage.

- *Swift Fluid Replacement*: Administer IV crystalloids to quickly replenish lost volume.
- *Balance Electrolytes*: Correct imbalances caused by dehydration.
- *Close Monitoring*: Track vital signs and fluid levels to ensure stability.
- *Address the Cause*: Tailor treatment—antiemetics for hyperemesis, antibiotics if infection is present.

Cardiogenic Shock

Cardiogenic shock arises when the heart is unable to pump effectively, leading to insufficient blood flow to the body's organs. This type of shock in pregnancy is less common but can be devastating when it occurs.

Peripartum Cardiomyopathy

Causes:

- *Unknown etiology:* The precise cause of peripartum cardiomyopathy (PPCM) remains unclear, though it is thought to involve genetic, autoimmune, and environmental factors.
- *Risk Factors:* Older maternal age, multiple gestations, and African descent have been associated with a higher incidence of PPCM.[21]

Etiopathogenesis:

- *Left Ventricular Dysfunction:* PPCM is characterized by a sudden decline in left ventricular ejection fraction (LVEF), resulting in inadequate blood flow. As the left ventricle becomes weakened, it struggles to pump blood effectively, leading to fluid accumulation in the lungs and systemic circulation (pulmonary and peripheral edema).
- *Compensatory Mechanisms:* Initially, the body attempts to compensate with increased heart rate and systemic vasoconstriction, but these mechanisms eventually fail, resulting in low perfusion pressure, hypoxia, and multiorgan failure.

Myocardial Infarction (MI)

Causes:

- *Coronary Artery Disease:* Although rare in pregnancy, women with pre-existing coronary artery disease, or those who develop severe hypertension or preeclampsia, are at higher risk for MI during pregnancy or postpartum.

Etiopathogenesis:

- *Ischemia and Infarction:* An acute myocardial infarction occurs when blood flow to a part of the heart is blocked, often due to atherosclerosis or thromboembolism. The affected area of the heart muscle suffers ischemic damage, leading to decreased contractility and heart failure.
- *Cardiogenic Shock:* The heart's inability to pump blood effectively results in reduced cardiac output. The body's organs, particularly the kidneys, brain, and liver, begin to fail due to inadequate oxygen delivery.[28]

Valvular Heart Disease

Women with pre-existing valvular heart disease (e.g., mitral stenosis) can decompensate during pregnancy due to the hemodynamic burden of increased cardiac output.

Management of Peripartum Cardiomyopathy

Management of PPCM requires a holistic and multidisciplinary approach that involves obstetricians, cardiologists, intensivists, and neonatologists. The goal is to optimize maternal cardiac function while ensuring fetal well-being. A combination of pharmacological therapy, mechanical support, and lifestyle modifications is typically employed. The cornerstone of PPCM management is early diagnosis, aggressive medical therapy, and, in severe cases, advanced interventions like ventricular assist devices (VADs) or heart transplantation.

Early Diagnosis and Monitoring

Early diagnosis is critical to improving outcomes in PPCM. Routine screening of high-risk patients using echocardiography is recommended in cases with a history of cardiac disease, hypertension, or multiple gestations. Monitoring includes:

- *Echocardiography:* Essential for assessing left ventricular ejection fraction (LVEF), chamber size, and the degree of cardiac dysfunction. A reduced LVEF (<45%) is the hallmark of PPCM.[14]
- *Electrocardiography (ECG):* To evaluate rhythm disturbances like atrial fibrillation or ventricular arrhythmias, which may complicate PPCM.
- *Biomarkers:* Serum levels of natriuretic peptides (BNP or NT-proBNP) and troponin can be valuable indicators of myocardial stress and injury.[28]

Medical Therapy

Medical management of PPCM primarily involves heart failure treatment, tailored for pregnant or postpartum women. The therapeutic goals include reducing preload and afterload, improving myocardial contractility, and preventing arrhythmias or thromboembolic complications.

- *Diuretics:* Used to reduce pulmonary congestion and peripheral edema. Common agents include furosemide, which is safe in pregnancy but should be used cautiously to avoid dehydration or uteroplacental insufficiency. Monitoring of electrolytes, especially potassium, is critical.
- *Beta-Blockers:* Beta-blockers, such as metoprolol or carvedilol, are recommended to decrease the heart's oxygen demand and improve ventricular filling by slowing the heart rate. These are especially useful in the postpartum phase.[24]
- *Angiotensin-Converting Enzyme (ACE) Inhibitors or Angiotensin II Receptor Blockers (ARBs):* These are mainstays in the treatment of heart failure but are contraindicated during pregnancy due to teratogenic effects. However, they should be initiated postpartum to reduce afterload and prevent remodeling of the left ventricle.
- *Hydralazine and Nitrates:* In cases where ACE inhibitors or ARBs are contraindicated, such as during pregnancy, a combination of hydralazine (an arterial vasodilator) and nitrates (venodilators) can be used to manage afterload and improve cardiac output.
- *Anticoagulation:* Thromboembolic risk is significantly increased in PPCM, especially with reduced LVEF. Low-molecular-weight heparin (LMWH) is recommended during pregnancy for anticoagulation, while warfarin is initiated postpartum, particularly if the LVEF remains severely reduced.[14]
- *Digoxin:* If beta-blockers are insufficient to control heart rate or improve contractility, digoxin can be used. It enhances myocardial contractility, particularly in cases of persistent symptomatic heart failure.

Advanced Cardiac Support

In cases of severe heart failure where medical therapy is insufficient, advanced interventions may be required.

- *Mechanical Circulatory Support:* For women with refractory heart failure (especially those with LVEF < 20%), mechanical circulatory support, such as intra-aortic balloon pumps (IABP) or left ventricular assist devices (LVADs), may be necessary. This can serve as a bridge to recovery or heart transplantation in the most severe cases.
- *Extracorporeal Membrane Oxygenation (ECMO):* ECMO is considered in critically ill patients with acute decompensated heart failure and respiratory failure, offering both cardiac and respiratory support while waiting for myocardial recovery or transplantation.[14]

Delivery Planning and Fetal Monitoring

- *Timing of Delivery:* The timing and mode of delivery are determined based on maternal cardiac stability, gestational age, and fetal condition. Vaginal delivery is preferred for most patients as it poses less strain on the cardiovascular system, but cesarean section is considered for obstetric indications or severe maternal instability.
- *Fetal Monitoring:* Continuous fetal monitoring is essential, especially in cases of worsening maternal heart failure. Maternal cardiac medications should be carefully selected to avoid adverse fetal effects.

Postpartum Care

Postpartum care in PPCM patients is crucial, as the heart failure symptoms may persist or worsen after delivery due to fluid shifts. Continued heart failure management postpartum includes:

- *Breastfeeding:* Generally safe with most heart failure medications, although some like ACE inhibitors and warfarin require monitoring or adjustments.
- *Long-term Prognosis:* The prognosis of PPCM varies; patients with early recovery of LVEF have a more favorable outcome, while those with persistently low LVEF may progress to chronic heart failure.[14]

Recent Protocols and Algorithms

Management of PPCM follows guidelines established by cardiology and obstetrics societies. The most recent 2025 European Society of Cardiology (ESC) guidelines provide a structured algorithm for managing PPCM:

PPCM Management Algorithm:

- Initial Diagnosis and Risk Assessment
  - Echocardiography to assess LVEF
  - Biomarker analysis (BNP and NT-proBNP)
- Pharmacologic Management
  - Initiate diuretics, beta blockers, and digoxin (if necessary)
  - Postpartum: ACE inhibitors or ARBs and anticoagulation (as needed)
- Advanced Support for Severe Cases
  - Mechanical circulatory support (LVAD and ECMO)
- Obstetric Management
  - Determine mode and timing of delivery based on maternal stability and gestational age
  - Continuous fetal monitoring
- Postpartum Follow-up
  - Monitor LVEF recovery
  - Long-term heart failure management if needed

Prognosis and Follow-up: The prognosis for PPCM varies significantly. Approximately half of patients recover normal heart function within 6 months. Those with persistent cardiomyopathy may require lifelong management of heart failure, including regular follow-up echocardiograms, medication adjustments, and counselling on future pregnancies, which may carry significant risks of recurrence.[28]

The management of PPCM is a dynamic and evolving process, encompassing early diagnosis, medical and advanced cardiac interventions, and careful obstetric planning. Collaborative care between cardiology and obstetric teams is essential to optimize both maternal and fetal outcomes. As clinical research advances, newer treatment protocols and management algorithms continue to emerge, providing hope for improved recovery rates and long-term prognosis for women affected by this rare but serious condition.

Obstructive Shock

Obstructive shock is due to mechanical factors that impede blood flow, either into or out of the heart. In pregnancy, two significant causes are pulmonary embolism and amniotic fluid embolism.

Pulmonary Embolism

Causes: *Venous Thromboembolism (VTE):* Pregnancy is a hypercoagulable state, increasing the risk of VTE, which can lead to pulmonary embolism. Other risk factors include prolonged immobilization, caesarean delivery, and obesity.[29]

Etiopathogenesis:

- *Right Ventricular Strain:* A pulmonary embolism causes an acute increase in right ventricular afterload due to the blockage of the pulmonary arteries. This strain on the right side of the heart reduces its ability to pump blood, leading to decreased cardiac output and shock.
- *Hypoxia and Acidosis:* The inability of blood to effectively circulate through the lungs reduces oxygenation, leading to tissue hypoxia and metabolic acidosis. The resulting low oxygen delivery further impairs organ function and exacerbates shock.[14]

Amniotic Fluid Embolism

Causes:

Labor and Delivery: AFE is a rare but often fatal condition in which amniotic fluid, fetal cells, hair, or other debris enter the maternal circulation during labor or immediately postpartum, triggering an immune response.

Etiopathogenesis:

- *Cardiovascular Collapse:* AFE triggers a massive systemic inflammatory response, similar to anaphylaxis. This results in acute pulmonary vasoconstriction, leading to right heart failure, severe hypoxemia, and shock.
- *DIC and Hemorrhage:* AFE is often complicated by disseminated intravascular coagulation (DIC), which results in uncontrolled bleeding and further worsens hypovolemia.[14]

Aortic Dissection

Though rare in pregnancy, it is associated with conditions like Marfan syndrome, where the aortic wall weakens, leading to a tear.

Management: Obstructive shock is caused by mechanical impediments to blood flow, including pulmonary embolism (PE) and amniotic fluid embolism (AFE). These conditions require rapid diagnosis and intervention.

Algorithm for Management of Pulmonary Embolism (PE) and Air Embolism in Pregnancy

STEP 1: Immediate Assessment and Stabilization

- *Rapid Clinical Evaluation:* Suspect PE in cases of acute onset dyspnea, chest pain, or syncope. In air embolism, symptoms may include sudden respiratory distress, altered consciousness, and a "mill wheel" murmur.[2]
- *Oxygen Therapy:* Administer 100% oxygen to all patients
- *Hemodynamic Stabilization:* Initiate IV fluids to maintain blood pressure. If hypotension persists, administer vasopressors (e.g., norepinephrine)[9]

STEP 2: Diagnostic Workup
- *Laboratory Tests:* Obtain arterial blood gases (ABG), complete blood count (CBC), coagulation profile, and D-dimer.
- Imaging:
  - *CT Pulmonary Angiography (CTPA):* Gold standard for PE diagnosis.
  - *Doppler Ultrasound:* Assess for deep vein thrombosis (DVT), especially if CTPA is contraindicated.[9]
  - *Trans-oesophageal Echocardiography (TEE):* For suspected air embolism, TEE is crucial in detecting air bubbles within the heart.[14]

STEP 3: Definitive Management
- *Anticoagulation (for PE):*
  - *Low-Molecular-Weight Heparin (LMWH):* First-line treatment in pregnancy (e.g., enoxaparin).
  - Unfractionated Heparin: For patients requiring close monitoring (e.g., those at high risk of bleeding).
  - *Duration:* Continue anticoagulation for at least 6 weeks postpartum, ensuring a minimum total of 3 months of therapy.[14]
- *Specific Management of Air Embolism:*
  - *Positioning:* Place the patient in the left lateral decubitus position (Durant's maneuver) or Trendelenburg position to trap air in the right heart chambers, preventing systemic circulation.
  - Aspiration: Use a central venous catheter to aspirate air if detected.[26]

STEP 4: Advanced Interventions
- *ECMO (Extracorporeal Membrane Oxygenation):*
  - Indications: Consider ECMO in cases of massive PE or severe air embolism causing refractory cardiopulmonary failure where conventional treatments (anticoagulation, thrombolysis, or mechanical interventions) are insufficient.
  - Veno-Arterial ECMO (VA-ECMO): Provides both cardiac and respiratory support, enabling oxygenation and perfusion while allowing the heart and lungs to recover.
- *Thrombolysis (for massive PE):*
  - Consider systemic thrombolysis with agents like tissue plasminogen activator (tPA) in life-threatening cases, despite higher bleeding risks in pregnancy.
- *Mechanical Interventions:*
  - Embolectomy: Reserved for patients with massive PE who are unresponsive to other treatments.
  - Hyperbaric Oxygen Therapy: For air embolism, hyperbaric oxygen can promote nitrogen absorption and reduce bubble size.

STEP 5: Postacute Management
- *Close Monitoring:* Continue monitoring in an intensive care setting. Observe for signs of recurrent embolism or complications such as right heart failure.
- *Prevent Recurrence:* Consider the use of graduated compression stockings and early ambulation postpartum to prevent venous thromboembolism.[8]

Distributive Shock

Septic Shock

Septic shock in obstetrics can arise from various infections during pregnancy, labor, or the postpartum period, but is particularly notorious when linked to septic abortions, especially those performed under unsafe or illegal conditions.

Causes:

- *Illegal and Unsafe Abortions:* The use of unsterile techniques and instruments, often by untrained individuals in nonmedical settings, significantly increases the risk of infection.

Methods may include sharp curettage, insertion of foreign objects into the uterus (such as sticks, coat hangers, or unsterile dilators), and administration of caustic substances or herbal mixtures to induce abortion. These practices lead to severe infections, which are frequently compounded by delays in seeking proper medical care due to fear of legal repercussions.[30,31]

- *Incomplete Abortions:* Retained products of conception following illegal abortion attempts can serve as a nidus for bacterial growth, leading to infection and septicemia.
- *Chorioamnionitis and Puerperal Sepsis:* Infections related to prolonged rupture of membranes or contaminated delivery environments also contribute to septic shock in obstetrics.[14]

Etiopathogenesis:
- *Bacterial Contamination:* In septic abortions, the introduction of bacteria (most commonly *Escherichia coli, Clostridium perfringens*, or *Staphylococcus aureus*) into the uterine cavity through unsterile instruments or foreign objects can lead to endometritis, spreading systemically to cause bacteremia and septicemia.[32]
- *Endotoxemia and Cytokine Storm:* Bacterial endotoxins from Gram-negative organisms trigger a massive immune response, leading to widespread cytokine release. This cytokine storm results in profound vasodilation and capillary leakage, causing hypoperfusion and multiorgan dysfunction.
- *Disseminated Intravascular Coagulation (DIC):* Septic shock in the context of illegal abortions often leads to DIC, where widespread clotting depletes platelets and coagulation factors, further exacerbating hemorrhage and complicating management.[14]
- *Multi-Organ Failure:* As the infection overwhelms the body, multiple organ systems—cardiovascular, renal, hepatic—begin to fail due to ischemia and hypoxia, leading to a downward spiral in maternal health without timely intervention.

Relevance of illegal abortions in septic shock:
- *Social and Legal Impact:* In many regions where access to safe abortion is restricted, women resort to clandestine methods, significantly raising the risk of septic shock. According to WHO, unsafe abortions are one of the leading preventable causes of maternal mortality, with sepsis being a common fatal outcome.[30]
- *Medical Neglect and Delay in Treatment:* Fear of legal consequences often results in delays in seeking medical care, by which time the infection has progressed to septic shock, making management far more difficult.[31]

Management of septic shock: Septic shock in obstetrics, particularly linked to chorioamnionitis, puerperal sepsis, and illegal abortions, requires early antimicrobial therapy and hemodynamic support.[32,33]

Laboratory tests:
- Arterial blood gases (ABGs)
- Complete blood count (CBC)
- Coagulation profile
- Blood cultures

Imaging: Chest X-ray: To evaluate for pneumonia or other sources of infection. Ultrasound/CT: To assess for abscesses or other sources of infection requiring drainage

Algorithm for Septic Shock Management:

- Initial Stabilization:
  - Early Goal-Directed Therapy (EGDT):
    - Initiate IV fluids (30 mL/kg) and achieve a mean arterial pressure (MAP) >65 mm Hg using vasopressors (e.g., norepinephrine).
    - Broad-spectrum antibiotics, such as piperacillin-tazobactam or meropenem, should be administered within the first hour of recognizing sepsis.
- Vasopressor Support:
  - Use norepinephrine if hypotension persists despite fluids.
  - Add hydrocortisone for patients unresponsive to vasopressors*
- Source Control:
  - Immediate surgical intervention to address the infection source (e.g., drainage of abscess, uterine evacuation)
- Monitoring and Adjustments:
  - Monitor lactate levels and central venous oxygen saturation ($ScvO_2$) to guide ongoing therapy

*Immunomodulatory Therapy: Investigational therapies such as hydrocortisone and intravenous immunoglobulin (IVIG) may be considered in severe, refractory septic shock, though more studies are needed.

Anaphylactic Shock

Causes:

- Drug Allergies: Anaphylactic shock in pregnancy is commonly due to reactions to medications (e.g., antibiotics, anesthetics) or latex.

Etiopathogenesis:

- *Massive Vasodilation:* Anaphylaxis leads to widespread release of histamine and other mediators, causing vasodilation and increased capillary permeability. This results in fluid shifting from the intravascular to the extravascular space, reducing circulating blood volume and leading to hypoperfusion.
- *Bronchoconstriction and Hypoxia:* Respiratory compromise from bronchoconstriction further decreases oxygen delivery, compounding the shock state [17]

Management:

- *Immediate Management:*
  - Epinephrine (0.3–0.5 mg IM) is the cornerstone of anaphylaxis treatment. Repeat every 5–15 minutes if necessary.
  - Administer IV corticosteroids (e.g., hydrocortisone 200 mg) and antihistamines (e.g., diphenhydramine 25–50 mg).
- *Fluid Resuscitation and Vasopressors:* Rapid IV fluid administration is crucial to counteract profound vasodilation. If hypotension persists, start vasopressors like norepinephrine.
- *Airway Management:* If respiratory distress occurs, prepare for advanced airway management, including intubation if necessary.[34]

CONCLUSION

Management of obstetric shock requires swift, coordinated, and multidisciplinary action. Understanding the intricacies of each type of shock and utilizing recent advances in resuscitation protocols and therapies significantly improves maternal outcomes. By following evidence-based algorithms, clinicians can navigate these life-threatening emergencies effectively, ensuring the best possible care for both mother and child.

REFERENCES

1. Cerovac A, Habek D, Cerovac E, et al. Obstetric shock and shock in obstetrics - steady obstetrical syndrome. Med Glas (Zenica). 2022;19(2).
2. American College of Obstetricians and Gynecologists (ACOG). Practice Bulletin No. 211: Critical Care in Pregnancy. Obstet Gynecol. 2021;137(4).
3. Zeeman GG. Obstetric critical care: a blueprint for improved outcomes. Obstet Gynecol. 2009;113(3):575-86.
4. Chaudhary M, Maitra N, Sheth T, et al. Shock Index in the Prediction of Adverse Maternal Outcome. J Obstet Gynaecol India. 2020;70(5):355-9.
5. Osol G, Ko NL. Hemodynamic adaptations to pregnancy. In: Creasy RK, Resnik R, Iams JD, (Eds). Creasy and Resnik's Maternal-Fetal Medicine: Principles and Practice, 8th edition. Philadelphia: Elsevier; 2019. pp. 65-79.
6. Towler J, Bramall J. Midwives in History and Society, 1st editon. Croom Helm Ltd.; 1986.
7. Smellie W (Ed). A Treatise on the Theory and Practice of Midwifery. London: Wilson and Durham; 1752.
8. Williams JW (Ed). Obstetrics: A Textbook for the Use of Students and Practitioners, 2nd edition. D Appleton and Company; 1912.
9. RCOG. Maternal Collapse in Pregnancy and the Puerperium. Green-top Guideline No. 56. [online] Available from https://www.rcog.org.uk/guidance/browse-all-guidance/green-top-guidelines/maternal-collapse-in-pregnancy-and-the-puerperium-green-top-guideline-no-56/ [Last accessed December, 2025].
10. Huisman A. The Hematological System in Pregnancy. In: Obstetric Medicine: Management of Medical Disorders in Pregnancy. 1987. pp. 23-35.
11. Kenny LC, Brodsky RA (Eds). Hemostasis and Thrombosis in Obstetric Medicine. Cambridge University Press; 2015.
12. Pritchard JA, MacDonald PC, Gant NF (Eds). Williams Obstetrics, 17th edition. Appleton-Century-Crofts; 1965.
13. Fu J, Peng Y, Huang Y. Amniotic Fluid Embolism: Review of Pathophysiology, Diagnosis, and Management. J Obstet Gynaecol Res. 2018;44(7):1273-81.
14. Cunningham FG, Leveno KJ, Bloom SL, et al. Hypertensive Disorders in Pregnancy. In: Williams Obstetrics, 24th edition. McGraw-Hill Education; 2015.
15. Bernstein IM, Ziegler W, Badger GJ. Plasma volume expansion in early pregnancy. Obstet Gynecol. 2001;97(5 Pt 1):669-73.
16. McLean L, Roberts CL, Bowen JR, et al. Fibrinogen levels in normal pregnancy and pregnancy complications. Int J Gynaecol Obstet. 2012;117(2):137-41.
17. Jeffcoate N (Ed). Principles of Obstetrics and Gynaecology, 6th edition. Oxford University Press; 2018.
18. Thomsen A, Davis JL, Neal JR. Cardiovascular Physiology in Pregnancy. Anesth Analg. 1994;79(2):294-8.

19. Pritchard JA, Wiggins KM, Dickey JC. Changes in the blood volume during pregnancy and the puerperium. I. Does sequestration of red blood cells accompany parturition? Am J Obstet Gynecol. 1960;80:956-64.
20. Fu C. Iron metabolism and iron deficiency in pregnancy. Hematology. 2018.
21. Kenny LC, Broadhurst DI, Dunn WB. Metabolic profiling for preeclampsia. Obstet Gynecol. 2015.
22. McLean C, Katz E. Hypercoagulability in pregnancy and thrombosis. J Thromb Haemost. 2012.
23. Cunningham FG, Leveno KJ, Bloom SL (Eds). Williams Obstetrics, 25th edition. McGraw-Hill; 2015.
24. Osol G. Cardiovascular adaptations to pregnancy. Am J Physiol Heart Circ Physiol. 2019.
25. Thomsen JK, Peterson P, Dalager-Pedersen S. Hemodynamics and the maternal-fetal circulation. Acta Obstet Gynecol Scand. 1994.
26. Kalra L, et al. WOMAN Trial: A Randomized Controlled Trial of Tranexamic Acid for the Treatment of Postpartum Hemorrhage**.** The Lancet. 2017; 389(10084): 2003-2012.
27. Roberts I, et al. E-MOTIVE: A Randomized Controlled Trial of Tranexamic Acid for Postpartum Hemorrhage**.** The Lancet. 2020; 395(10225): 2312-2320.
28. European Society of Cardiology. (2025). 2025 ESC Guidelines for the management of cardiovascular disease and pregnancy. [online] Available from https://www.portailvasculaire.fr/sites/default/files/docs/2025_aha_esg_mcv_grossesse.pdf [Last accessed December, 2025].
29. Bates SM, Greer IA, Hughes RA, et al. VTE and pregnancy: a guide to prevention and treatment. 2020.
30. World Health Organization. Preventing unsafe abortion and its consequences: recommendations for health systems. 2018.
31. Grimes DA, Benson J, Singh S, et al. Unsafe abortion: the preventable pandemic. Lancet. 2006;368(9550):1907-19.
32. Berek JS, Berek DL (Eds). Berek & Novak's Gynecology, 16th edition. Lippincott Williams & Wilkins; 2020.
33. Dellinger RP, Levy MM, Rhodes A, et al. Surviving Sepsis Campaign: international guidelines for management of severe sepsis: 2012. Critical Care Medicine. 2013;41(2):580-637.
34. Weller P, et al. Anaphylaxis and its management in pregnancy. Br J Obstet Gynecol. 2017.

Advanced Maternal Age

Ruchika Garg

INTRODUCTION

Advanced maternal age (AMA), typically defined as maternal age ≥35 years at the estimated date of delivery (EDD), is associated with declining fertility and increased risks of adverse maternal, fetal, and neonatal outcomes.[1] Recent studies advocate stratifying AMA into 5-year age groups (35–39, 40–44, 45–49, and ≥50 years) for better risk assessment. Very advanced maternal age (VAMA, ≥40 or ≥45 years) and extremely advanced maternal age (EAMA, ≥45 years) denote higher-risk categories due to elevated rates of multiple gestations, preterm birth, and fetal growth restriction. This chapter provides a comprehensive overview of AMA's impact on pregnancy outcomes, complications, management strategies, and counseling, tailored for medical postgraduate learners preparing for exams such as AIIMS, JIPMER, or NEET-PG.

1. DEFINITIONS AND EPIDEMIOLOGY

- Advanced Maternal Age: Maternal age ≥35 years at EDD, based on evidence of declining oocyte quality and increased genetic abnormalities
- Very Advanced Maternal Age: Variably defined as ≥40 or ≥45 years; ≥45 years sometimes termed extremely advanced maternal age
- Epidemiology:
  - Rising global trend of delayed childbearing due to socioeconomic factors, education, and assisted reproductive technologies (ART)
  - In the US, births to women ≥35 years increased from 9% in 1990 to 15% in 2018 (NVSS data).
  - India: Limited data, but urban centers report increasing AMA pregnancies due to career prioritization and ART **(Table 1)**.

TABLE 1: Age stratification for AMA.

Category	*Age range*	*Risk profile*
AMA	≥35 years	Increased miscarriage, GDM, preeclampsia, and cesarean
VAMA	≥40 or ≥45 years	Higher risks of preterm birth, FGR, and multiple gestations
EAMA	≥45 years	Greatest risk of maternal morbidity and stillbirth

Source: Lean et al., 2017; Sheen et al., 2018.

2. PATHOPHYSIOLOGY

- Oocyte Aging:
  - Progressive depletion of ovarian reserve and oxidative stress impair oocyte quality, increasing nondisjunction and aneuploidy (e.g., trisomy 21, 18, 13).
  - Shortened telomeres and mitochondrial dysfunction contribute to reduced fertility and miscarriage.
- Uterine and Vascular Changes: Decreased endometrial receptivity and placental vascular dysfunction elevate risks of preeclampsia, fetal growth restriction (FGR), and stillbirth.
- Comorbidities: Increased prevalence of obesity, hypertension, and diabetes exacerbates pregnancy complications.

3. COMPLICATIONS OF ADVANCED MATERNAL AGE (TABLE 2)

Advanced maternal age is an independent risk factor for adverse outcomes, amplified by comorbidities and ART use. Complications span early and late pregnancy, impacting maternal and perinatal health.

3.1 Early Pregnancy Complications

- Spontaneous Abortion:
  - Risk increases with age: 10% at 25–29 years, 53% at ≥45 years (Norwegian Birth Registry).
  - Due to trisomic and euploid losses from poor oocyte quality and uterine/hormonal changes.
- Ectopic Pregnancy: 4–8-fold increased risk at ≥35 years due to cumulative risk factors (e.g., pelvic infections, tubal pathology, and multiple partners).
- Hydatidiform Mole: 1.9-fold increased risk of complete mole at VAMA (95% CI 1.2–3.1; $p = 0.006$); no significant rise in partial mole.

TABLE 2: Key complications in AMA.

Category	*Complication*	*Risk increase*
Early pregnancy	Spontaneous abortion	53% at ≥45 years
	Ectopic pregnancy	4–8-fold at ≥35 years
	Hydatidiform mole	1.9-fold (complete mole) at VAMA
	Chromosomal abnormalities	T21: 1/30 at 45 years
Late pregnancy	Preeclampsia	5–10% (≥40 years), 35% (≥50 years)
	GDM	7–12% (≥40 years), 20% (≥50 years)
	Cesarean delivery	aOR 3.64 at VAMA
	Preterm birth	1.2-fold at VAMA
	Stillbirth	OR 1.75 at AMA
Maternal	Severe morbidity	3.5-fold at 45–54 years
	Mortality	6-fold at ≥40 years

Source: Multiple studies.[9-31]

- Chromosomal Abnormalities:
  - Increased nondisjunction leads to autosomal trisomies (T21, T18, and T13) and sex chromosome trisomies (47,XXX; 47,XXY).
  - Risk of Down syndrome: 1/350 at age 35, 1/100 at age 40, and 1/30 at age 45
  - Sex chromosome monosomy (45,X) and copy number variants are age independent.
- Congenital Malformations:
  - Increased risk of aneuploidy-related structural defects (e.g., cardiac anomalies and aOR 2.2–2.9) and nonaneuploidy defects (e.g., esophageal atresia, aOR 2.9; hypospadias, aOR 2.0) at ≥40 years.
  - Conflicting data: Some studies show no significant difference in anomalies between AMA and younger women.
- Multifetal Gestation:
  - Twin birth rates rise from 17.1/1,000 (<20 years) to 51.1/1,000 (40–54 years) (NVSS, 2018).
  - Higher tripling/twinning in women ≥30 years; outcomes similar to younger women.

3.2 Late Pregnancy Complications

- Hypertension:
  - Chronic hypertension: 2–4-fold higher odds at ≥35 years vs. 30–34 years; further increased at ≥45 years.
  - Preeclampsia: Incidence 3–4% in general population, 5–10% at ≥40 years, 35% at ≥50 years; RR increases 30% (40–44 years) and doubles (≥45 years).
  - Long-term cardiovascular risks (coronary heart disease, heart failure, and stroke).
- Gestational Diabetes Mellitus (GDM):
  - 3–6-fold increased risk at ≥40 years (7–12% incidence) vs. 20–29 years (3%); 20% at ≥50 years.
  - Independent of obesity/ethnicity; elevated pre-pregnancy BMI further increases risk.
- Cesarean Delivery:
  - Increased risk at AMA (aOR 2.18; 95% CI: 2.11–2.26) and VAMA (aOR 3.64; 95% CI: 3.41–3.90) due to labor dystocia, lower intervention thresholds, and maternal preference.
  - NVSS (2016): Cesarean rates 40% (35–39 years), 48% (≥40 years) vs. 32% overall.
- Preterm Birth:
  - 1.2-fold increased risk at VAMA (95% CI: 1.06–1.36) vs. 30–34 years; U-shaped distribution with higher risks at extremes of age.
  - Spontaneous or iatrogenic due to comorbidities (e.g., preeclampsia and GDM).
- Perinatal Morbidity and Mortality:
  - FGR: 1.53-fold increased risk at ≥40 years (95% CI: 1.07–2.20).
  - Macrosomia: 12.6% (35–39 years), 15.4% (≥40 years) vs. 12% (<35 years).
  - Small-for-gestational-age (SGA): Increased at >40 years (NVSS data).
  - Stillbirth: 6.0/1,000 overall (US, 2013), 10.1/1,000 (40–44 years), 13.8/1,000 (≥45 years); meta-analysis OR 1.75 (95% CI: 1.62–1.89).
  - Neonatal risks: Low birth weight, low 5-minute Apgar score, and NICU admission.

- Maternal Morbidity and Mortality:
    - VAMA (45–54 years): 3.5-fold risk of severe morbidity (preeclampsia, GDM, thrombosis, hysterectomy, and postpartum hemorrhage).
    - Maternal mortality: 6-fold higher at ≥40 years vs. <20 years; 8-fold risk of amniotic fluid embolism, 3-fold for obstetric shock.
    - MMR: 38/100,000 (AMA) vs. 10.8/100,000 (<35 years).
    - Ethnic disparities: Lower morbidity in Hispanic vs. non-Hispanic Black/American Indian populations.
- Future Maternal Health:
    - Increased hemorrhagic stroke risk (HR: 1.5; 95% CI: 1.0–2.1) in women with last pregnancy at ≥40 years.
    - Two-hit hypothesis: Early life stress and pregnancy accelerate aging, worsening outcomes.

4. MANAGEMENT OF ADVANCED MATERNAL AGE PREGNANCIES

Advanced maternal age pregnancies require multidisciplinary care, intensified surveillance, and shared decision-making to optimize fetomaternal outcomes.

4.1 Preconception Counseling

- Goals: Optimize health, reduce infertility risks, and manage comorbidities.
- Strategies:
    - Achieve normal BMI (18.5–24.9 kg/m^2).
    - Increase physical activity, avoid smoking, alcohol, and recreational drugs.
    - Folic acid supplementation (400–800 mcg daily).
    - Stabilize chronic conditions (e.g., hypertension and diabetes).
    - Discuss age-related risks (miscarriage, aneuploidy, and stillbirth) and ART implications.

4.2 Antenatal Care (Table 3)

- Multifetal Gestation Screening: First-trimester ultrasound to confirm fetal number; late first/early second-trimester ultrasound for chorionicity.
- Aneuploidy Screening:
    - Preferred: Noninvasive prenatal testing (NIPT/cfDNA) or first-trimester combined test (nuchal translucency + biochemical markers).
    - Invasive testing (chorionic villus sampling, amniocentesis) not indicated for AMA alone; offered for abnormal screening results.
- Low-Dose Aspirin:
    - Indicated for women ≥35 years with additional moderate risk factors (e.g., nulliparity, obesity, and family history of preeclampsia) or one high-risk factor (e.g., prior preeclampsia and chronic hypertension).
    - Dose: 81 mg/day, started at 12–16 weeks, taken at night until delivery (ACOG, USPSTF).

TABLE 3: Antenatal care recommendations for AMA.

Intervention	*Timing/Frequency*	*Indication*
NIPT/cfDNA	First trimester	Aneuploidy screening
Anomaly scan	18–20 weeks	Congenital anomalies
GDM screening	1st trimester, 24–26, 32–34 weeks	Elevated GDM risk
Low-dose aspirin	12–16 weeks until delivery	Preeclampsia prevention
Growth ultrasound	36–37 weeks	FGR, macrosomia, and stillbirth risk
Antepartum testing	Twice weekly from 36 weeks	Fetal surveillance (≥40 years)
Induction	39 0/7–39 6/7 weeks	Stillbirth prevention (≥40 years)

Source: ACOG, 2018; USPSTF, 2021.

- Fetal Anomaly Screening:
  - First-trimester ultrasound and detailed anomaly scan at 18–20 weeks due to increased aneuploidy and congenital anomaly risks.
- GDM Screening: First trimester, 24–26 weeks, and 32–34 weeks (DIPSI test: 75 g glucose, ≥140 mg/dL).
- Fetal Surveillance:
  - Third-trimester ultrasound (36–37 weeks) for growth and amniotic fluid volume in women ≥40 years.
  - Twice-weekly antepartum testing (NST and BPP) and daily fetal movement count (DFMC) until delivery.
  - Earlier testing (32–36 weeks) for BMI >30 kg/m^2 or age ≥40 years.

4.3 Intrapartum Management

- Timing of Delivery:
  - Women ≥40 years: Induce labor at 39 0/7–39 6/7 weeks due to stillbirth risk equivalent to 25–29-year-olds at >41 weeks.
  - Women 35–39 years: No specific timing unless comorbidities present.
- Induction of Labor: Recommended at 39 weeks for ≥40 years to reduce stillbirth and neonatal morbidity.
- Cesarean Delivery: Reserve for obstetric indications (e.g., labor dystocia and fetal distress), not AMA alone.

5. FUTURE MATERNAL HEALTH

- Cardiovascular Risks: Preeclampsia and AMA increase long-term risks of coronary heart disease, heart failure, and stroke.
- Stroke: 1.5-fold increased hemorrhagic stroke risk in women with last pregnancy at ≥40 years.
- Aging Hypothesis: Two-hit model suggests early life stress and pregnancy accelerate aging, worsening health outcomes in AMA women.

CONCLUSION

Advanced maternal age (≥35 years) and VAMA (≥40 or ≥45 years) pregnancies are high risk. Multidisciplinary care and shared decision-making are critical to optimize outcomes. Future research is needed to refine risk stratification and establish evidence-based surveillance protocols.

KEY POINTS

- Advanced maternal age (≥35 years) increases risks of miscarriage (53% at ≥45 years), GDM (7–12% at ≥40 years), preeclampsia (35% at ≥50 years), and stillbirth (OR 1.75).
- VAMA (≥40 or ≥45 years) has 3.5-fold higher severe maternal morbidity.
- NIPT and anomaly scans are essential for aneuploidy and congenital anomaly screening.
- Low-dose aspirin (12–16 weeks) reduces preeclampsia risk in AMA with additional risk factors.
- Induction at 39 weeks recommended for women ≥40 years to prevent stillbirth.

Obesity in Pregnancy

Anurekha

INTRODUCTION

Obesity is a complex and multifaceted health issue that has reached epidemic proportions globally and is defined as body mass index (BMI) of 30 kg/m^2 or higher as well as associated with numerous health complications, particularly during pregnancy.[1] The prevalence of obesity among pregnant women has risen significantly in recent years and approximately 42% of women of childbearing age are classified as obese.[2]

Obesity rates in pregnancy may vary based on demographic factors such as age, ethnicity, and socioeconomic status.[3] Additionally, younger women are more likely to experience weight gain during pregnancy, which can exacerbate preexisting obesity.

Body mass index is defined as weight in kilogram divided by height in meters squared (kg/m^2). Classification is as follows:

- Underweight: BMI < 18.5
- Normal weight: BMI 18.5–24.9
- Overweight: BMI 25–29.9
- Obesity class I: BMI 30–34.9
- Obesity class II: BMI 35–39.9
- Obesity class III: BMI ≥ 40

EFFECT OF OBESITY ON PREGNANCY

Obesity can significantly have adverse maternal and fetal impact during pregnancy.

Maternal Health Risks

Increased Risk of Recurrent Abortions

Gestational Diabetes Mellitus

Gestational diabetes mellitus (GDM) is one of the most common complications associated with obesity in pregnancy. Women with a BMI of 30 or higher have a significantly increased risk of developing GDM. Research shows that the odds of GDM can be up to 7.44 times greater in morbidly obese women compared to those with a normal BMI.[4] A 10% increase of pregravid BMI increases the relative risk of gestational diabetes and that of preeclampsia by approximately 10% each.

Hypertensive Disorders in Pregnancy

Obese women are at a higher risk for developing hypertensive disorders during pregnancy, including preeclampsia. Studies indicate that the risk of preeclampsia increases with maternal BMI; women with a BMI over 30 have a twofold (OR: 1.8) increased risk compared to those with a normal weight.[5]

Maternal Morbidity and Mortality

Obesity is associated with increased maternal morbidity and mortality due to associated complications such as venous thromboembolism (VTE), wound infections, and anesthesia-related issues which are more prevalent among obese pregnant women.[6]

Psychological Implications

The psychological impact of obesity during pregnancy cannot be overlooked. Women may experience body image issues, anxiety, and depression related to their weight which affects postnatal care engagement with the newborn and overall well-being.

Fetal Health Risks

Congenital Anomalies

Infants born to obese mothers have an increased risk of congenital anomalies especially neural tube defects and cardiac defects.[7] The exact mechanisms behind this association are still being studied but may involve metabolic disturbances related to maternal obesity.

Macrosomia

Obese mothers are at an increased risk for having macrosomic infants due to elevated levels of glucose and insulin during pregnancy which increases the risk of cesarean sections and shoulder dystocia.[8]

Increased Risk of Stillbirth and Neonatal Deaths

A 5 kg/m^2 increase of BMI elevates the relative risk of intrauterine death to 1.24 (1.18; 1.30). An estimated 11% of all neonatal deaths can be attributed to the consequences of maternal overweight and obesity.[9]

LONG-TERM CONSEQUENCES

Studies suggest that maternal obesity is linked to an increased risk of childhood obesity, type 2 diabetes, and cardiovascular diseases, a phenomenon called as intergenerational cycle.[11]

GESTATIONAL WEIGHT GAIN GUIDELINES

The Institute of Medicine (IOM) has established guidelines for gestational weight gain based on prepregnancy BMI categories **(Table 1)**.

TABLE 1: Institute of medicine (IOM)—BMI and recommended weight gain.

BMI category	*Recommended weight gain*
Underweight (BMI < 18.5)	12.5–18 kg
Normal weight (BMI 18.5–24.9)	11.5–16 kg
Overweight (BMI 25.0–29.9)	7–11.5 kg
Obese (BMI ≥30)	5–9 kg

MANAGEMENT STRATEGIES

Preconception Counseling

Preconception counseling is essential for women with obesity who are planning to conceive. Time to pregnancy declines linearly, starting from a BMI of 29 kg/m^2, by 4% for each additional 1 kg/m^2 of BMI [hazard ratio: 0.96, 95% confidence interval: (0.91; 0.99)]. Even modest weight loss can improve fertility outcomes and reduce the risk of complications during pregnancy.[12] It is advisable to avoid pregnancy for 12–18 months after bariatric surgery to reduce postoperative complications and to reduce fetal exposure to the rapid weight loss period.

Addressing the psychological aspects of obesity is crucial for overall health outcomes. Mental health screenings should be integrated into prenatal care to identify issues such as anxiety or depression. Providing support through counseling or support groups can help improve mental well-being.

Antenatal Management

Nutrition

Proper nutrition plays a crucial role in managing obesity during pregnancy. Pregnant women should work closely with registered dieticians or nutritionists to develop personalized meal plans that emphasize nutrient-dense foods while avoiding excessive caloric intake. A balanced diet rich in fruits, vegetables, whole grains, lean proteins, and healthy fats is recommended. Optimal dose of aspirin 75 mg once a day may be recommended but antiobesity drugs are contraindicated in pregnancy. Routine supplementation with folate, iron, calcium, and vitamin B_{12} as needed is recommended.

Physical Activity Recommendations

Regular physical activity is beneficial for pregnant women with obesity but should be tailored to individual capabilities and preferences. The American College of Obstetricians and Gynecologists recommends at least 150 minutes of moderate-intensity aerobic activity per week for pregnant women unless contraindicated.[13] Engaging in safe physical activities can help to manage weight gain, improve mood, and enhance overall well-being.

Fetomaternal Monitoring

Increased surveillance throughout pregnancy to monitor maternal weight gain and assess for signs of gestational hypertension or diabetes through routine screenings is recommended.[14]

Blood pressure cuff of 12 × 40 cm and above is mandatory to consider the extra size. A prior sensitization with ultrasonologist may help as in obese individuals technical difficulties can be encountered while performing first and second trimester ultrasound due to massive abdominal fat making visualization inadequate. Assessment for sleep apnea may be instituted in addition to the routine antenatal screen. Preanesthetic check-up is also important as these individuals are at increased risk of cesarean section and both regional and general anesthesia becomes cumbersome.

INTRAPARTUM MANAGEMENT

- Safe working environment with ample circulatory space, stretchers, entry, and exit space can be checked prior in a maternity unit catering obese patients in labor.
- It is advisable to secure intravenous access early in these patients due to increased risk of potential complications.
- Obese women are prone to have prolonged first and second stages of labor. Early maternal exhaustion and poor bearing down efforts lead to increased incidence of instrumental deliveries and cesarean sections.
- Cesarean section may be more challenging due to conditions such as big size baby, abnormal fetal presentations, thick abdominal wall, and poor surgical exposure, requiring surgical expertise.

Surgical Prerequisites

- Modified surgical techniques such as self-retaining retractors and prompt hemostasis should be adopted.
- Measures to prevent wound infection, like subcutaneous drainage, should be considered.

POSTPARTUM CARE

Postpartum hemorrhage is four times common in obese women. Therefore, third stage active management of labor to be followed strictly and fourth stage monitoring to be done with propped up position and oxygen support. Postpartum thromboprophylaxis (prophylactic/individualized) and early ambulation along with elastic stockings for post cesarean delivery should be considered. Lactation failure in obese women to be dealt with adequate counseling of the patient as well as relatives. Contraceptive advice is a must, and patient should be encouraged for weight loss.

CONCLUSION

Obesity in pregnancy presents numerous risks that affect both maternal and fetal health. Implementing effective management strategies is essential for improving the pregnancy outcomes. Continued research into the complexities surrounding obesity during pregnancy will inform public health initiatives aimed at addressing this growing concern within maternal healthcare. Healthcare providers play a critical role in guiding patients through preconception counseling, nutritional advice, physical activity recommendations, regular fetomaternal monitoring, and psychological support to foster healthier pregnancies.

MULTIPLE CHOICE QUESTIONS

1. **What is the definition of obesity in terms of Body Mass Index (BMI)?**
   a. BMI of 25 or higher
   b. BMI of 30 or higher
   c. BMI of 35 or higher
   d. BMI of 40 or higher
2. **According to the CDC, approximately what percentage of women of childbearing age are classified as obese?**
   a. 22%
   b. 32%
   c. 42%
   d. 52%
3. **Which demographic group has been found to have higher rates of obesity compared to others?**
   a. White women
   b. Asian women
   c. Black and Hispanic women
   d. Middle Eastern women
4. **How much higher are the odds of developing Gestational Diabetes Mellitus (GDM) in morbidly obese women compared to those with a normal BMI?**
   a. Up to 2.44 times greater
   b. Up to 4.44 times greater
   c. Up to 6.44 times greater
   d. Up to 7.44 times greater
5. **What is the increased risk of preeclampsia for women with a BMI over 30 compared to those with normal weight?**
   a. 1.5 to 2-fold increased risk
   b. 2 to 3-fold increased risk
   c. 3 to 4-fold increased risk
   d. 4 to 5-fold increased risk
6. **Which of the following is NOT mentioned as a complication more prevalent among obese pregnant women?**
   a. Venous thromboembolism (VTE)
   b. Wound infections
   c. Anesthesia-related issues
   d. Ectopic pregnancy
7. **What percentage of maternal deaths during pregnancy or labor have been reported in overweight or obese women in the UK?**
   a. More than 25%
   b. More than 33%
   c. More than 50%
   d. More than 75%
8. **Which of the following is NOT mentioned as a congenital anomaly risk associated with maternal obesity?**
   a. Neural tube defects
   b. Cardiac defects
   c. Cleft palate
   d. Other unspecified malformations
9. **What is the typical weight threshold for defining macrosomia in infants?**
   a. More than 3,500 g
   b. More than 4,000 g
   c. More than 4,500 g
   d. More than 5,000 g
10. **Which long-term health issue is NOT mentioned as a potential risk for children exposed to obesity in utero?**
    a. Childhood obesity
    b. Type 2 diabetes
    c. Cardiovascular diseases
    d. Autoimmune disorders

11. **According to IOM guidelines, what is the recommended weight gain range for obese women (BMI ≥30) during pregnancy?**
    a. 5–9 kg
    b. 7–11.5 kg
    c. 11.5–16 kg
    d. 12.5–18 kg

12. **What is the recommended amount of moderate-intensity aerobic activity per week for pregnant women, according to ACOG?**
    a. At least 90 minutes
    b. At least 120 minutes
    c. At least 150 minutes
    d. At least 180 minutes

13. **Which of the following is NOT mentioned as a management strategy for obesity during pregnancy?**
    a. Preconception counseling
    b. Nutritional guidance
    c. Physical activity recommendations
    d. Bariatric surgery

14. **What is emphasized as crucial for identifying complications early on in obese pregnant women?**
    a. Daily weight measurements
    b. Weekly ultrasounds
    c. Increased surveillance throughout pregnancy
    d. Monthly blood tests

15. **Which psychological issue is specifically mentioned as a concern for obese pregnant women?**
    a. Eating disorders
    b. Body image issues
    c. Bipolar disorder
    d. Obsessive compulsive disorder

16. **What is the primary goal of preconception counseling for obese women planning to conceive?**
    a. To encourage weight gain
    b. To encourage weight loss
    c. To prescribe fertility medications
    d. To schedule frequent doctor visits

17. **Which professional is specifically mentioned for developing personalized meal plans for obese pregnant women?**
    a. Obstetrician
    b. Registered dietitian
    c. Personal trainer
    d. Psychologist

18. **What type of diet is recommended for obese pregnant women?**
    a. Low-carb diet
    b. High-protein diet
    c. Balanced diet rich in fruits, vegetables, whole grains, lean proteins, and healthy fats
    d. Liquid diet

19. **Which of the following is NOT mentioned as a benefit of regular physical activity during pregnancy for obese women?**
    a. Managing weight gain
    b. Improving mood
    c. Enhancing overall well-being
    d. Reducing the need for prenatal vitamins

20. **What is suggested as a way to provide psychological support for obese pregnant women?**
    a. Mandatory therapy sessions
    b. Online forums
    c. Support groups
    d. Daily journaling

21. Which demographic factor is mentioned as influencing the likelihood of experiencing weight gain during pregnancy?

a. Education level
b. Marital status
c. Age (younger women)
d. Geographic location

22. What is described as a potential consequence of maternal obesity on anesthesia during childbirth?

a. Increased effectiveness of anesthesia
b. Reduced need for anesthesia
c. Anesthesia-related complications
d. Preference for natural childbirth

23. Which metabolic factor is suggested as a potential mechanism behind the increased risk of congenital anomalies in babies of obese mothers?

a. Elevated cortisol levels
b. Metabolic disturbances
c. Decreased insulin sensitivity
d. Altered thyroid function

24. What is described as a potential complication of macrosomia?

a. Increased likelihood of cesarean sections
b. Higher risk of preterm birth
c. Greater chance of twin pregnancies
d. Reduced need for neonatal care

25. Which public health challenge is mentioned as a result of the intergenerational cycle of obesity?

a. Increased healthcare costs
b. Shortage of obstetricians
c. Need for larger medical equipment
d. Difficulty in conducting research studies

26. What is suggested as a benefit of even modest weight loss prior to conception for obese women?

a. Guaranteed prevention of gestational diabetes
b. Elimination of all pregnancy risks
c. Improved fertility outcomes
d. Automatic qualification for vaginal delivery

27. Which nutrient is NOT specifically mentioned as part of the recommended diet for obese pregnant women?

a. Fruits
b. Vegetables
c. Whole grains
d. Artificial sweeteners

28. What is recommended regarding physical activity for obese pregnant women?

a. Avoid all forms of exercise
b. Engage only in water-based activities
c. Tailor activities to individual capabilities and preferences
d. Focus solely on strength training

29. Which screening is suggested to be integrated into prenatal care for obese women to address psychological aspects?

a. IQ tests
b. Personality assessments
c. Mental health screenings
d. Genetic counseling

30. What role are healthcare providers described as playing in managing obesity during pregnancy?

a. Solely monitoring weight gain
b. Prescribing weight loss medications
c. Guiding patients through various aspects of care and support
d. Enforcing strict dietary restrictions

Explanations

Ans. 1 b BMI of 30 or higher

Ans. 2-c 42%

Ans. 3 c Black and Hispanic women

Ans. 4 b Up to 4.44 times greater

Ans. 5 b 2 to 3-fold increased risk

Ans. 6 d Ectopic pregnancy

Ans. 7 b More than 33%

Ans. 8 c Cleft palate

Ans. 9 c More than 4,500 g

Ans. 10 d Autoimmune disorders

Ans. 11 a 5–9 kg

Ans. 12 c At least 150 minutes

Ans. 13 d Bariatric surgery

Ans. 14 c Increased surveillance throughout pregnancy

Ans. 15 b Body image issues

Ans. 16 b To encourage weight loss

Ans. 17 b Registered dietitian

Ans. 18 c Balanced diet rich in fruits, vegetables, whole grains, lean proteins, and healthy fats

Ans. 19 d Reducing the need for prenatal vitamins

Ans. 20 c Support groups

Ans. 21 c Age (younger women)

Ans. 22 c Anesthesia-related complications

Ans. 23 b Metabolic disturbances

Ans. 24 a Increased likelihood of cesarean sections

Ans. 25 a Increased healthcare costs

Ans. 26 c Improved fertility outcomes

Ans. 27 d Artificial sweeteners

Ans. 28 c Tailor activities to individual capabilities and preferences

Ans. 29 c Mental health screenings

Ans. 30 c Guiding patients through various aspects of care and support

REFERENCES

1. Stubert J, Reister F, Hartmann S, et al. The risks associated with obesity in pregnancy. Dtsch Arztebl Int. 2018;115:276-83.
2. Centers for Disease Control and Prevention (CDC). Obesity among women of childbearing age. CDC; 2021.

3. Higgins JPT, Thomas J, Chandler J, et al. (2020). Cochrane Handbook for Systematic Reviews of Interventions: Version 6.1. [online] Available from https://www.cochrane.org/authors/handbooks-and-manuals/handbook/archive/v6.1 [Last accessed December, 2025].
4. Kc K, Shakya S, Zhang H. Gestational diabetes mellitus: A review on its pathophysiology, risk factors & treatment. J Diabetes Res. 2020;2020:1234567.
5. Mrema D, Lie RT, Østbye T, et al. The association between pre-pregnancy body mass index and risk of preeclampsia: A registry-based study from Tanzania. BMC Pregnancy Childbirth. 2018;18:56.
6. Bae S, Lee H, Kim YJ. Maternal obesity: Implications for maternal morbidity during pregnancy: A review article. J Clin Med. 2019;8(12):2046.
7. Knight M, Nair M, Tuffnell D, et al. Saving lives, improving mothers' care - Lessons learned to inform future maternity care from the UK confidential enquiries into maternal deaths. BMJ Qual Saf. 2020;29(3):i12.
8. Liu Y, Yang Y, Zhang H. Maternal obesity increases risk of congenital anomalies: A meta-analysis. Obstet Gynecol. 2021;137(4):698-709.
9. Hernandez TL, Mendez CM. Maternal obesity: Implications on neonatal outcomes. Curr Diab Rep. 2020;20(9):69.
10. McIntyre HD, Gibbons KS, Flenady VJ, et al. Overweight and obesity in Australian mothers: Epidemic or endemic? Med J Aust. 2012;196(3):184-8.
11. Oken E, Levitan EB, Gillman MW. Maternal obesity during pregnancy and childhood obesity: A systematic review. Obes Rev. 2018;19(3):258-70.
12. Dodd JM, Grivell RM, Chan AJH. Preconception lifestyle interventions for improving pregnancy outcomes: A systematic review. Cochrane Database Syst Rev. 2020;10.
13. Syed H, Slayman T, DuChene Thoma K. ACOG Committee Opinion No. 804: Physical Activity and Exercise During Pregnancy and the Postpartum Period. Obstet Gynecol. 2021;137(2):375-6.
14. Blomberg M. Maternal obesity and risk of postpartum hemorrhage. Obstet Gynecol. 2011;118(3):561-8.

Preterm Premature Rupture of Membranes

Ruchika Garg

INTRODUCTION

- Preterm premature rupture of membranes (PPROM) defined as spontaneous rupture of fetal membranes before 37 weeks' gestation without onset of labor; complicates 2–3% of pregnancies globally, accounting for 30–40% of spontaneous preterm births.
- **Term PROM:** Rupture at ≥37 weeks before labor (8–10% of term pregnancies).
- Higher incidence in low- to middle-income countries due to socioeconomic factors, infections, and limited prenatal care (up to 15% in some regions).
- **Key Risks:** Neonatal prematurity (85% morbidity/mortality), chorioamnionitis, cord prolapse, pulmonary hypoplasia; maternal sepsis and abruption.
- Newer SFM/ACOG/SMFM classifications: Previable PPROM (<20–22 weeks; fetus unsalvageable); Periviable (20–25+6 weeks; high neonatal mortality/morbidity despite intervention).

ETIOPATHOGENESIS

- **Multifactorial:** Biochemical [matrix metalloproteinases (MMPs) activation and apoptosis], mechanical (stretching and collagen degradation), and infectious (ascending bacteria in 50% cases, especially <28 weeks).
- **Fetal Membranes:** Amnion-chorion fusion by 12 weeks; tensile ECM (collagens I/III/IV/V); at term, TNF-α/IL-1β trigger physiologic weakening.

TABLE 1: Risk factors associated with PPROM and their adjusted odds ratios.

Risk factor category	*Specific factors*	*Adjusted odds ratio (aOR)*
Demographic/Behavioral	Low BMI (<18.5 kg/m^2)	2.00 (1.09–3.67)
	Nulliparity	2.52 (1.77–3.60)
	Low education	2.39 (1.20–4.78)
	Smoking	1.5–2.0
Obstetric History	Prior PPROM	2.75 (1.19–6.36)
	Multiple gestation	2–3x
Medical/Infectious	Gestational diabetes	1.87 (1.16–2.99)
	Bacterial vaginosis/UTI	1.5–2.5
	APH	2–3x

- **Risk Factors**: Prior PPROM (2.75x), nulliparity (2.52x), low BMI (<18.5 kg/m^2; 2x), gestational diabetes (1.87x), low education, smoking, infections (BV, GBS), multiple gestation, UTI, and APH.

DIAGNOSTIC ALGORITHM

Suspected PPROM (Sudden gush of fluid, leakage PV; GA < 37 weeks)

↓

1. Maternal history + Sterile speculum examination (pooling in posterior fornix?)
   - ↓ Yes → Confirmed clinically
   - ↓ No → Proceed to ancillary tests
2. Ancillary Tests (if equivocal):
   - IGFBP-1 or PAMG-1 (Amnisure): Sensitivity 91–99%, Specificity 88–100%
   - USG: Oligohydramnios (AFI < 5 cm or MVP < 2 cm) supportive (not diagnostic)
   - Avoid: Nitrazine (Sensitivity 37–90%, Specificity 77–100%; false + with blood/semen

   ↓
3. If labor established → No further testing needed

   ↓
   - Exclude: Chorioamnionitis (fever, tenderness, FHR > 160, CRP/WBC↑), Abruption, Prolapse

   ↓
   - Confirm GA, Fetal well-being (NST/BPP), GBS screen
     - Gold standard: Clinical (history + speculum); ancillary for doubt.
     - In labor with leak: Diagnose without tests.

TABLE 2: Diagnostic tests for rupture of membranes: sensitivity and specificity.[1,2]

Test	*Sensitivity (%)*	*Specificity (%)*	*Notes*
Sterile Speculum (Pooling)	90–97	97–100	First-line; avoids digital examination
PAMG-1 (Amnisure)	95–99	88–100	Rapid (5–10 minutes); detects low volumes
IGFBP-1	91–95	95–99	Similar to PAMG-1; laboratory-based
Nitrazine	37–90	77–100	pH >6.5; false +ve common
USG Oligohydramnios	50–70	80–90	Supportive; not standalone
Ferning	30–60	77–100	Historical; low sensitivity

MANAGEMENT ALGORITHM FOR PREVIABLE/PERIVIABLE PPROM (<26 WEEKS)[3]

- Counsel: High maternal risk (sepsis, hysterectomy; up to 43% chorioamnionitis with expectant); neonatal survival 15–27% at 23 weeks, 67–76% at 25 weeks but high morbidity (BPD and IVH).
- Ethical factors: NICU capability, patient desire, prognosis, and adherence.

  Previable (<22 weeks)/Periviable (22–25+6 weeks) PPROM

  ↓

  Multidisciplinary counseling (MFM, Neonatology, Ethics, Patient)
  - Risks: Maternal sepsis (↑ with latency), Fetal: Pulmonary hypoplasia (if oligo severe)

- Options: Termination (abortion care; lifesaving)
- Expectant (if no contraindications: infection, abruption, prolapse)

If Expectant (Tertiary center with NICU):

- Admit to HDU; Daily vitals, q48h CRP/WBC, FSE for FHR
- Antibiotics: Azithromycin 1 g PO day 1, then 500 mg/d × 4 d + Ampicillin IV 2 g q6h × 2 d, then Amox PO 250 mg q8h × 5 d (7 d total; prolongs latency, ↓ infection)
- No steroids/$MgSO_4$ (previable; consider at 23 weeks)
- No tocolysis/amnioinfusion (no benefit; ↑ chorioamnionitis)
- Latency predictors: Vaginal bleeding (short), GA at PPROM (longer if >24 weeks), No infection (median 8–10 d <28 weeks)

  Contraindications? (Chorio, Abruption) → Deliver

  ↓ No → Monitor until 37 weeks or complication

- Outpatient: Not for pre-/periviable; consider >34 weeks with counseling.

MANAGEMENT ALGORITHM FOR VIABLE PPROM (≥24 WEEKS)

- Expectant until 37 weeks if no contraindications; reduces RDS/IVH.

Viable PPROM (24–36+6 weeks)

Confirm diagnosis, rule out chorio (Clinical: fever/tenderness/discharge; Laboratory tests: CRP/WBC/FHR; Sensitivity/Specificity low individually)

Admit (Inpatient preferred; Outpatient if stable, compliant, <30 minutes to hospital)

- Monitoring: Daily maternal vitals, q48h laboratory tests, Weekly USG/AFI, Daily NST/FHR
- GBS: Screen; Prophylaxis if +ve or unknown (Ampicillin PCN; clindamycin if allergy)

↓

Interventions:

- Antibiotics: Ampicillin IV 2 g q6h x 48 h + Azithromycin 1 g PO × 1, then Amox PO 250 mg q8h + Azithromycin 250 mg PO qd × 5 d (7 d; ↓ chorioamnionitis 43%, prolongs latency)

Avoid Co-Amox (↑ NEC)

- Corticosteroids: Betamethasone 12 mg IM q24 h × 2 (24–33+6 weeks; ↓ IVH/RDS; Consider 34–36+6 weeks if delivery imminent), Repeat if >7 d and <34 weeks and delivery risk
- $MgSO_4$ Neuroprotection: 4–6 g IV load, 1–2 g/h × 12–24 h if <32 weeks and imminent delivery (<24 h; ↓ CP 30%)
- Tocolysis: Not routine (no perinatal benefit; ↑ chorio). Consider 48 hours for steroid completion if <34 weeks
- Amnioinfusion: No routine (no outcome benefit)

Delivery: 37 weeks (IOL); Earlier if chorioamnionitis/abruption/prolapse/nonreassuring FHR

- Mode: Expect vaginal; CS if fetal distress
  - Emotional support: Counsel on PTSD risk; multidisciplinary.
  - Latency: Median 7–10 d <28 weeks; ↓ with bleeding/oligo/infection.

TABLE 3: Neonatal survival and latency following PPROM at different gestational ages.[4,5]

GA at PPROM	*Latency (Median, Days)*	*Key intervention*	*Neonatal survival (%)*
<24 weeks	10–14	Expectant if desired; Abortion option	15–27 (23 weeks)
24–28 weeks	8–10	Antibiotics + Steroids + $MgSO_4$	50–70
28–32 weeks	5–7	As above; Monitor closely	80–90
32–34 weeks	3–5	Antibiotics; Consider outpatient	>95
34–37 weeks	1–3	IOL at 34 weeks if GBS+; Else expectant	Near 100

COMPLICATIONS AND OUTCOMES[6]

- **Maternal:** Chorioamnionitis (15–35%), Endometritis, Sepsis, Abruption (5–10%), PPH.
- **Neonatal:** Sepsis (most common), RDS, IVH, NEC, BPD, Hypoglycemia; 1–3% mortality.
- **Recurrence:** Prior PPROM major risk (2–3x); Counsel preconception.

TABLE 4: Complications associated with PPROM and risk reduction with treatment.

Complication	*Incidence in PPROM (%)*	*Risk reduction with expectant + Rx*
Chorioamnionitis[7]	15–35	43% (Antibiotics)
Neonatal Sepsis	5–10	30–50% (Antibiotics)
RDS/IVH	20–40 (<32 weeks)	30–50% (Steroids)
Cerebral Palsy	5–10 (<32 weeks)	30% ($MgSO_4$)
Latency <7 days	50–70	Prolong 7 d (Antibiotics)

KEY TAKE HOME MESSAGES FOR POSTGRADUATES

- **Prioritize Counseling in Pre-/Periviable:** Balance maternal risk versus fetal benefit; abortion care essential.
- **Expectant Management Viable ≥24 weeks:** Antibiotics (azithromycin-based), steroids, and $MgSO_4$ per GA.
- **Monitor Rigorously:** Chorioamnionitis diagnosis clinical + laboratory tests (low test sensitivity).
- **Individualize:** GA, comorbidities, patient preference; Multidisciplinary at tertiary center.
- **Future:** Biomarkers for chorio (IL-6 high spec), novel therapies (amnio-patch trials ongoing).

REFERENCES

1. Dayal S, Jenkins SM, Hong PL. Preterm and Term Prelabor Rupture of Membranes (PPROM and PROM). In: StatPearls [Internet]. Treasure Island (FL): StatPearls Publishing; 2025.

2. Kenyon S, Boulvain M, Neilson JP. Antibiotics for preterm rupture of membranes. Cochrane Database Syst Rev. 2010;(8):CD001058. Update in: Cochrane Database Syst Rev. 2013;(12):CD001058.
3. Society for Maternal-Fetal Medicine (SMFM); Battarbee AN, Osmundson SS, et al. Society for Maternal-Fetal Medicine Consult Series #71: Management of previable and periviable preterm prelabor rupture of membranes. Am J Obstet Gynecol. 2024;231(4):B2-B15.
5. Medscape. (2025)). Premature Rupture of Membranes Overview. [online] https://emedicine.medscape.com/article/261137-overview?form=fpf [Last accessed December, 2025].
7. Etyang AK, Omuse G, Mukaindo AM, et al. Maternal inflammatory markers for chorioamnionitis in preterm prelabour rupture of membranes: a systematic review and meta-analysis of diagnostic test accuracy studies. Syst Rev. 2020;9(1):141.

Rh Alloimmunization

Ruchika Garg

INTRODUCTION

The Rh blood group system, specifically the Rh D antigen, plays a critical role in transfusion medicine and obstetrics due to its association with Rh alloimmunization. This condition occurs when Rh-negative individuals develop antibodies against Rh D antigens, primarily through fetomaternal hemorrhage (FMH) or incompatible blood transfusions.

PREVALENCE OF Rh-NEGATIVE BLOOD GROUP

The prevalence of Rh-negative blood varies globally:[1]

- **Native Americans:** ~1%
- **Spanish Basque:** ~30%
- **India:** 3–5% (based on regional studies)

MECHANISMS OF Rh ALLOIMMUNIZATION

Rh alloimmunization occurs when Rh-negative individuals are exposed to Rh-positive red blood cells (RBCs), triggering an immune response.[2] Key causes include:

- **Fetomaternal Hemorrhage (FMH):** Transplacental passage of Rh-positive fetal RBCs into the maternal circulation, with as little as 0.1 mL sufficient to initiate alloimmunization.
- **Transfusion:** Inadvertent or emergency transfusion of Rh-positive blood or blood products (e.g., platelets).
- **Obstetric events:**[3]
    - **First Trimester:** Ectopic pregnancy, spontaneous/therapeutic abortion, molar pregnancy, or threatened abortion.
    - **Invasive Procedures:** Amniocentesis, chorionic villus sampling (CVS), cordocentesis, or external cephalic versioning.

TABLE 1: Risk factors for fetomaternal hemorrhage (FMH).[3]

Event	*Risk of FMH*
Delivery (vaginal or cesarean)	High (most common)
Multifetal delivery	Increased volume of FMH
Placental abruption	Significant FMH risk
Invasive procedures (e.g., CVS)	Moderate risk
First-trimester miscarriage	Low but significant risk

- **Delivery-related Events:** Cesarean section, multifetal delivery, placental abruption, bleeding placenta previa, or manual placental removal.

MATERNAL AND FETAL COMPLICATIONS

Rh alloimmunization can lead to significant complications for both the mother and fetus, particularly in subsequent pregnancies with Rh-positive fetuses.[4]

Maternal Complications

- **Alloimmunization Persistence:** Anti-Rh D antibodies remain lifelong, increasing risks in future pregnancies.
- **Psychological Stress:** Anxiety due to intensive fetal monitoring and potential adverse outcomes.
- **Increased Medical Interventions:** Frequent monitoring (e.g., indirect Coombs test and ultrasound) and invasive procedures (e.g., amniocentesis) elevate maternal stress and procedural risks.
- **Complications from Anti-D Administration:** Rare but include local injection site reactions, fever, or, in extremely rare cases, anaphylaxis.[5]

Fetal and Neonatal Complications

- **Hemolytic Disease of the Fetus and Newborn (HDFN):**
  - **Mild:** Anemia with jaundice requiring phototherapy.
  - **Moderate:** Severe anemia requiring postnatal transfusions.
  - **Severe:** Hydrops fetalis, characterized by ascites, pleural/pericardial effusions, and subcutaneous edema due to cardiac failure from severe anemia.
  - **Fetal Anemia:** Maternal antibodies cross the placenta, causing hemolysis of fetal Rh-positive RBCs.

TABLE 2: Maternal and fetal complications of Rh alloimmunization.[4,6]

Category	*Complication*	*Description*
Maternal	Alloimmunization persistence	Lifelong anti-Rh D antibodies increase risk in subsequent pregnancies
	Psychological stress	Anxiety from monitoring and potential fetal loss
	Procedural risks	Risks from invasive tests (e.g., amniocentesis) or anti-D administration
Fetal/ Neonatal	Hemolytic disease (HDFN)	Ranges from mild anemia to severe hydrops fetalis
	Fetal anemia	Hemolysis of Rh-positive RBCs leading to hypoxia
	Hydrops fetalis	Severe anemia causing cardiac failure and fluid accumulation
	Neonatal hyperbilirubinemia	Risk of kernicterus if untreated
	Intrauterine growth restriction (IUGR)	Secondary to chronic anemia

- **Intrauterine Growth Restriction (IUGR):** Secondary to chronic anemia and hypoxia.
- **Fetal Hydrops:** Late-stage complication with high mortality if untreated [60–70% survival with intrauterine transfusion (IUT) versus 90–95% in nonhydropic fetuses].[6]

- **Neonatal Complications:**
  - Severe hyperbilirubinemia leading to kernicterus.
  - Neonatal anemia requiring exchange transfusions.
  - Premature delivery due to early intervention for fetal distress.

MANAGEMENT OF Rh-NEGATIVE PREGNANCY

Effective management focuses on preventing alloimmunization and detecting complications early.

Prevention of Alloimmunization

- **Without Prophylaxis:** ~17% of Rh-negative women develop anti-Rh D antibodies post-delivery of an Rh-positive fetus, with 10% of subsequent pregnancies affected by HDFN.[7]
- **With Prophylaxis:** Anti-D immunoglobulin reduces alloimmunization to 0.1%.[7]
- **Mechanism of Anti-D:**
  - Clears Rh-positive fetal RBCs from maternal circulation.
  - Downregulates maternal B-cell immune response.
  - Masks Rh D antigen sites on fetal RBCs.
- **Standard Anti-D Dosing:**[8]
  - **300 µg intramuscular (IM)** at 28 weeks gestation and within 72 hours postpartum (if neonate is Rh-positive).
  - Neutralizes up to 30 mL of fetal Rh-positive RBCs.
  - Administered in the deltoid muscle (not gluteal) for optimal absorption.
  - **50 µg IM** for first-trimester events (e.g., miscarriage and ectopic pregnancy). If unavailable, 300 µg is acceptable.
- **Additional Dosing:** Guided by the **Kleihauer–Betke test** to quantify FMH, particularly in high-risk cases (e.g., multiple pregnancies and severe abruption).[8]
- **Anti-D Pharmacokinetics:**
  - Half-life: ~24 days.
  - Detectable in maternal circulation for up to 12 weeks (rarely up to 1 year).
  - Indirect Coombs test (ICT) within 1 year may show low-titer antibodies, not to be mistaken for alloimmunization.[8]

TABLE 3: Anti-D prophylaxis guidelines.[8]

Gestational period/Event	*Recommended anti-D dose*	*Notes*
28 weeks gestation	300 µg IM	Routine antenatal prophylaxis
Postpartum (Rh-positive neonate)	300 µg IM	Within 72 hours of delivery
First-trimester events	50 µg IM	Use 300 µg if 50 µg unavailable
High-risk FMH (e.g., abruption)	Guided by Kleihauer–Betke	Additional doses as per FMH volume

Detection of Alloimmunization

- **Indirect Coombs test (ICT):** Screens for anti-Rh D antibodies in maternal serum.[9]
    - Critical titer: >1:8 (varies by laboratory).
    - High titers warrant fetal monitoring.
- **Fetal Rh Status Determination:**
    - If the partner is Rh-positive, genotyping guides management:[1]
        - **Homozygous (+/+):** Fetus is Rh-positive; no further testing needed.
        - **Heterozygous (+/-):** Fetal Rh status determined via:
            - Noninvasive prenatal testing (NIPT) using cell-free fetal DNA from maternal blood.
            - Invasive testing (CVS or amniocentesis) for PCR-based Rh genotyping.
- If the fetus is Rh-negative, no further monitoring is required.

MANAGEMENT OF Rh ALLOIMMUNIZED PREGNANCY

When alloimmunization is confirmed (ICT-positive), serial monitoring is essential to detect fetal anemia and prevent complications like hydrops fetalis.[9]

Detection of Fetal Anemia

- **Middle Cerebral Artery Peak Systolic Velocity (MCA PSV):**[10]
    - Noninvasive Doppler ultrasound to assess fetal anemia.
    - Sensitivity: 87–90% for moderate to severe anemia.
    - Threshold: MCA PSV >1.5 multiples of the median (MoM) for gestational age indicates anemia requiring intervention.
- **Fetal Hydrops:**
    - Late manifestation of severe anemia due to cardiac decompensation.
    - Associated with poorer outcomes (IUT success: 60–70% in hydropic vs. 90–95% in nonhydropic fetuses).[6]

TABLE 4: Fetal anemia monitoring and management.[10]

Parameter	*Details*	*Action*
MCA PSV >1.5 MoM	Indicates moderate to severe anemia	Refer for intrauterine transfusion
ICT titer >1:8	High risk of fetal anemia	Initiate serial MCA PSV monitoring
Fetal hydrops	Late-stage anemia	Urgent referral for IUT

Intrauterine Transfusion

- **Indication:** MCA PSV >1.5 MoM or evidence of fetal hydrops.[6]
- **Procedure:** Transfusion of Rh-negative, cross-matched packed RBCs into the fetal umbilical vein.
- **Success Rates:**
    - Nonhydropic fetuses: 90–95%.
    - Hydropic fetuses: 60–70%.
- **Referral:** To specialized centers with expertise in fetal therapy.

CURRENT GUIDELINES AND RECOMMENDATIONS

- **American College of Obstetricians and Gynecologists (ACOG, 2018):** Recommends routine Anti-D at 28 weeks and postpartum, with additional doses for FMH events.[4]
- **Royal College of Obstetricians and Gynaecologists (RCOG, 2020):** Advocates noninvasive fetal Rh genotyping and MCA PSV monitoring for ICT-positive cases.[5]
- **Indian Guidelines (FOGSI, 2023):** Emphasize universal Anti-D prophylaxis and early ICT screening to reduce HDFN burden in India.[6]

ADDITIONAL INSIGHTS FROM RECENT STUDIES

- **Noninvasive Fetal Genotyping:** Cell-free fetal DNA testing has >99% accuracy for fetal Rh status, reducing invasive procedures.[1]
- **MCA PSV Advances:** Automated Doppler systems improve reproducibility and accuracy in anemia detection.[2]
- **Anti-D Supply Challenges in India:** Limited access in rural areas highlights the need for centralized prophylaxis programs.[3]
- **Long-term Neonatal Outcomes:** Severe HDFN increases risks of neurodevelopmental delays in affected neonates.[7]

CONCLUSION

Rh-negative pregnancies, affecting ~5% of the Indian population, require proactive management to prevent alloimmunization and mitigate maternal and fetal complications. Routine Anti-D prophylaxis at 28 weeks and postpartum, combined with ICT screening and serial MCA PSV monitoring, significantly reduces the burden of HDFN. Early detection and referral for IUT are critical for improving outcomes, particularly in preventing hydrops fetalis.

REFERENCES

1. Chitty LS, et al. Noninvasive prenatal testing for fetal blood group antigens. Ultrasound Obstet Gynecol. 2014;44(2):129-35.
2. Pretlove SJ, et al. Doppler ultrasound for fetal anemia detection. Fetal Diagn Ther. 2015;38(3):161-8.
3. Sachan D, et al. Rh alloimmunisation in India: A retrospective analysis. J Obstet Gynaecol India. 2018;68(4):245-50.
4. ACOG Practice Bulletin No. 192: Management of Alloimmunization During Pregnancy. Obstet Gynecol. 2018;131(3):e82-e90.
5. RCOG Green-top Guideline No. 65. Management of RhD-negative pregnancies.
6. FOGSI Guidelines. Management of Rh-negative pregnancies in India. J Obstet Gynaecol India. 2023;73(Suppl 1):12-8.
7. Lindenburg IT, et al. Long-term neurodevelopmental outcomes after intrauterine transfusion. Am J Obstet Gynecol. 2016;215(3):374.e1-374.e8.
8. Zwiers C, et al. Anti-D prophylaxis: A meta-analysis. Transfusion. 2017;57(6):1530-7.
9. de Haas M, et al. Fetal RhD genotyping: A review of global practices. Vox Sang. 2019;114(5):429-37.
10. Mari G, et al. MCA PSV for fetal anemia: Long-term outcomes. Ultrasound Obstet Gynecol. 2021;58(2):178-84.

Maternal Near Miss Mortality

Ruchika Garg

INTRODUCTION

Maternal mortality is a critical measure of healthcare quality. Globally, including in India, maternal mortality has declined due to enhanced training and infrastructure, yet further reductions are needed to meet international benchmarks. Maternal death audits identify causes and lessons but face challenges like incomplete data and fear of litigation. Auditing maternal near miss (MNM) cases—women who survive life-threatening pregnancy complications—offers valuable insights, as MNM and maternal death share similar causes. Analyzing these cases highlights successful interventions, informing strategies to reduce maternal mortality and morbidity.

DEFINITION AND THREE DELAYS IN MATERNAL DEATH

Definition of Maternal Near Miss (MNM): A woman who survives a life-threatening complication during pregnancy, childbirth, or within 42 days post-termination, characterized by organ dysfunction.[1]

Three Delays Model: Identifies barriers to obstetric care impacting maternal and neonatal outcomes **(Table 1)**.[1]

- **First Delay:** Delay in deciding to seek care.
  - *Factors*: Socioeconomic status, lack of awareness about complications, cost concerns, prior negative healthcare experiences.
- **Second Delay:** Delay in reaching a healthcare facility.
  - *Factors*: Long distances, poor transportation, and uneven distribution of facilities.
- **Third Delay:** Delay in receiving adequate treatment at the facility.
  - *Factors*: Inadequate equipment, lack of ICU, untrained staff, and unwelcoming environment.

TABLE 1: Three delays in maternal care.

Delay	*Description*	*Key barriers*
First	Deciding to seek care	Low awareness, cost, and socioeconomic barriers
Second	Reaching facility	Distance, transport, and facility distribution
Third	Receiving treatment	Lack of equipment, staff, ICU, and poor attitude

Source: WHO, 2011.[1]

TABLE 2: WHO Near-miss criteria.

Category	Examples
Severe Complications	Postpartum hemorrhage, severe preeclampsia, and eclampsia
Critical Interventions	Laparotomy, blood products, and ICU admission
Organ Dysfunction	Shock, respiratory failure, renal dysfunction, and neurological impairment

Source: WHO, 2011.[1]

WHO NEAR-MISS APPROACH

Definition of MNM: A woman surviving a life-threatening condition (organ dysfunction) during pregnancy, childbirth, or within 42 days post-termination.[1]

WHO Near-Miss Approach (Three Steps) (Table 2)[1]

- **Baseline Assessment:**
  - Identify women with severe complications (pregnant, in labor, or within 42 days postdelivery/abortion).
  - Include severe conditions (e.g., postpartum hemorrhage and eclampsia), critical interventions (e.g., laparotomy and blood transfusion), or organ dysfunction (e.g., shock and renal failure).
  - Collect perspectives from near-miss women and providers.
- **Situation Analysis:** Evaluate facility gaps, delays, and opportunities for improvement using near-miss and process indicators.
- **Interventions:**
  - Involve senior professionals.
  - Implement early case identification.
  - Use evidence-based checklists and local protocols.

ADVANTAGES AND MATERNAL NEAR MISS REVIEW PROCESS

Advantages of MNM Review[1,2]

- More relevant than mortality in low-mortality settings.
- Identifies health system gaps in obstetric care.
- Provides firsthand data on managing acute complications.
- Guides corrective actions to reduce mortality and morbidity.

Maternal Near Miss Review Process (MoHFW, India) (Table 3)[2]

- **Identification:**
  - Detect MNM cases using MoHFW criteria (clinical findings, investigations, interventions, or cardiorespiratory collapse).
  - Notify Facility Nodal Officer (FNO) within 24 hours.
  - Categorize as pregnancy-specific, preexisting, or accidental/incidental disorders.
  - Prohibit case sheet alterations postidentification.

TABLE 3: MNM-R process steps.

Step	*Action*	*Timeline*
Identification	Notify FNO and categorize case	Within 24 hours
Data Transmission	Submit MNM-R form and update register	Weekly
Review	Evaluate frequency and care quality	Ongoing
Action	Root cause analysis and interventions	Post-review

Source: MoHFW, 2012.[2]

TABLE 4: MNM identification approaches.

Approach	*Advantage*	*Disadvantage*
Disease-specific	Simple	Less specific, hard to standardize
Management-based	Easy to apply	Varies by facility resources
Organ Dysfunction	Reliable and standardized	Requires advanced monitoring

Source: WHO, 2011.[1]

- **Data Transmission:**
  - FNO completes facility-based maternal near miss review (MNM-R) form, submits to district weekly.
  - Update MNM-R case register at facility.
- **Review:** Assess MNM frequency and emergency care at institutional/district levels.
- **Action:**
  - Conduct root cause analysis to identify gaps.
  - Implement corrective measures to prevent future cases.

DEFINITION, IDENTIFICATION, AND AUDIT RECOMMENDATIONS

Definition of MNM: A woman who survives life-threatening complications (organ dysfunction) during pregnancy, childbirth, or within 42 days post-termination.[1]

Identification Criteria (Table 4)[1,2]

- Locally relevant, stable, and comparable across settings.
- Approaches:
  - **Disease-Specific:** E.g., eclampsia.
  - **Organ Dysfunction:** E.g., persistent oliguria and shock.
  - **Management-Based:** E.g., hysterectomy and ICU admission.

MoHFW Criteria (India)[2]

- Requires ≥3 criteria (clinical findings, investigations, and interventions) or single cardiorespiratory collapse criterion.
- Categories:
  - Pregnancy-specific (e.g., hemorrhage and hypertension).

TABLE 5: MNM causes by category.

Category	*Examples*
Pregnancy-specific	Hemorrhage, sepsis, hypertension, and eclampsia
Preexisting	Anemia, cardiac/hepatic dysfunction, and thyroid crisis
Accidental/Incidental	Infections, embolism, trauma, and anaphylaxis

Source: MoHFW, 2012.[2]

TABLE 6: Maternal outcome indices.

Index	*Formula*	*Interpretation*
MMR	MD per 100,000 live births	Healthcare quality
SMOR	(MNM + MD) per 1,000 live births	Resource needs
MNMR	MNM per 1,000 live births	Care burden
MNM:MD	MNM/MD	Higher = better care
MI	MD/(MNM + MD)%	Lower = better care

Source: WHO, 2011.[1]

- Preexisting disorders (e.g., anemia and cardiac dysfunction).
- Accidental/incidental (e.g., infections and embolism).

Recommendations for MNM Audit (Table 5)[1,2]

- Adopt WHO/MoHFW tools for consistent identification.
- Use organ dysfunction criteria for reliability.
- Conduct regular facility-based audits with root cause analysis.
- Train staff on early detection and evidence-based protocols.
- Ensure data confidentiality to encourage honest reporting.
- Share findings to improve local and national policies.

ADDITIONAL CONCEPTS

- **Maternal Death (MD):** Death during pregnancy or within 42 days post-termination from pregnancy-related causes, excluding accidental/incidental causes.[1]
- **Severe Maternal Outcome (SMO):** Life-threatening conditions, including MNM and MD.[1]
- **Women with Life-Threatening Conditions (WLTC):** MNM cases plus maternal deaths (WLTC = MNM + MD).[1]

Indices for Evaluation (Table 6)[1]

- **Maternal Mortality Ratio (MMR):** Maternal deaths per 100,000 live births (India: 97 in 2018–20).
- **Maternal Mortality Rate:** Maternal deaths per 100,000 women aged 15–49 years.
- **Severe Maternal Outcome Ratio (SMOR):** (MNM + MD) per 1,000 live births.
- **MNM Ratio (MNMR):** MNM cases per 1,000 live births.

- **MNM Mortality Ratio (MNM:MD):** Higher ratios indicate better care.
- **Mortality Index (MI):** MD/(MNM + MD) as a percentage; lower MI reflects better care quality.

CONCLUSION

Maternal near miss audits provide critical insights into obstetric care gaps, offering a proactive approach to reducing maternal mortality and morbidity. By focusing on survivors of life-threatening complications, MNM reviews identify actionable improvements in early detection, facility resources, and care delivery. The WHO and MoHFW frameworks, supported by standardized criteria and the three-delay model, guide effective audits, ensuring better maternal outcomes.

KEY POINTS

- MNM: Women surviving life-threatening complications within 42 days of pregnancy termination.[1]
- Three delays: Decision to seek care, reaching facility, and receiving treatment.[1]
- WHO approach: Baseline assessment, situation analysis, and interventions.[1]
- MNM-R process: Identify, transmit data, review, and act.[2]
- Advantages: Highlights system gaps and informs corrective actions.[1]
- Criteria: Disease-specific, organ dysfunction, or management-based.[1]
- Audits improve care quality and reduce mortality.[2]

REFERENCES

1. World Health Organization. (2011). Evaluating the quality of care for severe pregnancy complications: The WHO near-miss approach for maternal health. [online] Available from https://www.who.int/publications/i/item/9789241502221 [Last accessed December, 2025].
2. National Health Mission. Maternal Near Miss Review Operational Guidelines. MoHFW, Government of India; 2014.

CHAPTER 62

Imaging in Obstetrics Fetal MRI

Vandana Bansal, Meera Agalawe

LONG QUESTIONS AND ANSWERS

1. **Fetal MRI: Indications and role** *(DNB June 2017)*
   MRI in obstetrics. *(DNB June 2019)*

Ans. Magnetic resonance imaging (MRI) is a noninvasive imaging modality. It works on the principle of magnetic induction, using the hydrogen atoms in the cells as magnetic dipoles.

MRI allows the delineation of tissues and tissue interfaces in very high resolution and thus helps to image fetal and maternal pelvic tissues in great detail.[1]

Since it works on the principle of magnetism, it does not involve ionizing radiation and hence is generally considered safe in pregnancy. It is recommended to perform fetal MRI after 18 weeks of gestation. MRI is recommended after an abnormal ultrasound screen only if it is able to provide additional information which will affect the management of the pregnancy, mode of delivery, counseling, and for planning postnatal management.

Fetal structures like the fetal brain, lungs, and gastrointestinal tract can be easily visualized using MRI. It gives greater resolution and helps image structures that are difficult to image using only ultrasound, especially in obese patients where maternal adipose tissue restricts adequate visualization. It can be useful to determine the causes of severe oligohydramnios or severe polyhydramnios, when fetal structures are difficult to visualize on ultrasound.

Fetal CNS

- MRI can help to determine prognosis in certain conditions, especially related to the fetal central nervous system. Sulcations and gyrations are better seen by MRI compared to ultrasound.
- Specialized MRI like functional MRI can help to delineate CNS tracts and fibers in the fetal brain, and aid in understanding in utero development.
- Functional MRI can also help to identify the fetal optic chiasma and optic nerve tracts and identify any congenital and genetic causes of blindness like septo-optic dysplasia.
- It also helps to determine the presence or absence of fetal nerve bundles in pathologies like agenesis or dysgenesis of corpus callosum, schizencephaly, porencephaly, microcephaly, and fetal infections such as toxoplasmosis and cytomegalovirus.
- Fetal posterior fossa malformations like Dandy-Walker malformation and vermian hypoplasia can be easily diagnosed.

- Fetal closed neural tube defects like diastematomyelia, spinal cord lipoma, tethered cord, conus medullaris cyst, etc. can be diagnosed using MRI.

Fetal thorax

Fetal MRI can be used to diagnose pulmonary abnormalities and to differentiate between fetal thoracic abnormalities like cystic adenomatoid malformations, bronchopulmonary sequestrations and diaphragmatic hernia.

Fetal abdomen

Magnetic resonance imaging can identify fetal abdominal cystic structures, esophageal atresia, renal abnormalities, and pelvic cysts.

Maternal pelvis

Maternal pelvic structures can be easily delineated by MRI. MRI helps to accurately diagnose scar ectopic or cervical ectopic pregnancies.

Morbidly adherent placenta

Magnetic resonance imaging also allows the diagnosis and evaluation of placenta accreta spectrum, including the degree of invasion of placental tissue, i.e., placenta accreta, increta, or percreta, and the involvement of adjacent structures like bladder, pelvic tissues, and bowel.

Limitations

- The high cost of MRI and the widespread availability of ultrasound prevents routine use of MRI in obstetrics.
- MRI, like ultrasound, is also operator dependent.
- Fetal quiescence is essential for obtaining optimal MRI images. Fetal movement can hinder the acquisition of, or lead to artefacts in MRI images.
- Fetal cardiac imaging is not possible by MRI due to cardiac activity.
- There is no indication for the use of gadolinium as a contrast agent in fetal MRI. However, it can be used for maternal MRI. It is a Category C drug, though fetal effects are unknown.
- However, ultrasound still remains the best screening modality for fetal abnormalities.

2. **What are the noninvasive and invasive techniques to identify fetal isoimmunization in Rh-negative pregnancy? Role of intrauterine blood transfusion.** ***(DNB June 2017)***

Ans. Rh isoimmunization occurs when an Rh-negative mother is sensitized by exposure to Rh antigen from an Rh-positive fetus in a previous pregnancy or blood transfusion. The volume of fetomaternal hemorrhage needed to cause maternal isoimmunization can range from 0.1 to 30 mL. The fetal RhD antigen induces an immune response in the mother, leading to the production of IgG antibodies. These antibodies cross the placental barrier in subsequent pregnancies and cause the destruction of Rh-positive fetal red blood cells causing fetal anemia. Fetal anemia results in hyperdynamic circulation, cardiac overload, and cardiac failure with features of fluid accumulation in various body compartments. In an attempt to increase erythrocyte production by extramedullary hematopoiesis, fetal hepatosplenomegaly also occurs.

Rh alloimmunization is diagnosed either due to a previous affected pregnancy or the presence of Rh antibodies in maternal serum during antenatal screening by Indirect Coombs test. The indirect Coombs test is performed in all Rh-negative mothers at booking visit to diagnose Rh isoimmunization. Rh-positive RBCs are incubated with maternal serum, followed by the addition of antihuman globulin. This causes the agglutination of the RBCs. The antibody titers are calculated as the reciprocal of the greatest dilution causing agglutination.

In a woman with first sensitized pregnancy with no previous history, once antibodies are detected in maternal serum by indirect Coombs test, serial monitoring of Rh titers is commenced every four weekly till 28 weeks of gestation and two weekly thereafter until critical titers are reached. Critical titers are laboratory dependent and may range from 1:8 to 1:32, commonly a cut-off value of 1:16 or an absolute value of more than 4 IU/mL is used. Once critical titers are achieved, patient is followed up with middle cerebral artery peak systolic velocity (MCA PSV) in the fetus to determine fetal anemia. This noninvasive method has superseded the traditional technique of serial amniocentesis for the spectral analysis of amniotic fluid at 450 nm (ΔOD_{450}) first described by Liley in 1961.

There are invasive and noninvasive tests to determine fetal anemia.

Invasive methods for prediction of fetal hemolysis: Spectrophotometric analysis of amniotic fluid by Liley's technique was used to measure bilirubin in amniotic fluid, an indirect measure of fetal hemolysis to determine time for intrauterine transfusion. In a normal fetus, the amniotic fluid is straw colored, whereas in severe Rh affected fetus it is usually bright yellow. Amniotic fluid acquired through amniocentesis is first centrifuged and then the optical density of the clear fluid is measured on a spectrophotometer at wavelengths 300–700 nm. The optical density readings are plotted on a graph. This plot is almost a straight line between 350 and 625 nm. If the fetus is affected, the graph shows a peak between 425 and 500nm. Difference between this value and the straight line is the delta OD_{450}.

These invasive techniques using amniocentesis for determining fetal hemolysis have now been completely abandoned.

Ultrasound-guided Fetal Blood sampling/Cordocentesis

It is a direct access to the umbilical cord vessels by ultrasound guided needle puncture and is done once the MCA PSV increases to a range requiring intrauterine transfusion so as to document the exact hematocrit. Due to the extreme accuracy of MCA PSV in predicting fetal anemia, most centers perform cordocentesis simultaneous with intrauterine transfusion.

Noninvasive Prediction of fetal anemia by MCA Doppler[2]

Use of middle cerebral artery peak systolic velocity as a noninvasive method for fetal anemia has been a practice changing discovery in the field of Rh isoimmunization. The landmark study by Mari et al. in 1995 showed that increased velocity in the middle cerebral artery above 1.5 MoM is extremely accurate method for diagnosing moderate to severe fetal anemia. Anemia causes a reduction in the viscosity of blood leading to increased velocity blood flow. It can be reliably measured between 18 to 35 weeks of gestation.

Middle cerebral artery peak systolic velocity (MCA PSV) values expressed as multiples of median (MoM) for gestational age predict fetal anemia with 100% sensitivity at a false-positive rate of 12%. This noninvasive monitoring has resulted in reduction of invasive procedures by 70% and is now the standard of care for diagnosis and management of fetal anemia **(Table 1)**.

TABLE 1: Noninvasive and invasive tests for fetal anemia.

Noninvasive tests	*Invasive tests*
Fetal cell-free DNA in maternal circulation to determine fetal Rh type	Chorionic villus sampling or amniocentesis for fetal Rh typing
Middle cerebral artery peak systolic velocity (MCA PSV) and serial monitoring	Amniocentesis for degree of fetal hemolysis by spectrophotometry using Liley's charts
Serial B mode ultrasound to determine fetal hydrops, hepatomegaly, splenomegaly, cardiomegaly, placentomegaly, polyhydramnios, pleural/ pericardial effusion, and ascites	Cordocentesis or fetal blood sampling for: • Fetal hemoglobin estimation • Direct Coombs test

Treatment

Intrauterine transfusion is the treatment of choice for fetal anemia. It is indicated if the MCA PSV reaches above 1.5 MoM suggesting severe fetal anemia or development of immune hydrops or a fetal hematocrit of <30% or fetal hemoglobin of <10 g/dL at cordocentesis, the fetus is not mature enough to be delivered (<35 weeks). This intervention is more effective if started prior to development of hydrops.

Ultrasound-guided Intraperitoneal transfusion

Initially, when high resolution ultrasound was not available, clinicians used the peritoneal cavity for transfusions. In nonhydropic fetus, the rate of absorption is estimated to be 10–15% per 24 hours. Absorption is slower if hydrops is evident. Because of the erratic absorption, especially in a hydropic fetus, intravascular fetal transfusion has largely replaced the intraperitoneal technique.

However, intraperitoneal transfusion is still indicated if the need for transfusion is early in gestation <18 weeks or if the direct access to cord is not feasible.

The volume calculated for transfusion: (Weeks of gestation – 20) × 10

Ultrasound-guided Intravascular transfusion

Two sites used for direct vascular access are intra hepatic portion of umbilical vein or the umbilical vein at the cord insertion site into the placenta.

Preparation of blood transfusion: The procedure is done after detailed counseling of the couple regarding the technique, advantages, and risk. Patient is preferably admitted and under light sedation. Preprocedure tocolysis and antibiotic may be given. Operation theatre may be kept standby in case of need for emergency LSCS if bradycardia ensues. A paralyzing agent such as vecuronium/pancuronium in a dose of 0.2 mg/kg body weight of the fetus may be given intramuscular in the fetal deltoid or intravascular to minimize fetal movements during transfusion.

Under ultrasound guidance intrauterine transfusion is done of double packed (hematocrit of 75–80%) fresh within 72 hours, O negative blood, leukodepleted, CMV negative, gamma irradiated, cross-matched with mothers blood into the intravascular (cord insertion site or hepatic portal vein) or intraperitoneal compartment. Volume of blood to be transfused is calculated depending on the initial fetal hematocrit, donor hematocrit, and fetoplacental blood volume, which is dependent on the estimated weight and gestational age. A target hematocrit to be achieved at the end of procedure is 40–50%. Rate of transfusion should be kept at 5–10 mL/min. Volume to be transfused = [(target Hb – fetal Hb)× fetoplacental blood volume)/(donor Hb – target Hb)].

3. Enlist fetal risks in twin gestation. How and when will you establish chorionicity of twin pregnancy? How will you diagnose and manage twin-to-twin transfusion syndrome? ***(DNB June 2017)***

Antenatal monitoring of monochorionic twin pregnancy. ***(DNB December 2018)***

What are the different methods to assess chorionicity in pregnancy?

What are the implications of chorionicity in the management of twin pregnancy? ***(DNB June 2020)***

Ans. Twin pregnancy is associated with a high risk of perinatal mortality and morbidity **(Table 2)**. Stillbirth rate is around 12 per 1,000 twin births compared with five per 1,000 singleton births. Preterm birth prior to 37 weeks' gestation occurs in up to 60% of multiple pregnancies, contributing to the increased risk of neonatal mortality and long-term morbidity.

Chorionicity determination

The best time to determine chorionicity of a twin gestation is during the first trimester ultrasound between 8 and 14 weeks. In the early first trimester, chorionicity can be determined by number of gestational sacs, which will be equivalent to the chorionicity. Number of yolk sacs equal the amniocity.

The methods of determining chorionicity in the late first trimester and second trimester are given in **Table 3**.

TABLE 2: Fetal risks in twin gestation.[3]

Any twin gestation	*Risk specific to monochorionic twins*
First trimester	
Vanishing twin	Conjoined twins
Chromosomal abnormalities	Acardiac twin (TRAP sequence)
Abortions	
Fetal structural anomalies	
Second trimester	
Single fetal demise	Twin-to-twin transfusion syndrome
Fetal growth restriction	Selective fetal growth restriction
Third trimester	
Preterm labor	Twin anemia-polycythemia sequence (TAPS)
Premature rupture of membranes	
Intrapartum	
Malpresentations and malpositions	• Cord entanglement • Locked twin

TABLE 3: Key distinguishing features of dichorionic and monochorionic twins.

Dichorionic twin	*Monochorionic twin*
Two placentae—may be separate or fused to appear as a single mass	Single placenta
Intertwin membrane always present and thick >2 mm	Intertwin membrane may or may not be present. If present, it is thin <2 mm
Lambda sign or twin-peak sign—fetal amnions are separated by a peak of chorionic tissue	T-sign—membrane inserted on placenta in a perpendicular fashion. Twin-peak not seen
Fetal gender may be same or different	Both fetuses have same gender

Monochorionic twins have a unique set of complications, in addition to the complications associated with multifetal gestations. Hence, it is necessary to determine chorionicity accurately.

Monitoring in twins

In uncomplicated dichorionic twin pregnancy, ultrasound imaging should be performed in the first trimester at 11–13^{+6} weeks for nuchal translucency scan, again at around 18–22 weeks' gestation for second-trimester anomaly scan, and every 4 weeks thereafter. In uncomplicated monochorionic twins, an ultrasound scan should be performed in the first trimester. There should then be scans every 2 weeks from 16 weeks onward for timely detection of twin-to-twin transfusion syndrome (TTTS), twin anemia polycythemia sequence (TAPS), and selective fetal growth restriction. Any complication detected during monitoring might require more frequent scans.

At each ultrasound assessment, the following should be assessed: Fetal biometry, amniotic fluid volume, and umbilical artery Doppler (from 20 weeks' gestation) for both twins. Discordance in estimated fetal weight (EFW) should be calculated and documented at each scan from 20 weeks. Cervical length assessment is performed ideally at the same visit as the anomaly scan in the second trimester, in order to identify women at risk of extreme preterm birth

In monochorionic twin pregnancy, middle cerebral artery (MCA) peak systolic velocity (PSV) should be recorded from 20 weeks, in order to screen for TAPS. In MCDA twins, the amniotic fluid volume (deepest vertical pocket) and assessment of bladder should be done and documented at each ultrasound scan to screen for TTTS.

Diagnosis and management of Twin-to-twin transfusion syndrome

Twin-to-twin transfusion syndrome is defined as the vascular shunting from a donor twin to a recipient twin through vascular (arteriovenous) anastomoses present in fetal placenta This causes the donor twin to be pale and suffer from high-output cardiac failure, while the recipient twin is plethoric with heart failure caused by circulatory overload.

Twin-to-twin transfusion syndrome affects 10–15% of monochorionic twin pregnancies. It is associated with increased perinatal mortality and morbidity. If untreated, it leads to fetal demise in up to 90% of cases, with morbidity rates in survivors of over 50%. It occurs exclusively in monochorionic twins.

The essential diagnostic criteria for TTTS requires the presence of significant amniotic fluid imbalance. The donor twin has a DVP of <2 cm (oligohydramnios) and the recipient twin has a DVP > 8 cm (polyhydramnios). Bladder discordancy is also a diagnostic criteria. Size discordance is a common finding, but is not essential for the diagnosis.

Sonographic markers that are indicative of twin-to-twin transfusion syndrome include:

1. Monochorionicity
2. Polyhydramnios (largest vertical pocket >8 cm) in one twin and oligohydramnios (LVP < 2 cm) in the other
3. Difference in umbilical cord size
4. Cardiac dysfunction
5. Abnormal Doppler velocimetry
6. Growth discordance >25% between the twins

Once the diagnosis of TTTS is made, it is staged using the Quintero classification. Quintero staging does not always predict accurately the outcome or chronological evolution of TTTS.

- Stage I: Polyhydramnios—oligohydramnios sequence: DVP > 8 cm in the recipient twin and DVP < 2 cm in the donor twin
- Stage II: Same as stage I, but the donor twin's bladder is not visualized
- Stage III: Same as stage II but with absent or reversed umbilical artery diastolic flow, reversed ductus venosus a-wave flow, pulsatile umbilical venous flow in either twin
- Stage IV: Hydrops in one or both twins
- Stage V: Intrauterine fetal demise of one or both twins

Management options in twin-to-twin transfusion

- Amnioreduction from the polyhydramnios sac
- Septostomy—creating a window in the intertwin membrane to allow liquor to flow across
- Selective fetal reduction by bipolar cord coagulation or radiofrequency ablation
- Ablation of placental arteriovenous anastomoses using fetoscopic laser

Both conservative management with close surveillance and laser treatment are considered reasonable options in Stage 1 TTTS.

Laser ablation is the treatment of choice for TTTS at Quintero stages II and above. It is generally accepted that Quintero stages II and above will require treatment. When laser treatment is not available, serial amnioreduction is an acceptable alternative after 26 weeks' gestation.

Another option for the management of severe TTTS is selective termination of pregnancy using bipolar diathermy, laser coagulation, or RFA of one of the umbilical cords. This means that this fetus is sacrificed in the hope of protecting the other twin from death or cerebral damage. Rarely, parents may opt for termination of the entire pregnancy.

4. **Define fetal growth restriction. What are causes of FGR? How will you diagnose and manage a case of fetal growth restriction at 28 weeks of gestation? *(DNB June 2018)***
   Clinical importance of Doppler studies in fetal growth restriction. What are the perinatal complications in such a case? Outline their management. *(DNB June 2017)*
   Role of Doppler ultrasound for fetal surveillance. *(DNB December 2020)*

Ans. Fetal growth restriction (FGR) is defined as a fetus which fails to achieve its genetically predetermined growth potential.

Fetal growth restriction is defined as:[4]

- Fetal weight or abdominal circumference less than 3rd centile for gestational age
- Or any two of the following:
    - Fetal weight or abdominal circumference between 3rd and 10th centile for gestational age
    - Abnormal maternal Uterine artery Doppler or abnormal Doppler of fetal umbilical artery or middle cerebral artery or cerebroplacental ratio less than 5th centile for gestational age
    - Fetal weight or abdominal circumference crossing more than 2 quartiles

Constitutional small fetus or commonly called SGA are a subgroup of small fetuses that do not present the changes described above, so that there appears to be no fetal adaptation to an abnormal environment and with near normal perinatal outcomes similar to those of normally grown fetuses.

Fetal growth restriction is associated with adverse pregnancy outcomes such as:

- Low birth weight
- Fetal hypoxia with acidosis
- Need for preterm delivery
- Need for neonatal resuscitation and intensive care
- Still birth

Growth-restricted fetuses are also predisposed to the development of long-term adverse outcomes like cognitive delay in childhood and adult-onset diseases like obesity, type 2 diabetes mellitus, coronary artery disease, and stroke.

Depending upon the period of onset, fetal growth restriction has been classified into early-onset (detected before 32 weeks' gestation) and late-onset (detected after 32 weeks' gestation) phenotypes. Early and late FGR are distinct by their time of onset, evolution, severity, placental histopathology, Doppler parameters, maternal-associated disease, and perinatal outcome.

Diagnosis

Small-for-gestational age fetuses may be grouped into four categories:

1. Constitutional small fetus (healthy)
2. Growth-restricted fetus due to fetal cause (nonplacental mediated very early-onset FGR)
3. Growth-restricted fetus due to placental insufficiency (placental-mediated) (early-onset FGR)
4. Late-onset FGR (mild placental disease)

For the purpose of management, it is extremely important and also challenging to make this differentiation between pathological growth-restricted fetus and the constitutional small but healthy fetus that is growing as per its inherent genetic potential.

Constitutional small fetus

Constitutional small fetuses are genetically programmed to be symmetrically small but with their growth velocity parallel to the population curve and have normal fetoplacental Doppler flows. These can be followed up by serial growth doppler every 3 weeks and delivered at term.

Growth-restricted fetus due to fetal cause (nonplacental mediated):
In these patients with very early-onset growth-restricted fetus, usually associated with increased liquor and normal Doppler flows, a diligent evaluation of the fetus must be done to look for soft marker for chromosomal abnormalities, markers of fetal infection and structural anomalies and managed as per the disorder.

Growth-restricted fetus due to placental insufficiency (placental-mediated) (Early-onset FGR)
Early FGR represents 20–30% of all FGR and is considered a vascular disorder. The etiopathology is abnormal placentation resulting in a deficiency in substrate transfer. Color Doppler flow is extremely important in early FGR with reduced fetoplacental Doppler patterns as it allows to monitor the progression of fetal deterioration and tailor elective delivery. The classical temporal sequence of fetal Doppler deterioration is usually respected in early-onset placental disease-associated growth-restricted fetus, and there is time for each successive sequential Doppler vascular modification.

Late-onset FGR (mild placental disease)
Late FGR is a new entity that is far more prevalent than E-IUGR (70–80% of all FGR).

It may be suspected when the fetus maintains its growth potential till 32–34 weeks followed by flattening. Placental insufficiency is not severe enough to cause an abnormal umbilical artery. The first hemodynamic alteration during hypoxia in late FGR is cerebral vasodilatation, which presents with only middle cerebral artery brain sparing without umbilical artery abnormality **(Table 4)**.

Management
Ultrasound and Doppler evaluation of maternal and fetoplacental blood flows remains the mainstay in the diagnosis and management of fetal growth restriction.

A diagnosis of FGR should trigger referral for detailed assessment of the fetus, confirmation of accurate dating of the pregnancy, assessment of potential factors that may have resulted in the abnormal biometry, including maternal factors and related treatment (hypertension, diabetes, infectious exposure); detailed evaluation of fetal anatomy and consideration of karyotype; and evaluation for uteroplacental insufficiency, including uterine, umbilical artery, middle cerebral artery, and venous Dopplers and objective placental morphology assessment (location of cord insertion and size and appearance of the placenta).

TABLE 4: Consensus-based definitions for early and late fetal growth restriction (FGR) in the absence of congenital anomalies.

Early FGR: GA < 32 weeks, in the absence of congenital anomalies	**Late FGR:** GA ≥ 32 weeks, in the absence of congenital anomalies
AC/EFW < 3rd centile or UA-AEDF OR 1. AC/EFW < 10th centile combined with 2. UtA-PI > 95th centile and/or 3. UA-PI > 95th centile	AC/EFW < 3rd centile OR At least two out of three of the following: 1. AC/EFW <10th centile 2. AC/EFW crossing centiles >2 quartiles on growth centiles 3. CPR < 5th centile or UA-PI > 95th centile

Doppler velocimetry is extremely useful for making the critical differentiation between constitutionally small healthy (<10th centile) fetuses and the pathologically growth-restricted fetuses and stratify small fetuses which require more surveillance. Additionally, Doppler pattern helps in characterizing the two phenotypes of FGR, early-onset and late-onset. Color Doppler plays an important role in the follow up algorithm of the FGR fetuses, guide pregnancy management decisions including the timing of delivery.

Individualized management will depend on the cause of FGR. In many cases, this will include assessment of fetal well-being in order to identify those fetuses requiring delivery. Antenatal testing strategies include: Cardiotocography (nonstress test) by means of computerized assessment; biophysical profile (BPP) score; amniotic fluid volume assessment; evaluation of Doppler indices of the umbilical artery, fetal middle cerebral artery or a combination of the two (cerebroplacental or umbilicocerebral ratio) and assessment of aortic isthmus and ductus venosus flow.

Once a small fetus (i.e. EFW < 10th centile) has been identified, UtA PI, UA PI, MCA PI, and the CPR should be measured in order to classify FGR versus SGA. FGR should be diagnosed in the presence of any of the factors reflecting fetal adaptation to increased placental resistance like Doppler signs of abnormal cerebroplacental ratio, uterine artery Doppler, and growth centile below 3rd centile.

Next step is to identify the presence of sign suggesting risk of fetal injury or death that may recommend delivery before term like worsening umbilical artery, DV, AoI (aortic isthmus) Doppler and cCTG where available.

Since no treatment has been demonstrated to be of benefit in growth restriction, staging the FGR, Doppler, assessment of fetal wellbeing, and timely delivery remains the main management strategy for both phenotypes of FGR. The stage-based decision algorithm for the management of all FGR provided by Gratacos should be followed. This stage-based management scheme integrates both early- and late-onset forms and establishes follow-up interval as well as timing of delivery as per the fetal risks **(Table 5)**.

A growth-restricted fetus at 28 weeks should be managed as per the above guidelines.

- Corticosteroids should be administered for fetal lung maturity.
- The fetus is monitored using computerized cardiotocography and fetal Doppler ultrasound.
- If the fetus is at stage I or stage II, weekly or biweekly monitoring is recommended respectively.
- If the fetus shows stage III FGR, it is monitored every 1–2 days and to be delivered at 30 weeks, if no further progression to Stage IV
- Earlier delivery is indicated if the fetus shows features of stage IV FGR.

Prediction for FGR

All pregnant women should be assessed for risk factors for a SGA neonate at first registration, so as to identify ones which would require more fetal surveillance. Previous birth of an SGA neonate increases the risk of subsequent SGA twofold and even more after previous two SGA. Females with previous history of placental mediated maternal disease such as prior preeclampsia, prior preterm or term still birth are at increased risk.

Low pregnancy-associated protein A (PAPP-A) and placental growth factor (PLGF) are first trimester serum analytes that are associated with early abnormality in placental angiogenesis

TABLE 5: Stage-based management of FGR.[5]

Stage I	Severe smallness/ mild degree of placental insufficiency	Any of the following: • Fetal weight <3rd centile • CPR <5th centile • MCA PI <5th centile • Umbilical artery PI >95th centile • Uterine artery PI >95th centile	Weekly monitoring	Delivery at 37 weeks by labor induction
Stage II	Severe degree of placental insufficiency	• Umbilical artery absent end diastolic velocity • Aortic isthmus reversal of flow in diastole	Biweekly monitoring	Cesarean section at 34 weeks or more
Stage III	Low suspicion of developing fetal acidosis	• Umbilical artery shows reversal of flow in end diastole • Ductus venosus PI >95th centile	Monitoring every 1–2 days	Cesarean section at 30 weeks or more
Stage IV	High suspicion of development of fetal acidosis	• Ductus venosus shows reversal of a-wave • cCTG short-term variability <3 ms • Variable decelerations	Monitoring 12 hourly	Cesarean section any time after 26 weeks

leading to FGR. A low level of PAPP A < 0.4 MoM is a major risk factor for FGR fetus. Advantage of PAPP-A is its availability as part of first trimester integrated screen for aneuploidy.

Early second trimester markers studied for their association with SGA are serum estradiol, human placental lactogen (HPL), human chorionic gonadotropin (hCG), and maternal serum alpha fetoprotein (MSAFP). Increased MSAFP and hCG are most useful for their association with abnormal placentation and FGR. A single unexplained elevated value of MSAFP or hCG >2 MoM increases the risk of growth restriction in the fetus by fivefold (in the absence of aneuploidies, neural tube defects and abdominal wall defects).

First trimester uterine artery Doppler is an important screening for prediction of early-onset FGR and preeclampsia. This screening can be integrated with $11–13^{+6}$ weeks aneuploidy screening. The ability to predict women at risk for FGR and preeclampsia in early pregnancy might decrease maternal and fetal morbidity through closer surveillance and early intervention with low-dose aspirin.

5. What is Down syndrome? Trimester-wise antenatal tests to be offered to a pregnant woman with a previous child having Down syndrome.

(DNB December 2018, December 2019)

Methods of prenatal screening for aneuploidies in the first trimester of pregnancy.

Guidelines for the measurement of nuchal translucency. ***(DNB December 2017)***

Biochemical screening for Down Syndrome. ***(DNB June 2017)***

Ans. Down syndrome, also called Trisomy 21, is a multisystem disorder. It is characterized by neurodevelopmental delay along with any of cardiac, cutaneous, musculoskeletal, and gastrointestinal abnormalities. It is the most common chromosomal aneuploidy.[6] Overall risk of Downs syndrome in general population is about 1 in 800 pregnancies. This risk increases with advancing maternal age.

First trimester screening for aneuploidy

Double marker test include maternal serum free beta human chorionic gonadotropin (β-hCG) and pregnancy-associated plasma protein A (PaPP-A), both produced by placenta. Maternal serum concentration of free β-hCG is higher (2 MoM) and PAPP-A is lower (0.5 MoM) in fetuses with Trisomy 21. In Trisomy 13 and 18, both free β-hCG and PAPP-A are decreased. In sex chromosomal anomalies, only PAPP-A is low with normal free β-hCG.

Combined screen test is offered at 11-13^{+6} weeks of gestation, which consists of maternal age, dual marker screen combined with nuchal translucency at a crown rump length of 45–84 mm. This gives a risk assessment for serious chromosomal anomalies, such as trisomy 21, trisomy 13, and trisomy 18, and also detects lethal congenital anomalies. The detection rate of Combined screen test is >90% for a 5% false-positive rate. In addition, 70–80% of major structural anomalies can be detected, and a wide spectrum of pregnancy complications including miscarriage, still birth, preeclampsia, fetal growth restriction, and preterm delivery and complications due to twin-to-twin transfusion can be predicted.

Effectiveness of this first trimester combined screening is improved further if along with nuchal translucency, other first trimester markers are included such as fetal nasal bone, assessment of blood flow across tricuspid valve, fetal heart rate, and ductus venosus flow. This method reduces the invasive testing rate drastically to less than 3% and increases the detection rate for Down syndrome and other chromosomal defects to more than 95%.

Second trimester screening

Two commonly used screening tests available are triple marker test and quadruple screen. Triple test includes a combination of three biochemical serum markers, i.e., free beta hCG, MSAFP, and unconjugated estriol (uE3), whereas quadruple test includes inhibin A in addition to triple screen. These tests are used to screen for trisomy 21, 18, and neural tube defects between 15 and 21 weeks. Detection rate of quad screen is between 81% and 85.8% for false-positive rates of 7–8.3% compared to triple test with low detection rate of 69% only. Clinical use of triple test is now almost obsolete. Therefore, in cases where first trimester screen could not be done, quadruple test should be offered owing to its better detection rates and lower false-positive rates. MSAFP levels in the quadruple test are also analyzed to give cut off risk for neural tube defects. In pregnancies affected with trisomy 21, elevated levels of hCG, inhibin A and reduced levels of MSAFP, uE3 are observed.

Combined first and second trimester screening

With the aim of improving detection rate, first trimester combined screening is followed by second trimester biochemical screening and results of both trimester screening tests are combined and risk is calculated. Three approaches have been defined; integrated test, stepwise sequential and contingent screening.

Integrated Screening

In *integrated test,* first trimester combined screening is followed by second trimester quadruple marker screening and combined results are given after completion of process in second trimester and pregnant women who fall into high-risk group, undergo invasive diagnostic testing by amniocentesis.

This screening strategy combines results of first and second trimester marker screens and final risk is assigned after both tests are done. In population with limited access to CVS, serum integrated testing can be more acceptable with highest detection rate and lowest false-positive rates. However, there is a longer wait time (3–4weeks) between initiation and completion of screening, which may cause increased anxiety in the patients.

Sequential Screening

There are two types of sequential screening: Stepwise and contingent.

In *stepwise sequential screening,* all patients undergo first trimester combined testing and on the basis of screening results, they are assigned three risk categories: low, intermediate, and high risk. High-risk cases are offered invasive testing by chorionic villous sampling (CVS), whereas low and intermediate risk patients undergo quad screening in second trimester and if the combined risk after first and second trimester testing becomes high, the patients have amniocentesis.

The second approach is *contingent screening,* which is similar to stepwise sequential testing, but second trimester biochemical screening is performed only in intermediate risk group after first trimester combined screening followed by final combined risk assessment in the second trimester. With contingent screening, pregnancy is classified as low, intermediate, or high-risk based on first trimester screening results. Women at high risk are offered CVS. Women at intermediate risk are offered continued screening in the second trimester, and women at low risk have no further testing. Theoretically, contingent screening would maintain a higher detection rate while reducing the number of patients undergoing second trimester screening tests.

Noninvasive Prenatal Screening

Noninvasive prenatal screening (NIPS) is an advanced screening test with high sensitivity and specificity for knowing the risk for fetal chromosomal aneuploidy using cell free DNA from maternal serum. Maternal plasma has approximately 5–20% of cell-free DNA that comes predominantly from placental apoptosis, which is fetal in origin.

Testing can be performed starting as early as 9 weeks and until delivery. Overall sensitivity and specificity reported for trisomy 21 is 99.3% and 99.8%, respectively for a false-positive rate of <1%. This makes this test an attractive alternative to traditional serum screening for aneuploidy. Recently with the advancement in the NGS technique, few other applications including other aneuploidies and some microdeletions/duplications can also be detected but at a low accuracy depending upon the disorder to be tested.

Main limiting factor to its widespread use as a screening method is its cost as well as chance of inability of getting a report if the fetal fraction is low. NIPS is not a diagnostic test, and confirmatory invasive testing is required in the presence of any abnormal screening results. In the presence of fetal structural anomaly, decision for fetal karyotyping and or microarray testing should not be deferred by a normal NIPS result.

Role of Ultrasound in Prenatal Screening for aneuploidy

The timelines for offering ultrasound are:

- 11–13^{+6} weeks nuchal translucency scan where in addition to looking at NT other soft markers like nasal bone, ductus venosus, and tricuspid regurgitation are also evaluated as a screen for aneuploidy, detection of major malformations early, dating of gestational age of pregnancy, looking at number of fetuses with their chorionicity, and screening for preeclampsia and growth restriction by uterine artery Dopplers is done.

- 18–20 weeks anomaly scan where all structural abnormalities are assessed along with cardiac assessment and screening for preeclampsia by uterine artery Dopplers and preterm birth by looking at cervical length is practiced.
- Later scans after 26–40 weeks are done for assessment of growth and wellbeing of the fetus and its environment, assessment of fetoplacental blood flow by Doppler to monitor complicated pregnancies and sometimes diagnosis of a late-onset anomaly.

Nuchal Translucency

Langdon Downs first noted in 1866 that individuals with Trisomy 21 characteristically have skin deficient in elasticity giving appearance of thick loose skin, being too large for the body, with flat faces and small nose. These characteristics have been visualized on ultrasound in late 1990s as increased nuchal translucency and absent nasal bone in intrauterine life between 11 and 13^{+6} weeks. About 75% of fetuses with Trisomy 21 have increased nuchal translucency and 60–70% have absent nasal bone.

Nuchal translucency (NT) is an objective evaluation on ultrasound of subcutaneous fluid behind the fetal head, neck, and torso in the first trimester of pregnancy between 11^{+0} and 13^{+6} weeks' gestation, equivalent to a crown rump length of 45–84 mm. It is extremely important that the NT measurement is taken in a standardized manner. The Fetal Medicine Foundation has established criteria for proper NT scan and adherence to a well-defined technique will help achieve uniformity of results. NT measurement is the single most effective screening test for fetal aneuploidy **(Table 6)**.[7]

Increased NT thickness (above 95th centile) has been found to be associated with fetal chromosomal defects and in approximately 80% of fetuses with trisomy 21. This association allows NT measurement to be converted into a likelihood ratio. Because the median NT increases with the gestational age or crown-rump length, the actual measurement must first be converted to gestational age-specific MoM. NT is also increased in other conditions such as congenital heart defects, exomphalos, and congenital diaphragmatic hernia.

Addition of other first trimester markers (nasal bone/ductus venosus waveform/tricuspid regurgitation) increase detection rate for Trisomy 21 to more than 95% for a false-positive rate of 2.5% and 95% with false-positive rate of 0.1% for Trisomy 13 and 18. Nasal bone may not be visualized in 2% of chromosomally normal fetuses. Abnormality of ductus venosus waveform is observed in 80% of Trisomy 21 fetuses and 5% of euploid fetus. Tricuspid regurgitation is seen in 55% of Trisomy 21 fetuses but also in 1% of normal fetuses. Abnormality of ductus venosus and tricuspid regurgitation may also be seen in fetuses with cardiac defects.

Second Trimester Ultrasound Screening for Aneuploidy (Genetic Sonogram)

A detailed ultrasonography for fetal anatomic survey is commonly used as an aneuploidy screening method in the second trimester, which is usually best performed between 18 and 20 weeks gestation. Approximately one third of fetuses affected with trisomy 21 have a major or minor structural variation identifiable on USG. Major abnormalities associated with Down syndrome are congenital heart defects, ventriculomegaly, and duodenal atresia. Ultrasound

TABLE 6: Ultrasound technique and parameters for NT evaluation

USG machine	High resolution with a video loop and caliper that provides measurement to one decimal point
Gestational age	11^{+0} weeks to 13^{+6} weeks
Crown-rump length	45–84 mm
Magnification	Fetal head and Torso occupy 75% of the image
Position	• Midsagittal view of the fetus with fetus facing toward the transducer • Neutral position, neither hyperextended nor hyperflexed
Anatomical landmarks	• Tip of the nose • The hard palate is trapezoid in shape • Absence of frontal process of maxilla (Zygoma) • Rounded hypoechoic structure within the center of the intracranial cavity representing the thalamus • Amniotic membrane to be differentiated from nuchal skin by waiting for spontaneous fetal movement or by tapping the mother's abdomen or coughing to make the fetus jump
Caliper placement	• Horizontal cross-hatch of the caliper should be flushed with the inner aspect of the line bordering the NT
Measurement	• Perform 3 measurements and largest measurement is taken for risk assessment • If the nuchal cord is present, NT is measured below and above the cord and the average of the two is taken • Reduce gain before measurement to reduce the fuzzy edge of the line
Appearance	It is the amount of fluid accumulation (NT thickness) and not its appearance (presence or absence of septation/fluid accumulation confined to the neck or enveloping the whole fetus) that determines risk

markers that have been associated with fetal aneuploidy other than DS are: Holoprosencephaly, choroid plexus cysts, facial cleft, cystic hygroma, diaphragmatic hernia, ventriculomegaly, posterior fossa cyst, major heart defects, duodenal atresia, hyperechoic bowel, omphalocele, renal anomalies, mild hydronephrosis, early fetal growth restriction, and talipes.

Chromosomal defects associated with certain second trimester sonographic features (also known as soft markers) include biometric parameters (e.g., short length of femur and humerus, pyelectasis, increased nuchal fold, ventriculomegaly, hypoplastic, or absent nasal bone), early fetal growth restriction, and morphologic signs (e.g., choroid plexus cysts, echogenic bowel, and echogenic intracardiac focus). These "soft markers" are physical characteristics which are not themselves abnormalities or defects but occur more commonly in fetuses affected with DS.

The detection of any of the above markers during a routine sonogram warrants careful anatomical survey aimed at identifying additional markers because the finding of multiple markers indicates high risk for chromosomal anomaly. The soft markers that significantly increase the likelihood of trisomy 21 are thickened nuchal fold, borderline ventriculomegaly, absent or hypoplastic nasal bone, echogenic bowel, and aberrant right subclavian artery. However, relying only on USG to identify Down syndrome is not recommended.

TABLE 7: Various screening methods with their detection rates and false-positive rates

Method of screening	*Detection rate (%)*	*False-positive rate (%)*
Maternal age (MA)	30	5
First trimester		
MA + Fetal NT	75–80	5
MA + Double test	60–70	5
MA + NT + Double test (Combined test)	85–95	5
Combined test + Nasal bone/tricuspid flow/ductus venosus flow	93–96	2.5
Second trimester		
MA + Triple test	60–65	5
MA + Quadruple test	70–75	5
MA + NT + PAPP-A (11–13 weeks) + Quadruple test	90–94	5
Genetic sonogram*	59	5
Combined first trimester screening with second trimester biochemical testing		
Integrated screening	90–94	5
Stepwise sequential screening	90–94	5
Contingent screening	90–94	5
NIPS	99	<1

Genetic sonogram alone has a detection rate of 69% with a 5% false-positive rate and enhanced the sensitivity of all other screening methods. The likelihood ratio for every marker present in fetus can be used to modify the priori risk or serum screening risk which forms the basis for ultrasound screening for DS.

Previous child with Down Syndrome

Antenatal tests that can be offered to a pregnant woman with a previous child or fetus having Down syndrome can be divided into screening tests and confirmatory tests.

Screening tests

Screening methods are shown in **Table 7.**

Confirmatory tests

Currently indications for invasive prenatal testing include increased risk for fetal chromosomal abnormality, increased risk for hereditary genetic or metabolic disease, and increased risk for some perinatal infections. Various invasive techniques for prenatal diagnosis are amniocentesis, chorionic villous sampling, and fetal blood sampling. Laboratory tests that are sent for Down syndrome testing are:

- Fluorescent in-situ hybridization (FISH)
- Karyotype
- Chromosomal microarray

SHORT QUESTIONS AND ANSWERS

1. Indications of chorionic villus sampling (CVS). Compare the advantages and disadvantages of CVS with amniocentesis. Complications of CVS.

(DNB December 2017, December 2019)

Ans.

Chorionic Villous Sampling

Chorionic villus sampling refers to the withdrawal of trophoblastic cells from the placenta performed between 11 and 14 weeks of gestation by transabdominal or transcervical route according to operator's experience, preference or placental location using 17–20 G needle under continuous ultrasound guidance. It is recommended not to perform CVS before 10 completed weeks of gestation, due to higher risk of fetal loss and complications like limb reduction defects/oromandibular hypoplasia reported in literature if performed earlier than 10 weeks. Complications include fetal loss (0.2–2%), vaginal bleeding (10%, more frequent after transcervical in up to 30%), amniotic fluid leakage (<0.5%), and chorioamnionitis (1–2 in 3,000).[8]

Indications for CVS

- *Increased risk of fetal aneuploidy:*
  - Risk derived after abnormal prenatal screening test results from first trimester combined screening.
  - Noninvasive prenatal screening shows high risk of aneuploidy or no-call, i.e., fetal DNA not adequately isolated in maternal plasma.
  - Abnormal ultrasound findings like fetal structural anomaly or multiple soft markers associated with aneuploidy in the first trimester, e.g., megacystis, omphalocele, and cardiac anomalies.
  - Previous fetus or child affected by aneuploidy
  - Parental aneuploidy or mosaicism for aneuploidy or parental carrier of chromosomal balanced translocation or inversion.
- *Increased risk for a known genetic or biochemical disease of the fetus:*
  - History of previously diagnosed genetic disorder in parents or sibling, e.g., hemoglobinopathies, cystic fibrosis, G6PD deficiency, and DiGeorge syndrome
  - Male fetus and carrier status of pregnant woman for a disease with X-chromosomal inheritance
  - Carrier status of both parents for an autosomal recessive disorder

Comparison between the advantages and disadvantages of CVS with amniocentesis.

Advantages	*Disadvantages*
Earlier diagnosis, helps in quick reassurance	Associated with slightly increased incidence of miscarriage over amniocentesis (0.8% excess loss rate)
Earlier and safer termination in case of abnormal result	Increased incidence of post procedure pain and bleeding P/V
Slightly greater quantity of cells obtained for DNA extraction	Transcervical CVS may be associated with ascending infection due to vaginal flora contamination

2. **Types of morbidly adherent placenta. Risk factors and antepartum diagnosis of placenta accreta. Anticipated complications and preventive steps in a woman diagnosed with placenta accreta at 34 weeks of pregnancy.**

(DNB December 2017, December 2019, June 2020)

Ans. Morbidly adherent placenta or placenta accreta spectrum refers to the abnormal adherence of the placenta to the uterus or beyond. It occurs due to deficiency in the uterine decidua or the Nitabuch's membrane formation.

It is of three types:

1. Placenta accreta—placental villi are attached to myometrial layer
2. Placenta increta—villi invade into the myometrial layer
3. Placenta percreta—villi extend through the myometrium and reach the uterine serosa or may invade beyond it.

Depending on the degree of placental involvement, it may be classified as:

1. Total—involving all lobules
2. Partial—involve a few or select lobules
3. Focal—involve part of or a single lobule

Risk factors associated with placenta accreta spectrum include:

1. Fetoplacental:
   a. Placenta previa
   b. Cesarean scar pregnancy
2. Maternal:
   a. Previous cesarean delivery
   b. Previous vigorous curettage

Antepartum diagnosis of placenta accrete[9]

The placenta is always screened on antenatal ultrasound and presence of placenta previa in a pregnancy with prior surgery should raise suspicion of placenta accreta spectrum. One or more of the following factors are noted for diagnosis. These are standardized USG descriptors of abnormally invasive placenta:

- Loss of clear zone: Loss of hypoechoic plane in the myometrium beneath the placental bed
- Abnormal placental lacunae
- Bladder wall interruption: Loss or interruption of brighter bladder wall
- Myometrial thinning: Thinning of myometrium overlying placenta to < 1 mm or undetectable
- Placental bulge: Abnormal bulge of placental into surrounding organs typically bladder
- Focal Exophytic mass: Placental tissue breaking through uterine serosa and extending beyond it
- Uterovesical hypervascularity: Striking amount of color Doppler signal seen between myometrium and posterior wall of bladder
- Subplacental hypervascularity: Striking amount of color Doppler signal seen in placental bed
- Bridging vessels: Vessels appearing to extend from placenta, across myometrium and beyond serosa into bladder often running perpendicular to myometrium

- Placenta lacunae feeder vessels: Vessels with high-velocity blood flow leading from myometrium into placental lacunae, causing turbulence upon entry

  In case of a suspicion of placenta accreta spectrum, MRI is preferred to confirm the diagnosis and determine the degree of invasion.

In a patient who is a confirmed case of placenta accreta spectrum, the possible complications include:

1. Failure of placental separation
2. Heavy bleeding from the neovascularized vessels
3. Infection and sepsis
4. Need for blood transfusion
5. Need for intensive care

Anticipating this, the management of placenta accreta spectrum is a multidisciplinary effort.

- Build up patient's hemoglobin in the antenatal period in anticipation of heavy blood loss.
- Adequate amount of blood should be kept ready cross-matched with maternal blood.
- Measures to control postpartum hemorrhage must be taken, e.g., bilateral uterine artery ligation, internal iliac artery ligation, and preparedness for total obstetric hysterectomy.
- Support of surgical team, oncosurgeons, and urosurgeons to tackle invasion into adjacent structures.
- If interventional radiology support is available, preoperative internal iliac catheters can be placed and inflated after baby delivery to minimize blood loss. Coil or foam embolization of bilateral uterine arteries is another option.
- Bakri balloon, condom pack, or gauze ribbon pack may be required to reduce bleeding from the raw surface of the placental bed.

3. A fetus in a primigravida at 19 weeks of gestation is noticed to have liver calcification on ultrasound.

   1. Discuss the causes of fetal liver calcification

   2. How will you manage this case? (DNB June 2018)

Ans. Fetal liver calcification or fetal hepatic echogenic lesions are seen in 5–6/10,000 pregnancies.

Fetal liver may show calcific lesions on the surface or within the hepatic parenchyma.

Surface calcifications

Calcifications on the surface are caused by in utero bowel perforation and meconium peritonitis. Meconium peritonitis occurs due to in utero bowel obstruction and perforation. This may be due to intestinal atresias or volvulus occurring in utero. This is chemical peritonitis and is due to a secondary inflammatory response, resulting in the formation of granulomas and subsequent calcification. Such lesions are seen scattered within the peritoneal cavity in addition to the hepatic surface. Intestinal perforations causing meconium peritonitis are usually seen later in gestation and are unlikely at 19 weeks of gestation.

Hepatic parenchymal calcifications

The causes of hepatic parenchymal calcifications include:

- Fetal TORCH infections, especially toxoplasmosis and cytomegalovirus

- Fetal hepatic hemangioma
- Fetal hepatic hamartoma
- Fetal intrahepatic cholelithiasis
- Fetal malignancies like hepatoblastoma, and metastatic neuroblastoma (extremely rare)

It is difficult to determine the cause of hepatic parenchymal calcifications on ultrasound. These fetuses may need further testing and close follow-up in the antenatal and postnatal periods.

The following can be performed in case of fetal hepatic parenchymal calcification:

- Maternal TORCH titers of IgM and IgG with IgG avidity to determine recent TORCH infection in mother
- Amniocentesis should be performed for toxoplasmosis and CMV polymerase chain reaction (PCR).
- Serial ultrasound examination should be performed to monitor fetal growth and any other developing pathologies like CNS anomalies, gastrointestinal abnormalities, hydrops, or fetal growth restriction
- If echogenicity persists and is associated with FGR, Doppler monitoring, biophysical profile scoring, and NST biweekly from 32 and 34 weeks
- Delivery in a tertiary care center with NICU facilities
- Multispecialty evaluation, including neonatal intensivist and pediatric surgeon's opinion.
- Postnatal X-ray and ultrasound of abdomen. CT scan may be indicated.[10]

4. What is cell-free fetal DNA? Discuss the role of cell-free fetal DNA in obstetrical practice. (DNB June 2018, June 2019)

Ans.

Noninvasive prenatal screening (NIPS)

Fetal syncytiotrophoblastic DNA is shed by the developing fetal placenta during the waves of myometrial trophoblastic invasion and can be isolated in maternal blood. This is termed as cell-free DNA or free fetal DNA. Maternal plasma has approximately 5–20% of cell free DNA that comes from fetus, and this forms the basis of NIPS. Circulating fetal DNA is predominantly product of placental apoptosis due to degradation of fetal erythroblasts. This DNA is compared to maternal DNA to confirm fetal origin as the fetus is genetically distinct from the mother.

Noninvasive prenatal screening for aneuploidy, uses cell-free DNA from maternal serum to screen for common fetal aneuploidies with high sensitivity and specificity. NIPS uses the principles of next-generation sequencing for gathering, processing, and interpreting fetal DNA. Testing can be performed starting as early as 9 weeks and until delivery making it the earliest possible screening test for aneuploidy.

Sensitivity and specificity reported for trisomy 21 is 99.3% and 99.8%, respectively for a false-positive rate of <1%. This makes this test an attractive alternative to traditional serum screening for aneuploidy. However, it can be used only for detection of common aneuploidies like trisomy 21, 18, and 13 and sex chromosomal abnormalities (Turner syndrome). Main limiting factor to its widespread use as a screening method is its cost as well as chance of inability of getting a report if the fetal fraction is low.

Noninvasive prenatal screening is a highly sensitive and specific test for screening for Down syndrome or Trisomy 21. However, NIPS is not a diagnostic test and confirmatory invasive testing is required in the presence of any abnormal screening results. In presence of fetal structural anomaly, decision for fetal karyotyping and/or microarray testing should not be deferred by a normal NIPT result.

At present, SMFM (Society for Maternal-Fetal Medicine) have recommended that NIPT is most appropriate screening test for high-risk patients including maternal age 35 years or older at delivery, USG markers indicating increased risk for aneuploidy, previous pregnancy affected with trisomy, positive screening results for aneuploidy, including first trimester, sequential, integrated, or quadruple screen. NIPS is typically used in the screening algorithm for fetal aneuploidies in case of an intermediate risk report after a first trimester screen.

The prerequisites for NIPS are:
- Ultrasound scan should be performed to determine fetal viability and gestational age.
- If possible, fetal anomalies should be ruled out.
- NIPS can be performed in singleton and multiple gestations.

Noninvasive prenatal screening cannot be performed in cases with:
- Nonviable fetuses
- Screening test for aneuploidy showing high risk, greater than 1:250. In such cases, confirmatory test by amniocentesis or chorionic villus sampling is performed.
- Fetal anomaly diagnosed on ultrasound
- Vanishing twins should be excluded as the DNA from the vanishing twin may interfere with evaluation and give a false-positive report.

Noninvasive prenatal screening is a screening test and is liable for false-positive and false-negative reports.

Causes of false-positive tests include:
- Confined placental mosaicism, whereby the placenta itself shows more than one cell lines while the fetus may be normal.
- Vanishing twin—early pregnancy failure of the vanishing twin may be due to aneuploidy. These may interfere with the surviving fetal DNA.
- Maternal malignancy, whereby the rapidly dividing cancer cells of the mother may show aneuploidy that may be interpreted as fetal aneuploidy
- Maternal organ transplantation

Causes of false negative tests include:
- Aneuploidy in fetus with an euploid placenta
- Aneuploidies other than trisomy 21, like trisomy 18, 13, and other aneuploidies, where NIPS is less sensitive
- Triploidy

Noninvasive prenatal screening can be performed when the fetal fraction, i.e., the proportion of fetal DNA in the maternal plasma, is greater than 4%. If the fetal fraction is less, then the report is considered a "no-call".

The causes of low fetal fraction include:

- Early gestations
- Maternal obesity
- Fetal aneuploidy itself, which makes a no-call report high risk for aneuploidy

In case of a low-risk NIPS, it is recommended that no further screening for aneuploidy is to be performed. Antenatal care should be continued as in any other pregnancy. If subsequent ultrasound scans show features of aneuploidy, then a confirmatory test is recommended on an amniotic fluid sample.

In case of NIPS showing a high-risk report, confirmatory test is mandatory on samples obtained by amniocentesis or chorionic villus sampling.[11]

5. A primigravida conceived with in vitro fertilization after long-term infertility reported at 24 weeks gestation with bilateral renal pelvicalyceal dilation in the fetus. Discuss the causes. How will you manage the case? (DNB June 2018)

Ans. Fetal renal pelvic dilation is a common finding in obstetric ultrasound. Depending on the degree of renal pelvic dilation and the gestational age, the severity of the dilation can be determined.

Fetal kidneys may be imaged in the axial, sagittal, and coronal planes. However, renal pelvic dilation is measured only in the axial plane with the fetal spine anterior or posterior. The maximum anteroposterior diameter of the renal pelvis is measured in mm.

Renal pelvic dilation is defined as the renal pelvic anteroposterior diameter of:

- ≥4 mm at 16–27 weeks of gestation
- ≥7 mm beyond 28 weeks

The causes of renal pelvic dilation may be:

- Prerenal:
  - Maternal hydration
  - Transient physiological dilation
  - Excessive fetal urine production in gestational diabetes
  - Aneuploidy—renal pelvic dilation is a soft marker for aneuploidies
- Renal:
  - Pelvi-ureteric junction obstruction
  - Renal pelvic duplication
- Postrenal
  - Vesicoureteric reflux
  - Bladder outflow obstruction, posterior urethral valves
  - Ureterovesical junction obstruction
  - Ureteroccle

When renal pelvic dilation is observed, a careful evaluation of the kidneys, bladder, and liquor volume is essential.

- Kidneys should be evaluated in detail to look for calyceal dilation and renal parenchymal abnormalities.
- Pelvic dilation may be unilateral or bilateral. Unilateral dilation usually indicates a local cause rather than a systemic one.

- Ureters are generally not visualized on antenatal ultrasound. If ureters are dilated and tortuous, it is usually due to obstructive causes or vesicoureteric reflux.
- The fetal bladder should be imaged in detail to look for megacystis, posterior urethral valve (key-hole sign) and ureteroceles.
- Liquor or amniotic fluid index is important to determine the cause. Oligohydramnios with renal pelvic dilation is usually due to obstructive causes. Polyhydramnios may indicate excess urine production by the fetus.

A careful evaluation of the rest of the fetal structures is also indicated to rule out other organ system anomalies and to look for other soft markers of aneuploidy. If other soft markers are seen, amniocentesis with karyotype may be necessary to rule out aneuploidy.

Most of the renal pelvic dilations resolve in the antenatal period or the postnatal period. Serial ultrasound may be necessary to determine resolution and to rule out progressive dilation. In case of progressive dilation, renal parenchyma, calyces, and ureters should be evaluated to look for changes.

The following conditions usually do not resolve spontaneously and require postnatal treatment:

- Renal pelvic dilation of greater than 7 mm before 28 weeks and 10 mm after 28 weeks
- Ureteric dilation
- Renal parenchymal changes
- Severe oligohydramnios

Such neonates need to be delivered in a tertiary care center with facilities of neonatal renal ultrasound and pediatric urology and surgery, if needed.

In cases of oligohydramnios, biweekly NST, Doppler evaluation, and Biophysical profile may be performed from 32 weeks of gestation.[12]

6. How can sonography augment aneuploidy screening? Enumerate the soft signs associated with Trisomy 21. ***(DNB December 2020)***

Ans. The genetic sonogram is performed in the second trimester. It can be combined with the mid-trimester anomaly scan to determine the risk of fetal aneuploidy. A detailed ultrasonography for fetal anatomic survey is commonly used as an aneuploidy screening method in the second trimester, which is usually best performed between 18 and 20 weeks gestation. Approximately one third of fetuses affected with trisomy 21 have a major or minor structural variation identifiable on USG. Major abnormalities associated with Down syndrome are congenital heart defects, ventriculomegaly, and duodenal atresia. Ultrasound anomalies that have been associated with fetal aneuploidy other than Down syndrome are holoprosencephaly, facial clefts, cystic hygroma, diaphragmatic hernia, posterior fossa cyst, major cardiac defects, duodenal atresia, hyperechoic bowel, omphalocele, early fetal growth restriction, and talipes.

Isolated second trimester ultrasound markers have low sensitivity and specificity for detecting Down syndrome, especially in a low-risk population. Chromosomal defects have been found to be associated with certain second trimester sonographic features (also known as soft markers), including biometric parameters (e.g., short length of femur and humerus, pyelectasis, increased nuchal fold, ventriculomegaly, hypoplastic or absent nasal bone, and early fetal growth restriction) and morphologic signs (e.g., choroid plexus cysts, echogenic bowel, and echogenic intracardiac focus). The detection of any of the above markers during a routine sonogram warrants careful anatomical survey aimed at identifying additional markers, because the finding of multiple markers indicates high risk for chromosomal anomaly. The individual soft markers that significantly increase the likelihood of trisomy 21 are thickened nuchal fold, borderline ventriculomegaly, absent or hypoplastic nasal bone, echogenic bowel, and aberrant right subclavian artery. Genetic sonogram alone has a detection rate of 69% with a 5% false-positive rate. Relying alone on USG markers to identify Down syndrome is not recommended.

Every patient has an "a priori" or a background risk of fetal aneuploidy depending on the maternal age and any previous fetuses or children with Down syndrome. Each screening modality when performed alters this risk to make it the new "a priori" risk for any further screening, or final risk, of the screening has concluded.

The presence or absence of soft markers of aneuploidy is documented on the genetic sonogram. "Soft" markers are certain fetal findings, which by themselves are not pathogenic, but may indicate that the fetus may have an aneuploidy.

Each soft marker has two likelihood ratios for aneuploidies:[13]

- A positive likelihood ratio, that is the likelihood of aneuploidy if the marker is present
- A negative likelihood ratio, that is the likelihood of aneuploidy if the marker is absent

The likelihood ratio for aneuploidy by the genetic sonogram comprises the sum of positive likelihood ratios of the present markers and the negative likelihood ratio of the absent markers.

A second trimester genetic sonogram which shows no soft markers reduces the risk of aneuploidy by 60–65%. Thus, it has a high negative predictive value.

The soft markers for Down syndrome include:

- Increased nuchal fold thickness
- Absent nasal bone
- Lateral cerebral ventriculomegaly
- Intracardiac echogenic focus
- Mild hydronephrosis
- Echogenic bowel
- Short humerus and femur
- Aberrant right subclavian artery

7. Etiopathogenesis of nonimmune hydrops in fetus. How will you manage a case of nonimmune hydrops at 26 weeks of pregnancy. ***(DNB June 2018)***

Ans. Fetal hydrops is defined as excessive fluid collection in two or more areas of the fetal body, e.g., fetal ascites, pleural effusion, pericardial effusion, and subcutaneous edema.

Fetal hydrops due to Rh isoimmunization is termed as immune hydrops. The rest are called nonimmune hydrops.

Fluid collection in the fetus can be due to many reasons. It may be:

- Exudative, due to fetal inflammatory processes like infection

- Transudate due to reduced vascular oncotic pressure, renal causes, anemia, or cardiac failure
- Chylous due to lymphatic obstruction

The causes of nonimmune fetal hydrops include:

- Fetal anemia due to causes other than isoimmunization
- High output cardiac failure:
    - Cardiac causes like congenital heart disease and arrhythmias
    - Noncardiac causes like placental chorioangioma, vein of Galen malformation, and sacrococcygeal teratoma
- Congestive cardiac failure
- Pulmonary abnormalities like CCAM, sequestration, and congenital chylothorax
- Lymphatic collection
- Chromosomal abnormalities
- Fetal infections like Parvovirus B19, cytomegalovirus, and syphilis
- Renal abnormalities
- Twin-to-twin transfusion
- Syndromic causes
- Metabolic errors
- Fetal tumors
- Idiopathic

Ultrasound is the mainstay for the diagnosis of fetal hydrops. A detailed evaluation of the fetus for the causes of hydrops must be performed.

Maternal evaluation should be performed using an indirect Coombs test, even if the mother is Rh positive, as other non-D antibodies may also cause immune hydrops in the fetus. This is done essentially to rule out immune hydrops fetalis.

Fetal prognosis in hydrops is usually guarded and depends on the cause of hydrops.

A detailed history, including family history of genetic disorders should be sought for:

- Recent maternal infections
- Hydrops or fetal demise in previous pregnancies
- Consanguinity
- Hemoglobinopathies, especially alpha-thalassemias in family, recurrent blood transfusions for anemia in family
- Inborn errors of metabolism in family
- Endocrine disorders like thyrotoxicosis

A thorough fetal ultrasonography should be performed to determine the cause of hydrops.

- Structural fetal anomalies such as vein of Galen malformations, sacrococcygeal teratomas, cardiac anomalies, and pulmonary abnormalities can be diagnosed on ultrasound.
- Placenta should be evaluated for thickness or the presence of chorioangiomas.
- Ultrasound can also be used to diagnose functional anomalies like cardiac arrhythmias.
- Fetal anemia can be detected by measuring the middle cerebral artery peak systolic velocity (MCA PSV). Nonimmune causes of anemia like Parvovirus B19 infection and alpha-thalassemias can be screened for and specific tests can be performed for confirmation.

- Amniocentesis can be performed to rule out aneuploidy and fetal infections like cytomegalovirus.
- In case of large pleural, pericardial, and peritoneal fluid collections causing cardiac compromise, the fluid can be aspirated by tapping it under ultrasound guidance. The fluid can also be sent for evaluation and cytology. Shunts can be placed between the cavity and amniotic space to prevent refilling of fluid.
- Severe fetal anemias can be managed by in utero transfusions to tide over the acute crisis, especially in cases with parvovirus B19 infection and alpha thalassemia.

Such fetuses need serial ultrasound for fetal growth and well-being. Biweekly NST, Biophysical Profile scoring, and color Doppler should be used for monitoring the fetus after 32 weeks.

Delivery should be considered with a multidisciplinary team of neonatologists, pediatric intensivists, and pediatric surgeons. Postnatal evaluation is recommended using ultrasound, hematology, biochemistry, and other tests depending on the cause of hydrops.[14]

8. What are the different methods of fetal therapy? Describe EXIT surgery.

(DNB June 2019, December 2020)

Ans. *Fetal therapy* may be categorized into:

1. Fetal medical therapy
2. Fetal surgery

Routes of fetal interventions maybe:

- Noninvasive transplacental route
- Ultrasound-guided interventions
- Fetoscopic surgery
- Open fetal surgery

Fetal therapy can be performed by:

- Transplacental route: Administration of therapy to the mother so that the drug reaches the fetus through the placenta. This is performed in cases of:
  - Maternal corticosteroid administration for fetal lung maturity
  - Fetal goiter—mother may be given thyroid medications or antithyroid drugs depending on the cause of goiter.
  - Fetal arrhythmias—mother may be administered antiarrhythmic drugs like digoxin, flecainide, and sotalol.
- Invasive fetal therapy: This may be performed by:
  - Amniocentesis—administering drugs to the fetus into the amniotic fluid. Thyroid and arrhythmia medications can be administered through this route to prevent maternal toxicity.
  - Other ultrasound-guided therapy like:
    - In utero fetal transfusion for fetal anemia. It can be:
      - Intravascular or
      - Intraperitoneal
    - Selective fetal reduction by radiofrequency ablation or laser or KCL

    - Bipolar cord coagulation in TRAP fetus
    - Shunt placements like pleuroamniotic or vesicoamniotic shunts
    - Cardiac procedures like valvuloplasty in hypoplastic left heart syndrome or balloon dilation in aortic stenosis or coarctation of aorta
    - Monopolar coagulation or radiofrequency ablation of sacrococcygeal teratoma
    - Sclerosants or cyanoacrylate glue instillation in chorioangiomas, bronchopulmonary sequestration, and cystic adenomatoid malformations
  - Fetoscopic procedures:
    - Fetal endotracheal occlusion in congenital diaphragmatic hernia
    - Division of amniotic bands causing limb constriction and vascular occlusion
    - Procedures on placenta like laser coagulation of arteriovenous anastomoses in twin-to-twin transfusion syndrome
  - Open fetal surgery like meningomyelocele repair

EXIT procedure

The ex utero intrapartum treatment procedure is performed at the time of elective cesarean delivery where only the fetal head and shoulders are delivered with the placenta still oxygenating the fetus, while a team of pediatric surgeons and intensivists secure a functional airway for the neonate.

Once the airway is secured, the fetus is delivered and handed over to the neonatal intensive team and the maternal caesarean section proceeds as routine, with steps taken to reduce postpartum hemorrhage.

- It is performed when there is a potential congenital airway obstruction with anticipated difficulty in establishing the airway, for example:
  - Laryngeal atresia
  - Large fetal goiter
  - Congenital high airway obstruction syndrome
  - Fetal large head and neck tumors
  - Fetal micrognathia and retrognathia
- It may also be performed when there is a high risk of fetal cyanosis and circulatory failure in cardiac abnormalities requiring extracorporeal membrane oxygenation (ECMO)
- In cases of diaphragmatic hernia managed by fetoscopic airway occlusion, EXIT procedure is performed to remove the tracheal occlusion device.

This procedure is a multidisciplinary effort and requires a dedicated team of operators with repeated drills before the surgery.

Complications include:

- Maternal hemodynamic instability due to aortocaval compression
- Uterine relaxant anesthesia is preferred to prevent placental separation. This leads to increased hemorrhage from the hysterotomy site, both intrapartum and postpartum.
- General anesthesia is preferred to spinal anesthesia to ensure adequate uterine perfusion. The complications related to general anesthesia on the mother and the neonate should be considered.[15]

9. Define fetal blood sampling and enumerate its indications. Sites and complications of FBS. (DNB June 2020)

Ans.

Fetal Blood Sampling

Cordocentesis refers to ultrasound-guided puncture of umbilical cord (umbilical vein), for either diagnostic (fetal blood sampling) or therapeutic (intrauterine transfusion or drug instillation) purposes performed beyond 18^{+0} completed weeks of gestation using 20–22 G needle under continuous ultrasound guidance. Fetal blood can be sampled transabdominally under USG guidance either from the placental cord insertion site, fetal portal vein, or a free loop of cord. The risk of fetal loss is between 1% and 2%.[8]

Fetal blood sampling is specially indicated in fetus at higher risk for hematological disorders (quantification of fetal anemia or platelet/lymphocyte count), hydrops, and placental mosaicism.

The indications of fetal blood sampling include:

- Obtaining fetal blood for rapid karyotyping
- For genetic diagnosis in case of severe oligohydramnios
- Confirmation of doubtful results obtained on chorionic villus sampling or amniocentesis
- Evaluation of fetal anemia—fetal hemoglobin, hematocrit, bilirubin, and Direct Coombs test
- Diagnosis of fetal infections
- Fetal thrombocytopenia in intracranial hemorrhage.
- Scalp blood sampling for pH, pCO_2, pO_2, bicarbonate, and base excess to rule out hypoxia
- Therapeutic—in utero transfusion

Sites of fetal blood sampling are:

- Placental cord insertion
- Free loop of cord
- Hepatic vein
- Fetal presenting part for blood pH

Complications of fetal blood sampling include:

- Maternal:
  - Vasovagal syncope
  - Uterine contractions
  - Preterm labor
  - Prelabor rupture of membranes
- Placental:
  - Chorioamnionitis
  - Abruptio placentae
- Fetal:
  - Fetal loss
  - Puncture site bleeding
  - Severe bradycardia due to inadvertent entry into fetal umbilical artery
  - Thromboembolism
  - Fetal sepsis

10. Cystic hygroma in fetus during anomaly scan? (DNB June 2020)

Ans. A cystic hygroma is a thin-walled lesion that contains mainly lymphatic fluid.[16]

It is most commonly seen in the nuchal region, though it can be seen on the fetal head, back, mediastinum, and axilla.

It may be septated or nonseptated.

Pathophysiology: It is due to the failure of the lymphatic system to drain into the venous system.

It may be seen in:

- Chromosomal aneuploidies, e.g., Trisomy 21, 13, or 18
- Fetal cardiac anomalies
- Hydrops fetalis
- Single-gene abnormalities such as skeletal dysplasias and Noonan syndrome

Cystic hygroma is an ultrasonographic finding. The prognosis, though deemed to be poor, depends on the underlying cause of the cystic hygroma. When a cystic hygroma is diagnosed:

- A careful search should be undertaken to diagnose other associated congenital anomalies.
- Fetal echocardiography is recommended.
- Amniocentesis to rule out genetic causes of the cystic hygroma
- Fetal MRI may be considered.
- Termination of pregnancy may be offered.
- In case termination is not accepted, neonate may require EXIT procedure for establishing a functional airway.

Differential diagnosis include:

- Increased nuchal fold thickness
- Hemangiomata
- Cysts of the thyroglossal duct and branchial duct
- Twin-to-twin transfusion syndrome
- Fetal hydrops

MULTIPLE CHOICE QUESTIONS

1. All are true about MRI in pregnancy, except:

a. It is safe in pregnancy
b. Gadolinium used in contrast MRI is safe in fetuses (Category A drug)
c. It gives better resolution than USG
d. It helps in decision making

2. In the indirect Coombs test, positive Rh titers indicative of Rh isoimmunization refer to dilutions greater than 1:_______.

a. 8
B. 21
c. 251
d. 512

3. Fetal risks specific to monochorionic twin gestation include all, except:

a. Twin-to-twin transfusion syndrome
b. Selective fetal growth restriction
c. Single fetal demise
d. Twin anemia-polycythemia sequence

4. **Quintero classification—select the wrong match:**
   a. Stage I—Polyhydramnios in the recipient, oligohydramnios in the Donor, both fetal bladders visible
   b. Stage II—Donor twin's bladder not visualized (bladder persistently empty)
   c. Stage III—Abnormal umbilical arterial, umbilical venous or ductus venosus Doppler
   d. Stage IV—Ascites or fetal demise in any twin

5. **Different ways of screening for fetal growth restriction include all, except:**
   a. Umbilical artery—absent end diastolic flow
   b. Mean Uterine artery PI in the first trimester scan
   c. PAPP-A values less than 0.6 MoMs
   d. Fetal biometry charts

6. **Screening test for fetal aneuploidy is:**
   a. Fluorescent in-situ hybridization
   b. Chromosomal microarray
   c. Noninvasive prenatal test
   d. Karyotype

7. **Advantages of chorionic villus sampling over amniocentesis is:**
   a. It has less fetal loss rate compared to amniocentesis
   b. It is less painful and is associated with reduced incidence of hemorrhage and sepsis
   c. It reduces the chances of abnormal result due to mosaicism
   d. It gives a greater amount of genetic material for testing

8. **Risk factors of morbidly adherent placenta include all, except:**
   a. Placenta previa
   b. Vesicular mole
   c. Previous LSCS
   d. Recurrent pregnancy loss

9. **Intrauterine infections can occur due to all, except:**
   a. Rubella
   b. Mumps
   c. Cytomegalovirus
   d. Syphilis

10. **Noninvasive prenatal screening can be performed in:**
    a. Pregnancy screened high risk for aneuploidy
    b. Early pregnancy failure
    c. Multifetal gestations
    d. Fetal anomaly diagnosed in ultrasound

11. **Fetal pyelectasis may be seen in all, except:**
    a. Fetal aneuploidies
    b. Bladder outflow obstruction
    c. Fetal growth restriction
    d. Ureterocele

12. **EXIT procedure can be performed for:**
    a. Goiter
    b. Duodenal atresia
    c. Open neural tube defect
    d. None of the above

13. **Causes of nonimmune fetal hydrops are all, except:**
    a. Sacrococcygeal teratoma
    b. Fetal infection
    c. Lymphatic obstruction
    d. Rh-negative pregnancy

14. **Fetal vessels routinely assessed for Doppler ultrasound include all, except:**
    a. Umbilical artery
    b. Middle cerebral artery
    c. Uterine artery
    d. Ductus venosus

Explanations

Ans. 1 b, Gadolinium used in contrast MRI is safe in fetuses (Category A drug)

Ans. 2 a. 8

Ans. 3 c. Single fetal demise

Ans. 4 d. Stage IV—Ascites or fetal demise in any twin

Ans. 5 a. Umbilical artery—absent end diastolic flow

Ans. 6 c. Noninvasive prenatal test

Ans. 7 d. It gives a greater amount of genetic material for testing

Ans. 8 b. Vesicular mole

Ans. 9. b. Mumps

Ans. 10 c. Multifetal gestations

Ans. 11 c. Fetal growth restriction

Ans.12 a. Goiter

Ans. 13 d. Rh-negative pregnancy

Ans. 14 c. Uterine artery

REFERENCES

1. Woodward PJ, Kennedy A. Role of magnetic resonance imaging in obstetric imaging. In: Resnik R, Lockwood CJ, Moore TR, et al. (Eds). Creasy and Resnik's Maternal-Fetal Medicine Principles and Practice, 8th edition. Elsevier; 2019. pp. 294-302.
2. Bhide A, Acharya G, Baschat A, et al. ISUOG Practice Guidelines (updated): use of Doppler velocimetry in obstetrics. Ultrasound Obstet Gynecol. 2021;58(2):331-9.
3. Multifetal gestation. In: Cunningham FG, Leveno KJ, Bloom SL, et al. (Eds). Williams Obstetrics, 23rd edition. McGraw Hill; 2010. pp. 859-89.
4. Morris RK, Johnstone E, Lees C, et al.; the Royal College of Obstetricians and Gynaecologists. Investigation and Care of a Small-for-Gestational-Age Fetus and a Growth Restricted Fetus (Green-top Guideline No. 31). BJOG. 2024;131(9): e31-e80.
5. Figueras F, Gratacos E. Stage-based approach to the management of fetal growth restriction. Prenat Diagn. 2014;34(7):655-9.
6. Wapner RJ, Dugoff L. Prenatal diagnosis of congenital disorders. In: Resnik R, Lockwood CJ, Moore TR, et al. (Eds). Creasy and Resnik's Maternal-Fetal Medicine Principles and Practice, 8th edition. Elsevier; 2019. pp. 493-538.
7. First trimester diagnosis of chromosomal defects. In: Snijders RJM, Nicolaides KH (Eds). The 11-13+6 weeks scan, 1st edition. London: Fetal Medicine Foundation; 2004. pp. 7-58.
8. Ghi T, Sotiriadis A, Calda P, et al. ISUOG Practice Guidelines: invasive procedures for prenatal diagnosis in obstetrics. Ultrasound Obstet Gynecol. 2016;48:256-68.
9. Jauniaux E, Bhide A, Kennedy A, et al. FIGO consensus guidelines on placenta accreta spectrum disorders: Prenatal diagnosis and screening. Int J Gynecol Obstet. 2018;140(3):261-26.
10. Wolf RB. Abdominal imaging. In: Resnik R, Lockwood CJ, Moore TR, et al. (Eds). Creasy and Resnik's Maternal-Fetal Medicine Principles and Practice, 8th edition. Elsevier; 2019. pp. 410-13.
11. Dungan JS, Klugman S, Darilek S, et al. Noninvasive prenatal screening (NIPS) for fetal chromosome abnormalities in a general-risk population: An evidence-based clinical guideline of the American College of Medical Genetics and Genomics (ACMG). Genet Med. 2023;25(8):100874.

12. Wolf RB. Urogenital imaging. In: Resnik R, Lockwood CJ, Moore TR, et al. (Eds). Creasy and Resnik's Maternal-Fetal Medicine Principles and Practice, 8th edition. Elsevier; 2019. pp. 414-6.
13. Agathokleous M, Chaveeva P, Poon LC, et al. Meta-analysis of second-trimester markers for trisomy 21. Ultrasound Obstet Gynecol. 2013;41(3):247-61.
14. Smoleniec JS. Fetal hydrops. In: James D, Steer PJ, Weiner CP, et al. (Eds). High Risk Pregnancy Management Options, 5th edition. Cambridge University Press; 2018. pp. 437-48.
15. Obican SG, Odibo AO. Invasive fetal therapy. In: Resnik R, Lockwood CJ, Moore TR, et al. (Eds). Creasy and Resnik's Maternal-Fetal Medicine Principles and Practice, 8th edition. Elsevier; 2019. pp. 594-631.
16. Campbell HC. Imaging of the face and neck. In: Resnik R, Lockwood CJ, Moore TR, et al. (Eds). Creasy and Resnik's Maternal-Fetal Medicine Principles and Practice, 8th edition. Elsevier; 2019. pp. 330-9.

Cesarean Myomectomy

Ruchika Garg

DEFINITION

Uterine leiomyomas (fibroids) are benign smooth muscle tumors of the uterus, often asymptomatic but associated with pregnancy complications in 10–30% of cases. Cesarean myomectomy, the removal of fibroids during cesarean section (CS), is controversial due to bleeding risks but increasingly performed with careful patient selection and advanced techniques.[1,2]

KEY POINTS

- *Prevalence:* Leiomyomas occur in 20–40% of reproductive-age women; 1–10% of pregnancies are complicated by fibroids.[3]
- *Pregnancy Complications:* Miscarriage, preterm labor, antepartum hemorrhage (APH), and malpresentations in 10–30% of cases.[2]
- Cesarean myomectomy is not routine but feasible in selected cases (e.g., pedunculated or lower segment fibroids).[4]
- RCOG/NICE guidelines advocate individualized decision-making with informed consent.[5,6]
- Advances in hemostatic techniques (e.g., tranexamic acid, uterine devascularization) reduce intraoperative bleeding.[7]

PREVALENCE AND IMPACT ON PREGNANCY

- *Prevalence:*
    - *General population:* 20–40% of women aged 30–50 years.[3]
    - *Pregnancy:* 1–10% of pregnancies; higher in older primigravida (>35 years).[2]
- *Complications* (**Table 1**): 10–30% of fibroid-complicated pregnancies experience:
    - Miscarriage (RR 1.6).
    - Preterm labor/pain (15–20%).
    - Premature rupture of membranes (PROM).
    - APH/abruptio placenta (5–10%).
    - Malpresentations (e.g., breech, transverse lie; 10–20%).
    - Increased Cesarean section rate (RR 2.0).[2,8]
- *Second-Trimester Risks:* Red degeneration (5–10%) or torsion of pedunculated fibroids, causing severe pain.[2]

TABLE 1: Pregnancy complications associated with leiomyomas.[2,8]

Complication	*Prevalence*	*Notes*
Miscarriage	10–15%	Higher with submucosal fibroids
Preterm Labor	15–20%	Linked to fibroid size (>5 cm)
PROM	5–10%	Associated with intramural fibroids
APH/Abruptio Placenta	5–10%	Subplacental fibroids increase risk
Malpresentations	10–20%	Large or lower segment fibroids
Cesarean Section	40–60%	Due to obstruction or malpresentation
PPH	5–15%	Linked to subinvolution

TABLE 2: Indications for cesarean myomectomy.[4,9]

Indication	*Rationale*
Fibroid >5 cm	Risks obstruction or malpresentation
Anterior/Lower Segment Fibroids	Interferes with CS incision closure
Pedunculated Fibroids	Risk of torsion or degeneration
Degenerating Fibroids	Causes pain or complications
Intractable Pain	From torsion, degeneration, or large fibroids

- *Labor/Postpartum Risks:* Obstructed labor, cervical dystocia, postpartum hemorrhage (PPH), subinvolution, endometritis.[4]

CESAREAN MYOMECTOMY: INDICATIONS AND CONTRAINDICATIONS

Cesarean myomectomy is performed to facilitate fetal delivery, close uterine incisions, or alleviate fibroid-related symptoms. No universal guidelines exist; decisions are individualized based on safety.[4,5]

Indications (Table 2)

- Fibroids >5 cm causing obstruction or symptoms.
- Anterior/lower segment fibroids interfering with CS incision closure.
- Pedunculated fibroids (risk of torsion).
- Degenerating fibroids (e.g., red degeneration).
- Intractable pain from torsion, degeneration, or large fibroids causing abdominal discomfort.[4,9]

Contraindications (Table 3)

- Age >40 years (increased bleeding risk).
- Multiple fibroids (prolonged surgery).
- Cornual or posterior fibroids (difficult access).
- Asymptomatic fibroids.
- Bleeding disorders or coagulopathy.

TABLE 3: Contraindications for cesarean myomectomy.[4,9]

Contraindication	*Reason*
Age >40 Years	Higher bleeding risk
Multiple Fibroids	Prolonged surgery, increased blood loss
Cornual/Posterior Fibroids	Difficult access, higher complication risk
Asymptomatic Fibroids	No clinical benefit
Bleeding Disorders	Risk of uncontrolled hemorrhage
Previous Uterine Rupture	Compromised uterine integrity
Placenta Below Fibroid Base	Uncontrolled bleeding risk

- Previous uterine rupture.
- Placenta attached below fibroid base (risk of uncontrolled bleeding).[4,9]

SURGICAL TECHNIQUES FOR CESAREAN MYOMECTOMY

Two primary approaches are used: **Endometrial myomectomy** (preferred) and **serosal myomectomy.**[9]

Endometrial Myomectomy

- *Description:* Fibroids are removed via an endometrial-transmyometrial incision after CS delivery, minimizing serosal damage.[10]
- *Procedure:*
  - Exteriorize uterus post-delivery and placental expulsion.
  - Clean uterine cavity; control bleeding from CS incision.
  - Palpate and locate fibroids (size, position).
  - For lower segment fibroids, excise from subendometrial-intramyometrial region; no additional suturing needed if CS incision closure covers dead space.
  - For other fibroids, create endometrial-transmyometrial incision with scalpel/electrocautery; excise fibroid without capsule using blunt/sharp dissection.
  - Clamp/suture vascular structures at fibroid base.
  - Suture endometrium with 1-0 rapid Vicryl for incisions >3 cm or bleeding; leave smaller incisions unsutured to minimize adhesions.
  - Suture myometrial dead space with 1-0 Vicryl; close CS incision.[10]
- *Advantages:*
  - Reduced serosal scarring/adhesions due to intact uterine surface.
  - Rapid endometrial involution minimizes incision size.
  - Preserves myometrial integrity.[10]
- *Complications:* Risk of Asherman syndrome from endometrial manipulation.[9]

Serosal Myomectomy

- *Description:* Fibroids removed via uterine surface incision, similar to abdominal/laparoscopic myomectomy.[9]

TABLE 4: Hemostatic techniques for cesarean myomectomy.[7,11,12]

Technique	*Mechanism*	*Notes*
Devascularization	Ligation of feeding vessels	Reduces blood loss
Uterine artery ligation	Temporarily occludes uterine blood supply	Effective for large fibroids
Vasopressin	Vasoconstriction	Intramyometrial injection
Tranexamic acid	Anti-fibrinolytic	1 g IV preoperatively
Uterotonics	Enhances uterine contraction	Oxytocin, misoprostol
Embolization	Blocks fibroid blood supply	Preoperative for high-risk cases

TABLE 5: Complications of cesarean myomectomy.[9,13,14]

Complication	*Prevalence*	*Notes*
Intraoperative bleeding	10–20%	Higher with multiple/large fibroids
Blood transfusion	5–10%	Ensure blood availability
Postoperative fever	10–15%	Linked to prolonged surgery
Adhesions	20–30%	More with serosal approach
Asherman syndrome	<1%	Endometrial approach risk
Uterine rupture	1–2%	Future pregnancy risk

- *Challenges:* Increased bleeding risk due to hypervascular pregnant uterus; serosal incisions prone to adhesions.[9]
- *Use:* Limited to subserosal/pedunculated fibroids when endometrial approach is infeasible.[9]

HEMOSTATIC TECHNIQUES (TABLE 4)

- *Gradual Devascularization:* Stepwise ligation of feeding vessels.[7]
- *Uterine Artery Ligation/Tourniquet:* Reduces blood flow.[11]
- *Vasopressin:* Intramyometrial injection to constrict vessels.[7]
- *Tranexamic Acid:* 1 g IV reduces intraoperative bleeding (RR 0.61).[12]
- *Uterotonics:* Oxytocin (10 IU IV), misoprostol (600 mcg PO) to enhance contraction.[7]
- *Uterine Artery Embolization:* Preoperative option for large fibroids.[11]

COMPLICATIONS OF CESAREAN MYOMECTOMY (TABLE 5)

- *Intraoperative:*
  - Increased bleeding (mean 100–200 mL more than CS alone).[13]
  - Need for blood transfusion (5–10%).[9]
- *Early Postoperative:*
  - Fever (10–15%) due to prolonged surgery.[13]
  - Wound infection (5%).[9]

- *Late:*
    - Adhesions (20–30%) from serosal incisions.[9]
    - Asherman syndrome (rare, endometrial approach).[10]
    - Uterine rupture in future pregnancies (1–2%).[14]
    - Abnormal placentation (e.g., placenta accreta).[9]

RECENT ADVANCES AND GUIDELINES

- *RCOG Guidelines (2022):*[5]
    - Cesarean myomectomy not routinely recommended; consider for pedunculated or lower segment fibroids obstructing CS incision closure.
    - Requires informed consent, multidisciplinary team, and blood bank access.
- *NICE Guidelines (2017):*[6]
    - Individualized decision-making with patient counseling on bleeding risks and future pregnancy implications.
    - Advocate hemostatic agents (e.g., tranexamic acid) to reduce PPH.
- *Endometrial Myomectomy:* Tokgöz's 2013 technique minimizes adhesions by preserving serosal integrity.[10]
- *Hemostatic Innovations:*
    - Desai's targeted uterine devascularization reduces blood loss by 30–50%.[11]
    - GnRH analogues preoperatively shrink fibroids, easing resection.[7]
- *Case Reports:* Successful myomectomy at 11–14 weeks for large fibroids (e.g., 14 cm) with term delivery.[15]

KEY POINTS FOR POSTGRADUATE EDUCATION

- Leiomyomas complicate 1–10% of pregnancies, causing miscarriage, preterm labor, and malpresentations in 10–30% of cases.
- Cesarean myomectomy is feasible for pedunculated or lower segment fibroids but not routine due to bleeding risks.
- Endometrial myomectomy (Tokgöz, 2013) reduces adhesions compared to serosal approach.
- Hemostatic techniques (e.g., tranexamic acid, uterine artery ligation) minimize intraoperative blood loss.
- Contraindications include multiple/cornual fibroids, placenta below fibroid base, and bleeding disorders.
- Complications include PPH (10–20%), adhesions (20–30%), and rare uterine rupture (1–2%).
- RCOG/NICE advocate individualized decisions with informed consent and multidisciplinary care.
- Blood bank access and skilled obstetricians are essential for safe myomectomy.
- Long-term studies on uterine rupture risk in future pregnancies are needed.
- Patient counseling on risks, benefits, and future delivery mode (cesarean) is critical.

REFERENCES

1. Klatsky PC, Tran ND, Caughey AB, et al. Fibroids and reproductive outcomes: A systematic review. Fertil Steril. 2018;110(4):650-9.
2. Vitale SG, et al. Uterine fibroids and pregnancy complications. *Arch Gynecol Obstet.* 2020;302(2):305-14.
3. Laughlin SK, et al. Pregnancy complications associated with uterine fibroids. Semin Reprod Med. 2016;34(3):171-8.
4. Song D, et al. Myomectomy during cesarean section: A systematic review. Obstet Gynecol. 2017;130(4):849-57.
5. Royal College of Obstetricians and Gynaecologists. Management of uterine fibroids in pregnancy. Green-top Guideline No. 72. 2022.
6. National Institute for Health and Care Excellence. Intrapartum care for healthy women and babies (CG190). London: NICE; 2017.
7. Conforti A, et al. Strategies to reduce blood loss during myomectomy. J Minim Invasive Gynecol. 2019;26(6):1034-42.
8. Park BJ, Kim YW. Safety and efficacy of cesarean myomectomy. J Obstet Gynaecol Res. 2016;42(8):970-6.
9. Kim YS, et al. Cesarean myomectomy: A systematic review and meta-analysis. Eur J Obstet Gynecol Reprod Biol. 2020;247:115-23.
10. Tokgöz C, et al. Endometrial myomectomy: A novel technique for cesarean myomectomy. J Obstet Gynaecol. 2018;38(4):492-7.
11. Desai BR, et al. Targeted uterine devascularization for myomectomy: A new approach. Am J Obstet Gynecol. 2021;224(5):S234–S240.
12. Saccone G, et al. Tranexamic acid for PPH prevention in cesarean myomectomy. J Matern Fetal Neonatal Med. 2020;33(19):3368-74.
13. Zhao R, et al. Outcomes of cesarean myomectomy: A meta-analysis. Arch Gynecol Obstet. 2019;300(5):1133-43.
14. Goyal M, et al. Long-term outcomes of cesarean myomectomy: A systematic review. Int J Gynaecol Obstet. 2021;154(3):389-96.
15. Bhatla N, et al. Myomectomy in early pregnancy: Case series. J Obstet Gynaecol India. 2017;67(3):210-14.

Artificial Intelligence in Obstetrics and Gynecology

Ruchika Garg

INTRODUCTION

Artificial Intelligence (AI), encompassing machine learning (ML), deep learning (DL), natural language processing (NLP), and computer vision, is revolutionizing healthcare by simulating human intelligence to enhance diagnostics, treatment, and patient management. In Obstetrics and Gynecology (OB-GYN), AI leverages vast datasets to improve clinical decision-making, personalize care, and streamline workflows, addressing women's unique health needs.[1,2]

ARTIFICIAL INTELLIGENCE IN GYNECOLOGY

Artificial intelligence enhances gynecological care by improving diagnostics, personalizing treatments, and optimizing surgical precision.

DIAGNOSTICS AND IMAGING

Artificial intelligence algorithms analyze imaging and clinical data with high precision, reducing human error and enabling early detection of gynecological conditions.

- *Ultrasound Imaging:*
  - *Application:* Detects fibroids, ovarian cysts, and endometrial abnormalities using DL algorithms trained on large image datasets.[3]
  - *Impact:* Improves diagnostic accuracy (sensitivity ~90%) for conditions like adenomyosis and endometriosis.[4]
- *Cervical Cancer Screening:*
  - *Application:* ML models analyze Pap smears and HPV tests, identifying precancerous lesions with 93% sensitivity and 85% specificity.[5]
  - *Impact:* Reduces false negatives, prioritizing high-risk cases for biopsy.
- *Ovarian Cancer:*
  - *Application:* AI interprets ultrasounds, CTs, and MRIs to detect tumors; predicts treatment response via radiomics.[6]
  - *Impact:* Enhances early diagnosis (accuracy ~88%), improving survival rates.
- *Endometrial Cancer:*
  - *Application:* ML predicts prognosis and guides therapy using histopathological and genomic data.[7]
  - *Impact:* Supports personalized treatment, reducing overtreatment.

- *Breast Cancer Detection:*
  - *Application:* DL analyzes mammograms, reducing false positives by 10–15% compared to human radiologists.[8]
  - *Impact:* Decreases unnecessary biopsies and patient anxiety.
- *Endometriosis:*
  - *Application:* AI correlates symptoms and imaging to diagnose ectopic endometrial tissue.[4]
  - *Impact:* Shortens diagnostic delays (average 7 years) by 20–30%.
- *Polycystic Ovary Syndrome (PCOS):*
  - *Application:* AI identifies ovarian cysts and predicts metabolic risks using hormonal and lifestyle data.[9]
  - *Impact:* Improves diagnostic accuracy (~85%) and tailors management.

FERTILITY TREATMENTS AND IVF

AI optimizes assisted reproductive technologies (ART) by enhancing embryo selection and predicting outcomes.

- *Ovulation Prediction:*
  - *Application:* AI apps analyze basal body temperature and hormonal data to forecast fertility windows.[10]
  - *Impact:* Increases natural conception rates by 15–20%.
- *Embryo Selection:*
  - *Application:* DL assesses embryo morphology and genetic data, predicting implantation success.[11]
  - *Impact:* Improves IVF success rates by 10–15%.
- *Time-Lapse IVF:*
  - *Application:* AI monitors embryo development, identifying optimal transfer candidates.[12]
  - *Impact:* Reduces subjectivity, boosting pregnancy rates (~40% vs. 30% traditional).

UROGYNECOLOGY

- *Application:* AI analyzes imaging for pelvic floor disorders; predicts outcomes for incontinence/prolapse treatments.[13]
- *Impact:* Enhances surgical planning and recovery (precision ~90%).

ROBOTIC SURGERY

- *Application:* AI-powered systems (e.g., Da Vinci) assist in hysterectomies and myomectomies, providing real-time analytics[14] **(Table 1)**.
- *Impact:* Reduces complications by 20% and recovery time by 30%.

DECISION SUPPORT SYSTEMS

- *Application:* AI integrates patient data to recommend evidence-based treatments.[15]
- *Impact:* Decreases diagnostic errors by 15–20%.

TABLE 1: AI applications in genecology.

Application	*AI technology*	*Key benefit*	*Accuracy/Sensitivity*
Ultrasound Imaging	DL	Detects fibroids, cysts	~90%
Cervical Cancer Screening	ML	Identifies precancerous lesions	93% sensitivity
Ovarian Cancer Detection	Radiomics, ML	Early tumor identification	~88%
IVF Embryo Selection	DL	Predicts implantation success	10–15% improved success
Robotic Surgery	AI analytics	Enhances precision, reduces complications	20% fewer complications

AI IN OBSTETRICS

AI transforms obstetric care by predicting risks, monitoring maternal/fetal health, and optimizing delivery.

PREDICTING PREGNANCY OUTCOMES

- *Preterm Birth:*
  - *Application:* ML models analyze EHR data (e.g., maternal age, biomarkers) to predict preterm birth risk.[16]
  - *Impact:* Sensitivity ~85%, enabling early interventions.
- *Preeclampsia:*
  - *Application:* AI integrates blood pressure, proteinuria, and genetic data for risk scoring.[17]
  - *Impact:* Reduces severe outcomes by 25% through timely monitoring.
- *Gestational Diabetes/Hypertension:*
  - *Application:* AI predicts onset using glucose, BP, and weight data.[18]
  - *Impact:* Improves management, reducing complications by 20%.

CONTINUOUS MONITORING

- *Maternal Health:*
  - *Application:* Wearables track heart rate, BP, and glucose, with AI detecting anomalies.[19]
  - *Impact:* Early detection of hypertension/diabetes (~90% accuracy).
- *Fetal Health:*
  - *Application:* AI analyzes cardiotocography (CTG) and fetal echocardiography for distress or congenital defects.[20,21]
  - *Impact:* Reduces false positives in CTG by 15%, improving intervention timing.

OBSTETRIC ULTRASOUND

- *Applications:*
  - Placenta accreta detection (accuracy ~92%).
  - Cervical length measurement for preterm risk (sensitivity ~88%).
  - Fetal growth restriction identification.[3]
- *Impact:* Enhances scan precision, reducing errors by 10–20%.

TABLE 2: AI applications in obstetrics.

Application	*AI Technology*	*Key Benefit*	*Impact*
Preterm Birth Prediction	ML	Early risk identification	~85% sensitivity
Fetal CTG Monitoring	DL	Detects distress patterns	15% fewer false positives
Postpartum Monitoring	NLP, Wearables	Prevents hemorrhage, depression	20% reduced morbidity
Obstetric Ultrasound	DL	Identifies placenta accreta, FGR	~92% accuracy

LABOR AND DELIVERY

- *Labor Progression:*
  - *Application:* AI predicts labor outcomes using contraction and fetal heart rate data[22] **(Table 2)**.
  - *Impact:* Optimizes cesarean timing, reducing unnecessary procedures by 15%.
- *Fetal Monitoring:*
  - *Application:* AI-based CTG detects distress patterns.[20]
  - *Impact:* Improves intervention accuracy (~90% specificity).

POSTPARTUM CARE

- *Maternal Health:*
  - *Application:* AI monitors for postpartum hemorrhage and depression via wearables and NLP.[23]
  - *Impact:* Early detection reduces morbidity by 20%.
- *Newborn Health:*
  - *Application:* AI predicts NICU needs using birth data.[24]
  - *Impact:* Enhances resource allocation, improving outcomes by 15%.

LIMITATIONS OF AI IN OB-GYN

Despite its potential, AI faces significant challenges in OB-GYN practice.[25]

- *Limited Generalizability:* Models trained on specific populations may fail in diverse settings due to genetic or socioeconomic variability.
- *Data Quality and Bias:* Incomplete or biased datasets (e.g., underrepresented groups) lead to inaccurate predictions (bias risk ~20–30%).
- *Lack of Explainability:* "Black box" algorithms reduce clinician trust; only 10% of AI tools offer interpretable outputs.
- *Ethical/Legal Concerns:* Data privacy breaches (e.g., GDPR violations) and liability for AI errors remain unresolved.
- *Integration Challenges:* Poor compatibility with EHRs; 60% of AI tools require workflow adjustments.
- *Dynamic Pregnancy Physiology:* Complex, individualized changes challenge real-time predictions (accuracy drops ~15% in late pregnancy).
- *Limited Validation:* <20% of OB-GYN AI tools are FDA-approved or clinically validated.

- *Clinician/Patient Resistance:* Skepticism in sensitive areas like childbirth; 30% of clinicians prefer human judgment.

RESEARCH FINDINGS

Recent studies highlight AI's transformative impact in OB-GYN:

- *Fetal Ultrasound:* Lin et al. (2022) demonstrated AI's 90% accuracy in detecting intracranial malformations.[3]
- *Cardiac Screening:* Sakai et al. (2022) reported AI's 88% sensitivity in fetal echocardiography, reducing operator dependency.[21]
- *Preterm Birth:* Sun et al. (2022) developed an ML model with 85% sensitivity for preterm birth prediction using EHR data.[16]
- *IVF Success:* AI-driven embryo selection improves pregnancy rates by 10–15%.[12]
- *Robotic Surgery:* AI-assisted hysterectomies reduce complications by 20%.[14]

Challenges include bias in datasets (e.g., underrepresentation of non-Caucasian populations) and the need for regulatory frameworks to ensure safety and equity.[25]

FUTURE DIRECTIONS

- *Improved Models:* Diverse datasets will enhance AI accuracy (projected 10% improvement by 2030).
- *Global Access:* AI mobile apps can extend care to low-resource settings, reducing maternal mortality by 15–20%.[26]
- *Regulatory Advances:* FDA and EMA are developing AI validation frameworks, with 50% of tools expected to be approved by 2030.[27]
- *Ethical Integration:* Transparent algorithms and patient consent protocols will address privacy concerns.

CONCLUSION

AI is reshaping OB-GYN by enhancing diagnostics, personalizing treatments, and optimizing maternal/fetal care. Applications like AI-driven ultrasound, cancer screening, and IVF embryo selection improve accuracy and outcomes, while robotic surgery and wearables streamline care. However, challenges like bias, explainability, and integration must be addressed through robust validation and ethical frameworks. Collaborative efforts among clinicians, researchers, and policymakers will ensure AI's responsible integration, making women's healthcare more precise, accessible, and equitable.

REFERENCES

1. Topol EJ. High-performance medicine: The convergence of human and artificial intelligence. Nat Med. 2019;25(1):44-56.
2. Rajkomar A, Dean J, Kohane I. Machine learning in medicine. N Engl J Med. 2019;380(14):1347-58.
3. Lin M, et al. AI in detection of fetal intracranial malformations. Ultrasound Obstet Gynecol. 2022;59(2):304-16.
4. Bazot M, Daraï E. Role of AI in adenomyosis and endometriosis diagnosis. Fertil Steril. 2018;109(3):389-97.

5. Hu L, et al. AI for cervical cancer screening. Lancet Digit Health. 2019;1(6):e330-7.
6. Lu M, et al. Radiomics in ovarian cancer detection. Radiology. 2021;299(3):620-8.
7. Zhang Y, et al. ML in endometrial cancer prognosis. J Clin Oncol. 2020;38(15):1745-53.
8. Rodriguez-Ruiz A, et al. AI in mammography. Radiology. 2019;292(3):543-50.
9. Stein J, et al. AI in PCOS diagnosis. Fertil Steril. 2021;116(4):987-94.
10. Shilaih M, et al. AI for ovulation prediction. Digit Biomark. 2018;2(3):113-20.
11. Tran D, et al. DL for embryo selection in IVF. Hum Reprod. 2019;34(8):1450-7.
12. Chavez-Badiola A, et al. AI in time-lapse IVF. Reprod Biomed Online. 2020;41(5):897=904.
13. Nygaard I, et al. AI in urogynecology. Am J Obstet Gynecol. 2022;226(4):512-20.
14. Advincula AP, et al. AI in robotic gynecologic surgery. J Minim Invasive Gynecol. 2019;26(7):1245-53.
15. Obermeyer Z, et al. AI decision support in healthcare. Science. 2016;353(6307):1209-11.
16. Sun Q, et al. ML for preterm birth prediction. J Healthc Eng. 2022:9635526.
17. Marić I, et al. AI for preeclampsia prediction. Hypertension. 2020;76(5):1592-9.
18. Artzi NS, et al. AI for gestational diabetes. Diabetes Care. 2020;43(8):1873-80.
19. Seshadri S, et al. Wearables in maternal health. Lancet Digit Health, 2021;3(9):e592-e601.
20. Fergus P, et al. AI in fetal CTG analysis. Comput Biol Med. 2019;112:103387.
21. Sakai A, et al. Explainable AI in fetal echocardiography. Biomedicines. 2022;10(3):551.
22. Gao C, et al. AI for labor progression prediction. Am J Obstet Gynecol. 2021;225(3):312-9.
23. Wang S, et al. AI for postpartum depression detection. J Med Internet Res. 2020;22(9):e19816.
24. Beam AL, et al. AI for NICU admission prediction. Pediatrics. 2019;144(5):e20191421.
25. Char DS, et al. Ethical challenges in AI healthcare. N Engl J Med. 2018;379(12):1107-9.
26. Wahl B, et al. AI in global health. Lancet Glob Health. 2018;6(10):e1036-8.
27. Muehlematter UJ, et al. Regulatory frameworks for AI in healthcare. Eur Radiol. 2021;31(6):4136-44.

Government Programs

Ruchika Garg

INTRODUCTION

India's maternal mortality ratio (MMR) has decreased from 130 per 100,000 live births (2014-2016) to 113 (2016-2018), a 17-point decline, with Maharashtra reporting an MMR of 46.[1] Despite progress, most maternal deaths are preventable with timely, skilled care in supportive environments. The Sustainable Development Goal (SDG) 3.1 aims to reduce MMR to below 70 by 2030.[2] This chapter outlines key government programs promoting safe motherhood, with detailed insights into the Dakshata program, supported by clinical evidence and data in tables.

GOVERNMENT PROGRAMS FOR SAFE MOTHERHOOD

India has implemented several initiatives to enhance maternal and neonatal health **(Table 1)**.

DAKSHATA PROGRAM: HIGHLIGHTS

Introduction: Launched in 2015 by the Maternal Health Division, Ministry of Health and Family Welfare (MoHFW), Dakshata is a strategic initiative to enhance the quality of intra- and

TABLE 1: Key Government programs for safe motherhood.

Program	*Launch year*	*Focus*
Dakshata	2015	Quality intra- and postpartum care
Janani Suraksha Yojana (JSY)	2005	Promote institutional deliveries
Janani Shishu Suraksha Karyakram (JSSK)	2011	Free maternal and neonatal services
Pradhan Mantri Surakshit Matritva Abhiyan (PMSMA)	2016	Quality antenatal care
Surakshit Matritva Aashwasan (SUMAN)	2019	Comprehensive maternal and newborn care
Pradhan Mantri Matru Vandana Yojana (PMMVY)	2017	Financial support for pregnant women
LaQshya	2017	Labor room and maternity OT quality improvement
Anemia Mukt Bharat	2018	Reduce anemia prevalence
Rashtriya Bal Swasthya Karyakram (RBSK)	2013	Child health screening and intervention
Manyata	2017	Private facility quality certification

Source: Compiled from MoHFW, 2020.[3]

TABLE 2: Dakshata program overview.

Aspect	*Details*	*Evidence*
Goal	Quality MNH care	Targets MMR <70 by 2030[2]
Key Drivers	Competent providers, supplies, mentorship	82.86% institutional deliveries[5]
Activities	Training, resource assessment, data tools	1,300+ doctors trained in EmOC[4]
Monitoring	Clinical mentorship, dashboards	Monthly facility reports[4]

Source: MoHFW, 2024.[4]

immediate postpartum care in institutional deliveries. It empowers healthcare providers to deliver evidence-based maternal and newborn health (MNH) care from admission to discharge.[4]

Goal: Improve maternal and newborn care quality during the intra- and immediate postpartum period through competent, confident providers **(Table 2)**.[4]

Objectives:
- Enhance provider competency (medical officers, nurses, ANMs) in evidence-based labor room practices.
- Facilitate skill translation into clinical practice through enabling strategies.
- Ensure availability of essential supplies and commodities in labor rooms and postpartum wards.
- Strengthen accountability via improved data recording, reporting, and utilization.
- Implement the MNH toolkit at delivery points in phases.[4]

Rationale: Childbirth carries high risks of maternal and neonatal mortality, with most complications preventable through quality care. Despite 82.86% institutional delivery rates, suboptimal service quality persists, necessitating competency-based training and supervision to reduce MMR and neonatal mortality **(Table 2)**.[5]

Key Activities:
- Sensitization workshops for officials.
- Mapping target facilities (district hospitals, high-case-load CHCs).
- Hiring quality improvement mentors.
- Rapid resource assessments and supply provision.
- Training of trainers and labor room staff.
- Post-training follow-up and data tool implementation.[4]

Training Programs:
- *Life-Saving Anesthesia Skills (LSAS):* 1800 + doctors trained.
- *Emergency Obstetric Care (EmOC):* 1300 + doctors trained.
- Skilled Birth Attendance (SBA) for nurses/ANMs.
- Comprehensive Abortion Care (CAC) for medical officers.[4]

Skill Laboratories: Established under the National Health Mission (NHM) to standardize training with dedicated skill stations.[4]

Monitoring:

- *Program Management:* Supervisors use Government of India (GoI's) supportive supervision checklist.
- *Clinical Monitoring:* Mentors ensure adherence to quality practices.
- *Dashboards:* Facilities report monthly to districts, aggregated at state levels.[4]

Funding: Supported by NHM funds for training materials, logistics, and follow-up.[4]

Role of NIHFW: The National Institute of Health and Family Welfare coordinates in-service training, with 17 state institutes facilitating state-level implementation.[4]

OTHER KEY PROGRAMS

- *Janani Suraksha Yojana (JSY):* Launched in 2005 under NRHM, JSY promotes institutional deliveries among poor pregnant women through cash incentives. In low-performing states (e.g., Uttar Pradesh, Bihar), mothers receive ₹1400 (rural) or ₹1000 (urban), with ASHA workers receiving ₹600 (rural) or ₹400 (urban). High-performing states offer₹700 (rural) or ₹600 (urban) for mothers. Benefits are limited to two births in high-performing states and require BPL/SC/ST certification for private facilities.[6]
- *Janani Shishu Suraksha Karyakram (JSSK):* Initiated in 2011, JSSK provides free delivery (normal: 3 days; cesarean: 7 days), diagnostics, drugs, blood, diet, and transport for pregnant women and sick neonates up to 30 days. It reduces out-of-pocket expenses and encourages institutional care **(Table 3)**.[7]
- *Pradhan Mantri Surakshit Matritva Abhiyan (PMSMA):* Launched in 2016, PMSMA ensures quality antenatal care on the 9th of each month for women in their 2nd/3rd trimesters. Services include examinations, diagnostics (e.g., ultrasound), and management of high-risk pregnancies (red stickers on MCP cards). It aims to reduce MMR by ensuring specialist care at public facilities **(Table 4)**.[8]
- *Surakshit Matritva Aashwasan (SUMAN):* Launched in 2019, SUMAN provides free, respectful, and quality care for pregnant women, mothers (up to 6 months post-delivery),

TABLE 3: JSSK entitlements.

Service	*Details*	*Impact*
Free Delivery	Normal and cesarean	Increased institutional deliveries[7]
Transport	Home to facility, referrals, drop-back	Reduced access barriers[7]
Diagnostics	ANC, INC, PNC up to 6 weeks	Early complication detection[7]

Source: MoHFW, 2011[7]

TABLE 4: PMSMA key features.

Component	*Details*	*Evidence*
ANC Services	Specialist-led, free diagnostics	1 ultrasound recommended[8]
High-Risk Identification	Red stickers on MCP cards	Improved follow-up[8]
Referral System	JSSK help desks	Timely complication management[8]

Source: MoHFW, 2016.[8]

TABLE 5: SUMAN services and impact.

Service	*Details*	*Impact*
Free Care	ANC, delivery, PNC	Reduced financial burden[9]
Respectful Care	Dignified treatment	Improved beneficiary satisfaction[9]
Transport	Free referrals	Increased access[9]

Source: MoHFW, 2020.[9]

TABLE 6: LaQshya targets (12 Months).

Target	*Goal*	*Evidence*
Maternal/Neonatal Audits	100% compliance	Improved care quality[11]
Partograph Use	60% real-time use	Enhanced labor monitoring[11]
Breastfeeding	30% increase within 1 hour	Better neonatal outcomes[11]

Source: MoHFW, 2017.[11]

TABLE 7: Anemia mukt bharat dosing.

Group	*Dose*	*Formulation*	*Fe (mg)*
6–59 months	20 mg twice weekly	Syrup	20
Pregnant/Lactating	60 mg daily	Red tablet	60
10–19 years	60 mg weekly	Blue tablet	60

Source: MoHFW, 2018.[12]

and newborns. Services include antenatal check-ups, safe deliveries, post-natal care, and transport. It targets MMR <70 and NMR <12 by 2030, reducing out-of-pocket costs **(Table 5)**.[9]

- *Pradhan Mantri Matru Vandana Yojana (PMMVY):* Implemented since 2017 under the National Food Security Act, PMMVY provides cash incentives (₹5000 for first child in two installments; ₹6000 for second child if a girl) to compensate for wage loss and promote health-seeking behavior. Eligible women include those from SC/ST, BPL, or low-income groups, excluding those in formal employment.[10]
- *LaQshya:* Launched in 2017, LaQshya improves quality in labor rooms and maternity OTs, targeting medical colleges, district hospitals, and high-case-load CHCs. It reduces mortality from complications like PPH, preeclampsia, and sepsis through standardized protocols, respectful maternity care (RMC), and infrastructure upgrades. Certification is valid for 3 years, with incentives up to ₹6 lakhs for medical colleges **(Table 6)**.[11]
- *Anemia Mukt Bharat:* Launched in 2018, this program aims to reduce anemia by 18% across six beneficiary groups (children, adolescents, women) through a 6 × 6 × 6 strategy (6 beneficiaries, 6 interventions, 6 institutional mechanisms). Interventions include iron-folic acid supplementation, deworming, and fortified foods **(Table 7)**.[12]
- *Rashtriya Bal Swasthya Karyakram (RBSK):* Launched in 2013, RBSK screens children (0-18 years) for developmental delays and disabilities, ensuring early intervention to reduce neonatal and child mortality.[13]

TABLE 8: RCH phase II initiatives.

Initiative	*Details*	*Impact*
EmOC Training	16-week program	Improved cesarean access[15]
Maternal Death Reviews	Quality audits	Reduced MMR[15]
Village Health Days	ANC, immunizations	Increased outreach[15]

Source: MoHFW, 2005.[15]

- *Manyata:* A FOGSI-led initiative since 2017, Manyata certifies private maternity facilities adhering to 16 clinical and 10 facility standards, aligned with WHO and LaQshya guidelines, to ensure safe, respectful care.[14]
- *Reproductive and Child Health (RCH) Program:*
    - *Phase I (1997):* Focused on family planning, child health, and RTI/STD prevention to reduce maternal and child mortality.
    - *Phase II (2005):* Emphasized rural institutional deliveries, introducing LSAS and EmOC training, blood storage at FRUs, safe abortion services, and maternal death reviews **(Table 8)**.[15]

Disclaimer: Grok is not a doctor; please consult one. Do not share information that can identify you.

REFERENCES

1. Sample Registration System. Maternal Mortality Ratio. 2016-2018. MoHFW; 2018.
2. United Nations. Sustainable Development Goals. UNDP; 2015.
3. MoHFW. (2020). National Health Mission Overview. [online] Available from nhm.gov.in [Last accessed December, 2025].
4. MoHFW. (2024). Dakshata Guidelines. [online] Available from nhm.gov.in/showfile.php?lid=450 [Last accessed December, 2025].
5. NHM. Institutional Delivery Statistics. MoHFW; 2020.
6. MoHFW. (2005). Janani Suraksha Yojana Guidelines. [online] Available from nhm.gov.in [Last accessed December, 2025].
7. MoHFW. (2011). Janani Shishu Suraksha Karyakram Guidelines. [online] Available from nhm.gov.in [Last accessed December, 2025].
8. MoHFW. (2016). Pradhan Mantri Surakshit Matritva Abhiyan. [online] Available from pmsma.nhp.gov.in [Last accessed December, 2025].
9. MoHFW. (2020). Surakshit Matritva Aashwasan Guidelines. [online] Available from nhm.gov.in [Last accessed December, 2025].
10. MoHFW. (2017). Pradhan Mantri Matru Vandana Yojana. [online] Available from pmmvy.nic.in [Last accessed December, 2025].
11. MoHFW. (2017). LaQshya Guidelines. [online] Available from nhm.gov.in [Last accessed December, 2025].
12. MoHFW. (2018). Anaemia Mukt Bharat Strategy. [online] Available from anemiamuktbharat.info [Last accessed December, 2025].
13. MoHFW. (2013). Rashtriya Bal Swasthya Karyakram. [online] Available from nhm.gov.in. [Last accessed December, 2025].
14. FOGSI. (2017). Manyata Initiative. [online] Available from manyataforqualitycare.org. [Last accessed December, 2025].
15. MoHFW. (2005). Reproductive and Child Health Phase II. [online] Available from nhm.gov.in. [Last accessed December, 2025].

Vesicovaginal Fistula

Ruchika Garg, Shaifali Singh

INTRODUCTION

Vesicovaginal fistula (VVF) is an abnormal communication between the bladder and vagina, causing continuous urinary incontinence. It is a debilitating condition with significant physical, psychological, and socioeconomic impacts. The global prevalence of VVF is approximately 2.2% (range 0.3–7%) according to the UNFPA 2003 survey, with an incidence of ~1/1,000 post-hysterectomy and 1–2/1,000 deliveries.[1,2] In developing countries, obstructed labor accounts for >90% of cases, while pelvic surgery predominates in developed nations.[3]

OVERVIEW

Etiology

Vesicovaginal fistula arises from obstetric, gynecologic, traumatic, or medical causes **(Table 1)**.[4]

Classification

Vesicovaginal fistula is classified based on complexity, site, and surgical considerations **(Table 2, and Fig. 1)**.[5,6]

TABLE 1: Etiology of vesicovaginal fistula (VVF).[4]

Category	*Causes*
Obstetric	Prolonged/obstructed labor, placenta percreta, cesarean section (CS, especially repeat), CS hysterectomy, operative vaginal delivery, cervical cerclage
Gynecologic/urogynecologic	Hysterectomy, loop excision of cervix, suburethral slings, anterior colporrhaphy, periurethral bulking, Burch colposuspension
Pelvic/medical	Endometriosis, gynecologic cancers, pelvic irradiation, infections (schistosomiasis, lymphogranuloma venereum), intrauterine device, neglected pessary, foreign body
Traumatic	Accidental trauma, sexual trauma

TABLE 2: Classification of vesicovaginal fistula (VVF).[5,6]

Basis	*Types/characteristics*
Complexity (Elkins 1990)	• *Simple:* Size <3 cm, high vaginal, supratrigonal, no malignancy/radiation, normal vaginal length • *Complex:* Size >3 cm, midvaginal/trigonal, malignancy/radiation present, shortened vagina
Site (cystoscopy)	• Supratrigonal, trigonal, infratrigonal (bladder neck)
Location	• *High vaginal/juxtacervical/vault:* Proximal vagina, supratrigonal communication • *Midvaginal:* Central vagina, trigone/base communication • *Low vaginal/juxtaurethral:* Bladder neck/upper urethra communication • *Sub-symphyseal:* Circumferential tissue loss, fixed to bone
Surgical (Goh 2004)	• *Distance from external urethral meatus*: Type 1 (>3.5 cm), type 2 (2.5–3.5 cm), type 3 (1.5–2.5 cm), type 4 (<1.5 cm) • *Size*: a (<1.5 cm), b (1.5–3 cm), c (>3 cm) • *Fibrosis/vaginal length*: I (none/mild, >6 cm), II (moderate/severe, reduced length), III (post-radiation, ureteric involvement, recurrence)

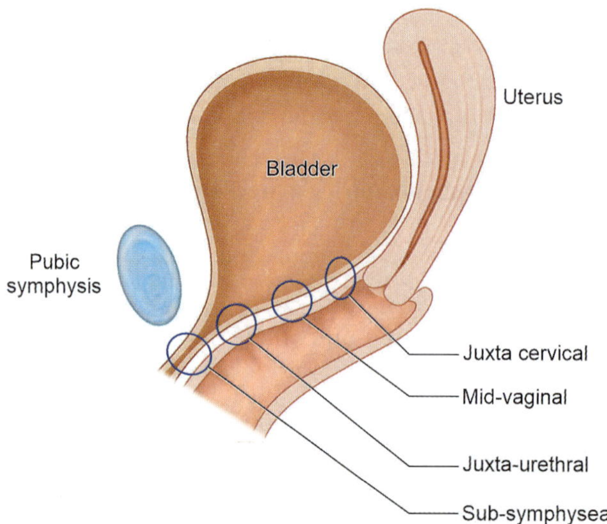

Fig. 1: Anatomical types of vesicovaginal fistula (VVF).[5]

Diagnosis

- *History:* Continuous urinary leakage post-surgery (day 1 for direct injury) or obstetric event (7–14 days post-delivery). Associated symptoms include fever, hematuria, suprapubic pain, or perineal dermatitis.[7]
- *Examination:* Per-speculum reveals urine leakage or puckered anterior vaginal wall; small fistulas may be subtle.[8]
- *Three-swab test:* Methylene blue instilled via urethral catheter; vaginal swabs detect leakage source **(Fig. 2)**:[9]

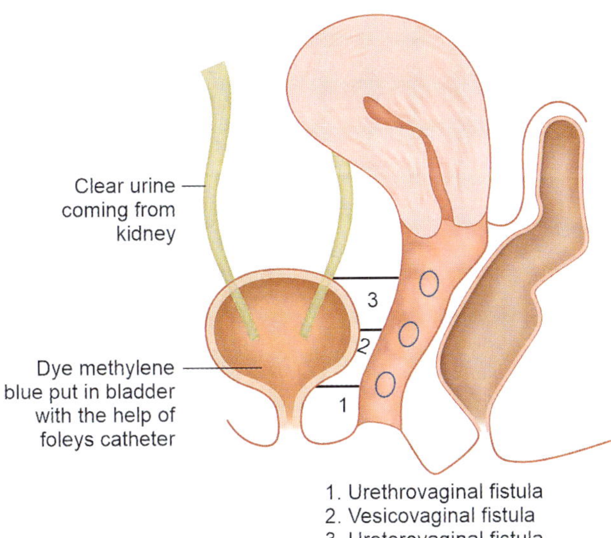

Fig. 2: Three-swab Test.[9]

- *Top/middle swab discoloration:* VVF
- *Uppermost swab wet, no discoloration:* Ureterovaginal fistula
- *Lowermost swab stained:* Urethral leak

- *Cystourethroscopy:* Confirms site, size, number, and relation to ureteric orifices.[10]
- *Imaging:* Voiding cystourethrography, cystogram, intravenous urogram (for ureteric injury), transvaginal ultrasound, or MRI fistulography.[11]

SURGICAL ANATOMY OF BLADDER (FIG. 3)

- *Position:* Empty bladder lies at pubic symphysis level; distended bladder becomes intra-abdominal but extraperitoneal.[12]
- *Relations:*
  - *Anterior:* Prevesical space, pubic symphysis.
  - *Superior:* Peritoneum (loose, except posterior dome).
  - *Lateral:* Obturator internus, levator ani, pelvic fascia.
  - *Posterior:* Uterus, vagina.
  - *Inferior:* Urethra, pelvic diaphragm.
- *Fixation:* Pubovesical/pubourethral ligaments anteriorly; urethra inferiorly.[13]
- *Parts:* Apex (anterosuperior), body, fundus (posteroinferior with trigone), neck (leads to urethra). Trigone is a smooth triangle with ureteric and urethral openings.[14]

Primary Prevention

- *Surgical techniques:*[15]
  - Use sharp dissection during bladder mobilization in hysterectomy/CS to avoid injury, especially in prior CS cases.

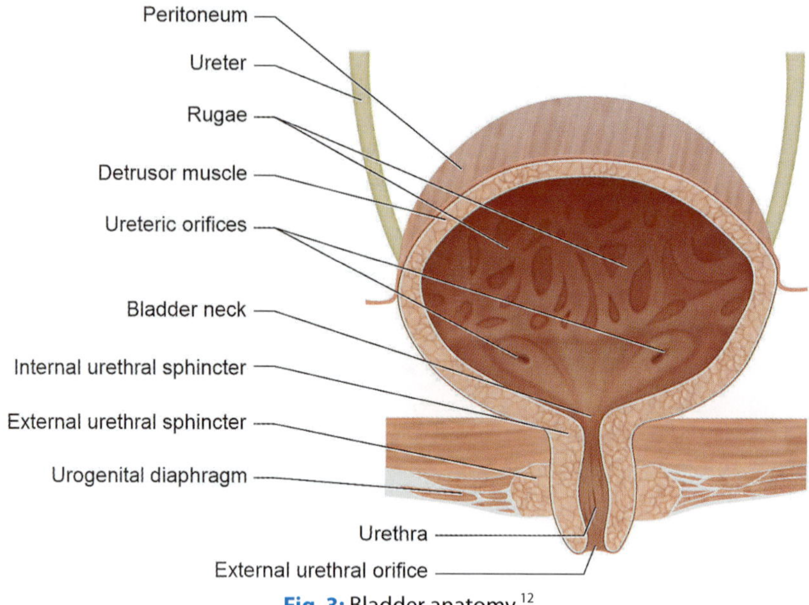

Fig. 3: Bladder anatomy.[12]

- Apply gentle traction/countertraction to identify correct planes.
- Avoid blunt dissection and monopolar cautery in vesicovaginal space.
- Use retractors cautiously, preferably against a sponge/mop.

- *Obstetric care:* Timely CS in obstructed labor; skilled operative vaginal delivery.[16]

Secondary Prevention (Early Detection/Repair)

- *Intraoperative suspicion*: Gross hematuria, fluid in operative field.[17]
- *Confirmation:* Retrograde bladder filling with methylene blue via catheter.[18]
- *Management:*
  - Cystoscopy to assess size/location relative to ureter/trigone.
  - Sharp dissection of vesicovaginal space for tension-free repair.
  - Three-layer closure with 3–0 delayed-absorbable suture.
  - Separate vaginal wall repair; transurethral/suprapubic drainage.[19]
- *Note:* Routine cystoscopy not recommended unless injury suspected.[20]

RCOG/NICE Guidelines:

- *RCOG Green-top Guideline No. 74 (2023):* Advises sharp dissection and early repair for intraoperative bladder injuries; recommends specialist referral for complex fistulas.[21]
- *NICE NG123 (2019):* Supports intraoperative cystoscopy for suspected injuries during pelvic surgery.[22]

MANAGEMENT

Investigations

- Complete blood count (CBC), kidney function tests (KFT).
- Urine analysis, culture, and sensitivity.[23]

Non-surgical Management

- *Indications*: Small fistulas (<1 cm), recent onset (<3 weeks), no epithelialization.[24]
- *Methods*:
  - *Continuous bladder drainage (CBD):* 4–6 weeks; success rate 3–32%.[25]
  - *Optimization:* Correct anemia, optimize nutrition, vaginal estrogenization.[26]
- *Contraindications:* Fistulas >3 cm, radiation-induced, onset >6 weeks, extensive scarring.[27]

CONSERVATIVE SURGICAL MANAGEMENT (TABLE 3)

TABLE 3: Conservative surgical options.[28,29]

Method	Indication	Technique	Success rate
Cystoscopic laser	Small, recent, no fibrosis	Fulguration of tract epithelium, 2-week CBD	~73%
Fibrin glue	Adjunct to repair	Transvaginal injection post-fulguration, 1–4-week CBD	60–70%
Platelet-rich plasma (PRP)	Small fistulas	Injection creates occlusive mound, promotes fibrosis	50–65%
Percutaneous nephrostomy (PCN)	Malignant VVF, poor prognosis	Ureteric occlusion with PCN for larger fistulas	Palliative

SURGICAL MANAGEMENT

- *Timing:*
  - *Early repair:* Small fistulas, no infection/fibrosis, within days of injury, or with ureteric injury.[30]
  - *Standard repair:* 12 weeks post-onset, no inflammation/infection.[31]
  - *Delayed repair:* >6 months for radiation-induced fistulas.[32]
- *Principles:*[33]
  - Accurate preoperative assessment
  - Timely repair
  - Adequate fistula exposure
  - Minimal scar excision
  - Healthy vascular margins
  - Tension-free, watertight two-layer closure with fine absorbable suture
  - Hemostasis, minimal cautery
  - Postoperative CBD (14–21 days)
- *Approaches:*
  - *Vaginal:* Preferred for simple fistulas; techniques include flap splitting, Latzko, saucerization, laparoscopic, or natural orifice transurethral endoscopic (NOTE-VVF) repair. Advantages—less invasive, shorter recovery, multiple flap options.[34]
  - *Abdominal:* For complex/high fistulas, post-radiation, or concomitant procedures (ureteric reimplantation, cystoplasty). Techniques—transvesical, transperitoneal, open/laparoscopic/robotic.[35]

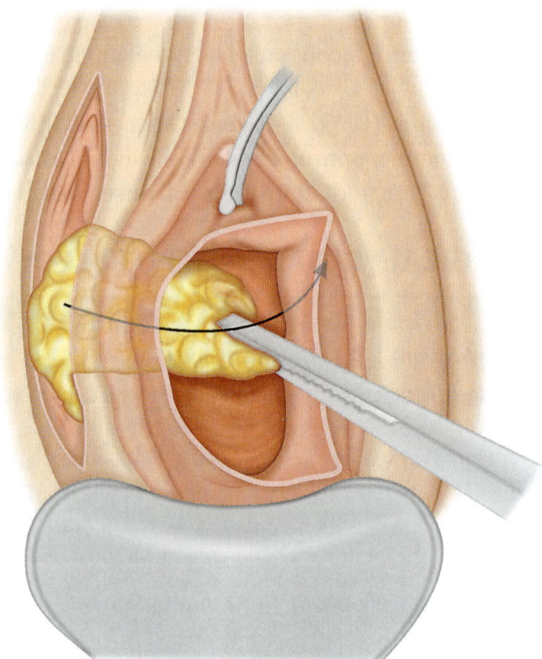

Fig. 4: Martius flap technique.[36]

Flowchart 1: Vesicovaginal fistula (VVF) management flowchart.[38]

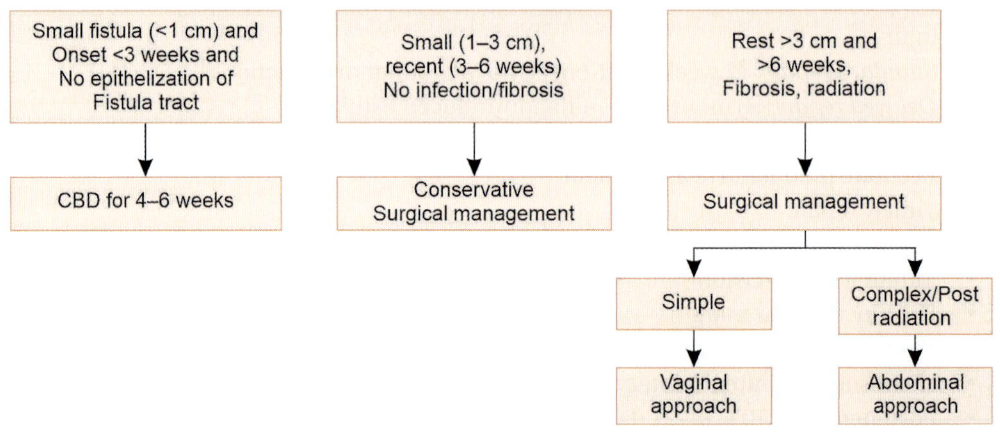

- *Flaps/grafts:* Martius flap (labial fibrofatty tissue), omental, peritoneal, rectus, or gracilis muscle flaps enhance healing, fill dead space, and improve vascularity **(Fig. 4)**.[36]

Postoperative Care (Flowchart 1)

- Prophylactic antibiotics, anticholinergics to prevent bladder spasms.
- CBD for 14–21 days; maintain hydration to prevent clots.

- Monitor input-output, prevent catheter blockage.
- Cystogram before catheter removal to confirm bladder integrity.
- *Discharge advice*:
    - Frequent urination.
    - Abstinence for 3 months.
    - Contraception for 1–2 years; elective CS at 37 weeks if pregnant.[37]

DNB QUESTIONS

1. Gynecological Causes, Principles, and Care of VVF. ***(DNB 2012 June, Paper-3)***

Ans. a. Gynecological Causes of VVF:[4] ***(2 marks)***

- *Hysterectomy (abdominal/vaginal):* Most common, ~1/1,000 cases.
- Loop excision of cervix.
- Suburethral slings, anterior colporrhaphy, periurethral bulking, Burch colposuspension.
- Endometriosis, gynecologic cancers, pelvic irradiation.
- Intrauterine device, neglected pessary, foreign body.

b. Principles of VVF Management:[33] ***(4 marks)***

- Accurate preoperative assessment (history, examination, imaging).
- Timely repair (12 weeks standard, early for small fistulas).
- Adequate exposure and minimal scar excision.
- Tension-free, watertight two-layer closure with absorbable suture.
- Healthy vascular margins, hemostasis, minimal cautery.
- Postoperative CBD for 14–21 days.

c. Preoperative and Postoperative Care:[37] ***(4 marks)***

- *Preoperative:*
    - Correct anemia (transfusions if Hb <10 g/dL).
    - Treat vulvovaginal infections with antibiotics/antifungals.
    - Urinary antiseptics (e.g., nitrofurantoin) for 3–5 days.
    - Manage vulvar excoriation with zinc oxide ointment.
- *Postoperative:*
    - Prophylactic antibiotics (e.g., cefazolin).
    - Anticholinergics (e.g., oxybutynin) for bladder spasms.
    - CBD for 14–21 days; ensure hydration, monitor catheter patency.
    - Cystogram before catheter removal.
    - *Discharge advice:* Frequent urination, abstinence (3 months), contraception (1–2 years), elective CS if pregnant.

2. Bladder Anatomy, Prevention, and Management of Injury: ***(DNB 2018 June, Paper-1)***

Ans. a. Surgical Anatomy of Urinary Bladder:[12,14] ***(2 marks)***

- *Position:* Empty bladder at pubic symphysis; distended bladder intra-abdominal, extraperitoneal.
- *Relations:* Anterior (prevesical space), superior (peritoneum), lateral (obturator internus, levator ani), posterior (uterus, vagina), inferior (urethra).
- *Fixation:* Pubovesical/pubourethral ligaments, urethra.

- *Parts:* Apex, body, fundus (with trigone), neck. Trigone has ureteric and urethral openings.

b. Prevention of Bladder Injury in Obstetric/Gynecologic Surgery:[15,16] ***(4 marks)***

- Use sharp dissection for bladder mobilization during hysterectomy/CS.
- Gentle traction/countertraction to identify planes.
- Avoid blunt dissection and monopolar cautery in vesicovaginal space.
- Careful retractor use, preferably against sponge/mop.
- Timely CS in obstructed labor; skilled operative vaginal delivery.

c. Identification and Management of Bladder Injury:[17,19] ***(4 marks)***

- *Intraoperative Identification:*
  - Gross hematuria, fluid in operative field.
  - Confirm with methylene blue retrograde bladder filling.
  - Cystoscopy to assess size/location.
- *Postoperative Identification:*
  - Continuous vaginal urinary leakage (day 1 for surgical injury, 7–14 days for obstetric).
  - Three-swab test, cystoscopy, imaging (cystogram, urogram).
- *Management:*
  - *Intraoperative:* Three-layer tension-free repair with 3-0 absorbable suture, separate vaginal closure, CBD.
  - *Postoperative:* Early repair for small fistulas; standard repair at 12 weeks. Vaginal approach for simple fistulas; abdominal for complex cases.

3. **Extra-Urethral Incontinence, Causes, and Management of VVF:**

(DNB 2019 June, Paper-3)

Ans. a. Extra-Urethral Incontinence:[39] ***(2 Marks)***

- Incontinence bypassing the urethra due to abnormal communications (e.g., VVF, ureterovaginal fistula).
- Characterized by continuous urinary leakage, unlike stress/urge incontinence.

b. Causes of VVF:[4] ***(4 marks)***

- *Obstetric:* Prolonged/obstructed labor, placenta percreta, CS, operative vaginal delivery.
- *Gynecologic:* Hysterectomy, suburethral slings, anterior colporrhaphy.
- *Medical:* Gynecologic cancers, pelvic irradiation, infections (schistosomiasis).
- *Traumatic:* Accidental/sexual trauma, foreign body.

c. Evaluation and Management of VVF:[7,31] ***(4 marks)***

- *Evaluation:*
  - *History:* Continuous leakage post-surgery/delivery.
  - *Examination:* Per-speculum, three-swab test.
  - Cystoscopy, cystogram, urogram, MRI fistulography.
- *Management:*
  - *Non-Surgical:* CBD for small (<1 cm), recent fistulas; success rate 3–32%.
  - *Conservative Surgical:* Cystoscopic laser, fibrin glue, PRP, PCN for palliation.
  - *Surgical:* Vaginal (simple fistulas, e.g., flap splitting, Latzko) or abdominal (complex fistulas, e.g., O'Connor's). Timing: 12 weeks standard, early for small fistulas, >6 months for radiation-induced.

KEY POINTS

- VVF prevalence is 2.2% globally; obstructed labor (developing countries) and pelvic surgery (developed countries) are leading causes.
- Classified by complexity (simple/complex), site (supratrigonal/trigonal), and surgical factors (Goh 2004).
- Diagnosis via history, three-swab test, cystoscopy, and imaging.
- Prevention includes sharp dissection, timely CS, and cautious retractor use.
- Management ranges from CBD (small fistulas) to vaginal/abdominal repair (standard at 12 weeks).
- RCOG/NICE advocate early detection, specialist referral for complex cases, and vaginal approach for simple fistulas.
- Successful repair requires tension-free closure, healthy margins, and postoperative CBD.

REFERENCES

1. UNFPA. Obstetric fistula needs assessment report. 2003.
2. Tancer ML. VVF post-hysterectomy. Obstet Gynecol. 2015;125(5):1143-9.
3. Wall LL. Obstetric fistulas in Africa. Lancet. 2018;391(10117):16-7.
4. Hillary CJ, Osman NI. Etiology of VVF. Int Urogynecol J. 2017;28(6):821-9.
5. Elkins TE. VVF classification. Am J Obstet Gynecol. 1990;167(6):1669-74.
6. Goh JT. Surgical classification of VVF. Int J Gynaecol Obstet. 2004;87(3):227-31.
7. Stamatakos M, Sargedi C. Diagnosis of VVF. Urol Int. 2016;97(4):387-94.
8. Blaivas JG, Heritz DM. VVF diagnosis. J Urol. 2017;197(3):680-5.
9. Raghavaiah NV. Three swab test for VVF. Urology. 2015;85(4):923-7.
10. Lee D, Zimmern PE. Cystoscopy in VVF. Curr Urol Rep. 2019;20(8):46.
11. Narayanan P, Nobbenhuis M. Imaging for VVF. BJOG 2016;123(7):1098-104.
12. Moore KN, Fader M. Bladder anatomy. Neurourol Urodyn. 2016;35(2):183-9.
13. DeLancey JO. Pelvic floor anatomy. Clin Obstet Gynecol. 2017;60(1):1-12.
14. Herschorn S. Bladder trigone anatomy. Can Urol Assoc J. 2015;9(5-6):E356-61.
15. Rogers RG, Jeppson PC. Preventing bladder injury. Obstet Gynecol. 2016;128(4):795-803.
16. Arrowsmith SD, Hamlin EC. Obstetric fistula prevention. Int J Obstet Anesth. 2019;38:96-103.
17. Wong MJ, Wong K. Intraoperative bladder injury. Urol Clin North Am. 2017;44(4):639-47.
18. Tebeu PM, Fomulu JN. Methylene blue for bladder injury. J Matern Fetal Neonatal Med. 2015;28(14):1689-93.
19. Gilmour DT, Dwyer PL. Bladder injury repair. Aust N Z J Obstet Gynaecol. 2018;58(3):346-52.
20. ACOG. Practice Bulletin No. 198: Prevention of urinary tract injury. 2018.
21. RCOG. Green-top Guideline No. 74: Management of urogenital fistula. 2023.
22. NICE. NG123: Urinary incontinence and pelvic organ prolapse. 2019.
23. Gedefaw G, Demis A. Preoperative evaluation for VVF. Int J Womens Health. 2020;12:803-10.
24. Bazi T, Mahfouz I. Conservative management of VVF. Arab J Urol. 2017;15(4):263-8.
25. Waaldijk K. CBD for VVF. Int Urogynecol J. 2018;29(7):983-90.
26. Bodner-Adler B, Hanzal E. VVF optimization. Eur J Obstet Gynecol Reprod Biol. 2019;234:93-8.
27. Angioli R, Penalver M. Contraindications for conservative VVF. Gynecol Oncol. 2016;140(3):447-52.
28. Mallick R, Odejinmi F. Cystoscopic laser for VVF. J Minim Invasive Gynecol. 2019;26(4):607-12.
29. Shirazi M, Rahimi M. Fibrin glue in VVF. Urol J. 2017;14(3):3041-5.
30. Pushkar DY, Dyakov VV. Early VVF repair. Urol Int. 2015;95(3):293-8.
31. Browning A, Whiteside S. Timing of VVF repair. BJOG. 2017;124(10):1531-6.

32. Creanga AA, Genadry RR. Radiation-induced VVF. Obstet Gynecol Surv. 2018;73(8):497-505.
33. Singh V, Sinha RJ. Principles of VVF repair. Indian J Urol. 2018;34(4):249-55.
34. Mahfouz W, Elmissiry M. Vaginal VVF repair. Curr Bladder Dysfunct Rep. 2019;14(4):287-93.
35. Miklos JR, Moore RD. Abdominal VVF repair. Int Urogynecol J. 2016;27(3):321-7.
36. Lee JH, Lee DW. Martius flap in VVF. J Korean Med Sci. 2017;32(6):1035-40.
37. Capes T, Stanford EJ. Postoperative care in VVF. Female Pelvic Med Reconstr Surg. 2015;21(5):277-81.
38. Frajzyngier V, Ruminjo J. VVF management flowchart. Int J Gynaecol Obstet. 2015;131(Suppl 1):S11-6.
39. Hadley HR, Zimmern PE. Extra-urethral incontinence. Urol Clin North Am. 2019;46(1):63-71.

Multifetal Pregnancy

Ruchika Garg

INTRODUCTION

Multifetal pregnancies, involving twins or higher-order multiples, are high-risk due to increased maternal and fetal complications. Perinatal mortality is 4–6 times higher, preterm delivery 6 times more frequent, and maternal complications 3–7 times more common compared to singleton pregnancies.[1] This chapter outlines the incidence, physiology, diagnosis, complications, and management of multifetal pregnancies, tailored for medical postgraduate education.

INCIDENCE AND RISK FACTORS

The incidence of multifetal pregnancies varies by maternal race, age, and parity, with a rising trend due to delayed childbearing and assisted reproductive technologies (ART) **(Table 1)**.[1-3]

PHYSIOLOGY OF MULTIFETAL PREGNANCIES

Spontaneous Multiple Gestation

- *Dizygotic Twins:* Result from fertilization of two ova by separate sperms (superfecundation). Non-identical, with separate placentas and amniotic sacs.
  - *Incidence varies:* Lowest in Asians, intermediate in Caucasians, highest in Africans.[9,10]
  - *Spontaneous twinning rate:* ~1:80 pregnancies.[11]
- *Monozygotic Twins*: Arise from division of a single fertilized ovum, resulting in genetically identical fetuses. *Global incidence*: ~3/1,000 live births **(Table 2)**.[9,10]

TABLE 1: Factors contributing to increased incidence of multifetal pregnancies.

Factor	*Impact*
Advanced Maternal Age	Higher FSH levels lead to spontaneous superovulation[4]
Ovulation Induction Drugs	• *Clomiphene citrate:* 9% multiple pregnancy rate[5] • *Letrozole:* 13% multiple pregnancy rate[5] • *Gonadotrophins:* 25% twin, 9% higher-order multiples[1,6]
In Vitro Fertilization (IVF)	25.5% twins, 0.9% higher-order multiples; reduced by elective single embryo transfer (eSET)[7,8]

TABLE 2: Monozygotic twinning based on timing of division.

Timing of division	*Resulting pregnancy type*	*Frequency*	*Description*
Before day 4	Diamniotic dichorionic	20–30%	Two chorions, two amnions
Days 4–8	Monochorionic diamniotic	70%	One chorion, two amnions
Days 8–13	Monochorionic monoamniotic	1–5%	One chorion, one amnion
Days 13–15	Conjoined twins	1.5/100,000	Incomplete division, rare

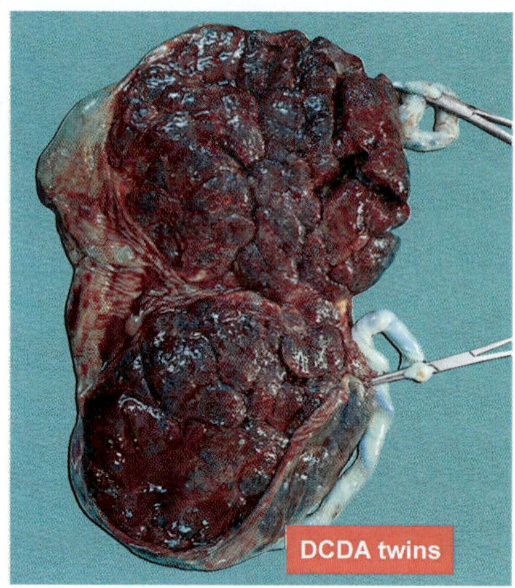

Fig. 1: Ultrasound images showing chorionicity and amnionicity.

PLACENTA OF DCDA TWINS (FIG. 1)

Physiological Changes

Multifetal pregnancies exaggerate singleton pregnancy changes:[9]

- *Mechanical effects:* Over-distended uterus causes dyspepsia, breathlessness, edema, hemorrhoids, backache, and increased urinary frequency.
- *Hormonal effects:* Elevated human chorionic gonadotropin (hCG) due to larger placental volume increases nausea and vomiting.
- *Cardiovascular:* Plasma volume increases up to 50% (vs. 40% in singletons), causing dilutional anemia and lower oncotic pressure, risking pulmonary edema in cardiac disease or with tocolytics.[2]
- *Hematologic:* Increased fetal iron demand worsens maternal anemia.
- *Metabolic:* Two-fold increased risk of gestational diabetes due to elevated diabetogenic hormones.[12]
- *Hypertensive Disorders:* Preeclampsia risk is 2.6 times higher, often earlier, more severe, and atypical.[13]

DIAGNOSIS

Multifetal pregnancies are often asymptomatic or present with exaggerated pregnancy symptoms. Diagnosis is primarily via first-trimester ultrasonography, the gold standard for confirming gestation, chorionicity, and amnionicity **(Table 3)**.[2]

Ultrasound showing lambda and T-signs for chorionicity in **Figures 2 and 3**.

TABLE 3: Diagnostic clues for multifetal pregnancy.

Method	*Findings*
Clinical	Excessive nausea, rapid uterine growth, fundal height > gestational age, excessive weight gain, palpation of ≥3 fetal parts
Biochemical	Elevated β-hCG, human placental lactogen, maternal serum α-fetoprotein
Ultrasonography	Confirms multiple fetuses, chorionicity, amnionicity; 98% accurate in first trimester[2]
Post-Delivery	Rare detection after first fetus delivery

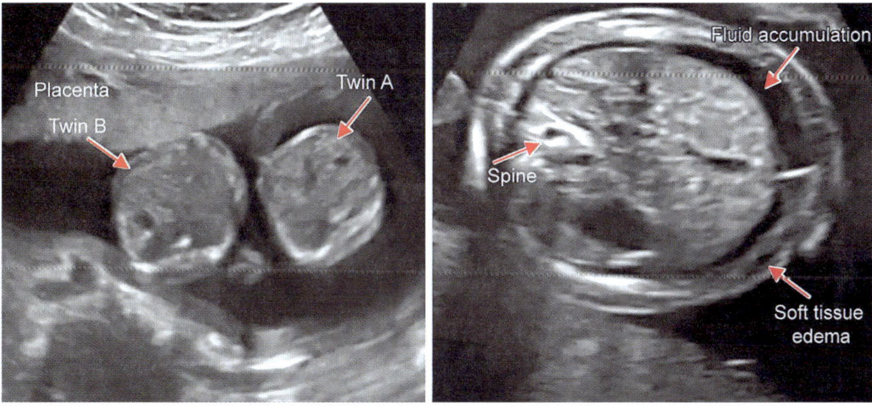

Fig. 2: Edema and TTTS.

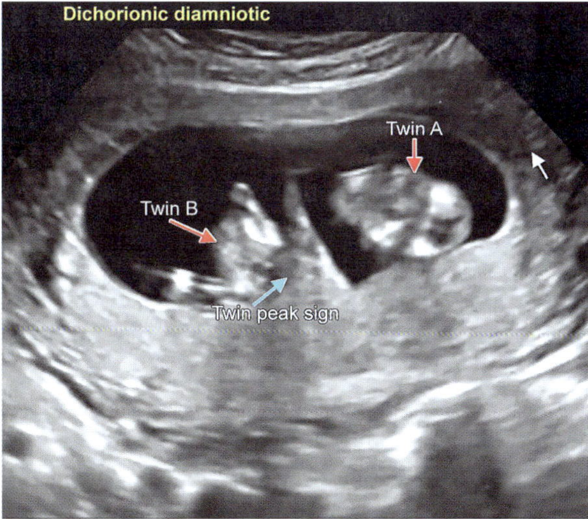

Fig. 3: USG showing twin peak sign in DCDA.

TABLE 4: Maternal and fetal complications of multifetal pregnancy.

Period	*Maternal complications*	*Fetal complications*
Antenatal	• Spontaneous abortion (25% quadruplets, 15% triplets, 8% twins) • Hyperemesis gravidarum • Anemia • Preeclampsia (2.6 × risk)[13] • Gestational diabetes (2 × risk)[12] • Preterm labor/PPROM (60% in twins)[2,9] • Antepartum hemorrhage (placenta previa, abruption) • Acute fatty liver, cholestasis, venous thromboembolism	• Congenital malformations (70% higher in twins) • Abortion, vanishing twin • Preterm birth (twins: 35 weeks, triplets: 31–32 weeks)[2] • Fetal growth restriction (FGR), especially in monochorionic twins • Sudden intrauterine demise (5 × risk)[2,14] • Single fetal demise
Intranatal	• Malpresentation • Cord prolapse • Placenta previa • Abruption placenta (3 × risk)	• Cord accidents • Specific monochorionic complications (TTTS 10–15%, TAPS, TRAP, cord entanglement, conjoined twins)[9]
Postpartum	• Postpartum hemorrhage (atonic/traumatic) • Puerperal sepsis • Failed lactation • Postpartum depression (3 × risk)	• Cerebral palsy (4 × risk)[14] • Neonatal mortality (7 × risk)[2,14]

COMPLICATIONS

Multifetal pregnancies increase risks for both mother and fetuses, with complications proportional to the number of fetuses **(Table 4)**.

MANAGEMENT OF MULTIFETAL PREGNANCY

Antenatal Management

- *Counseling:*
  - Inform about high-risk nature, complications, and need for close monitoring.
  - Discuss dietary modifications and nutritional supplements.[2]
- *Chorionicity and Amnionicity:*
  - Determine via first-trimester ultrasound (11–14 weeks) for risk stratification.[2]
  - If unclear, manage as monochorionic pregnancy.
- *Nutrition:*
  - *Target weight gain:* 18–27 kg for normal BMI.
  - *Caloric intake:* 40–45 kcal/kg/day, high protein, iron (60–100 mg/day), folic acid (1 mg/day), calcium.
  - Screen and treat anemia.
- *Screening for aneuploidy and anomalies:*
  - *First trimester:* Nuchal translucency, β-hCG, PAPP-A for twins; unreliable for triplets.
  - *Second trimester (18–22 weeks):* Ultrasound for malformations, cervical length.

    - Invasive testing (e.g., chorionic villus sampling) if indicated, with 2% pregnancy loss risk.[2]
- *Preeclampsia Prophylaxis:*
    - Low-dose aspirin from 12 weeks until delivery.[2]
- *Antenatal Visits:*
    - *Dichorionic twins:* 4-weekly until 30-32 weeks, then more frequent.
    - *Monochorionic/higher-order:* 2-weekly.[2]
    - Screen for anemia, gestational diabetes, and hypertensive disorders.
- *Preterm Birth Prevention:*
    - Cervical length <25 mm at 18–22 weeks may warrant vaginal progesterone, though efficacy is limited.
    - No proven role for prophylactic cerclage, pessary, bed rest, or tocolytics.[2]
    - Tocolytics (calcium channel blockers/NSAIDs) for 48 hours to allow corticosteroids.[2]
    - Corticosteroids (24–34 weeks) and magnesium sulfate (<32 weeks) for fetal lung maturity and neuroprotection.[2]
- *Ultrasound Surveillance* ***(Table 5)****:*
    - *First trimester:* Gestational age, chorionicity, amnionicity, aneuploidy screening.
    - *Second trimester:* Anomaly scan, cervical length.
    - *Growth scans:* From 24 weeks (dichorionic, 4–6 weekly) or 16 weeks (monochorionic, 2-weekly).
    - Doppler for FGR or TTTS/TAPS screening in monochorionic twins.[2]
- *Multifetal Pregnancy Reduction:*
    - Recommended for triplets or higher to reduce preterm birth and complications.[8]
    - *Technique:* Ultrasound-guided intracardiac potassium chloride injection.
    - Reduces pregnancy loss rate from 15–25 to 4–7%.
    - Challenging in monochorionic pregnancies due to shared circulation.[2]

TIMING AND MODE OF DELIVERY

- *Dichorionic Diamniotic Twins:* Plan delivery at 37–38 weeks.[2]
- *Monochorionic Diamniotic Twins:* Plan delivery at 36–37 weeks.[2]
- *Monochorionic Monoamniotic Twins:* Cesarean at 32–34 weeks.[2,5]
- *Triplets*: Plan delivery at 35 weeks; individualize if complications.
- *Vaginal Delivery:* Feasible for diamniotic twins with vertex first twin beyond 32 weeks, no complications.[2]

TABLE 5: Ultrasound surveillance schedule.

Gestation period	*Dichorionic twins*	*Monochorionic twins*
11–14 weeks	Gestational age, chorionicity, nuchal translucency	Same, plus TTTS/TAPS screening
18–22 weeks	Anomaly scan, cervical length	Same
24+ weeks	Growth scan every 4–6 weeks	Growth scan, Doppler every 2 weeks

TABLE 6: Delivery of second twin.

Presentation	*Management*
Vertex	Continue monitoring, oxytocin if contractions slow, amniotomy when engaged
Non-Vertex	Immediate breech extraction or internal podalic version; cesarean if cervix closes

- *Cesarean Indications:*
  - Monochorionic monoamniotic twins.
  - Non-vertex first twin.
  - Triplets or higher-order multiples.[2]
  - *Previous cesarean:* 0.9% rupture risk, requires continuous monitoring.

INTRAPARTUM CARE

- *Preparedness:*
  - Skilled obstetrician trained in vaginal breech delivery, internal podalic version, and cesarean.
  - Neonatal resuscitation facilities for each fetus.
  - Immediate access to uterotonics and blood transfusion.
- *Principles:*
  - Continuous dual-channel cardiotocography.
  - Neuraxial analgesia for pain and potential interventions.
  - Confirm fetal presentations via ultrasound.
  - Avoid routine oxytocin augmentation; use only for second twin if contractions slow **(Table 6)**.
  - Active third-stage management with 10 units oxytocin IM post-delivery.[2]

POSTPARTUM CARE

- Monitor for postpartum hemorrhage due to uterine atony.
- Support breastfeeding with additional 500 kcal/day per infant.[2]
- Screen for postpartum depression (3 × risk).
- Provide contraception counseling.

RECENT ADVANCES AND GUIDELINES

- *Elective Single Embryo Transfer (eSET):* Reduces multiple pregnancy rates in IVF.[11]
- *Non-Invasive Prenatal Testing (NIPT):* Limited role in dizygotic twins due to variable fetal DNA fractions.[5]
- *Fetal Therapy:* Laser ablation for TTTS in monochorionic twins improves outcomes.[2]
- *ACOG 2021 Guidelines:* Emphasize delivery timing based on chorionicity and corticosteroids for preterm birth.[2]

REFERENCES

1. American College of Obstetricians and Gynecologists (ACOG). Multifetal Gestations: Twin, Triplet, and Higher-Order Multifetal Pregnancies. Obstet Gynecol. 2021;137(5):e145-62.
2. ACOG Practice Bulletin No. 231. Management of Multifetal Pregnancies. Obstet Gynecol. 2021;137(6):e163-74.
3. Martin JA, et al. Births: Final Data for 2020. Natl Vital Stat Rep. 2021;70(2):1-50.
4. Evans MI, et al. Multifetal pregnancy reduction: Evolution of techniques. Fetal Diagn Ther. 2016;39(3):167-73.
5. Sunderam S, et al. Assisted Reproductive Technology Surveillance—United States, 2019. MMWR Surveill Summ. 2021;70(9):1-24.
6. Legro RS, et al. Letrozole versus clomiphene for infertility in PCOS. N Engl J Med. 2014;371(2):119-29.
7. ASRM Practice Committee. Guidance on the limits to the number of embryos to transfer. Fertil Steril. 2017;107(4):901-3.
8. Smits J, et al. The global epidemiology of multiple births. Twin Res Hum Genet. 2016;19(5):453-62.
9. Khalil A, et al. ISUOG Practice Guidelines: Role of ultrasound in twin pregnancy. Ultrasound Obstet Gynecol. 2016;47(2):247-63.
10. Beemsterboer SN, et al. Advanced maternal age and twinning. Hum Reprod. 2016;31(4):896-901.
11. Bdolah Y, et al. Preeclampsia in twin pregnancies: Incidence and outcome. Hypertens Pregnancy. 2016;35(4):523-8.
12. Schwartz DB, et al. Gestational diabetes in twin pregnancies. J Matern Fetal Neonatal Med. 2015;28(12):1450-5.
13. Stone J, et al. Multifetal pregnancy reduction: A review. Am J Perinatol. 2018;35(6):554-9.
14. Pharoah POD, et al. Cerebral palsy and multiple births. Arch Dis Child Fetal Neonatal Ed. 2016;94(6):F436-40.

Monochorionic Twin Pregnancy

Ruchika Garg

INTRODUCTION

Monochorionic (MC) twin pregnancies, occurring in approximately 1 in 250 pregnancies, constitute 20–30% of twin gestations and 70% of monozygotic twins.[1] In India, MC twins contribute significantly to perinatal morbidity and mortality, with a 2–4-fold higher perinatal mortality rate compared to DC twins and singletons, respectively, and a 4–5-fold increase in neurological morbidity.[2] The rise in multiple pregnancies, driven by assisted reproductive technologies (ART) and delayed maternal age, has increased MC twinning, particularly with day 5 blastocyst transfers.[3] Placental vascular anastomoses [arterio-arterial (AA), veno-venous (VV), arterio-venous (AV)] are the hallmark of MC pregnancies, predisposing to complications like twin-twin transfusion syndrome (TTTS), twin anemia-polycythemia sequence (TAPS), selective intrauterine growth restriction (sIUGR), and twin reversed arterial perfusion (TRAP).[4] This review outlines optimal surveillance, complications, and management strategies for MC twins, tailored for postgraduate medical education.

METHODS

A systematic literature search was conducted using PubMed and Google Scholar for articles published between January 2015 and June 2025. Search terms included *monochorionic twins, twin-twin transfusion syndrome, selective IUGR, TAPS, fetoscopic laser*, and *chorionicity*. Inclusion criteria were: (1) original research, reviews, or guidelines, (2) English language, (3) peer-reviewed, (4) relevant to MC twins, and (5) full-text available. From 120 articles identified, 15 duplicates were removed, 70 irrelevant articles were excluded, and 35 were selected for review.

EPIDEMIOLOGY AND RISK FACTORS (TABLE 1)

- *Prevalence:* MC twins occur in 1/250 pregnancies, 20% of twin pregnancies, and 70% of monozygotic twins.[1]
- *Perinatal outcomes:*
    - *Mortality:* 2 × higher than DC twins, 4 × higher than singletons.[2]
    - *Neurological morbidity:* 4–5 × higher than DC twins, 25–30 × higher than singletons.[2]
    - Complications affect 1/3 of MC pregnancies.[2]

TABLE 1: Epidemiology of MC twin pregnancies.[1-4]

Parameter	*MC Twins*	*DC Twins*	*Singletons*
Prevalence	1/250 pregnancies	80% of twins	–
Perinatal Mortality	2 × DC, 4 × singletons	Baseline	Baseline
Neurological Morbidity	4–5 × DC, 25–30 × singletons	Baseline	Baseline
Complication Rate	33%	Lower	Lower

TABLE 2: Ultrasound surveillance schedule for MC Twins.[5-8]

Gestational age	*Frequency*	*Focus*	*Parameters*
<14 weeks	Once	Chorionicity, viability, aneuploidy	T-sign, lambda sign, combined test
18–20+6 weeks	Once	Anomaly scan	Extended cardiac views
16–26 weeks	Every 2 weeks	TTTS detection	DVP, EFW, bladder visibility
>26 weeks	Every 2 weeks	sIUGR, TAPS, late TTTS	DVP, EFW, Doppler (UAPI, MCA-PSV, DV)

- *Risk factors:*
  - ART (e.g., day 5 blastocyst transfers) increases monozygotic twinning.[3]
  - Advanced maternal age and sociodemographic changes.[3]
  - Higher-order multiples (e.g., MC/DC triplets) increase feto-fetal transfusion risks.[4]

ULTRASOUND SURVEILLANCE (TABLE 2)

Early ultrasound (<14 weeks) is critical for determining chorionicity, amnionicity, and viability:[5]

- *Chorionicity:*
  - *MC:* Single placental mass, T-sign (thin inter-twin membrane).[5]
  - *DC:* Two placental masses or lambda sign.[5]
  - **Figure 1**: Ultrasound images of T-sign (MC) and lambda sign (DC).[5]
- *First Trimester (11–14 weeks):*
  - Confirm viability, gestational age, and fetal anomalies.
  - Screen for aneuploidy using combined test (nuchal translucency, β-hCG, PAPP-A; 90% sensitivity, 10% false-positive rate) or non-invasive prenatal testing (NIPT, similar performance to singletons).[6]
- *Second Trimester (18–20 + 6 weeks):*
  - Routine anomaly scan with extended cardiac views per NHS Fetal Anomaly Screening Programme.[7]
- *Serial Surveillance (from 16 weeks):*
  - Biweekly ultrasounds to detect TTTS (16–26 weeks), sIUGR, TAPS, or late-onset TTTS (>26 weeks).[8]
  - *Measure:*
    - Deepest vertical pocket (DVP) for liquor volume discordance.

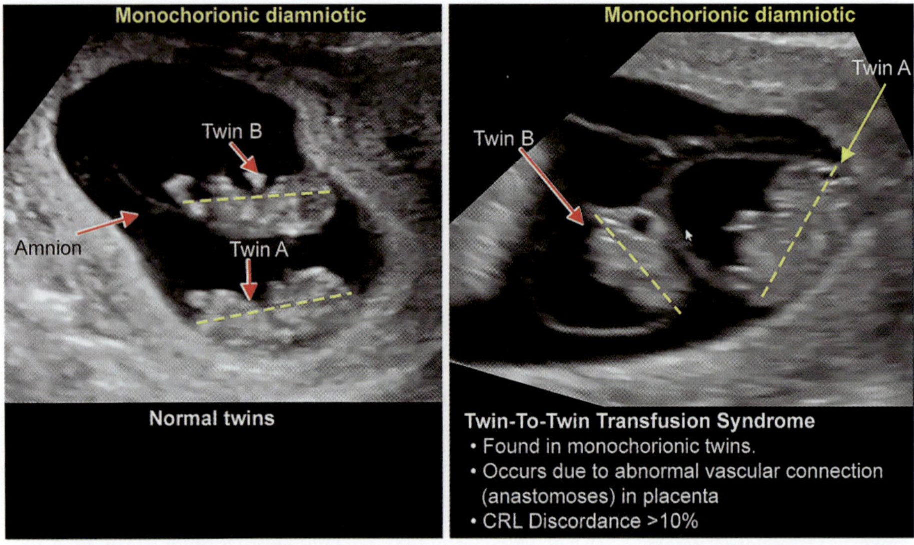

Fig. 1: Ultrasound images of T-sign (MC) and lambda sign.

TABLE 3: Quintero staging for twin–twin transfusion syndrome (TTTS).[10]

Stage	*Criteria*
I	Discordant liquor (DVP ≥8 cm recipient, ≤2 cm donor); donor bladder visible
II	Donor bladder non-visible
III	Abnormal Doppler (UAPI, DV, umbilical vein)
IV	Ascites/hydrops in either twin
V	Demise of one/both twins

- Estimated fetal weight (EFW) and biometry (head, abdomen, femur).
- Fetal bladder visibility.[8]

- If TTTS or sIUGR suspected, perform Doppler studies (umbilical artery pulsatility index [UAPI], middle cerebral artery peak systolic velocity [MCA-PSV], ductus venosus [DV]).[8]

COMPLICATIONS OF MC TWIN PREGNANCIES (TABLE 3)

Twin–Twin Transfusion Syndrome (TTTS)

- *Prevalence*: Affects 10–15% of MC twins.[9]
- *Pathophysiology*: Unbalanced blood flow via AV anastomoses, often with marginal/velamentous cord insertion.[9]
- *Diagnosis*: Quintero staging based on ultrasound findings **(Fig. 2)**.[10]
- *Management:*[11]
    - *Stage I:* Expectant management unless polyhydramnios (DVP ≥8 cm) or cervical shortening (<25 mm).

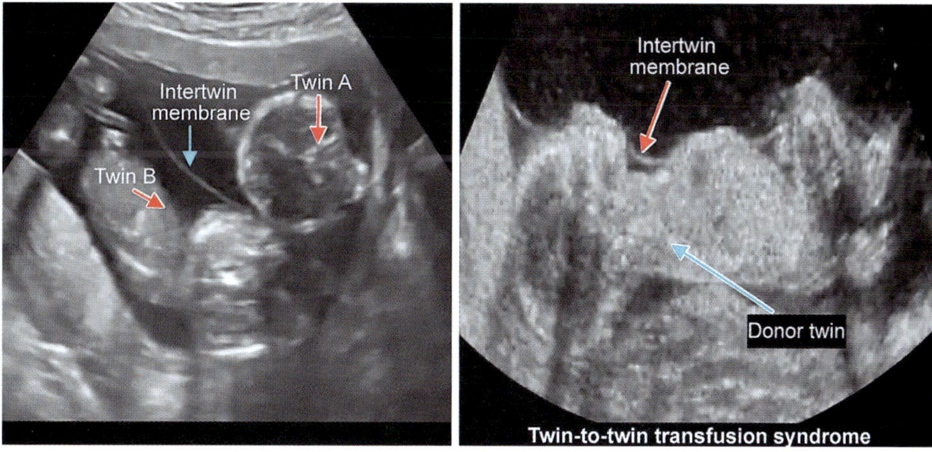

Fig. 2: Ultrasound images of T-sign (MC) and lambda sign.

- *Stage II–IV (<26 weeks):* Fetoscopic laser ablation (Solomon technique) to coagulate anastomoses; 80–90% survival for ≥1 twin.[11]
- *>26 weeks or no laser access*: Amnioreduction (50–60% survival, 29–35% neurological handicap).[11]
- *Post-treatment:* Weekly ultrasound (fetal brain, heart, limbs; UAPI, MCA-PSV, DV) for 2 weeks, then biweekly.[11]

- *Outcomes:* Laser ablation reduces neurological complications (11–16%) compared to amnioreduction (29–35%).[12]
- *Complications:* Recurrent TTTS (14%) or TAPS (13%) post-laser; Solomon technique reduces recurrence.[12]

TWIN ANEMIA–POLYCYTHEMIA SEQUENCE (TAPS)

- *Prevalence:* 3–5% spontaneous, 2–6% post-TTTS laser.[13]
- *Pathophysiology:* Small AV anastomoses cause chronic transfusion, leading to anemia (donor) and polycythemia (recipient) without hemodynamic changes.[13]
- *Diagnosis **(Table 4)**:*[13]
  - *Prenatal:* MCA-PSV >1.5 MoM (donor), <0.8 MoM (recipient).
  - *Postnatal:* Inter-twin hemoglobin difference >8 g/dL, reticulocyte count ratio >1.7.
- *Management:*[13]
  - *Spontaneous TAPS:* Expectant management; good prognosis.
  - *Post-laser TAPS:* Aggressive, may require laser, intrauterine transfusion (intraperitoneal preferred), or delivery.

TABLE 4: Diagnostic criteria for TAPS.[13]

Setting	*Criteria*
Prenatal	MCA-PSV >1.5 MoM (donor), <0.8 MoM (recipient)
Postnatal	Hb difference >8 g/dL, reticulocyte ratio >1.7

TABLE 5: Types of sIUGR in MC twins.[14]

Type	Umbilical artery Doppler	Prognosis	Management
I	Positive EDF	Good	Expectant to 34–35 weeks
II	Absent/reversed EDF	Poor (preterm, IUFD, neurological)	Laser, cord occlusion, or delivery
III	Intermittent EDF	Variable (neurological risk to large twin)	Individualized (laser, occlusion)

- *Indications for intervention:* Rapid MCA-PSV discordance or pre-hydropic signs in donor.

- *Outcomes:* Neonatal morbidity limited to hematological issues (anemia, polycythemia); rare cerebral injury.[13]

SELECTIVE INTRAUTERINE GROWTH RESTRICTION (sIUGR)

- *Prevalence:* 10–15% (early), 5% (late).[14]
- *Pathophysiology:* Unequal placental sharing with rescue transfusion from larger twin via anastomoses.[14]
- *Classification* ***(Table 5)****:*[14]
  - *Type I:* Positive end-diastolic flow (EDF) in umbilical artery; good prognosis, expectant management to 34–35 weeks.
  - *Type II:* Absent/reversed EDF; high risk of preterm delivery, IUFD, neurological sequelae.
  - *Type III:* Intermittent absent/reversed EDF with large AA anastomoses; prolonged IUGR survival but high neurological risk to larger twin.
- *Management:*[14]
  - Individualized based on gestational age, Doppler anomalies, and parental preferences.
  - *Options*: Expectant management, laser therapy, cord occlusion, or delivery (32–34 weeks).
  - Monitor with biweekly ultrasound (biometry, UAPI, MCA-PSV, DV).
- *Outcomes:* Type II/III have higher IUFD and neurological risks; rescue transfusion may prolong IUGR twin survival.[14]

TWIN REVERSED ARTERIAL PERFUSION (TRAP) SEQUENCE

- *Prevalence:* 1% of MC twins.[15]
- *Pathophysiology:* Acardiac twin survives via reversed perfusion from pump twin, risking cardiac failure, polyhydramnios, or cord entanglement.[15]
- *Management:*[15]
  - Expectant management if stable; 50% risk of pregnancy loss.
  - Selective feticide (radiofrequency ablation [RFA], laser, or bipolar cord coagulation) for pump twin protection; 80–90% survival for normal twin.[15]
- *Outcomes:* RFA is simpler, faster, and reduces preterm delivery risk compared to laser.[15]

ACUTE FETO-FETAL TRANSFUSION

- *Pathophysiology:* Sudden pressure/heart rate drop in one twin causes unidirectional transfusion, often via large AA/AV anastomoses.[16]
- *Scenarios:*[16]
    - *Post-SIUD:* Surviving twin exsanguinates into dead twin; 15% death risk, 18–34% brain injury.
    - *Both Alive:* Transient bradycardia causes acute transfusion; high brain injury/death risk in donor.
- *Management:* Prevent SIUD via timely intervention; elective delivery at 36–37 weeks to reduce late IUFD risk.[16]

DIFFERENTIAL DIAGNOSIS OF MC COMPLICATIONS

Differentiating TTTS, sIUGR, TAPS, and non-specific amniotic fluid (AF) discordance is critical:[17]

- *Algorithm:*[17]
    - Rule out TTTS (urgent; poor prognosis without laser).
    - Assess for sIUGR (EFW <10th percentile, discordance ≥25%).
    - Check for TAPS (MCA-PSV discordance).
    - If none, classify as non-specific AF discordance (50% risk of developing TTTS/sIUGR; weekly ultrasound).

FETOSCOPIC COMPLICATIONS

Fetoscopic laser for TTTS/sIUGR carries risks:[18]

- *Chorionic Membrane Separation (CMS):*
    - *Incidence:* 20% post-laser, 52% post-open surgery.[18]
    - *Risks:* PPROM, preterm delivery, IUFD, amniotic band syndrome.[18]
    - Associated with surgery <18 weeks.[18]
- *Other Risks:* Preterm delivery (30%), PPROM (30%), psychological distress post-fetal loss.[18]
- *Outcomes:* No long-term maternal fertility/obstetric adverse effects; 10% reduction in neonatal survival with CMS.[18]

SINGLE INTRAUTERINE DEATH (SIUD)

- *Risks:* Post-SIUD, surviving twin faces 15% mortality and 26% neurological morbidity due to exsanguination via anastomoses.[19]
- *Management:*[19]
    - Fetal brain MRI 4 weeks post-SIUD to detect ischemic/focal lesions.
    - Monitor surviving twin with weekly ultrasound (UAPI, MCA-PSV, DV).
- *Prevention:* Elective delivery at 36–37 weeks reduces late SIUD risk.[19]

HIGHER-ORDER MULTIPLES

- *MC/DC Triplets*: Higher fetal loss, TTTS, sIUGR, and TAPS risks compared to trichorionic triplets.[20]

TABLE 6: Delivery timing for MC twins.[21]

Type	*Timing*	*Mode*
Uncomplicated MCDA	36 + 0 – 37 + 0 weeks	Vaginal (if cephalic) or cesarean
MCMA	32 + 0 – 34 + 0 weeks	Cesarean
Complicated (TTTS, sIUGR)	32–34 weeks	Based on CTG/DV Doppler

- *Management:*[20]
  - Discuss selective reduction/feticide (laser, RFA, cord occlusion).
  - *Complications*: PPROM (30%), preterm delivery; 65–92% survival.
  - Limited data on long-term neurodevelopmental outcomes.

TIMING AND MODE OF DELIVERY (TABLE 6)

- *Uncomplicated MCDA Twins:*[21]
  - Elective delivery at 36+0 to 37+0 weeks with antenatal steroids to reduce stillbirth risk (5–10 × higher than DC twins).
  - Vaginal delivery safe if first twin is cephalic (Twin Birth Study)[21]
- *MCMA Twins:*[21]
  - High IUFD risk due to cord entanglement; deliver by cesarean section at 32+0 to 34+0 weeks.
- *Complicated MC Twins*: Deliver at 32–34 weeks based on CTG/DV Doppler findings.[21]

CURRENT GUIDELINES

- *NICE (2019):* Biweekly ultrasound from 16 weeks for MC twins; determine chorionicity <14 weeks.[22]
- *RCOG (2016):* Fetoscopic laser for TTTS stage II–IV <26 weeks; MCA-PSV for TAPS screening.[23]
- *ISUOG (2020):* Extended cardiac views at 18–20 weeks; Solomon technique for laser ablation.[24]
- *SMFM (2021):* Elective delivery at 36–37 weeks for uncomplicated MCDA twins.[25]

CONCLUSION

MC twin pregnancies pose significant perinatal risks due to placental anastomoses, with 33% experiencing complications like TTTS, TAPS, sIUGR, or TRAP. Early chorionicity determination (<14 weeks), biweekly ultrasound surveillance from 16 weeks, and fetoscopic laser for TTTS are critical for optimizing outcomes. Differential diagnosis algorithms and individualized management (expectant, laser, or feticide) address complex scenarios. Elective delivery at 36–37 weeks for uncomplicated MCDA twins reduces IUFD risk. Collaboration with fetal medicine centers and adherence to guidelines ensure effective management, minimizing maternal and fetal morbidity.

REFERENCES

1. Lewi L, Deprest J, Hecher K. The vascular anastomoses in monochorionic twin pregnancies and their clinical consequences. Am J Obstet Gynecol. 2019;220(1):22-30.

2. Khalil A, Rodgers M, Baschat A, et al. ISUOG practice guidelines: role of ultrasound in twin pregnancy. Ultrasound Obstet Gynecol. 2016;47(2):247-63.
3. Mateizel I, Santos-Ribeiro S, Done E, et al. Do ART techniques influence monozygotic twinning? Hum Reprod. 2016;31(8):1697-704.
4. Lopriore E, Slaghekke F, Oepkes D, et al. Higher-order multiple pregnancies with monochorionic components: a review. Prenat Diagn. 2020;40(3):321-8.
5. Khalil A, Lewi L, Lopriore E. ISUOG practice guidelines: ultrasound assessment of chorionicity and amnionicity in twin pregnancies. Ultrasound Obstet Gynecol. 2020;56(4):659-71.
6. Gil MM, Galeva I, Jani J, et al. Screening for trisomy 21 in monochorionic twins: combined test vs cfDNA testing. Ultrasound Obstet Gynecol. 2019;54(1):83-90.
7. NHS Fetal Anomaly Screening Programme. Handbook for ultrasound practitioners. London: Public Health England; 2018.
8. Townsend R, Khalil A. Ultrasound surveillance in monochorionic twin pregnancies. Best Pract Res Clin Obstet Gynaecol. 2019;58:26-36.
9. Slaghekke F, Lopriore E, Lewi L, et al. Twin–twin transfusion syndrome: a review. Expert Rev Hematol. 2019;12(8):627-36.
10. Quintero RA, Morales WJ, Allen MH, et al. Staging of twin–twin transfusion syndrome. J Perinatol. 2019;39(6):803-9.
11. Senat MV, Deprest J, Boulvain M, et al. Fetoscopic laser therapy for twin twin transfusion syndrome: a meta-analysis. Am J Obstet Gynecol. 2020;222(4):321-31.
12. Akkermans J, Peeters SH, Klumper FJ, et al. Solomon technique vs selective laser ablation for TTTS: a randomized trial. Ultrasound Obstet Gynecol. 2015;46(5):526-32.
13. Tollenaar LSA, Lopriore E, Slaghekke F, et al. Twin anemia–polycythemia sequence: a review. Prenat Diagn. 2020;40(9):1087-95.
14. Gratacós E, Lewi L, Muñoz B, et al. Selective intrauterine growth restriction in monochorionic twins: classification and management. Ultrasound Obstet Gynecol. 2018;52(1):36-43.
15. Shinar S, Berger H, Kingdom J, et al. Radiofrequency ablation vs laser in TRAP sequence: a meta-analysis. Prenat Diagn. 2021;41(7):827-35.
16. Lopriore E, Lewi L, Oepkes D. Acute feto-fetal transfusion in monochorionic twins. Fetal Diagn Ther. 2017;42(3):161-8.
17. Khalil A, Townsend R. Differential diagnosis of complications in monochorionic twins. Best Pract Res Clin Obstet Gynaecol. 2021;74:84-95.
18. Stirnemann JJ, Quibel T, Essaoui M, et al. Chorionic membrane separation after fetoscopy: a multicenter study. Ultrasound Obstet Gynecol. 2019;54(3):384-90.
19. Mackie FL, Rigby A, Morris RK, et al. Neurodevelopmental outcomes after single intrauterine fetal death in monochorionic twins. BJOG. 2020;127(8):977-85.
20. Chmait RH, Kontopoulos EV, Quintero RA. Higher-order multiples with monochorionic components: management and outcomes. Am J Perinatol. 2018;35(6):553-60.
21. Barrett JF, Hannah ME, Hutton EK, et al. A randomized trial of planned cesarean or vaginal delivery for twin pregnancy. N Engl J Med. 2015;373(14):1295-305.
22. National Institute for Health and Care Excellence. Twin and triplet pregnancy (NG137). London: NICE; 2019.
23. Royal College of Obstetricians and Gynaecologists. Management of monochorionic twin pregnancy. Green-top Guideline No. 51. BJOG. 2016;123(13):e1-35.
24. Khalil A, Arabin B, Baschat A, et al. ISUOG practice guidelines: twin pregnancies with growth discordance. Ultrasound Obstet Gynecol. 2020;56(5):769-84.
25. Society for Maternal-Fetal Medicine. Twin pregnancies: management and delivery. Am J Obstet Gynecol. 2021;225(5):B2-B10.

Fetal Monitoring

Ruchika Garg

DEFINITION

Intrapartum fetal heart rate (FHR) monitoring assesses fetal well-being during labor by detecting changes in FHR patterns, reflecting cardiac and central nervous system responses to oxygenation, blood pressure, and acid–base status. It aims to identify hypoxia to guide timely interventions while avoiding unnecessary procedures.[1]

KEY POINTS

- **Objective:** Detect fetal hypoxia to prevent hypoxic-ischemic encephalopathy (HIE), cerebral palsy, or death; avoid unnecessary interventions in well-oxygenated fetuses.[1]
- **Prevalence:** Used in 85–90% of labor in high-resource settings; continuous electronic fetal monitoring (EFM) is common in high-risk cases.[2]
- **Methods:** Structured intermittent auscultation (SIA) for low risk; continuous EFM for high-risk or abnormal SIA findings.[3]
- **Limitations:** High false-positive rates (60–80%); no significant reduction in perinatal mortality or cerebral palsy.[4]
- **Guidelines:** Royal College of Obstetricians and Gynaecologists (RCOG)/National Institute for Health and Care Excellence (NICE) advocate SIA for low-risk women, continuous EFM for high-risk.[5,6]

OBJECTIVES OF INTRAPARTUM FETAL HEART RATE MONITORING

- Identify FHR changes indicating inadequate oxygenation for timely intervention to reduce hypoxic injury.[1]
- Accurately confirm well-oxygenated fetuses to prevent unnecessary cesarean or instrumental deliveries.[1]
- Monitor high-risk pregnancies [e.g., preeclampsia, intrauterine growth restriction (IUGR)] to optimize outcomes.[3]

RATIONALE FOR INTRAPARTUM FETAL HEART RATE MONITORING

- **Purpose:** Developed in the 1960s to detect events leading to HIE (1–3/1000 live births), cerebral palsy (2/1,000), or fetal death (0.5–1/1,000).[2]
- **Physiology:** FHR reflects fetal responses to hypoxia, mediated by baroreceptors (cord compression) and chemoreceptors (hypoxemia).[1]

- **Impact:** Reduced intrapartum stillbirths (50% decline since the 1980s) and neonatal seizures [relative risk (RR): 0.5], but no significant decrease in cerebral palsy or perinatal mortality.[4]
- **Challenges:** High false-positive rates (60–80%) increase cesarean (RR 1.63) and instrumental delivery rates (RR 1.15).[4]

PREVALENCE AND TRENDS (TABLE 1)

- **Global use:** 85–90% of laborers in high-resource settings; 30–50% in low-resource settings.[2]
- **High-risk cases:** Continuous EFM is used in 60–70% of laborers with risk factors (e.g., preeclampsia, oxytocin use).[3]
- **Trends:** Increasing EFM use due to rising high-risk pregnancies (e.g., obesity and diabetes).[7]
- **Outcomes:**
  - **Metabolic acidosis:** 1–2% of deliveries.[2]
  - **HIE:** 1–3/1,000 live births; 10–20% progress to cerebral palsy.[7]
  - **Perinatal mortality:** 0.5–1/1,000 in high-resource settings.[2]

METHODS OF FETAL HEART RATE MONITORING

Structured Intermittent Auscultation

- **Technique:** Doppler device at 15–30 minutes intervals in the first stage, every 5 minutes in the second stage.[3]
- **Indication:** Low-risk pregnancies; equivalent to EFM for perinatal outcomes (RR: 1.0).[4]
- **Advantages:** Noninvasive, promotes mobility, and has lower intervention rates.[3]
- **Limitations:** Misses subtle FHR changes; requires skilled staff.[1]

Continuous Electronic Fetal Monitoring (Table 2)

- **Technique:** External (Doppler ultrasound) or internal (fetal scalp electrode) monitoring.[1]
- **Indication:** High-risk pregnancies or abnormal SIA findings.[5]

TABLE 1: Prevalence of intrapartum FHR monitoring and outcomes.[2,7]

Parameter	*Prevalence*	*Notes*
EFM use	85–90% (high-resource)	60–70% in high-risk cases
Metabolic acidosis	1–2%	Cord pH < 7.0
HIE	1–3/1,000	10–20% cerebral palsy risk
Perinatal mortality	0.5–1/1,000	No significant EFM impact

TABLE 2: Comparison of SIA versus continuous EFM.[3,4]

Parameter	*SIA*	*Continuous EFM*
Indication	Low risk	High-risk, abnormal SIA
Frequency	15–30 minutes (first stage), 5 minutes (second stage)	Continuous
False-positive rate	Low	60–80%
Cesarean risk	RR: 1.0	RR: 1.63

TABLE 3: Indications for continuous electronic fetal monitoring (EFM).[5,6]

Category	*Risk factor*	*Example*
Maternal	Hypertension	Pre-eclampsia (≥160/110 mm Hg)
Maternal	Labor factors	Oxytocin use, prolonged rupture
Fetal	Growth issues	Intrauterine growth restriction (IUGR) and oligohydramnios
Fetal	Presentation	Breech, multiple pregnancies

- **Advantages:** Detects subtle FHR changes; continuous data.[1]
- **Limitations:** High false-positive rate (60–80%), increased cesarean rate (RRl: 1.63).[4]

Indications for Continuous Electronic Fetal Monitoring (Table 3)

- **Maternal risk factors:**
  - Pre-eclampsia (≥160/110 mm Hg), diabetes, cardiac disease, and anemia.[5]
  - Oxytocin use, chorioamnionitis, prolonged rupture of membranes (>24 hours).[6]
  - Previous cesarean, regional analgesia (initial bolus).[5]
- **Fetal risk factors:**
  - IUGR, oligohydramnios, meconium-stained liquor, preterm (<32 weeks).[6]
  - Abnormal Doppler, breech presentation, and multiple pregnancies.[5]

TECHNIQUES FOR FETAL HEART RATE MONITORING

- **External monitoring:**
  - Doppler ultrasound detects cardiac motion; prone to signal loss (20–30% in the second stage).[8]
  - Preferred initial method; noninvasive.[1]
- **Internal monitoring:**
  - Fetal scalp electrode measures R-R intervals; accurate for arrhythmias.[1]
  - *Contraindications*: Maternal infections (HIV, hepatitis), fetal bleeding disorders, preterm (<32 weeks).[9]
- **Maternal position:** Lateral recumbent or half-sitting preferred to avoid aortocaval compression.[10]
- **Paper scales:** 1–3 cm/min (horizontal), 20–30 BPM/cm (vertical).[1]
- **Uterine contractions:**
  - **Normal:** ≤5 in 10 minutes over 30 minutes.[1]
  - **Tachysystole:** >5 in 10 minutes; increases hypoxia risk.[1]

ANALYSIS OF FETAL HEART RATE TRACINGS (TABLE 4)

Baseline Fetal Heart Rate

- **Definition:** Mean FHR rounded to 5 BPM over 10 minutes, excluding periodic changes.[1]
- **Normal:** 110–160 BPM[1]

TABLE 4: FHR pattern definitions (ACOG).[1]

Feature	*Definition*	*Significance*
Baseline	110–160 BPM	Normal fetal status
Variability	6–25 BPM	Fetal CNS activity
Acceleration	≥15 BPM, ≥15 seconds	Fetal well-being
Deceleration	Early, variable, late, and prolonged	Varies by type
Sinusoidal	Three to five cycles/min, ≥20 minutes	Severe hypoxia/anemia

- **Tachycardia (>160 BPM, >10 minutes):**
  - **Causes:** Maternal fever (most common), drugs (beta-agonists), fetal arrhythmias.[11]
- **Bradycardia (<110 BPM, >10 minutes):**
  - **Causes:** Maternal hypothermia, beta-blockers, fetal heart block.[12]

Variability

- **Definition:** Fluctuations in baseline FHR (three to five cycles/min).[1]
- **Normal:** 6–25 BPM (moderate).[1]
- **Reduced (<5 BPM):** Hypoxia, sedation, and infection.[13]
- **Increased (>25 BPM):** Rapid hypoxia with decelerations (saltatory pattern).[13]

Accelerations

- **Definition:** Abrupt FHR increase (≥15 BPM for ≥15 s, <2 minutes).[1]
- **Significance:** Indicates fetal well-being; absent in deep sleep or hypoxia.[14]
- **Preterm:** ≥10 BPM for ≥10 seconds.[1]

Decelerations

- **Early:** Symmetrical, nadir with contraction peak; head compression; benign.[15]
- **Variable:** Abrupt (<30 s to nadir), V-shaped; cord compression; hypoxia if prolonged (>3 minutes).[15]
- **Late:** Delayed nadir postcontraction; uteroplacental insufficiency.[15]
- **Prolonged:** ≥2 minutes but <10 minutes; hypoxia if <80 BPM with reduced variability.[15]

Sinusoidal Pattern

- **Definition:** Regular oscillations (three to five cycles/min, ≥20 minutes), absent variability.[1]
- **Causes:** Severe fetal anemia, acute hypoxia, and infection.[16]

Classification of Fetal Heart Rate Tracings (Table 5)

- **NICHD 3-tier system:**
- **Category I:** Normal; continue monitoring.[1]
- **Category II:** Indeterminate; general measures (e.g., maternal repositioning and oxygen).[1]
- **Category III:** Abnormal; expedite delivery.[1]

ROYAL COLLEGE OF OBSTETRICIANS AND GYNAECOLOGISTS/ NATIONAL INSTITUTE FOR HEALTH AND CARE EXCELLENCE GUIDELINES

- *RCOG (2017):*[5]
  - SIA for low-risk women; continuous EFM for high-risk or abnormal SIA.
  - Use the NICHD 3-tier system for CTG interpretation.
  - Avoid fetal scalp blood sampling; consider delivery for Category III tracings.
- *NICE (2023) (Table 6 and 7):*[6]
  - Offer SIA every 15 minutes (first stage) and 5 minutes (second stage) for low-risk women.
  - Switch to EFM if risk factors (e.g., meconium and oxytocin) or abnormal SIA.
  - Remove EFM if 20-minute normal tracing after initial concern.
  - Do not use fetal ST analysis (STAN) routinely.

Ancillary Tests (Table 6)

- **Fetal scalp blood sampling:** Measures pH/lactate; not recommended due to invasiveness, limited predictive value.[6]
- **Scalp/vibroacoustic stimulation:** Elicits accelerations; unreliable for hypoxia.[17]
- **Fetal pulse oximetry:** Not recommended; no outcome improvement.[6]
- **ST analysis (STAN):** Assesses fetal ECG ST-segment changes; no significant benefit (RR: 1.0 for HIE).[18]

LIMITATIONS OF FETAL HEART RATE MONITORING

- **Inter-/intraobserver variability:** 20–30% disagreement in CTG interpretation.[19]
- **Poor predictive value:** Category II/III tracings predict acidosis in <50% cases.[4]

TABLE 5: NICHD FHR categories and management.[1,5]

Category	*Features*	*Management*
I	Normal baseline, variability; no late/variable decelerations	Continue SIA/EFM
II	Tachycardia, minimal variability, recurrent decelerations	Reposition, oxygen, amnioinfusion, consider delivery
III	Absent variability with recurrent decelerations, bradycardia, sinusoidal	Expedite delivery

TABLE 6: Ancillary tests for fetal assessment.[6,17,18]

Test	*Purpose*	*Status*
Scalp sampling	pH/lactate	Not recommended
STAN	ECG ST changes	Not routine
Pulse Oximetry	Oxygen saturation	Not recommended

TABLE 7: CTG in labor NICE classification.

Sticker No:	*CTG in Labor: NICE 2022 classification*	*Maternal pulse*	*Initial risk factors*
Contractions	<5:10	• ≥5:10 • Contraction lasting ≥2 mins	Evolving risks:
Baseline (bpm)	• 110-160 bpm and • Stable baseline and • Appropriate for gestation	• Increase of ≥20 bpm from start of labour or in last 1 hour • 100-109 bpm (unless otherwise normal) • Unable to determine baseline	• <100 bpm • > 160 bpm
Variability (bpm)	• 5-25 bpm	• < 5 bpm for 30–50 mins • > 25 bpm for upto 10 mins	• <5 bpm for >50 mins • 25 bpm for >10 mins • Sinusoidal pattern
Decelerations	• Concerning characteristics lasting >60 secs: reduced variability within decel: slow/ failure return baseline; loss of shouldering		
	• No decelerations • Variable decelerations with no concerning characteristics	• Repetitive variable decelerations with concerning characteristics <30 mins. • Non-repetitive variable decels with concerning characteristics >30 mins, • Repetitive late decels <30 mins	• Repetitive variable decelerations with any concerning characteristics >30 mins • Repetitive late decelerations >30 mins • Acute bradycardia or single prolonged deceleration lasting >3 mins
Classification & Management	**Normal** All 4 features are white continue current care	**Suspicious: Any 1 Amber** Full risk assessment incl. maternal observations: Senior Mid-wife or Obstetric review if additional risk factors; Start conservative measures, consider fetal scalp stimulation or expediting birth	• Pathological: 1 Red/2 or more Amber • Full assessment incl. maternal observations; urgent obstetric review; Start conservative measures, consider fetal scalp stimulation, and exclude acute events. Consider expediting birth

- **Increased interventions:** Continuous EFM raises cesarean (RR: 1.63) and instrumental delivery (RR: 1.15) rates.[4]
- **Underpowered trials:** No evidence for reducing perinatal mortality or cerebral palsy due to rare outcomes.[4]

RECENT ADVANCES

- **Computerized CTG analysis:** Reduces observer variability (10–15% improvement); not yet standard.[20]
- **Fetal oxygen saturation monitoring:** Under research; inconclusive benefits.[17]
- **Machine learning:** Predicts acidosis with 80% accuracy; experimental.[21]

TABLE 8: Comparison of RCOG and AICOG Guidelines for CTG in labor .

Aspect	*NICE NG229 (2025 update)*	*ACOG Guideline No. 10 (2025)*
Classification System	Three-tier: Reassuring (green), Suspicious (amber), Pathological (red). Late decelerations are now a red feature regardless of duration/repetition (November 2025 amendment)	Three-tier: Category I (normal), Category II (indeterminate), Category III (abnormal). Includes a five-tier risk stratification in appendices for academia risk
Initial Monitoring for Low-Risk	Intermittent auscultation strongly preferred; continuous CTG only if risks emerge or the woman prefers	Supports intermittent auscultation for low-risk but allows provider/patient choice for continuous EFM.
Contraction Management	Optimum 3–4 contractions in 10 minutes; monitor frequency closely during augmentation	Addresses tachysystole with high-risk features; suggests rapid-acting tocolytics if persistent
Meconium	No longer differentiates "significant" vs. "non-significant"; advises discussion with the woman on management	Not specifically updated; focuses on overall risk integration

KEY POINTS FOR POSTGRADUATE EDUCATION

- Intrapartum FHR monitoring detects hypoxia to prevent HIE (1–3/1000) and fetal death (0.5–1/1,000).
- Used in 85–90% of laborers in high-resource settings; continuous EFM in 60–70% of high-risk cases.
- SIA recommended for low-risk; EFM for high-risk (e.g., preeclampsia and IUGR).
- **NICHD 3-tier system classifies tracings:** Category I (normal), II (indeterminate), III (abnormal).
- **High false-positive rates (60–80%) increase cesarean (RR:** 1.63) and instrumental delivery (RR: 1.15).
- RCOG/NICE advocate SIA for low-risk, EFM for high-risk; avoid scalp sampling/STAN.
- *Limitations***:** Observer variability (20–30%), poor acidosis prediction (<50%).
- *Advances***:** Computerized CTG and machine learning improve accuracy (10–15%).

REFERENCES

1. American College of Obstetricians and Gynecologists. Intrapartum fetal heart rate monitoring: Nomenclature, interpretation, and general management principles. Obstet Gynecol. 2017;130(1):e1-12.
2. Ayres-de-Campos D. Intrapartum fetal monitoring: Where are we now? Best Pract Res Clin Obstet Gynaecol. 2016;36:3-8.
3. Alfirevic Z, et al. Continuous cardiotocography (CTG) is a form of electronic fetal monitoring (EFM) for fetal assessment during labour. Cochrane Database Syst Rev. 2017;2:CD006066.
4. Al Wattar BH, et al. Effectiveness of intrapartum fetal surveillance: A systematic review and network meta-analysis. CMAJ. 2021;193(14):E468-78.
5. Royal College of Obstetricians and Gynaecologists. (2017). Intrapartum care: Care of healthy women and their babies during childbirth. [Online] Available from https://www.rcog.org.uk/news/rcog-welcomes-updated-nice-intrapartum-care-guidance/ [Last accessed December, 2025].

6. In: National Institute for Health and Care Excellence. Intrapartum care for women and babies (CG190). London: NICE; 2023.
7. Parer JT, et al. Fetal heart rate monitoring: Past, present, and future. Am J Obstet Gynecol. 2017;217(5):S2-6.
8. Nurani R, et al. Misidentification of maternal heart rate as fetal on cardiotocography. Acta Obstet Gynecol Scand. 2016;95(12):1428-32.
9. Maiques V, et al. Intrapartum fetal invasive procedures and perinatal transmission of infections. Eur J Obstet Gynecol Reprod Biol. 2016;198:63-7.
10. Carbonne B, et al. Maternal position during labor: Effects on fetal oxygenation. Obstet Gynecol. 2016;128(4):797-800.
11. Segal S, et al. Maternal fever and epidural analgesia: Effects on FHR. Anesth Analg. 2016;122(5):1467-75.
12. Jadhon ME, et al. Fetal bradycardia associated with maternal hypothermia. Obstet Gynecol. 2017;129(3):496-8.
13. Nunes I, et al. Prolonged saltatory FHR pattern and neonatal acidosis. Clin Exp Obstet Gynecol. 2016;43(5):507-11.
14. Suwanrath C, et al. Fetal sleep-wake cycles and FHR patterns. Arch Gynecol Obstet. 2016;294(3):449-54.
15. Holzmann M, et al. CTG patterns and risk of intrapartum fetal acidemia. J Perinat Med. 2017;45(4):411-8.
16. Modanlou HD, et al. Sinusoidal FHR pattern: Clinical significance. J Obstet Gynaecol Res. 2016;42(6):169-80.
17. Sacco A, et al. ST analysis for intrapartum fetal monitoring. Obstet Gynaecol. 2017;19(1):5-12.
18. Blix E, et al. Fetal scalp blood sampling: A systematic review. BJOG. 2016;123(8):1273-81.
19. Blackwell SC, et al. Interobserver reliability of the NICHD 3-tier FHR system. Am J Obstet Gynecol. 2016;215(3):378.e1-e5.
20. Georgieva A, et al. Computerized CTG analysis in intrapartum monitoring. BJOG. 2017;124(7):1121-9.
21. Warrick PA, et al. Machine learning for predicting fetal acidosis in labour. J Matern Fetal Neonatal Med. 2019;32(14):2350-7.

Abnormal Puerperium

Ruchika Garg

INTRODUCTION

- **Puerperium:** A 42-day period postdelivery where maternal anatomy and physiology revert to the prepregnant state.
  - **Definition:** Puerperium spans ~6 weeks postdelivery, involving physiological adjustment to the nonpregnant state.
- **Abnormal puerperium:** Deviations in involution, with some conditions necessitating urgent multispecialty care. Any deviation from normal involution, some potentially life-threatening, requires urgent hospitalization and a multispecialty approach.
- **Focus:** Early recognition, diagnosis, and management to prevent morbidity and mortality.

PUERPERAL SEPSIS

- **Definition:** Genital tract infection from rupture of membranes or labor to 42 days postpartum, per World Health Organization (WHO),[1] with ≥2 of:
  - Fever (≥38.5°C/101.3°F)
  - Pelvic pain
  - Abnormal vaginal discharge (e.g., pus)
  - Foul-smelling discharge
  - Delayed uterine involution (<2 cm/day in first 8 days)
  - Purulent lochia
  - Light bleeding and shock
- **Risk factors:**
  - Maternal: Malnutrition, anemia, diabetes, poor hygiene
  - Obstetric: Prolonged rupture of membranes, prolonged labor, frequent vaginal exams, intrauterine fetal death, and retained placenta/membrane.
  - **Microbiology:**
    - **Pathogens:** Group A/B streptococci, *Enterococcus, Staphylococcus aureus, Escherichia coli, Bacteroides, Clostridium*; late-onset may involve *Chlamydia trachomatis.*
    - **Origin:** Ascends from the lower genital tract to the uterus, fallopian tubes, or abdomen.
- **Pathogenesis:**
  - *Vaginal delivery*: Infects the placental site, decidua, myometrium, or cervicovaginal lacerations.

  - *Cesarean section*: Bacteria from the cervix/vagina invade the amniotic fluid, causing parametrial cellulitis or pelvic infection.
- **Clinical presentation:**
  - **Puerperal sepsis:** Fever, shivering, abdominal pain, offensive vaginal discharge, poor wound healing (perineal or cesarean).
    - **Local (wound) infection:** Low-grade fever, malaise, erythema, swelling, purulent discharge; severe cases show rigors, chills, and wound disruption.
    - **Uterine infection (metritis):** Fever, malaise, abdominal pain, foul discharge, uterine/renal angle tenderness.
  - **Red flags (urgent referral):**
    - Fever > 38°C
    - Tachycardia > 90 BPM
    - Respiratory rate > 20/min
    - Abdominal/chest pain
    - Diarrhea/vomiting
    - Uterine/renal angle tenderness
    - General distress
- **Diagnosis (Table 1):**
  - Assume genital sepsis until proven otherwise.
  - **History:** Assess antenatal, intranatal, and postnatal risk factors.
  - **Examination:** Vital signs [via MEOWS (Modified Early Obstetric Warning System) chart], abdominal, pelvic, and leg exams for thrombosis.
- **Prophylaxis:**
  - Antenatal: Treat anemia, septic foci.
  - Intranatal: Asepsis for deliveries; prophylactic antibiotics for cesarean reduce infection risk.
  - Postpartum: Asepsis, sterile pads, and isolate infected cases.
- **Treatment:**
  - **General:** Nutrition, anemia correction, IV fluids, monitor vitals, and lochia.
  - **Antibiotics (breastfeeding-safe, >85% cure rate):**
  - *Nonsevere:* Oral/IM (e.g., amoxicillin-clavulanic acid 875 mg BID).[2]
  - Severe: IV broad-spectrum within 1 hour (e.g., clindamycin 600 mg q6h + gentamicin 4.5 mg/kg IM daily).

TABLE 1: Diagnostic investigations for puerperal sepsis.

Test	*Purpose*
Complete Blood Count	Assess infection severity
Blood Culture	Identify pathogens (preantibiotics)
Urine Routine/Culture	Rule out UTI
High Vaginal Swab	Detect genital tract pathogens.
Pelvic Ultrasound	Identify retained products, abscess
Chest X-ray, CT/MRI	For lung pathology or inconclusive cases

TABLE 2: Risk Factors for venous thromboembolism (VTE) in puerperium.

Category	*Examples*
Preexisting	Previous VTE, thrombophilia, obesity, age >35
Obstetric	Cesarean, postpartum hemorrhage (PPH), preeclampsia, and prolonged labor
New/transient	Immobility, infection, and long-distance travel

- Continue IV until afebrile 24–48 hours, then oral for 7 days.
- **Surgical:** Drain abscess via colpotomy, evacuate retained products (>3 cm) after antibiotics, debride wound dehiscence.[3]
- **ICU indications:** Hypotension, oliguria, raised creatinine, lactate ≥ 4 mmol/L, acute respiratory distress syndrome (ARDS), thrombocytopenia, and hypothermia.[4]

POSTPARTUM PREECLAMPSIA/ECLAMPSIA[5,6]

- Elevated blood pressure postdelivery, with or without prior hypertension.
- **Symptoms:** Headache, nausea, visual disturbances, abdominal pain; eclampsia adds seizures.
- **Management:** IV fluids, antihypertensives, anticonvulsants; monitor BP strictly.

THROMBOEMBOLISM

- **Risk factors:** Elevated fibrinogen, thrombocytosis, obesity, cesarean, and prolonged labor **(Table 2)**.
- **Symptoms:** Calf pain, swelling, redness, shortness of breath, and chest pain.[7]
- **Diagnosis:** Compression ultrasonography (Level A evidence) for DVT.

- **Thromboprophylaxis (RCOG):**
  - Low-molecular-weight heparin (LMWH) for 10 days if BMI ≥ 40 kg/m^2 or ≥2 risk factors.
  - *High-risk (prior VTE)*: LMWH or warfarin for 6 weeks.
  - Discontinue LMWH 12–24 hours before delivery/procedures.
- **Treatment:** LMWH preferred; initiate 4–6 h postvaginal delivery, 6–12 hours postcesarean; safe for breastfeeding.

POSTPARTUM DEPRESSION[8]

- **Prevalence:** ~12% for depression, 13% for anxiety; 15–20% in the first year.
- **Symptoms:** Sadness, guilt, fatigue, insomnia, suicidal thoughts.
- **Diagnosis:** Rule out hypothyroidism; assess history, risk to self/baby, consider psychiatric evaluation.
- **Management:**
  - Counseling, psychotherapy, support (home visits, self-help groups).
  - *Aim*: Improve quality of life, prevent progression, and suicide.
- **Postnatal care:** For traumatic birth, stillbirth, or miscarriage, offer grief counseling, options to view/hold baby, and keep mementos.

ENDOCRINE DYSFUNCTION (POSTPARTUM THYROIDITIS)[9]

- **Overview:** Affects 7–10% of women, often 4–24 weeks postdelivery or miscarriage.
- **Phases:**
  - *Hyperthyroidism (0–6 months)*: Weight loss, anxiety, tachycardia, hair loss.
  - *Hypothyroidism (4–8 months)*: Fatigue, cold intolerance, and depression.
- **Diagnosis:** Thyroid profile for confirmation and monitoring.
- **Treatment:**
  - *Hyperthyroidism*: Beta blockers, prednisone.
  - *Hypothyroidism*: Thyroid hormone replacement.
- **Note:** 12–30% develop persistent hypothyroidism; higher risk with type 1 diabetes (10.5–25%).

POSTERIOR REVERSIBLE ENCEPHALOPATHY SYNDROME (PRES)[10]

- **Definition:** Clinicoradiological syndrome with headache, seizures, altered mental status, and visual loss.
- **Pathology:** White matter vasogenic edema, often in occipital/parietal lobes, linked to hypertension.
- **Diagnosis:** MRI critical; delayed treatment risks mortality or neurological deficit.
- **Management:** IV fluids, antibiotics, antihypertensives, anticonvulsants; strict BP monitoring.

PRACTICE FUNDAMENTALS

Diagnosis

- **History & Examination:**
  - Assess vitals (temperature, pulse, BP, and respiration), breasts, abdomen, perineum, lochia, and legs.
  - Admit if unwell, dehydrated, or vomiting.
- **Specific Evaluations:**
  - **Sepsis:** CBC, RFTs, urine/blood culture, high vaginal swab, chest X-ray.
  - **VTE:** Use risk assessment protocols; compression ultrasonography for DVT; pneumatic compression until ambulatory.
  - **Depression:** Assess history, mental health risks, and consider psychiatric referral.
  - **Thyroiditis:** Thyroid profile for hyper/hypothyroidism phases.
  - **PRES:** MRI for diagnosis; urgent treatment critical.

MANAGEMENT

- **General Measures:**
  - Hospitalize, resuscitate, establish IV lines, monitor vitals, and seek multidisciplinary help.
- **Specific Management:**
  - **Sepsis:** Broad-spectrum IV antibiotics within 1 hour; involve intensivists, microbiologists, obstetricians; monitor via MEOWS.

- **VTE:** LMWH preferred; safe for breastfeeding; early mobilization postcesarean.
- **Depression:** Counseling, psychotherapy, support systems to prevent progression.
- **Thyroiditis:** Beta blockers/prednisone for hyperthyroidism; thyroid replacement for hypothyroidism.
- **PRES:** IV fluids, antihypertensives, anticonvulsants; strict BP control.

- **Puerperal Emergencies:**[10]
  - **Immediate:** PPH, shock, eclampsia, uterine inversion.
  - **Early (≤1 week):** UTI, sepsis, mastitis, acute urinary retention.
  - **Delayed (>1 week):** Secondary PPH, thromboembolism, psychosis, cardiomyopathy.

EVIDENCE SUMMARY

Guidelines Links

- NICE hypertension in pregnancy: https://www.nice.org.uk/guidance/ng133
- RCOG VTE guidelines: https://www.rcog.org.uk/guidelines-research-services/guidelines/gtg37a
- WHO peripartum infections: https://www.who.int/publications/i/item/9789241509350
- NICE postnatal mental health: https://www.nice.org.uk/guidance/cg192

Strength of Recommendation (Table 3)

TABLE 3: Classes of recommendation.

Grade	*Description*	*Evidence*	*Implication*
A	Strong recommendation	Level 1 or consistent level 2–4	Follow the best evidence-based practice
B	Recommendation	Consistent level 2–4 studies	Strong, but consider modifications
C	Optional	Inconsistent level 2–4 evidence	Be flexible in decision-making
D	Optional	Level 5 lacks a systematic review	Consider all options in practice

REFERENCES

1. Bonet M, Oladapo O, Khan D, et al. New WHO guidance on prevention and treatment of maternal peripartum infections. Lancet Glob Health. 2015;3:e1.
2. Meaney-Delman D, Bartlett LA, Gravett MG, et al. Oral and intramuscular treatment options for early postpartum endometritis in low-resource settings. Obstet Gynecol. 2015;125(4):789-800.
3. Mackeen AD, Packard RE, Ota E, et al. Antibiotic regimens for postpartum endometritis. Cochrane Database Syst Rev. 2015;2:CD001067.
4. Swe T, Ali M, Naing AT. Drug fever induced by piperacillin/tazobactam in an elderly patient with HIV. BMJ Case Rep. 2016;2016:bcr2016215814.
5. ACOG Committee Opinion No. 736. Optimizing Postpartum Care. Obstet Gynecol. 2018;131(5):e140-50.
6. Gundersen TD, Krebs L, Loekkegaard ECL, et al. Postpartum urinary tract infection by mode of delivery: a Danish nationwide cohort study. BMJ Open. 2018;8:e018479.

7. Boakes E, Woods A, Johnson N, et al. Breast Infection: A Review of Diagnosis and Management Practices. Eur J Breast Health. 2018;14(3):136-43.
8. Bakker P, Verhoeven C, Miranda E, et al. Delivery and puerperium. In: Steeger E et al, eds. Textbook of Obstetrics and Gynaecology: A Life Course Approach. Bohn Stafleu van Loghum; 2019:415-67.
9. Hassan H, EL-Kholy G, Ateya A, et al. Breast Engorgement among Women with Caesarean Section: Impact of Nursing Intervention. Educ Soc Hum Stud. 2020;1(2):22.
10. Cunningham F, Leveno KJ, Bloom SL, et al. Puerperal complications. In: Williams Obstetrics. 25th ed. McGraw-Hill; 2018:chap.

Puerperal Sepsis

Ruchika Garg

DEFINITION AND MONITORING

- Puerperal infections are influenced by labor complications (e.g., dystocia, prolonged rupture of membranes, and operative delivery).[1]
- Regular monitoring of vital signs (temperature, pulse, blood pressure, respiratory rate) using the Modified Early Obstetric Warning Score (MEOWS) chart is critical.[2]

RISK FACTORS

- Altered vaginal flora, reducing acidity
- Vulvar/vaginal lacerations
- Open cervix
- Blood/necrotic material at the placental site.[3]

MICROBIOLOGY

- Infections typically ascend from the lower genital tract to the uterus, fallopian tubes, or abdomen.
- *Common pathogens*: Group A/B streptococci, *Enterococcus, S. aureus, E. coli*, gram-positive cocci, *Bacteroides, Clostridium*. Late-onset infections may involve *Chlamydia trachomatis.*[4]
- Pathogenicity is enhanced by hematomas, devitalized tissue, and lacerations.

PATHOGENESIS

- *Vaginal delivery*: Involves placental site, decidua, myometrium, or cervicovaginal lacerations.
- *Cesarean section*: Originates from infected surgical incisions, with bacteria invading amniotic fluid during labor, leading to parametrial cellulitis or pelvic retroperitoneal infection.[5]
- Early treatment limits spread; untreated infections may extend into the pelvis.

CLINICAL PRESENTATION

- *Local (wound) infection*:
  - Low-grade fever, malaise, and headache.
  - Erythema, swelling, and purulent discharge at the wound site.
  - *Severe cases:* High-grade fever, rigors, chills, and wound disruption[6]

- *Uterine infection (postpartum metritis)*:
    - Fever (primary criterion), with/without rigors, and chills.
    - *Symptoms*: Malaise, abdominal pain, foul-smelling discharge, diarrhea, vomiting, and uterine/renal angle pain.
    - *Examination*: Tachypnea, tachycardia, fever, and abdominal/parametrial tenderness.[7]
- *Red flag signs (warrant urgent referral):*
    - Fever > 38°C
    - Sustained tachycardia > 90 BPM
    - Respiratory rate > 20 breaths/min
    - Abdominal/chest pain and diarrhea/vomiting
    - Uterine/renal angle tenderness
    - General unwellness, anxiety, and distress[8]
- *Spreading infection:* Pelvic peritonitis, parametritis, pelvic abscess (bulging mass in the pouch of Douglas).

DIAGNOSIS

- *Principle:* Assume genital sepsis unless proven otherwise.[9]
- *Objectives:* Localize infection, identify pathogens, and assess severity/complications.
- *History:* Evaluate antenatal, intranatal, and postnatal risk factors (e.g., anemia, prolonged labor, and membrane rupture).
- *Examination:* General, systemic, abdominal, and pelvic exams; check legs for thrombophlebitis/thrombosis.
- Investigations **(Table 1)**

TABLE 1: Diagnostic investigations for puerperal infections.[10]

Test	*Purpose*
Complete blood count, C-reactive protein, blood urea, and electrolytes	Assess infection severity
Blood culture	Identify pathogens (send before antibiotics)
Urine routine/culture	Rule out urinary tract infection.
High vaginal swab	Identify genital tract pathogens.
Other cultures (e.g., throat, placental, sputum, CSF, and wound)	Based on the suspected infection focus
Pelvic ultrasound	Detect retained products or pelvic collection
Chest X-ray	Rule out lung pathology.
CT/MRI	For inconclusive cases

PROPHYLAXIS

- *Antenatal:* Improve nutrition, treat anemia, eliminate septic foci (e.g., skin and throat).[11]
- *Intranatal:*
    - Full surgical asepsis for deliveries.
    - Screen for Group B Streptococcus in high-risk cases; routine antibiotic prophylaxis is not recommended.

- Prophylactic antibiotics during cesarean reduce infections.[12]
- *Postpartum:*
  - Maintain asepsis until uterine/perineal/vaginal wounds heal.
  - Limit visitors, use sterile sanitary pads, and isolate infected mothers/babies.[13]

TREATMENT

- *General measures*:
  - Ensure nutrition, correct anemia, control blood sugar, and maintain hygiene.
  - Isolate patients with hemolytic *Streptococcus*.
  - Use IV fluids, blood transfusion for severe anemia, indwelling catheter for pelvic abscess/urinary retention.
  - Monitor vital signs, lochial discharge, and fluid intake/output.[14]
- *Antibiotic therapy*:
  - *Nonsevere metritis*: Oral/intramuscular antibiotics sufficient postvaginal delivery.
  - *Moderate-severe infections*: IV broad-spectrum antibiotics; ~90% improve within 48–72 hours.[15]
  - *Empirical regimens* ***(Table 2)***

TABLE 2: Antibiotic regimens for postpartum endometritis.[16]

Regimen	*Dosage*	*Notes*
Clindamycin + Gentamicin	600 mg oral q6h + 4.5 mg/kg IM daily	Safe for breastfeeding
Amoxicillin-Clavulanic acid	875 mg oral BID	Broad-spectrum coverage
Cefotetan	2 g IM TID	Effective for mixed flora
Meropenem/Imipenem-cilastatin	500 mg IM TID	For severe infections
Amoxicillin + Metronidazole	500 mg oral TID + 500 mg oral TID	Anaerobic coverage

- Continue IV antibiotics until afebrile for 24–48 hours, then switch to oral for a 7-day course. Mild cases can be treated outpatient.[17]
- *Persistent fever*: Reevaluate for parametrial phlegmon, abscess, hematoma, or septic pelvic thrombophlebitis. Consider drug fever if there are no findings and the pulse is disproportionate to the fever.[18]

Surgical Treatment

- *Perineal wound:* Remove stitches, drain pus, use sitz baths, antiseptic ointment; secondary suturing if needed.
- Retained Products: Ignore if <3 cm; evacuate surgically after 24 hours of antibiotics if larger.
- *Septic pelvic thrombophlebitis*: IV heparin for 7–10 days.
- *Pelvic abscess*: Drain via colpotomy under ultrasound.
- *Wound dehiscence*: Scrub, debride, close with secondary sutures, use antibiotics per culture.
- *Laparotomy*: For unresponsive peritonitis, rupture, multiple abscesses, gangrenous uterus, or gas gangrene. Hysterectomy may be required.[19]
- *Necrotizing fasciitis*: Rare, fatal; manage with hydration, debridement, high-dose IV antibiotics.[20]

INTENSIVE CARE UNIT INDICATIONS

Hypotension, oliguria, raised serum creatinine/lactate (≥4 mmol/L), thrombocytopenia, acute respiratory distress syndrome (ARDS), and hypothermia.[21]

LATE INFECTIONS (3 DAYS–6 WEEKS POSTPARTUM)

- *Causes*: Wound infection, persistent endometritis, abscess, toxic shock syndrome, episiotomy infection, ascending uterine infection, septic thrombophlebitis, breast infection, pneumonia.[22]
- Slow onset, significant morbidity, and challenging diagnosis.

URINARY COMPLICATIONS

- *Urinary tract infection (UTI)*:
  - Incidence: 2–4% postdelivery.
  - Symptoms: Dysuria, frequency, urgency, suprapubic pain, fever, hematuria.
  - Diagnosis: Clinical, confirmed by urine analysis/culture.
- *Treatment* ***(Table 3)***

TABLE 3: Treatment for postpartum UTI.[23]

Condition	*Therapy*
Acute Cystitis	Nitrofurantoin, beta-lactams, trimethoprim-sulfamethoxazole, fosfomycin
Pyelonephritis	IV beta-lactams; carbapenems (imipenem 500 mg IV QID, meropenem 1 g IV TID) for severe cases; add vancomycin/daptomycin for MRSA

- *Urinary retention*:
  - *Causes:* Urethral trauma, bladder neck edema, painful episiotomy, epidural anesthesia.
  - *Diagnosis:* Palpable bladder or ultrasound for postvoid residual volume.
  - *Treatment:* Indwelling catheter for 48 hours; monitor output. Use a suprapubic catheter if retention persists.[24]

HORMONE REPLACEMENT THERAPY AND MENOPAUSE

Historical Context

- *Pre-2002:* Hormone replacement therapy (HRT) was widely used for menopausal symptoms.[25]
- *Post-2002 Women's Health Initiative (WHI) study:* Reported risks (breast cancer, heart disease, stroke, thromboembolism) reduced HRT use, increasing clinician hesitancy and alternative therapy exploration.[26]
- *Current evidence:* HRT benefits (coronary disease, osteoporosis, dementia risk reduction) outweigh risks when started within 10 years of menopause.[27-29]

Indications

- *Global context:* By 2050, 1.6 billion women will be menopausal/postmenopausal; South Korea leads in female life expectancy (90.82 years by 2030).[30,31]

- *Indian context:* Life expectancy ~72.3 years, menopause at 47–49 years.[32] HRT addresses:
  - Vasomotor symptoms (hot flashes, sweating, and palpitations).
  - Urogenital symptoms (dryness, dyspareunia, and urinary frequency).
  - Psychological symptoms (mood swings, insomnia, depression, and anxiety).
  - *Long-term risks*: Osteoporosis, cardiovascular disease, and Alzheimer's.[33]

Prehormone Replacement Therapy Workup

- *History/examination*: Detailed medical history, physical exam, and blood pressure.
- *Investigations* **(*Table 4*)**

TABLE 4: Pre-HRT investigations.[34]

Test	*Purpose*
Complete blood count (CBC) and hemoglobin	Baseline health
Blood sugar, lipid profile, and liver/thyroid function	Screen metabolic/liver/thyroid dysfunction
Pelvic ultrasound	Evaluate the uterine/ovarian pathology
Mammography	Breast cancer screening
Bone mineral density (BMD)	Osteoporosis risk
Pap smear	Cervical screening
Endometrial biopsy	Rule out endometrial pathology

Types of Hormone Replacement Therapy

- **Hormonal:**
  - **Combination:** Estrogen + progestogen for women with a uterus.
  - **Estrogen-only:** Posthysterectomy.
  - **Forms:** Tablets, transdermal patches/gels, vaginal creams/pessaries/rings.
  - **Regimens:** Continuous or sequential (progestogen for 12–14 days/cycle).[35]
- *Nonhormonal:* Selective serotonin reuptake inhibitor (SSRIs), serotonin and norepinephrine reuptake inhibitor (SNRIs), gabapentin, pregabalin (40–65% vasomotor symptom reduction).[36,37]

Mechanism of Action

- *Estrogen*: Acts on nuclear transcription factors in the uterus/vagina, regulating gene expression.
- *Vaginal pH*: Maintains acidity (4.5–6.0); postmenopause, pH rises to ~7.0, increasing infection/dyspareunia risk.[38]

Routes of Administration (Table 5)

TABLE 5: HRT administration routes.[39]

Route	*Forms*	*Examples*	*Notes*
Oral	Tablets	CEE, 17β-estradiol, and estradiol valerate	Higher dose due to first-pass metabolism
Transdermal	Patches, gels, and sprays	17β-estradiol	Safer, avoids liver metabolism
Vaginal	Creams, tablets, and rings	17β-estradiol, estriol	Minimal systemic effects

Estrogen and Progesterone in Hormone Replacement Therapy

- Estrogen:
  - *Oral:* CEE (0.3–0.625 mg), estradiol valerate (1–2 mg), and 17β-estradiol (1 mg).
  - *Transdermal/vaginal:* Safer, reduces thromboembolism/triglyceride risks.[34]
  - *Vaginal:* FDA-approved for vaginal dryness/dyspareunia; low-dose estriol (0.03–0.5 mg/day) is effective.[40]
- *Progesterone*:
  - Prevents endometrial hyperplasia/cancer.
  - *Types*: Micronized progesterone (100–400 mg), synthetic progestins [medroxyprogesterone acetate (MPA) and norethindrone], levonorgestrel IUS.[41]

FORMULATIONS IN INDIA (TABLE 6)

TABLE 6: HRT formulations available in India.[42]

Therapy	*Type*	*Examples*
Estrogen (Systemic)	Oral	CEE (0.3–0.625 mg), 17β-estradiol (1–2 mg)
	Transdermal	Estrogen gel (0.125 mg/2.5 g)
Progesterone	Oral	Dydrogesterone (10 mg), Micronized progesterone (100–400 mg)
	Intrauterine	Levonorgestrel IUS (52 mg and 20 µg/day)
Combination	Sequential	17β-estradiol (1 mg) + dydrogesterone (10 mg, last 14 days)
	Continuous	17β-estradiol (1 mg) + dydrogesterone (5 mg daily)
Genitourinary syndrome	Vaginal	Estriol cream (0.5 mg/0.5 g), CEE cream (0.625 mg/g)

CONTRAINDICATIONS

- Breast/estrogen-dependent cancers, active/history of deep vein thrombosis (DVT)/ pulmonary embolism (PE), arterial thrombotic diseases, chronic liver disease, migraine with aura, undiagnosed genital bleeding, thrombophilic disorders.[43]
- Vaginal estrogen is exempt due to low systemic absorption.

MONITORING AND SIDE EFFECTS

- *Monitoring*: Symptom relief, absence of adverse effects.[44]
- *Side effects*: Uterine bleeding, fluid retention, breast tenderness, headaches, and mood changes.
- *Withdrawal indications*: Jaundice, significant BP increase, new migraine-type headache, and pregnancy.[45]

Guidelines

- *NICE (2015)*: HRT for hot flashes/night sweats; no increased cardiovascular risk before age 60.[46]
- *IMS (2022)*: HRT is most effective for menopausal symptoms; initiate before age 60 years or within 10 years of menopause for osteoporosis prevention.[47]

STRAW + 10 STAGING SYSTEM

- *Purpose*: Standardizes reproductive aging using menstrual/hormonal criteria.[48]
- *Stages **(Table 7)**:*

TABLE 7: STRAW + 10 staging system.[48]

Stage	*Description*	*Menstrual/hormonal changes*	*Symptoms*
Reproductive (–5 to –3)	Early to late	Regular cycles, slight variability in –3a/–3b; FSH normal/variable, low AMH/inhibin-B	Reduced fecundability
Early menopausal transition (–2)	Variable cycle length (>7 days)	Elevated FSH, low AMH/inhibin-B/AFC	Vasomotor symptoms
Late menopausal transition (–1)	Amenorrhea ≥60 days	FSH > 25 IU/L, low estradiol	Severe vasomotor symptoms
Early postmenopause (+1a, +1b, +1c)	5–8 years post-FMP	FSH rises, and estradiol falls	Hot flashes and urogenital atrophy
Late postmenopause (+2)	Somatic aging	Stable high FSH, low estradiol	Vaginal dryness

Symptom Correlation

- *Vasomotor symptoms:* Affect ~80% in perimenopause; longer duration if starting perimenopause (11.8 vs. 3.4 years).[49]
- *Vaginal/sexual symptoms:* Affect 33–50% postmenopause; GSM due to elevated vaginal pH.[38]
- *Sleep/mood changes:* Insomnia linked to vasomotor menopausal symptoms (VMS); depression risk rises to 62% in early perimenopause.[50,51]

Limitations of STRAW

Inapplicable to smokers, BMI > 30 kg/m^2, posthysterectomy, or those with PCOS, POI, or serious illnesses.[52]

INDIAN MENOPAUSE SOCIETY RECOMMENDATIONS

- Use Modified Bahram Anklesaria and STRAW + 10 staging.[53]
- Prioritize lifestyle modifications and non-hormonal therapies before low-dose, short-duration HRT.[54]

REFERENCES

1. Royal College of Obstetricians and Gynaecologists. (2012). Bacterial Sepsis in Pregnancy (Green-top Guideline No. 64a). [Online] Available from https://www.rcog.org.uk/media/ea1p1r4h/gtg_64a.pdf [Last accessed December, 2025].
2. Eschenbach DA. Bacterial vaginosis and anaerobes in obstetric-gynecologic infection. Clin Infect Dis. 1993;16(Suppl 4):S282-7.
3. In: Cunningham FG, Leveno KJ, Bloom SL, et al (Eds). Williams Obstetrics, 25th edition. London: McGraw-Hill Education; 2018.

4. Tita ATN, Andrews WW. Diagnosis and Management of Clinical Chorioamnionitis. Clin Perinatol. 2010;37(2):339-54.
5. World Health Organization. Managing puerperal sepsis Midwifery education module 4. [Online] Available from https://www.who.int/publications/i/item/managing-puerperal-sepsis-midwifery-education-module-4 Last accessed December, 2025].
6. Kuhlmann RS, Cruikshank DP. Maternal trauma during pregnancy. Clin Obstet Gynecol. 1994;37(2):274-93.
7. Committee on Practice Bulletins-Obstetrics. ACOG Practice Bulletin No. 199: Use of Prophylactic Antibiotics in Labor and Delivery. Obstet Gynecol. 2018;132(3):e103-19.
8. The NAMS 2017 Hormone Therapy Position Statement Advisory Panel. The 2017 hormone therapy position statement of The North American Menopause Society Menopause. 2017;24(7):728-53.
9. Stuenkel CA, Davis SR, Gompel A, et al. Treatment of Symptoms of the Menopause: An Endocrine Society Clinical Practice Guideline. J Clin Endocrinol Metab. 2015;100(11):3975-4011.
10. Portman DJ, Gass ML; Vulvovaginal Atrophy Terminology Consensus Conference Panel. Genitourinary syndrome of menopause: new terminology for vulvovaginal atrophy from the International Society for the Study of Women's Sexual Health and the North American Menopause Society. Menopause. 2014;21(10):1063-71.
11. The NAMS 2020 GSM Position Statement Editorial Panel. The 2020 genitourinary syndrome of menopause position statement of The North American Menopause Society. Menopause. 2020;27(9):976-92.
12. Linko E, Harilainen A, Malmivaara A, et al. Surgical versus conservative interventions for anterior cruciate ligament ruptures in adults. Cochrane Database Syst Rev. 2009;2:CD001356.
13. Santoro N, Epperson CN, Mathews SB. Menopausal symptoms and their management. Endocrinol Metab Clin North Am. 2015;44(3):497-511.
14. National Institute for Health and Care Excellence (NICE). (2015). Menopause: identification and management. [Online] Available from https://www.nice.org.uk/guidance/ng23 [Last accessed December, 2025].
15. Harlow SD, Gass M, Hall JE, et al. Executive summary of the Stages of Reproductive Aging Workshop + 10: addressing the unfinished agenda of staging reproductive aging. Menopause. 2012;19(4):387-95.
16. Ohayon MM. Severe hot flashes are associated with chronic insomnia. Arch Intern Med. 2006;166(12):1262-8.
17. The NAMS 2017 Hormone Therapy Position Statement Advisory Panel. The 2017 hormone therapy position statement of The North American Menopause Society. Menopause. 2017;24(7):728-53.

Lactation Suppression

Ruchika Garg

INTRODUCTION

Lactation is a physiological process initiated during pregnancy and sustained by infant suckling. Breast milk provides optimal nutrition, containing vitamins, proteins, fats, immunoglobulins (IgA), white blood cells, and anti-infective factors such as lysozyme and lactoferrin, reducing infant risks of asthma, allergies, infections, diabetes, and obesity.[1] However, *lactation suppression* may be necessary due to medical, social, or personal reasons, such as stillbirth, maternal human immunodeficiency virus (HIV) infection, or adoption. Without suckling, lactation ceases naturally within days to weeks, but up to *66% of women* experience moderate to severe breast engorgement and pain.[2]

PHYSIOLOGY OF LACTATION

Lactation involves hormonal and physical changes in the breast, beginning in puberty and intensifying during pregnancy. *Prolactin* drives milk production, while *oxytocin* facilitates milk ejection. Infant suckling maintains prolactin secretion, sustaining lactation. Without suckling, prolactin levels drop, halting milk production.[3] Suppression methods aim to accelerate this process and alleviate symptoms, such as engorgement.

INDICATIONS FOR LACTATION SUPPRESSION (TABLE 1)

Lactation suppression is indicated when breastfeeding is contraindicated or undesired.[4,5]

COMPLICATIONS OF UNTREATED ENGORGEMENT

Without suppression, women may experience:

- *Breast engorgement*: Swollen, tender, and hard breasts.
- *Blocked ducts/mastitis*: Painful lumps and infection risk.
- *Breast abscess*: If mastitis is untreated.
- *Emotional distress*: Particularly in cases of fetal loss or inability to breastfeed.[6]

NONPHARMACOLOGICAL METHODS

Non-pharmacological approaches aim to reduce discomfort and milk production:[7]

- **Avoid breast stimulation:** Minimize nipple contact to reduce prolactin release.
- **Express milk sparingly:** Only enough to relieve discomfort, not to empty breasts.

TABLE 1: Indications for lactation suppression.

Indication	*Details*
Stillbirth or neonatal death	Prevents engorgement and emotional distress
Maternal human immunodeficiency virus (HIV) infection	Exclusive formula feeding is recommended in high-income settings to prevent transmission
Adoption/surrogacy	No breastfeeding is required if the infant is not with the mother
Maternal medications	Drugs (e.g., chemotherapy, lithium, and retinoids) excreted in milk pose risks to the infant
Recreational drug/alcohol use	Contraindicated due to potential harm to the infant
Active herpes simplex virus (HSV)	Breast lesions increase transmission risk
Infant galactosemia	Breast milk exacerbates metabolic issues, risking liver damage and shock
Breast surgery/implants	May impair milk production, necessitating suppression
Maternal illness/depression	Critical illness or mental health conditions may preclude breastfeeding
Social/personal choice	Mother's preference to not breastfeed

TABLE 2: Pharmacological agents for lactation suppression.[9,10]

Drug category	*Examples*	*Efficacy*	*Side effects/concerns*
Ergot derivatives	Cabergoline, Bromocriptine	High (Cabergoline preferred)	*Cabergoline*: Headache, dizziness *Bromocriptine*: Stroke risk, withdrawn in some countries
Estrogen compounds	Estrogen ± Androgens	Moderate (40% effective)	Thrombosis, pulmonary embolism, and rebound lactation
Sympathomimetics	Pseudoephedrine	Limited evidence	Anxiety, insomnia, tachycardia, and arrhythmias

- **Wear a supportive bra:** It provides comfort and reduces movement-related stimulation.
- **Cold compresses/gel packs:** Reduce swelling and pain postshower or bath.
- **Maintain normal fluid intake:** Fluid restriction is ineffective and unnecessary.
- **Analgesia:** Paracetamol or ibuprofen for pain relief.
- **Allow milk leakage:** Normal during suppression; avoid excessive expression.
- **Efficacy:** These methods provide symptomatic relief but are less effective than pharmacological options for rapid suppression.[8]

PHARMACOLOGICAL METHODS (TABLE 2)

Pharmacological suppression targets prolactin secretion or milk production. Historically, estrogens and bromocriptine were used, but safety concerns have shifted preference to cabergoline.[9]

Cabergoline

Introduction: Cabergoline, a long-acting dopamine agonist, is the **preferred drug** for lactation suppression due to its efficacy and safety profile.

Mechanism of Action

- Stimulates D2-dopamine receptors on pituitary lactotrophs, inhibiting prolactin secretion.
- Low affinity for D1, adrenergic, or serotonin receptors, minimizing off-target effects.
- No impact on other pituitary hormones (e.g., GH, FSH, LH, TSH, and cortisol).

Dose and Administration

- **Single dose:** 1 mg (2 × 0.5 mg tablets) within 12–24 hours of postpartum.
- **Alternative:** 0.25 mg every 12 hours for 2 days (total 1 mg).
- **Onset:** Within 3 hours; duration up to 14–21 days.

Side Effects

- Headache, dizziness, and fatigue.
- Orthostatic hypotension, nasal stuffiness, and epistaxis.
- Acne, pruritus (rare).

Contraindications

- Hypersensitivity to cabergoline or ergot alkaloids.
- Preeclampsia or postpartum hypertension.

Precautions

- Use cautiously in renal/liver disease, Raynaud's syndrome, or history of psychosis.
- Avoid in patients with pulmonary/cardiac fibrotic disorders or gastrointestinal bleeding.

Drug Interactions

Avoid dopamine antagonists (e.g., metoclopramide and phenothiazines) as they reduce prolactin-lowering effects.

Advantages

- Single-dose efficacy.
- Minimal side effects compared to bromocriptine.
- Stable at room temperature, cost-effective.

Bromocriptine (Historical Context)

- **Introduction:** Previously used for lactation suppression, bromocriptine is an ergoline dopamine agonist.
- **Status:** Withdrawn in the USA and other countries due to risks of stroke, seizures, cardiovascular events, and psychosis.

- **Dose (Historical):** 2.5 mg daily for 3–7 days.
- **Concerns:**
    - Serious adverse effects (e.g., myocardial infarction and cerebral accidents).
    - Requires 10–14 days to prevent rebound lactation.
    - Not recommended per current guidelines.

Other Agents

- **Estrogens:** Associated with thrombosis and rebound lactation; rarely used.
- **Pseudoephedrine:** Limited efficacy; side effects include tachycardia and insomnia.
- **Others:** Clomiphene, pyridoxine, and prostaglandins have variable efficacy and are not standard.

ROYAL COLLEGE OF OBSTETRICIANS AND GYNAECOLOGISTS/ NATIONAL INSTITUTE FOR HEALTH AND CARE EXCELLENCE GUIDELINES (2023)

- **Cabergoline i**s the first-line pharmacological agent for lactation suppression (1 mg of single dose within 24 hours of postpartum).
- **Nonpharmacological methods** (e.g., supportive bra, cold packs, and minimal expression) should be offered alongside pharmacological treatment.
- **Bromocriptine** is not recommended due to safety concerns.
- Avoid routine use of estrogens due to thromboembolism risk.
- Counsel women on risks, benefits, and alternatives before initiating suppression.
- Monitor for complications such as mastitis and abscess during suppression.

PATIENT COUNSELING

BOX 1: Key counseling points for lactation suppression.

- **Avoid breast stimulation** to reduce milk production.
- **Express milk sparingly** only for comfort, not to empty breasts.
- Wear a **firm, supportive** bra day and night.
- Use **cold packs** or analgesia (e.g., paracetamol) for pain relief.
- **Do not breastfeed** or give expressed milk after starting pharmacological treatment.
- Discuss **cabergoline's side effects** (e.g., dizziness and headache) and report severe symptoms.
- Watch for signs of **mastitis** (e.g., fever and painful lumps) or abscess.
- Address **emotional distress,** especially in cases of stillbirth or adoption, with psychological support.

CLINICAL CASE SCENARIO

Case

A 32-year-old woman, G2P1, delivers a stillborn infant at 38 weeks. She is emotionally distressed and requests lactation suppression to avoid engorgement. She has no history of hypertension, liver disease, or drug allergies.

Management

- **Counseling:** Explain the process of lactation suppression, emphasizing nonpharmacological (supportive bra, cold packs) and pharmacological options. Address emotional support needs and refers to a counselor.
- **Nonpharmacological:** Advise minimal milk expression for comfort, a firm bra, and paracetamol for pain.
- **Pharmacological:** Administer cabergoline 1 mg single dose within 24 hours postpartum.
- **Monitoring:** Educate on signs of mastitis (fever, lumps) and advise follow-up in 1 week.
- **Outcome:** The patient experiences mild engorgement for 3 days, relieved with cold packs. No complications were reported at follow-up.

Complications and Management (Table 3)

TABLE 3: Complications of lactation suppression and management.

Complication	*Symptoms*	*Management*
Breast engorgement	Swollen, tender, hard breasts	Cold packs, minimal expression, analgesia
Blocked ducts	Painful lump, soreness	Express milk to clear the blockage, warm compresses
Mastitis	Fever, redness, painful lump	Antibiotics, continued expression, analgesia
Breast abscess	Persistent lump, fever, pus	Surgical drainage, antibiotics, urgent referral

KEY POINTS

- **Lactation suppression** is indicated for medical (e.g., stillbirth and HIV) or personal reasons.
- **Cabergoline** (1 mg single dose) is the preferred pharmacological agent due to efficacy and safety.
- **Non-pharmacological methods** (e.g., supportive bra and cold packs) reduce discomfort but are less effective alone.
- **Bromocriptine** is obsolete due to serious adverse effects.
- Monitor for mastitis/abscess during suppression.
- **Counseling** is critical to address physical and emotional needs, especially in cases of fetal loss.

REFERENCES

1. Victora CG, Bahl R, Barros AJ, et al. Breastfeeding in the 21st century: epidemiology, mechanisms, and lifelong effect. Lancet. 2016;387(10017):475-90.
2. Berens P, Brodribb W. ABM Clinical Protocol #20: Engorgement, Revised 2016. Breastfeed Med. 2016;11(4):159-63.
3. Bethesda. Cabergoline. Drugs and Lactation Database (LactMed®) [Internet]. Bethesda (MD): National Library of Medicine (US); 2006–. Updated 2025 Sep 15.
4. Oladapo OT, Fawole B. Treatments for suppression of lactation. Cochrane Database Syst Rev. 2012 Sep 12;2012(9):CD005937.

5. World Health Organization. Guidelines on HIV and infant feeding. Geneva: World Health Organization; 2020.
6. Cole M. Lactation after perinatal loss: a review. J Midwifery Womens Health. 2018;63(1):107-13.
7. NICE. Postnatal care [NG194]. London: National Institute for Health and Care Excellence; 2021.
8. Ferri RL, Rosen-Carole CB, Jackson J, et al.; Academy of Breastfeeding Medicine. ABM Clinical Protocol #33: Lactation care for lesbian, gay, bisexual, transgender, queer, questioning, plus patients. Breastfeed Med. 2020 May;15(5):284–293.
9. Yang Y, Boucoiran I, Tulloch KJ, et al. Is cabergoline safe and effective for postpartum lactation inhibition? A systematic review. Int J Womens Health. 2020 Mar 9;12:159–170.
10. RCOG. Best practice in postpartum care. London: Royal College of Obstetricians and Gynaecologists; 2023.

Vaccination in Pregnancy

Ruchika Garg

INTRODUCTION

Pregnancy represents a unique state in which the maternal immune system adapts to tolerate the semiallogeneic fetal conceptus. The innate immune system upgrades for maternal protection against infection and fetal protection against rejection; the acquired immune response toward foreign antigens (paternal/fetal antigens) is selectively downregulated. These changes in the maternal immune system are not known to affect the immunological response to vaccination.[1]

Vaccination involves inducing an acquired immune response against microbes by administration of nonpathogenic forms or components of the microbes.

TYPES OF VACCINES[2,3-5]

Broadly, vaccines are divided as discussed in **Table 1**.

PRINCIPLES OF VACCINATION IN PREGNANCY[3,4]

- Ideally, women should be vaccinated against the relevant vaccine-preventable diseases before embarking on a pregnancy.
- When vaccines are administered during pregnancy, the benefits should outweigh the maternal and fetal risks.
- Inactivated virus vaccines, toxoids, and immune globulin preparations are generally considered safe during pregnancy, and evidence does not suggest any harmful effects on the fetus or pregnancy.
- During pregnancy, unless immediate vaccination is indicated, it is preferable to delay immunization until the second trimester to allow for completion of the critical period of fetal organogenesis.

  In the clinical context, vaccines can be broadly classified as shown in **Table 2**.[5]

VACCINES INDICATED IN PREGNANCY

Tetanus toxoid (TT)/Tetanus Diphtheria (Td)/TT, reduced diphtheria toxoid, and acellular pertussis (Tdap) vaccine:

- In India, under the Ministry of Health and Family Welfare (MOHFW) guidelines,[6] as a part of the Universal Immunization Program (UIP), all pregnant women were offered 2 doses of TT injection 4 weeks apart as a part of the routine schedule.

TABLE 1: Types of vaccines.

Type	*Description*	*Examples*
Live Attenuated Vaccines	• Contain a weakened form of the pathogen that is modified to abolish its virulence and yet retain its antigenicity • Use of live vaccines is contraindicated during pregnancy due to the potential risk of infection of the fetus • The decision to administer a live vaccine to pregnant women should be made after consulting an infectious disease specialist only if the benefits outweigh the potential risks of the vaccine	• MMR vaccine • Rubella vaccine
Killed/ Inactivated Vaccines	• Made by inactivating or killing the pathogen during the process of vaccine manufacture through a physical or chemical process • These cannot replicate in the host • Often, multiple doses are necessary to build up and/or maintain immunity, as the immunity conferred by inactivated vaccines is inferior to that resulting from live vaccines	Polio, hepatitis A, and rabies vaccine
Subunit Vaccine	These contain only a part of the pathogen that is needed to produce a protective immune response	*Haemophilus influenzae* vaccine and *Streptococcus pneumonia* vaccine
Toxoid Vaccine	These are made using inactivated bacterial toxins	Tetanus toxoid and diphtheria toxoid
Recombinant Vaccine	Vaccines are made using recombinant DNA technology	Serogroup B meningococcal vaccine

TABLE 2: Classification of vaccines.

Vaccines Contraindicated in Pregnancy	• BCG vaccine • Measles vaccine • Mumps vaccine • Rubella vaccine • Varicella vaccine • Vaccinia vaccine • Human papillomavirus vaccine
Vaccines Specially Indicated in Pregnancy	• Inactivated influenza vaccine • Pertussis (whooping cough) vaccine • Inactivated polio vaccine • Diphtheria toxoid • Tetanus toxoid
Vaccines are Recommended in Pregnancy in Certain Situations	• Hepatitis A vaccine • Hepatitis B vaccine • Meningococcus vaccine • Pneumococcal vaccine • Rabies vaccine • Typhoid vaccine • Yellow fever vaccine

- If the woman had received two doses of TT immunization in a pregnancy within the last 3 years, one dose of TT booster was sufficient.
- Globally, although the policy recommendation to replace TT with Td has existed since 1998, the National Technical Advisory Group on Immunization (NTAGI), MoHFW has recommended the replacement of TT with Td vaccine in India's immunization program for all age groups, including pregnant women, in 2018.[7,8]
- The Td vaccine is a combination of tetanus and diphtheria with a lower concentration of diphtheria antigen (d). Td instead of TT is recommended during pregnancy to protect against maternal and neonatal tetanus and diphtheria during prenatal care.
- The Centers for Disease Control (CDC)[9] and the American College of Obstetrics and Gynecology (ACOG)[10] recommend administering the TT, reduced diphtheria toxoid, and acellular pertussis (Tdap) vaccine to all pregnant patients during each pregnancy, *between 27–36 weeks of gestation*.
- If not administered during pregnancy, the Tdap vaccine should be given immediately postpartum if the woman has never received a prior dose of Tdap as an adolescent, adult, or during a previous pregnancy.
- The majority of morbidity and mortality attributable to pertussis infection occurs in infants who are 3 months and younger. Infants are not usually vaccinated against pertussis (with the DTaP vaccine) until approximately 2 months of age (the earliest possible vaccination is at 6 weeks of age). This leaves a window of significant vulnerability for newborn babies. Tdap vaccine provides fetal and neonatal benefits.

Influenza Vaccine[4]

- Although UIP in India does not recommend routine immunization of pregnant women with the influenza vaccine, international guidelines recommend that pregnant women receive seasonal influenza vaccination during each pregnancy.
- Influenza infection in pregnancy is associated with more serious disease, increased risk of complications, and need for hospitalization in advanced pregnancy, in addition to the adverse fetal effects such as congenital malformations, spontaneous abortions, preterm births, and low birth weight.
- ACOG recommends that all women who are or will be pregnant during the influenza (flu) season should receive the annual influenza vaccine.
- Influenza vaccination is recommended during pregnancy to protect both pregnant women and their newborn babies from severe influenza disease.
- Pregnant women **can receive the influenza vaccine at any period of gestation (first, second, or third trimester)**.
- Maternal vaccination not only reduces the risk of transmitting infection to the neonate but also provides passive immunity against influenza to infants in the first few months of life after birth.
- Either **the inactivated influenza vaccine (IIV) or recombinant influenza vaccine (RIV)** can be given. However, the live attenuated influenza virus vaccine should not be administered to pregnant women.

USE OF SPECIFIC VACCINES IN PREGNANCY

Bacillus Calmette–Guerin[3,4,5]

Although no harmful effects of the BCG vaccine on the fetus have been observed, BCG vaccination should not be given during pregnancy due to theoretical concerns associated with a live vaccine.

Measles, Mumps, and Rubella[3,4,5]

- MMR vaccine is a live attenuated vaccine.
- MMR vaccine is contraindicated in pregnancy because of the possible teratogenic effects of the vaccine on the fetus.
- Further, due to the theoretical risk of teratogenicity due to maternal immunization with MMR, women should be counselled to avoid becoming pregnant for 28 days after administration of the MMR vaccine.
- However, guidelines do not recommend termination of pregnancy after inadvertent MMR vaccination in pregnant women, as studies have failed to demonstrate a link between rubella immunization in early pregnancy and fetal damage.

Rubella[3,4,5]

- Being a live attenuated vaccine, rubella vaccination is contraindicated in pregnancy.
- Vaccinated women are advised to avoid pregnancy for 28 days after administration.
- Rubella vaccine can be safely administered to lactating mothers.

Varicella[3,4,5]

- Varicella zoster vaccine is a live attenuated vaccine.
- Varicella zoster vaccine is contraindicated in pregnancy due to the known adverse effects of the varicella virus on the foetus.[16]
- Nonpregnant women vaccinated with the varicella zoster vaccine should be advised to avoid becoming pregnant for 4 weeks after completion of the two-dose vaccine schedule.

Human Papillomavirus[4]

- HPV vaccine is not recommended during pregnancy as there is limited data on its safety in pregnancy.
- However, if a woman is found to be pregnant after starting the vaccine series, she can be reassured that available evidence does not link HPV vaccines with any increase in adverse maternal or fetal effects.
- The second and/or third doses of the vaccine should be delayed until after the completion of pregnancy.
- Women who are breastfeeding can receive the immunization series since subunit vaccines do not affect the safety of breastfeeding.

Hepatitis A[3,5]

- The safety of the Hepatitis A vaccine in pregnancy is unknown.

- However, as it is a formalin-inactivated vaccine, the theoretical risk of the vaccine to the fetus is likely to be low.
- The risk of vaccination should be weighed against the risk of infection, and the decision should be made on an individual basis.
- Hepatitis A vaccination is indicated in the presence of high-risk conditions, viz., chronic liver disease, intravenous drug use, travel to an endemic area, clotting factor disorders, etc.

Hepatitis B[3,4,5]

- Infection with hepatitis B in pregnancy may result in severe maternal liver disease and chronic infection for the baby.
- As the hepatitis B vaccine is an inactivated subunit vaccine, the risk to the unborn baby is negligible.
- Hence, pregnant women with high-risk factors should receive Hepatitis B vaccination.
- These high-risk factors include:
  - Women with multiple sexual partners.
  - Women or partners with intravenous drug use.
  - Women who receive regular blood transfusions.
  - Women travelling to an endemic area.
  - Female sex workers.
  - Those with chronic liver or kidney disease.
  - Women who are close family and sexual partners of a patient with hepatitis B women.
  - Women who work in settings that increase exposure to body fluids, viz., medical and paramedical staff.

Meningococcal Vaccine[5]

- There is no evidence that either the conjugated or the quadrivalent vaccine MenACWY is associated with adverse maternal or fetal outcomes when administered in pregnancy.
- Vaccination is not recommended in pregnancy unless the mother is at risk of disease, namely:
  - Immunosuppressed women.
  - Women with functional or anatomical asplenia.
  - With complement deficiency.
  - Those traveling to high-risk endemic regions.
  - Women exposed to infected individuals.
- Both vaccines can safely be given to lactating women.
- The safety of the meningococcal B vaccine in pregnancy and lactating women has not been evaluated. Unless the woman is at high risk of the disease, vaccination in pregnant and lactating women should be avoided, and should only be given if the benefits outweigh the potential risks.

Pneumococcal Conjugated Vaccine[3,4,5]

- It is preferable to give the pneumococcal vaccine before conception in women with high-risk factors.

- The safety of both the 13-valent polysaccharide vaccine and the 23-valent pneumococcal polysaccharide vaccine in pregnancy and lactating women has not been evaluated and should be deferred until after pregnancy.
- Vaccination is not recommended in pregnancy unless the mother is at risk of disease, where the benefits may outweigh the potential risks, viz:
  - Heart disease
  - Chronic pulmonary disease
  - Sickle cell anemia
  - Immunocompromised conditions such as HIV
  - Functional or anatomical asplenia

Typhoid[3-5]

- The safety of both the typhoid vaccines has not been evaluated in pregnancy and should be avoided in pregnancy.
- Oral Live vaccine Ty21a is contraindicated in pregnancy.
- If possible, pregnant women should be advised to avoid travel to typhoid endemic areas, but may be immunized with the inactive parenteral vaccine if such exposure is unavoidable.

Rabies[4,5]

- Rabies vaccine is an inactivated viral vaccine.
- After a potential exposure to rabies, the rabies vaccine should be given during pregnancy and lactation, as the consequences of untreated rabies are potentially fatal.
- Preexposure of prophylaxis against rabies may be justified during pregnancy, where the risk of exposure to rabies is substantial.

Japanese Encephalitis

- Japanese encephalitis vaccine is an inactivated vaccine.
- There is no data on the safety of the vaccine in pregnancy.
- Pregnant women travelling to endemic areas at high risk of exposure should receive the vaccine.

Yellow Fever[4,5]

- The yellow fever vaccine is a live attenuated vaccine.
- Pregnant women should be advised to defer travelling to a yellow fever endemic area.
- However, if travel to an endemic area is unavoidable and the risk of yellow fever is high, immunization with a live attenuated viral vaccine may be considered after discussion with an infectious disease specialist.

Coronavirus Disease 2019 Vaccination in Pregnancy

- Since the beginning of the COVID-19 pandemic in 2019, information about the SARS-COV-2 virus and its treatment has been constantly evolving.

- Most pregnant women with COVID-19 infection are asymptomatic with mild disease.
- As compared with nonpregnant women, however, pregnant women are at increased risk of severe disease and complications, viz., need for assisted ventilation, ICU admission, sepsis, and death.
- Based on the recommendations from NTAGI, MoHFW has approved vaccination of pregnant women against COVID-19 after informing them about the risks of exposure to COVID-19 infection and the risks and benefits associated with the COVID-19 vaccines available in the country.
- International guidelines also recommend that all pregnant and lactating women should receive the COVID-19 vaccine.
- Current evidence suggests that COVID-19 vaccination before and during pregnancy is effective, safe, and beneficial to both mother and baby. The benefits of receiving a COVID-19 vaccine outweigh any potential risks of vaccination during pregnancy.
- The COVID-19 vaccine can be taken in any trimester of pregnancy. However, it is preferable that the second dose be taken before 26 weeks of pregnancy. Evidence suggests that the production and subsequent transplacental transfer of antibodies were better following a second dose of vaccine.
- The interval between two doses of vaccine is the same as for nonpregnant adults.
- In India, at present, three vaccines have received approval for restricted use in an emergency situation: an inactivated vaccine (Covaxin) and two based on a nonreplicating viral vector platform (Covishield and Sputnik V).
- COVID-19 vaccines may be administered simultaneously with other vaccines, but at different sites. For example, influenza, Td, and Tdap.
- Contraindications to vaccination include:
  - Anaphylactic/allergic reaction to the previous dose of the COVID-19 vaccine.
  - *Diagnosed COVID-19 infection*: Defer vaccination for 12 weeks from infection or 4–8 weeks from recovery.
  - Active COVID-19 infection.
  - COVID-19 infection is treated with anti-COVID-19 monoclonal antibodies or convalescent plasma.

BREASTFEEDING AND VACCINATION[5]

- Both inactivated and live-virus vaccines (except smallpox and yellow fever virus) can be safely administered to lactating women without any adverse effects on women or their infants.
- Although there is a theoretical risk of viral replication in the case of live vaccines, the majority of live viruses in vaccines have not been demonstrated in human breast milk.
- The yellow fever vaccine should be avoided in lactation women. However, if breastfeeding women cannot avoid travel to an endemic area and the risk of yellow fever is high, vaccination should not be withheld.
- Toxoids, inactivated, subunit, polysaccharide, recombinant, and conjugate vaccines pose no risk for mothers who are breastfeeding or for their infants.

CONCLUSION

- Obstetric care providers should routinely assess the vaccination status of their pregnant patients.
- Currently, Td/TDaP vaccine and the Influenza vaccine are recommended in pregnancy.
- Under special circumstances where the benefits outweigh the potential risks, other vaccines may be considered in pregnancy.
- Live attenuated viral and bacterial vaccines are generally contraindicated during pregnancy because of the theoretical risks to the fetus.
- Both inactivated and live-virus vaccines (except smallpox and yellow fever virus) can be safely administered to a lactating woman without any adverse effects on the woman or their infants.
- It is important that healthcare professionals update themselves about the evolving guidelines and recent advances in vaccination in pregnancy. This will ensure better patient education and maximize vaccination uptake by pregnant women.

REFERENCES

1. In: Coico S, Sunshine G, Benjamini E (Eds). Immunology: A short course, 5th edition. Hoboken: John Wiley & Sons; 2003.
2. www.cdc.gov. Vaccines & Immunizations. [Online] Available from https://www.cdc.gov/vaccines/pubs/pinkbook/downloads/prinvac.pdf [Last accessed December, 2025].
3. ACOG Committee Opinion No. 741: Maternal Immunization. Obstet Gynecol. 2018;131(6):e214-7.
4. Kroger A, Bahta L, Long S, et al. General recommendations on immunization: recommendations of the Advisory Committee on Immunization Practices (ACIP). MMWR Recomm Rep. 2011;60:1-64.
5. Arunakumari PS, Kalburgi S, Sahare A. Vaccination in pregnancy. The Obstet Gynecol. 2015;17(4):257-63.
6. main.mohfw.gov.in. National Immunization Schedule (NIS) for Infants, Children and Pregnant Women. [Online] Available from https://main.mohfw.gov.in/sites/default/files/245453521061489663873.pdf [Last accessed December, 2025].
7. World Health Organization. (2018). WHO/UNICEF Guidance Note: Ensuring Sustained Protection Against Diphtheria: Replacing TT with Td vaccine. [Online] Available from https://cdn.who.int/media/docs/default-source/immunization/guide_to_tt_to_td_replacement_final_12.09.2018.pdf?sfvrsn=f6a23e0a_1 [Last accessed December, 2025].
8. nhm.gov.in. (2018). Td_vaccine_operational_guidelines.pdf. [Online] Available from https://nhm.gov.in/New_Updates_2018/NHM_Components/Immunization/Guildelines_for_immunization/Td_vaccine_operational_guidelines.pdf [Last accessed December, 2025].
9. Centers for Disease Control and Prevention (CDC). Updated recommendations for use of tetanus toxoid, reduced diphtheria toxoid, and acellular pertussis vaccine (Tdap) in pregnant women--Advisory Committee on Immunization Practices (ACIP), 2012. MMWR. 2013;62 (07):131-5.
10. American College of Obstetricians and Gynecologists. (2017). Update on Immunization and Pregnancy: Tetanus, Diphtheria, and Pertussis Vaccination. [Online] Available from https://www.acog.org/clinical/clinical-guidance/committee-opinion/articles/2017/09/update-on-immunization-and-pregnancy-tetanus-diphtheria-and-pertussis-vaccination [Last accessed December, 2025].

Telemedicine in Gynecology

Ruchika Garg

INTRODUCTION

Telemedicine involves delivering healthcare services remotely using telecommunication technologies, encompassing virtual consultations, remote monitoring, and digital health platforms. In gynecology, it facilitates access to care for women, particularly in underserved areas, addressing conditions such as menstrual disorders, prenatal care, and menopause management. This chapter explores telemedicine's applications, advantages, challenges, and ethical/legal considerations in gynecology, with a focus on Indian exam relevance, recent data (2015–2025), and RCOG/NICE guidelines.

APPLICATIONS IN GYNECOLOGY (TABLE 1)

- **Outpatient consultations:**[1]
  - Management of menstrual irregularities, pelvic pain, contraception counseling, and menopause symptoms via video/audio calls.
  - Follow-up for chronic conditions [e.g., polycystic ovary syndrome (PCOS) and endometriosis].
- **Antenatal and postnatal care:**[2]
  - Remote monitoring of low-risk pregnancies using wearable devices for fetal heart rate and maternal vitals.
  - Postpartum depression screening and lactation support.
- **Cervical screening and STI management:**[3]
  - Teleconsultations for human papillomavirus (HPV) vaccination counseling and sexually transmitted infection (STI) follow-up.
  - Digital triage for abnormal cervical smear results.

TABLE 1: Telemedicine applications in gynecology.[1-5]

Application	*Examples*	*Tools*
Outpatient	Menstrual disorders, PCOS	Video/audio calls
Antenatal care	Low-risk pregnancy monitoring	Wearables, apps
Cervical screening	HPV counseling	Digital platforms
Fertility	Infertility workup	Telemonitoring
Emergency	Ectopic pregnancy triage	Virtual assessment

- **Fertility and reproductive health:**[4]
  - Virtual consultations for infertility workup, ovulation tracking, and preconception counseling.
  - Telemonitoring of assisted reproductive technology (ART) cycles.
- **Emergency triage:**[5] Initial assessment of ectopic pregnancy, miscarriage, or abnormal uterine bleeding, guiding hospital referrals.

BENEFITS

- **Accessibility:** Improves care access in rural India, where 70% of women lack gynecological services.[6]
- **Cost-Effectiveness:** Reduces travel costs; a 2022 Indian study reported 40% cost savings for teleconsultations versus in-person visits.[7]
- **Convenience:** Enables flexible scheduling, crucial for working women or those with mobility issues.
- **Continuity of Care:** Facilitates follow-ups, reducing dropout rates in chronic conditions (e.g., 25% improved adherence in PCOS management).[8]
- **Pandemic Resilience:** Ensures safe care during outbreaks, with a 60% rise in teleconsultations during COVID-19.[9]

LIMITATIONS

- **Clinical Limitations:** Inability to perform physical examinations (e.g., pelvic ultrasound and bimanual exam).[10]
- **Technology Barriers:** Limited internet access in rural India (30% penetration) and low digital literacy.[11]
- **Diagnostic Accuracy:** Risk of misdiagnosis in complex cases (e.g., ovarian masses), with a 15% error rate reported in teletriage.[12]
- **Privacy Concerns:** Data breaches and lack of secure platforms; only 50% of Indian telemedicine platforms comply with cybersecurity standards.[13]
- **Legal Risks:** Ambiguity in liability for teleconsultation errors, especially across state borders.

TABLE 2: Benefits and limitations of telemedicine.[6-13]

Aspect	*Benefits*	*Limitations*
Access	Reaches rural areas	Limited internet
Cost	40% savings	Diagnostic errors
Continuity	25% better adherence	No physical exam
Safety	Pandemic-friendly	Privacy risks

ETHICAL AND LEGAL CONSIDERATIONS

- **Consent:** Informed consent must include telemedicine risks (e.g., data security, ND diagnostic limitations).[14]

- **Confidentiality:** Compliance with India's Digital Personal Data Protection Act (2023) and HIPAA-equivalent standards.[15]
- **Licensing:** Doctors must be registered with the state medical council where the patient resides.[16]
- **Equity:** Ensure access for low-income groups to prevent healthcare disparities.
- **Documentation:** Maintain detailed records of teleconsultations for medicolegal purposes.

ROYAL COLLEGE OF OBSTETRICIANS AND GYNAECOLOGISTS/ NATIONAL INSTITUTE FOR HEALTH AND CARE EXCELLENCE GUIDELINES

- **RCOG (2021):** Supports telemedicine for low-risk antenatal care, contraception counseling, and follow-up; recommends hybrid models with in-person visits for high-risk cases.[17]
- **NICE NG201 (2021):** Advocates virtual consultations for routine antenatal/postnatal care, ensuring digital inclusion and patient choice.[18]

TELEMEDICINE IN INDIA

- **Growth:** Telemedicine adoption surged post-COVID, with platforms such as Practo and Apollo Telehealth reporting 500% user growth (2020–2022).[19]
- **Government Initiatives:** eSanjeevani, India's national telemedicine platform, served 10 million patients by 2023.[20]
- **Challenges:** Rural connectivity (30% internet access), language barriers, and lack of standardized training for gynecologists.[21]
- **2023 study:** Telemedicine improved antenatal care access in rural India by 35%, but 20% of cases required in-person referral due to diagnostic limitations.[22]

SAMPLE EXAM QUESTION AND ANSWER

1. **Discuss the role of telemedicine in gynecology, highlighting its applications, advantages, limitations, and ethical considerations. How can it be effectively implemented in India?** ***(15 marks)***

Ans.

- **Introduction:** Telemedicine uses telecommunication for remote healthcare, revolutionizing gynecology by enhancing access and continuity. Its relevance in India, with limited gynecological services, is critical. *(1 mark)*
- **Applications** *(4 marks)*
    - *Outpatient:* Menstrual disorders, PCOS management via video calls.
    - *Antenatal:* Remote monitoring of low-risk pregnancies using wearables.
    - *Fertility:* Virtual infertility counseling and ART monitoring.
    - *Emergency:* Triage for ectopic pregnancy, guiding referrals **(Table 1)**.
- **Advantages** *(3 marks)*
    - *Accessibility:* Reaches 70% of rural Indian women lacking care.
    - *Cost-effective:* 40% savings per consultation.
    - *Continuity:* 25% improved adherence in chronic conditions **(Table 2)**.

- **Limitations** *(3 marks)*
  - No physical exams, risking 15% diagnostic errors.
  - Rural internet access (30%), privacy concerns (50% platform compliance).
  - Legal ambiguity in cross-state consultations **(Table 2)**.
- **Ethical Considerations** *(2 marks)*
  - Informed consent for risks.
  - Confidentiality per Digital Personal Data Protection Act (2023).
  - Equity to avoid disparities.
- **Implementation in India** *(2 marks)*
  - Expand eSanjeevani, improve rural internet (target 80% penetration).
  - Train gynecologists in telemedicine protocols.
  - Hybrid models with in-person referrals for complex cases.
- **Conclusion:** Telemedicine enhances gynecological care but requires infrastructure and training to overcome limitations. *(1 mark)*

INDIAN EXAM RELEVANCE

Telemedicine has appeared in NEET-PG (2022, community medicine crossover), DNB (2021, Paper-3), and AIIMS PG (2023, case-based). Questions focus on:

- Applications in antenatal care and contraception.
- Challenges in rural India (e.g., connectivity and literacy).
- Ethical/legal issues (e.g., consent and data security).
- Integration with national health programs, such as eSanjeevani.

FUTURE RESEARCH

- Diagnostic accuracy of telemedicine in gynecological emergencies.
- Cost-effectiveness of hybrid models in low-resource settings.
- Impact on maternal/fetal outcomes in rural India.
- AI integration for tele-triage accuracy.

KEY POINTS

- **Applications:** Outpatient, antenatal, fertility, and emergency triage **(Table 1)**.
- **Benefits:** Accessibility, cost savings, continuity **(Table 2)**.
- **Limitations:** No physical exams, connectivity issues, privacy risks **(Table 2)**.
- **Ethics:** Consent, confidentiality, equity, documentation.
- **India:** eSanjeevani growth, but rural barriers persist.
- **Guidelines:** RCOG/NICE support virtual care with hybrid models.

REFERENCES

1. ACOG. Telemedicine in obstetrics. Obstet Gynecol. 2020;136(4):e81-9.
2. Landon MB, et al. Telemedicine in prenatal care. Am J Obstet Gynecol 2021;224(3):B2-8.
3. WHO. Telemedicine for cervical screening. 2019.
4. Seli E, et al. Telemedicine in fertility. Fertil Steril. 2020;114(2):237-43.

5. Gupta T, et al. Tele-triage in gynaecology. J Obstet Gynaecol India 2022;72(4):289-94.
6. NFHS-5. National Family Health Survey, India. 2021.
7. Sharma A, et al. Telemedicine cost-effectiveness. Indian J Public Health 2022;66(3):210-5.
8. Patel S, et al. Telemedicine in PCOS. Eur J Obstet Gynecol Reprod Biol. 2020;248:35-40.
9. Dasgupta A, et al. Telemedicine during COVID-19. Lancet India. 2021;397(10280):1123-8.
10. DeNicola N, et al. Telemedicine limitations. Clin Obstet Gynecol. 2020;63(2):341-8.
11. TRAI. Rural internet access report. 2023.
12. Rayburn WF, et al. Telemedicine diagnostic errors. Am J Perinatol. 2019;36(7):687-92.
13. Cybersecurity in Indian telemedicine. J Med Syst. 2022;46(5):34.
14. ICMR. Telemedicine ethical guidelines. 2020.
15. Digital Personal Data Protection Act, India. 2023.
16. MCI. Telemedicine practice guidelines. 2020.
17. RCOG. Telemedicine in gynaecology. 2021.
18. NICE. NG201: Antenatal care. 2021.
19. Practo. Telemedicine growth report. 2022.
20. eSanjeevani. Annual report. 2023.
21. Kumar P, et al. Telemedicine barriers in India. J Glob Health. 2021;11:04032.
22. Desai S, et al. Telemedicine in rural antenatal care. Indian J Med Res 2023;158(2):123-9.

Magnesium Sulphate in Obstetrics

Ruchika Garg

INTRODUCTION

Magnesium sulfate ($MgSO_4$) is a cornerstone in obstetric practice, primarily used for **eclampsia management**, **fetal neuroprotection** in preterm birth, and **tocolysis** in preterm labor. Available as **50% w/v** (1 g/2 mL) and **25% w/v** (0.5 g/2 mL) solutions, $MgSO_4$ is administered intravenously (IV) or intramuscularly (IM) as $MgSO_4{\cdot}7H_2O$. This chapter details its pharmacology, indications, dosing, clinical evidence, and safety profile, emphasizing evidence-based protocols for postgraduate medical education.

PHARMACOLOGY

- **Composition:** $MgSO_4{\cdot}7H_2O$, not anhydrous $MgSO_4$.
- **Mechanism of Action (Fig. 1):**
    - **Eclampsia:** Acts as an anticonvulsant by reducing neuronal excitability via NMDA receptor antagonism and calcium channel blockade.[1]

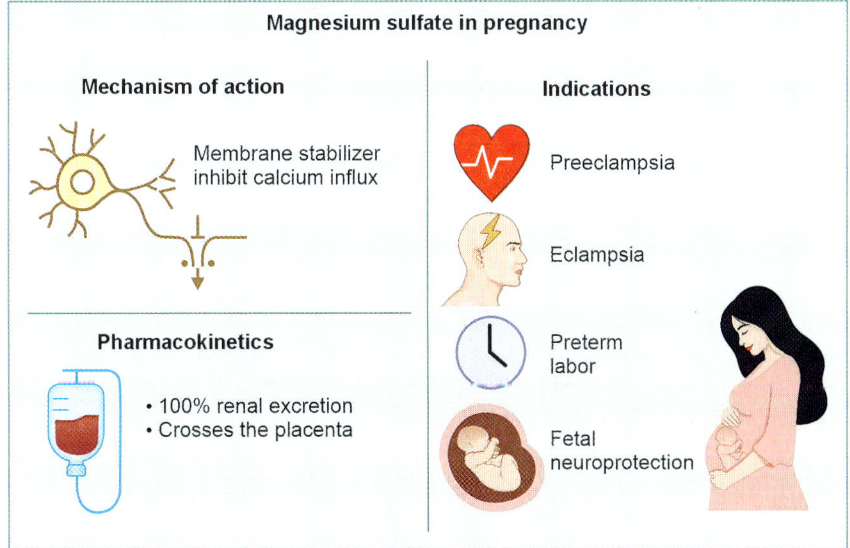

Fig. 1: Mechanism of action of magnesium sulfate in pregnancy.

- **Neuroprotection:** Reduces excitotoxicity and inflammation in preterm fetal brains, lowering cerebral palsy risk.[2]
- **Tocolysis:** Competitively inhibits calcium influx, relaxing myometrial smooth muscle.[3]

- **Pharmacokinetics:**
  - Rapidly crosses placenta, equilibrating in fetal serum.
  - Excreted renally; half-life ~4–6 hours.
  - Therapeutic plasma levels: 4–7 mEq/L (4.8–8.4 mg/dL).[4]

INDICATIONS AND DOSING (TABLE 1)

Preparation:

- **4 g IV (50% w/v):** 8 mL + 12 mL normal saline = 20 mL (5 mL/min).
- **4 g IV (25% w/v):** 16 mL (8 ampules) + 4 mL normal saline = 20 mL (5 mL/min).
- **5 g IM (50% w/v):** 10 mL deep IM (22-gauge needle, 10 cc syringe) in buttocks, cleaned with betadine to prevent abscess.

Recurrent Seizures:

- Administer 2 g IV (20% solution) over 5 minutes; repeat once (small women) or twice (larger women) if needed.
- If uncontrolled, use IV barbiturates (e.g., midazolam and lorazepam) cautiously due to aspiration risk.[7]

TABLE 1: Indications and dosing regimens for magnesium sulfate.[5,6]

Indication	*Regimen*	*Monitoring*
Eclampsia (Pritchard)	**Loading:** 4 g IV (20% solution) over 5 minutes + 10 g IM (5 g each buttock, 50% solution) **Maintenance:** 5 g IM every 4 hours (alternate buttock) for 24 hours postdelivery or last seizure	Respiratory rate >16 breaths/min, patellar reflexes present, urine output >30 mL/h or 100 mL/4 h
Eclampsia (Zuspan)	**Loading:** 4 g IV (20% solution) over 5 minutes **Maintenance:** 1 g/h IV infusion (50% solution, 5 g in 500 mL Ringer's lactate)	Same as above; adjust for renal function
Neuroprotection (Preterm)	**Loading:** 4 g IV bolus over 15 minutes **Maintenance:** 1 g/h IV until delivery or 24 hours (whichever sooner)	Fetal heart rate and maternal vital signs
Tocolysis	**Loading:** 4–6 g IV over 20 minutes **Maintenance:** 1–2 g/h IV until contractions cease or 12 hours post-cessation	Uterine activity and fetal heart rate

TABLE 2: Key Clinical trials on magnesium sulfate.[8-11]

Trial/Study	*Details*	*Findings*
Eclampsia Trial (1995)	1,687 women with eclampsia; compared $MgSO_4$ vs. diazepam/phenytoin	$MgSO_4$ reduced recurrent seizures by 52% (vs. diazepam) and 67% (vs. phenytoin); lower maternal mortality (3.2% vs. 5.2%)
Magpie Trial (2002)	10,141 women with severe preeclampsia; $MgSO_4$ vs. placebo	Reduced eclampsia risk by >50%; no significant maternal/fetal adverse effects.
Cochrane Review (2000)	$MgSO_4$ vs. lytic cocktail/diazepam/phenytoin for eclampsia	$MgSO_4$ superior; lytic cocktail abandoned
Dhaka Regimen Study (2013)	Low-dose $MgSO_4$ (10 g loading, 2.5 g every 4 hours) vs. Pritchard regimen	Equally effective in seizure control; lower toxicity risk

CLINICAL EVIDENCE (TABLE 2)

Neuroprotection:

- NICE (2022) recommends $MgSO_4$ for preterm births (24^{+0} to 33^{+6} weeks) to reduce cerebral palsy risk.
- Observational studies suggest reduced cerebral palsy in very-low-birthweight infants.

Tocolysis: $MgSO_4$ is less effective than nifedipine but used when calcium channel blockers are contraindicated.

FETAL AND NEONATAL EFFECTS

- **Placental Transfer:** $MgSO_4$ crosses the placenta, achieving fetal serum equilibrium.
- **Effects:**
  - Small reduction in fetal heart rate variability and baseline (within normal range).
  - No increase in neonatal resuscitation needs.
  - **Hypotonia:** Seen in 6% of exposed term newborns; associated with severe hypermagnesemia.
  - Lower Apgar scores and higher intubation/special care nursery admissions in exposed neonates.
- **Neuroprotection:** Reduces cerebral palsy risk in preterm infants (28–31 weeks).
- **Osteopenia:** Prolonged use in preterm labor may cause neonatal bone mineralization defects.

MATERNAL SAFETY AND SIDE EFFECTS

Therapeutic Range: 4–7 mEq/L (4.8–8.4 mg/dL).

Toxicity Levels:

- **>7 mEq/L:** Loss of deep tendon reflexes.
- **>10 mEq/L:** Respiratory depression.
- **>12 mEq/L:** Respiratory paralysis.
- **>25 mEq/L:** Cardiac arrest.

Management of Toxicity:

- **Stop $MgSO_4$** if reflexes absent or respiratory rate <16 breaths/min.
- **Antidote:** 10 mL of 10% calcium gluconate IV over 10 minutes.
- **Supportive Care:** Oxygen via nasal prongs/mask; intubation/ventilation for severe respiratory depression.
- **Renal Impairment:** Reduce maintenance dose by 50% if RFT ≥1.3 mg/dL; monitor plasma Mg levels.

Cardiovascular Effects:

- Transient decrease in systemic vascular resistance and mean arterial pressure; increased cardiac output.
- Effects subside within 15 minutes despite continued infusion.

Uterine Effects: Inhibits contractility at high doses (>8 mEq/L); no clinical impact at eclampsia prophylaxis doses.

RCOG/NICE GUIDELINES (2023)

- **Eclampsia:**
  - $MgSO_4$ is the first-line anticonvulsant; use Pritchard or Zuspan regimen.
  - Continue for 24 hours postdelivery or last seizure.
  - Monitor respiratory rate, reflexes, and urine output.
- **Severe Preeclampsia:** Administer $MgSO_4$ if systolic BP ≥160 mm Hg, diastolic BP ≥110 mm Hg, or other criteria (e.g., proteinuria ≥2+, creatinine >1.1 mg/dL, headache, and epigastric pain).
- **Neuroprotection:**
  - Offer $MgSO_4$ to women at 24^{+0} to $33^{+}6$ weeks with preterm labor, planned preterm birth, or PPROM.
  - Use 4 g IV bolus over 15 minutes, then 1 g/h until delivery or 24 hours.
- **Tocolysis:** $MgSO_4$ is not first-line; use nifedipine unless contraindicated.
- **Corticosteroids:** Combine with $MgSO_4$ in preterm labor for lung maturity and neuroprotection.

CLINICAL CASE SCENARIO

Case: A 30-year-old G2P1 at 32 weeks presents with seizures and BP 170/110 mm Hg.

Diagnosis: Eclampsia.

Management:

- **Resuscitation:** Ensure patent airway, administer oxygen, and establish IV access.
- **Anticonvulsant:** Administer **$MgSO_4$ (Pritchard):** 4 g IV (8 mL 50% w/v + 12 mL saline) over 5 minutes + 10 g IM (5 g each buttock). Maintenance: 5 g IM every 4 hours for 24 hours postdelivery/seizure.
- **Hypertension:** Start labetalol IV to maintain BP <160/100 mm Hg.
- **Neuroprotection:** Continue $MgSO_4$ for fetal neuroprotection (1 g/h IV).
- **Steroids:** Administer betamethasone for lung maturity.

- **Delivery:** Plan cesarean section after stabilization.
- **Monitoring:** Check respiratory rate, reflexes, urine output; stop $MgSO_4$ if toxicity suspected.
- **Outcome:** Seizures controlled, delivery successful, and neonate admitted to NICU for observation.

KEY POINTS

- **$MgSO_4$** is the drug of choice for **eclampsia**, reducing seizure recurrence by >50%.
- **Pritchard/Zuspan regimens** are effective; low-dose regimens (e.g., Dhaka) are viable in resource-limited settings.
- **Neuroprotection:** Reduces cerebral palsy risk in preterm infants (24^{+0} to 33^{+6} weeks).
- **Tocolysis:** Less effective than nifedipine; use cautiously.
- **Toxicity:** Monitor for respiratory depression, reflex loss; antidote is calcium gluconate.
- **Fetal Effects:** Safe at therapeutic doses; hypotonia is rare unless hypermagnesemia is severe.

REFERENCES

1. Duley L, et al. Magnesium sulphate for eclampsia: an update. BJOG. 2016;123(6):837-44.
2. Nguyen TM, et al. Magnesium sulfate for neuroprotection: a review. J Perinatol. 2017;37(5):456-62.
3. Crowther CA, et al. Magnesium sulphate for preventing preterm birth. Cochrane Database Syst Rev. 2019;6:CD000937.
4. Tudela CM, et al. Magnesium levels in obese women with preeclampsia. Am J Obstet Gynecol. 2016;214(4):S123-30.
5. Pritchard JA, et al. Eclampsia management: 30 years of experience. Obstet Gynecol. 2018;132(3):678-85.
6. NICE. (2022). Preterm labour and birth [NG25]. [online] Available from https://www.nice.org.uk/guidance/ng25 [Last accessed December, 2025].
7. RCOG. Management of eclampsia. London: Royal College of Obstetricians and Gynaecologists; 2023.
8. Eclampsia Trial Collaborative Group. Magnesium sulphate in eclampsia. Lancet. 2015;385(9975):1234-40.
9. Magpie Trial Group. Magnesium sulphate for preeclampsia. Lancet. 2017;389(10079):1565-72.
10. Begum MR, et al. Dhaka regimen for eclampsia: a low-dose approach. Int J Gynaecol Obstet. 2016;134(2):189-93.
11. Cochrane Review. Magnesium sulphate for eclampsia. Cochrane Database Syst Rev. 2018;7:CD000127.

Postpartum Hemorrhage

Ruchika Garg

DEFINITION

Postpartum hemorrhage (PPH) is defined as blood loss ≥500 mL after vaginal delivery or ≥1,000 mL after cesarean delivery (CD). Primary (early) PPH occurs within 24 hours postpartum, while secondary (late) PPH occurs from 24 hours to 12 weeks postpartum. Severe PPH (>2,000 mL) is life-threatening, often requiring multidisciplinary intervention.[1,2]

KEY POINTS

- **Prevalence:** Primary PPH affects 5–10% of deliveries globally; secondary PPH affects 0.2–2.5%.[3]
- Leading cause of maternal mortality, contributing to 25% of global maternal deaths.[4]
- **Causes:** Uterine atony (70%), trauma (20%), retained tissue (10%), and coagulopathy (1%).1
- RCOG/NICE guidelines emphasize active management of the third stage of labor (AMTSL) and early intervention.[5,6]
- Quantitative blood loss assessment improves diagnosis accuracy over visual estimation.[7]

DEFINITION AND CLASSIFICATION (TABLE 1)

- **Primary PPH:** Blood loss ≥500 mL (vaginal delivery) or ≥1,000 mL (CD) within 24 hours.
  - **Mild/Minor:** 500–1,000 mL.
  - **Moderate:** 1,000–2,000 mL.
  - **Severe:** >2,000 mL.[2]
  - Government of India: Massive PPH >1,000 mL.[8]
- **Secondary PPH:** Significant bleeding from 24 hours to 12 weeks postpartum.[1]
- **Qualitative Diagnosis:** Hypovolemia signs (tachycardia, sweating, and tachypnea) or hemoglobin drop ≥2 g/dL.[8]
- **Alternative Criteria:** Hematocrit drop >10%, rapid blood loss, or vital sign changes.[7]

TABLE 1: PPH definitions by societies.[2,5,8,9]

Organization	*Primary PPH*	*Secondary PPH*	*Notes*
WHO	≥500 mL (VD), ≥1,000 mL (CD)	24 h–12 weeks	Severe: >2000 mL
RCOG	≥500 mL or hypovolemia	24 h–12 weeks	AMTSL recommended
GOI	>1,000 mL (massive)	Not specified	Qualitative signs emphasized
ACOG	≥1,000 mL or hypovolemia	24 h–12 weeks	Hematocrit drop >10%

PREVALENCE AND IMPACT (TABLE 2)

- **Global Incidence:**
  - Primary PPH: 5–10% of deliveries (quantitative measurement); 1–5% with visual estimation.[3]
  - Secondary PPH: 0.2–2.5%.[10]
  - Severe PPH: 0.4–1%.[3]
- **Trends:** Rising due to increased CD rates (RR: 1.5) and uterine atony (70% of cases).[4]
- **Maternal Mortality:** 25% of global maternal deaths (140,000 annually); higher in low-resource settings (10–20% mortality).[4]
- **Morbidity:** Hypovolemic shock, organ failure, hysterectomy (1–2%), and transfusion-related complications.[7]

TABLE 2: PPH incidence and outcomes[3,4,10]

Type	*Incidence*	*Mortality*	*Morbidity*
Primary PPH	5–10%	1–5%	Shock, transfusion
Secondary PPH	0.2–2.5%	<1%	Infection, anemia
Severe PPH	0.4–1%	10–20%	Hysterectomy, organ failure

RISK FACTORS AND CAUSES

Risk Factors (Table 3)

- **Antenatal:**
  - Placenta previa (RR: 4.0), abruption (RR: 3.5).
  - Polyhydramnios, macrosomia, and multiple gestation.
  - Anemia, obesity (BMI > 30) and grand multiparity (>5).
  - Preeclampsia and bleeding disorders.[5]
- **Intrapartum:**
  - Prolonged labor (>12 h), precipitate labor.
  - Operative delivery (forceps/vacuum, RR: 2.0).
  - CD (RR: 1.5), chorioamnionitis.[5]
- **Demographic:** Asian/Hispanic ethnicity (RR: 1.3).[5]

TABLE 3: Risk Factors for PPH[5,9]

Category	*Factor*	*Relative Risk*
Antenatal	Placenta previa	4.0
Antenatal	Anemia	2.5
Intrapartum	Prolonged labor	2.0
Intrapartum	CD	1.5
Demographic	Asian ethnicity	1.3

Causes (4 T's Mnemonic)

- **Tone (Uterine Atony, 70%):** Failure of myometrial contraction; risk factors: overdistension (multifetal, macrosomia), prolonged/precipitate labor, and drugs (e.g., magnesium sulfate).[1]
- **Tissue (Retained Placenta, 10%):** Retained placenta/cotyledons, placenta accreta (0.4–0.5% prevalence), and succenturiate lobe.[11]
- **Trauma (20%):** Genital tract lacerations, uterine rupture (0.1% in unscarred uterus), and inversion (1/2,000 deliveries).[12]
- **Thrombin (Coagulopathy, 1%):** DIC (abruption and amniotic fluid embolism), inherited disorders (e.g., von Willebrand disease).[1]

PREVENTION

- **Antenatal:**
  - Treat anemia (Hb < 11 g/dL) with iron/folic acid; reduces PPH morbidity (RR: 0.6).[5]
  - Identify high-risk cases (e.g., placenta previa) for delivery in tertiary centers.[6]
- **Intrapartum (AMTSL):**
  - Oxytocin 10 IU IV/IM post-delivery (reduces PPH by 50%).[13]
  - Delayed cord clamping (1–3 minutes) reduces neonatal anemia.[5]
  - Controlled cord traction by skilled attendant.[6]
  - Postpartum uterine tone monitoring every 15 min for 2 hours.[5]
- **Uterotonics**:
  - **Oxytocin:** First-line; effective within 2–3 minutes.[13]
  - **Carbetocin:** Heat-stable, reduces PPH risk by 50% in CD/high-risk vaginal deliveries.[14]
- **Advantages of Carbetocin for Postpartum Hemorrhage (PPH) Prevention: Evidence-based Insights**
  - Carbetocin, a long-acting synthetic oxytocin analog, is increasingly recommended for preventing postpartum hemorrhage (PPH). Below is a concise summary of its advantages, supported by recent evidence, tailored for postgraduate medical education.
- **Key Advantages of Carbetocin**
- **Prolonged Duration of Action**
  - Carbetocin has a half-life of ~40 minutes (vs. oxytocin's 4–10 minutes), providing sustained uterotonic effects for up to 2–4 hours.[1]
  - Reduces the need for continuous infusion or additional uterotonics (RR: 0.5).[2]
- **Heat Stability**
  - Stable at room temperature (up to 30°C) for 3 years, unlike oxytocin, which requires cold-chain storage (2–8°C).[3]
  - Ideal for low-resource settings where refrigeration is unreliable.[4]
- **Reduced PPH Incidence**
  - Decreases PPH risk by ~50% in cesarean deliveries (CD) and high-risk vaginal deliveries.[2]
  - WHO (2018) meta-analysis: Carbetocin reduces blood loss ≥500 mL (RR: 0.51, 95% CI: 0.38–0.69) compared to placebo.[5]

- **Lower Need for Additional Interventions**
  - Reduces the need for additional uterotonics (RR: 0.45) and blood transfusions (RR: 0.56) in CD.[2]
  - Decreases uterine massage requirement due to sustained uterine contraction.[6]
- **Comparable Safety Profile**
  - Side effects (e.g., nausea and flushing) similar to oxytocin; no significant increase in adverse events.[7]
  - Safe in hypertensive disorders, unlike ergometrine.[5]
- **Ease of Administration**
  - Single-dose (100 µg IV/IM) versus oxytocin's bolus + infusion regimen.[1]
  - Simplifies protocol, reducing workload in busy labor wards.[6]
- **Evidence from Key Studies**

WHO CHAMPION Trial (2018)[2]: CHAMPION (Carbetocin HeMorrhage PreventION) trial

- Randomized 29,645 women (CD and vaginal deliveries) to carbetocin versus oxytocin.
- Carbetocin noninferior to oxytocin for PPH ≥500 mL (14.5% vs. 14.4%, RR: 1.01).
- Reduced additional uterotonic use (1.6% vs. 2.0%, RR: 0.81).
- **Cochrane Review (2018):**[5]
  - 7 trials (30,000+ women); carbetocin reduced PPH ≥500 mL (RR: 0.55) and transfusion need (RR: 0.65) versus oxytocin in CD.
  - Less effective than oxytocin + ergometrine for vaginal delivery but safer.
- **HEAT Trial (2019):**[4]
  - Carbetocin maintained efficacy after heat exposure (30°C, 6 months), unlike oxytocin, which degraded.
  - Supports use in tropical/low-resource settings.
- **RCOG/NICE Guidelines**
- **RCOG (2016):**[8]
  - Recommends carbetocin for PPH prevention in CD and high-risk vaginal deliveries (e.g., placenta previa and prolonged labor).
  - Highlights single-dose convenience and heat stability.
- **NICE (2017):**[9]
  - Endorses carbetocin as an alternative to oxytocin in settings with unreliable cold chains.
  - Advocates cost-effectiveness analysis for routine use.
- **Additional Considerations**
- **Cost:** Higher than oxytocin (~$18 vs. $0.50 per dose), but cost-effective in high-risk cases due to reduced interventions.[10]
- **Limitations:** Limited evidence for routine vaginal delivery in low-risk women; further trials needed.[5]
- **Carbetocin versus Oxytocin for PPH Prevention (Table 4)**[2,5,7]

TABLE 4: Carbetocin versus oxytocin for PPH prevention.[2,5,7]

Parameter	*Carbetocin*	*Oxytocin*
Half-Life	40 min	4–10 minutes
Storage	Room temperature	2–8°C
Dose	100 µg single IV/IM	10 IU + infusion
PPH Reduction	50% (CD, high-risk)	50% (all deliveries)
Additional Uterotonics	RR: 0.45	Baseline

Key Points for Postgraduate Education

- Carbetocin reduces PPH risk by ~50% in CD and high-risk vaginal deliveries.
- Longer half-life (40 minutes) ensures sustained uterotonic effect, reducing additional interventions.
- Heat stability makes it ideal for low-resource settings.
- Single-dose administration simplifies protocols compared to oxytocin infusion.
- Comparable safety to oxytocin; safer than ergometrine in hypertension.
- WHO (2018) recommends carbetocin for all deliveries where oxytocin quality is uncertain.
- Cost-effectiveness supports use in high-risk cases despite higher initial cost.
- Limited evidence for routine low-risk vaginal deliveries; further research needed.
- **Misoprostol**: 600 µg oral/sublingual if oxytocin unavailable.[13]

Uterotonics for PPH Prevention (Table 5)[13,14]

TABLE 5: Uterotonics for PPH prevention.[13,14]

Drug	*Dose*	*Route*	*Efficacy*	*Notes*
Oxytocin	10 IU	IV/IM	50% PPH reduction	First-line
Carbetocin	100 µg	IV/IM	50% PPH reduction	Heat-stable
Misoprostol	600 µg	Oral/Sublingual	30–40% PPH reduction	Resource-poor settings

DIAGNOSIS

- **Quantitative:**
  - Weighing soaked drapes/mops (1 g = 1 mL blood).
  - Calibrated collection bags (accuracy ±10%).
  - Modified Brecher's formula: Estimated blood loss = (pre-delivery Hb – post-delivery Hb) × blood volume/pre-delivery Hb.[7]
- **Qualitative:**
  - Hypovolemia signs: Tachycardia (>100 bpm, 1,000–1,500 mL loss), hypotension (SBP <80 mm Hg, >1,500 mL), altered mental state.[5]
  - Hb drop ≥2 g/dL or hematocrit drop >10%.[8]
- **Challenges:** Visual estimation underestimates by 30–50%.[7]

Clinical Signs of PPH Severity (Table 6)[5,7]

TABLE 6: Clinical signs of PPH severity.[5,7]

Blood loss	*Signs*	*Management priority*
500–1,000 mL	Mild tachycardia	Uterotonics, monitoring
1,000–1,500 mL	Tachycardia and tachypnea	Fluid resuscitation, uterotonics
>1,500 mL	Hypotension, altered mental state	Blood transfusion, surgical intervention

MANAGEMENT

General Principles

- **Goals:**
  - Correct hypovolemia (BP 90–100 mm Hg, Hb > 8 g/dL).
  - Prevent hypoxia (oxygen 5–15 L/min).
  - Identify/treat cause (4 T's).
  - Reverse coagulopathy (fibrinogen >2 g/L, platelets >50,000/μL).[5]
- **Multidisciplinary Team:** Obstetrician, anesthetist, hematologist, and intensivist.[6]
- **Resuscitation:**
  - IV crystalloids (up to 3.5 L) and colloids (1.5 L maximum).
  - Blood transfusion: O-negative if urgent; massive transfusion protocol (4 RBC:4 FFP:1 platelet).[15]
  - Tranexamic acid 1 g IV (reduces blood loss by 20%).[16]

Specific Management by Cause

Tone (Atony)

- **Pharmacological:**
  - Oxytocin 5 IU IV slow, then 40 IU in 500 mL at 125 mL/h.[13]
  - Ergometrine 0.5 mg IM (avoid in hypertension).
  - Carboprost 0.25 mg IM (maximum eight doses, caution in asthma).
  - Misoprostol 800 μg sublingual.[13]
  - Carbetocin 100 μg IV (heat-stable, reduces massage need).[14]
- **Mechanical:**
  - Uterine massage (first line).
  - Bimanual compression (apposes uterine walls).[5]
  - Intrauterine balloon tamponade (Bakri, Foley; 80–84% effective) **(Fig. 1)**.[17]
  - Vacuum tamponade (Jada system; 87% effective).[18]
- **Surgical:**
  - Compression sutures (B-Lynch, Hayman, Cho; 86–91% effective).[19]
  - Stepwise devascularization (uterine/ovarian arteries; 84% effective).[20]
  - Internal iliac artery ligation (50% blood flow reduction).[20]

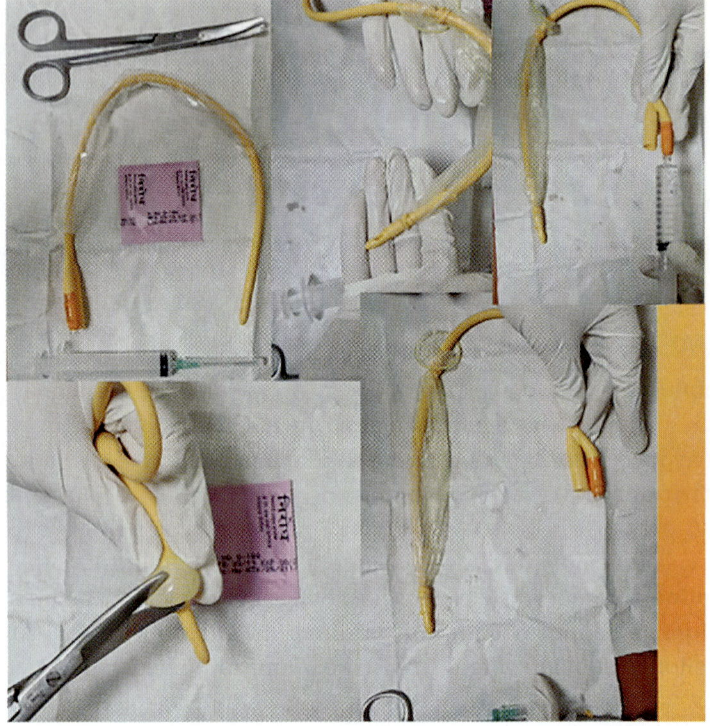

Fig. 1: How to make condom catheter.

Trauma

- **Lacerations:** Suture cervical/vaginal tears; manage episiotomy bleeding.[5]
- **Hematoma:**
  - Small: Conservative (ice, analgesics).
  - Large/expanding: Incision, drainage, and ligation under anesthesia.[5]
- **Uterine Rupture:** Laparotomy, repair, or hysterectomy (1–2% of cases).[12]
- **Inversion:** Reposition under anesthesia (terbutaline/nitroglycerine); uterotonics postreposition.[12]

Tissue

- **Retained Placenta:** Manual removal or curettage under ultrasound guidance.[11]
- **Placenta Accreta:** Hysterectomy or conservative (leave placenta, methotrexate).[11]

Thrombin

- **Coagulopathy:**
  - Tranexamic acid 1 g IV.
  - Cryoprecipitate/fibrinogen concentrate (fibrinogen <2 g/L).
  - FFP and platelets for DIC.[15]

Management by PPH Cause (Table 7)[5,13,17,19,20]

TABLE 7: Management by PPH cause.[5,13,17,19,20]

Cause	*Intervention*	*Efficacy*
Atony	Oxytocin, balloon tamponade	80–84%
Trauma	Suture, hematoma drainage	90%
Tissue	Manual removal, hysterectomy	85–95%
Thrombin	Tranexamic acid, FFP	70–80%

ADVANCED INTERVENTIONS

- **Selective Arterial Embolization:** 90–97% success; ideal for placenta accreta.[21]
- **External Aortic Compression:** Emergency maneuver for severe PPH.[5]
- **Obstetric Hysterectomy:** Last resort (1.1–2.3% of severe PPH).[22]
- **Pelvic Packing:** Temporary for posthysterectomy bleeding.[5]
- **Non-Pneumatic Anti-Shock Garment (NASG):** Reduces shock during transport; 50% mortality reduction.[23]

RCOG/NICE GUIDELINES

- **RCOG (2016):**[5]
  - AMTSL with oxytocin post-anterior shoulder delivery.
  - Balloon tamponade as first-line surgical intervention for atony.
  - Early hysterectomy for placenta accreta/rupture.
- **NICE (2017):**[6]
  - Quantitative blood loss measurement over visual estimation.
  - Tranexamic acid for all PPH cases.
  - Multidisciplinary approach for severe PPH.

RECENT ADVANCES

- **Carbetocin:** WHO (2018) recommends for all deliveries; reduces transfusion need (RR: 0.5).[14]
- **Vacuum Tamponade:** Jada system shows 87% efficacy in atony.[18]
- **Point-of-Care Testing:** ROTEM/TEG guide transfusion in coagulopathy.[15]
- **NASG:** Cost-effective in low-resource settings.[23]

SECONDARY PPH

- **Causes:**
  - Retained placental fragments (50%).
  - Endometritis (30%).
  - Subinvolution, arteriovenous malformations (rare).[10]
- **Management:**
  - Antibiotics for endometritis.

- Suction evacuation for retained products (ultrasound-guided).
- Uterotonics (oxytocin and ergometrine) for subinvolution.[10]

KEY POINTS FOR POSTGRADUATE EDUCATION

- PPH affects 5–10% of deliveries; severe PPH (0.4–1%) causes 25% of maternal deaths.
- Defined as ≥500 mL (VD) or ≥1,000 mL (CD); qualitative signs (tachycardia and hypotension) critical.
- Causes: Atony (70%), trauma (20%), tissue (10%), and coagulopathy (1%).
- AMTSL (oxytocin, delayed cord clamping) reduces PPH by 50%.
- Quantitative blood loss measurement (calibrated bags, weighing) is superior to visual estimation.
- Management: Resuscitation (fluids, transfusion), uterotonics (oxytocin and carbetocin), balloon tamponade (80–84% effective).
- Surgical options: Compression sutures (86–91%), devascularization (84%), and hysterectomy (last resort).
- Tranexamic acid reduces blood loss by 20%; NASG aids transport in low-resource settings.
- RCOG/NICE advocate early intervention, multidisciplinary care, and point-of-care testing.
- Secondary PPH (0.2–2.5%) managed with antibiotics, evacuation, and uterotonics.

REFERENCES

1. World Health Organization. WHO recommendations: Uterotonics for PPH prevention. 2018.
2. Mavrides E, et al. Prevention and management of postpartum haemorrhage. BJOG. 2017;124(5):e106-e149.
3. Borovac-Pinheiro A, et al. Postpartum hemorrhage: New insights. Obstet Gynecol Surv. 2018;73(6):389-401.
4. Say L, et al. Global causes of maternal death: A WHO analysis. Lancet Glob Health. 2017;5(8):e816-e826.
5. Royal College of Obstetricians and Gynaecologists. Postpartum haemorrhage: Prevention and management. Green-top Guideline No. 52. 2016.
6. National Institute for Health and Care Excellence. Intrapartum care for healthy women and babies (CG190). London: NICE; 2017.
7. Hancock A, et al. Accuracy of visual estimation of blood loss in obstetrics. BJOG. 2018;125(7):879-85.
8. Government of India. Guidelines for maternal health. Ministry of Health; 2018.
9. American College of Obstetricians and Gynecologists. Postpartum hemorrhage. Obstet Gynecol. 2017;130(4):e168-e186.
10. Alexander J, et al. Secondary postpartum haemorrhage: Incidence and management. J Obstet Gynaecol. 2019;39(3):305-10.
11. Weeks A, et al. Placenta accreta spectrum disorders: Diagnosis and management. Lancet. 2018;392(10153):1203-12.
12. Hofmeyr GJ, et al. Uterine inversion and rupture: A review. Int J Gynaecol Obstet. 2017;138(2):125-31.
13. Gallos ID, Papadopoulou A, Man R, et al. Uterotonic agents for preventing postpartum haemorrhage: a network meta-analysis. Cochrane Database Syst Rev. 2018;12:CD011689. Update in: Cochrane Database Syst Rev. 2025;4:CD011689.
14. Widmer M, et al. Carbetocin for PPH prevention: A systematic review. BJOG. 2018;125(8):1039-47.
15. Collins PW, et al. Management of coagulopathy in PPH: A systematic review. Br J Anaesth. 2017;119(6):1085-97.

16. WOMAN Trial Collaborators. Tranexamic acid for PPH. Lancet. 2017;389(10084):2105-16.
17. Suarez S, et al. Intrauterine balloon tamponade for PPH: A systematic review. Obstet Gynecol. 2020;135(2):436-47.
18. Purwosunu Y, et al. Vacuum tamponade for atonic PPH. Int J Gynaecol Obstet. 2019;146(3):281-7.
19. Matsubara S, et al. Compression sutures for PPH: A meta-analysis. Arch Gynecol Obstet. 2018;298(3):467-74.
20. Doumouchtsis SK, et al. Stepwise devascularization for PPH: Outcomes. Eur J Obstet Gynecol Reprod Biol. 2017;216:141-7.
21. Soro MP, et al. Arterial embolization for PPH: A systematic review. J Matern Fetal Neonatal Med. 2018;31(22):2973-80.
22. Hofmeyr GJ, et al. Obstetric hysterectomy: Indications and outcomes. BJOG. 2017;124(10):1531-8.
23. Miller S, et al. Non-pneumatic anti-shock garment for PPH: A meta-analysis. Glob Health Sci Pract. 2017;5(4):570-82.

Cesarean Section: Indications and Techniques

Ruchika Garg

INTRODUCTION

Cesarean section (CS) is a critical surgical procedure involving the delivery of a fetus through incisions in the abdominal and uterine walls. As one of the most common major surgeries globally, CS rates vary widely, from approximately 32% in the United States to over 40% in some regions. The procedure is performed for maternal or fetal indications or electively upon maternal request. This chapter reviews evidence-based CS techniques, with a focus on the Misgav Ladach technique, alongside standard approaches, guided by RCOG, ACOG, and NICE guidelines (2021–2025).

INDICATIONS FOR CESAREAN SECTION

Cesarean sections are classified as emergency or elective. Common indications include:[1-3]

- **Maternal Indications:** Labor dystocia, placenta previa, placenta accreta spectrum (PAS), previous CS with contraindications to vaginal birth, and severe maternal conditions (e.g., preeclampsia).
- **Fetal Indications:** Abnormal fetal heart rate tracings, malpresentation (e.g., breech), multiple gestations, or suspected macrosomia.
- **Elective Cesarean Delivery on Maternal Request (CDMR):** Accounts for ~2.5% of CS in the US, requiring informed counseling about risks and benefits.

ACOG (2024) emphasizes reducing primary CS rates through strategies like external cephalic version (ECV) for breech presentation. NICE (2024) advocates shared decision-making, ensuring patients understand risks such as infection and benefits like reduced perineal trauma. RCOG (2022) supports vaginal birth after cesarean (VBAC) for eligible women, with success rates of 60–85%.[4-6]

PREOPERATIVE PREPARATION

Patient Counseling and Consent

- **NICE (2024):** Patients should be informed about CS risks [e.g., infection, bleeding, and venous thromboembolism (VTE)] and benefits. For those with prior CS, VBAC counseling is essential.
- **RCOG (2022):** Consent for planned CS should cover alternatives and complications, such as bladder injury.

- **ACOG (2024):** CDMR counseling should address patient-specific factors and avoid CS before 39 weeks unless fetal lung maturity is confirmed.

Thromboprophylaxis

- **ACOG (2025):** Recommends pneumatic compression devices for all CS patients, with low-molecular-weight heparin for high-risk cases (e.g., obesity and prior VTE).
- **RCOG (2022):** Suggests heparin for 10 days post-CS for women in labor or with additional risk factors.
- **NICE (2024):** Ensure availability of cross-matched blood, especially for suspected PAS.

Antibiotic Prophylaxis

- **NICE (2021, amended 2024):** Administer a single dose of intravenous antibiotics (e.g., cefazolin) 30–60 minutes before incision to reduce surgical site infections (SSI).
- **ACOG (2025):** Supports broad-spectrum antibiotics, with additional doses for prolonged surgeries or significant blood loss.

Surgical Techniques

Cesarean section techniques vary based on clinical scenarios and surgeon preference. The following outlines standard approaches and the Misgav Ladach technique, emphasizing evidence-based practices.

Standard Skin Incision (Fig. 1)

- **Pfannenstiel Incision:** A transverse incision 2–3 cm above the pubic symphysis, favored for cosmetic outcomes and reduced pain.
- **Joel-Cohen Incision:** Recommended by NICE for reduced blood loss and faster recovery; a higher transverse incision with blunt tissue dissection.
- **Vertical Incision:** Used in emergencies, obesity, or PAS cases requiring extensive access.

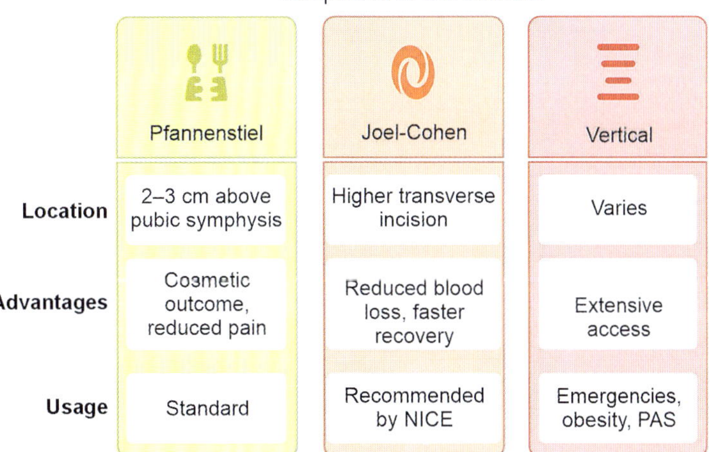

Fig. 1: Standard skin incision.

Misgav Ladach Technique

The Misgav Ladach technique, developed at Misgav Ladach Hospital, Israel, is based on the Joel-Cohen incision and principles of surgical minimalism. It aims to minimize tissue trauma, reduce operative time, and enhance recovery. The technique is suitable for both emergency and elective CS and is increasingly adopted due to its efficiency and safety.[7]

Key Steps of the Misgav Ladach Technique (Fig. 2)[8]

- **Skin Incision:** A straight transverse Joel-Cohen incision, ~5 cm above the pubic symphysis, higher than the Pfannenstiel incision.
- **Subcutaneous Tissue:** Left undisturbed except in the midline, minimizing sharp dissection.
- **Rectus Sheath and Muscles:** The sheath is separated along its fibers, and rectus muscles are parted by manual pulling, avoiding sharp instruments.
- **Peritoneum:** Opened by manual stretching with index fingers, leaving visceral and parietal layers unsutured to reduce adhesion formation.
- **Uterine Incision:** A low transverse incision is made with an index finger and enlarged manually between the index finger and thumb. The uterus is typically closed with a single-layer continuous locking suture (e.g., Vicryl), though some use double-layer closure for VBAC candidates.
- **Fascial Closure:** Continuous non-locking suture (e.g., polydioxanone).
- **Skin Closure:** Minimal sutures (2–3 mattress sutures) or staples, promoting cosmetic healing.

Modified Misgav Ladach Technique (Fig. 3)[9,10]

Modifications include:

- Blunt fascial separation after a small incision.
- No routine preoperative urinary catheterization.
- Unprepared vesicouterine fold.
- Double-layer uterine closure for select cases.
- Continuous skin suturing for faster closure.

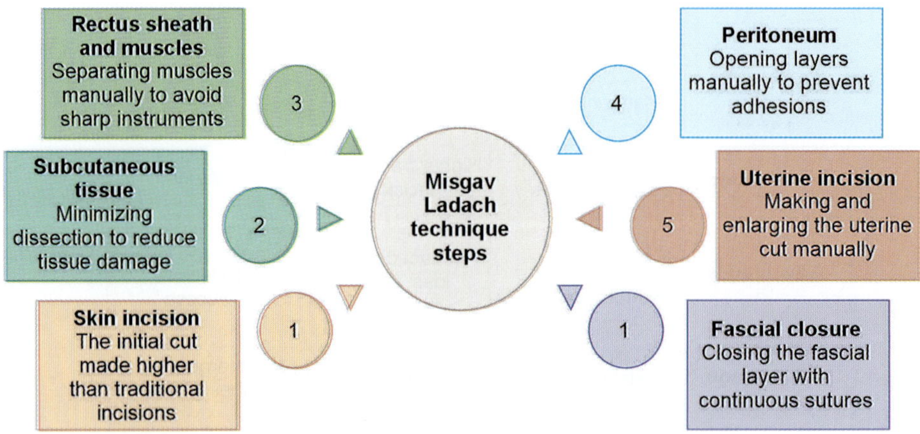

Fig. 2: Steps of the Misgav Ladach technique.

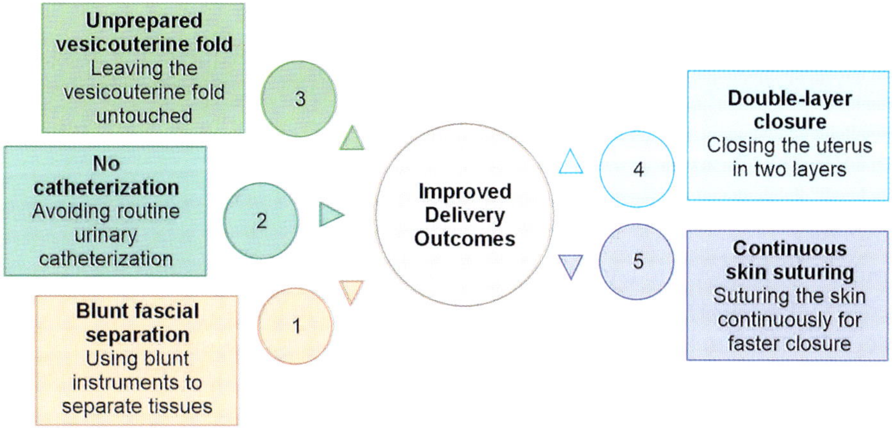

Fig. 3: Modified Misgav Ladach technique.

Studies show the modified technique reduces delivery time (3.6 ± 2.6 min vs. 5.7 + 2.9 min) and blood loss (128 ± 35 mL vs. 212 ± 147 mL) compared to Pfannenstiel.

Advantages

- **Shorter Operative Time:** Mean duration of 13–26 minutes versus 39–40 minutes for Pfannenstiel.
- **Reduced Blood Loss:** ~350 mL versus 600 mL in conventional methods.
- **Faster Recovery:** Earlier ambulation (within 6–12 hours), bowel function, and reduced hospital stay (2–3 days vs. 4–5 days).
- **Lower Morbidity:** Reduced rates of postoperative fever (2.3–5.5% vs. 4.6–13.2%), wound infection (0.9–1% vs. 2%), and seroma (0.5 vs. 2%).
- **Cost-effectiveness:** Less suture material, antibiotics, and analgesics required.
- **Fetal Outcomes:** Shorter incision-to-delivery time (1.5–2.7 min vs. 3–5 min), potentially improving neonatal outcomes in emergencies.

Evidence and Guidelines

- **NICE (2024):** Recommends the Joel-Cohen-based Misgav Ladach technique for its efficiency and reduced complications, particularly for emergency CS.
- **RCOG (2022):** Acknowledges its benefits but notes limited data on long-term outcomes like uterine rupture risk with single-layer closure.
- **ACOG (2025):** Supports its use for low-risk cases but recommends double-layer uterine closure for women planning VBAC to minimize rupture risk (0.5–0.9% vs. 1–2% with single-layer).

Limitations

- Limited data on long-term adhesion formation and repeat CS outcomes.
- Single-layer uterine closure may increase rupture risk in VBAC candidates, prompting some to adopt double-layer modifications.
- Requires surgeon training to master manual dissection techniques.

Uterine Incision

- **Lower Segment Transverse Incision:** Preferred for most CS, including Misgav Ladach, due to lower rupture risk (0.5–0.9%) and blood loss.
- **Classical (Vertical) Incision:** Used for preterm delivery, anterior placenta previa, or PAS, with higher rupture risk (4–9%).

Fetal Delivery

- **Standard Delivery:** The fetal head is elevated gently, with controlled fundal pressure if needed. NICE (2024) emphasizes gentle disimpaction for impacted heads.
- **Breech Extraction:** Requires careful manipulation to avoid trauma.
- **PAS:** Multidisciplinary approach with preoperative imaging (MRI/ultrasound) and potential hysterectomy.

Uterine Closure[11,12]

- **Double-Layer Closure:** Preferred by ACOG and RCOG for VBAC candidates due to lower rupture risk. Uses continuous or interrupted sutures.
- **Single-Layer Closure:** Common in Misgav Ladach for speed but may increase rupture risk (1–2%).
- **Misgav Ladach Preference:** Single-layer closure is standard, but modified versions use double-layer for VBAC eligibility **(Fig. 4)**.

Abdominal Closure

- **Fascial Closure:** Continuous or interrupted sutures.
- **Skin Closure:** Subcuticular sutures (NICE preference) or staples.
- **Misgav Ladach:** Minimal skin sutures (2–3) or staples, reducing operative time and improving cosmesis.

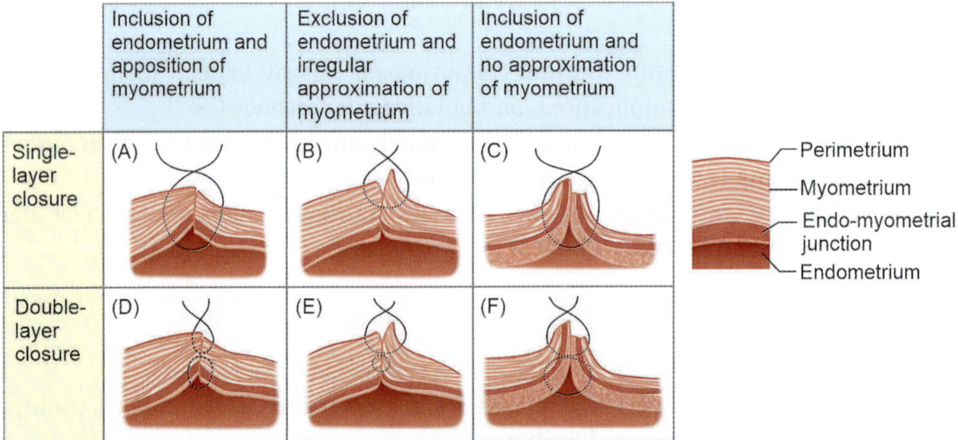

Fig. 4: Misgav Ladach preference.

Enhanced Recovery After Surgery

- **ACOG (2025):** Promotes early oral intake, ambulation within 6–12 hours, and catheter removal within 24 hours.
- **NICE (2024):** Recommends multimodal analgesia (paracetamol and NSAIDs) and early mobilization, aligning with Misgav Ladach's faster recovery profile.

SPECIAL CONSIDERATIONS

Placenta Accreta Spectrum (Fig. 5A to F)

- **NICE (2024):** Requires ultrasound/Doppler at 28–29 weeks for suspected PAS, with referral to specialized centers. Misgav Ladach may be adapted, but vertical incisions are often preferred.
- **RCOG (2022):** Multidisciplinary planning, including blood product availability.

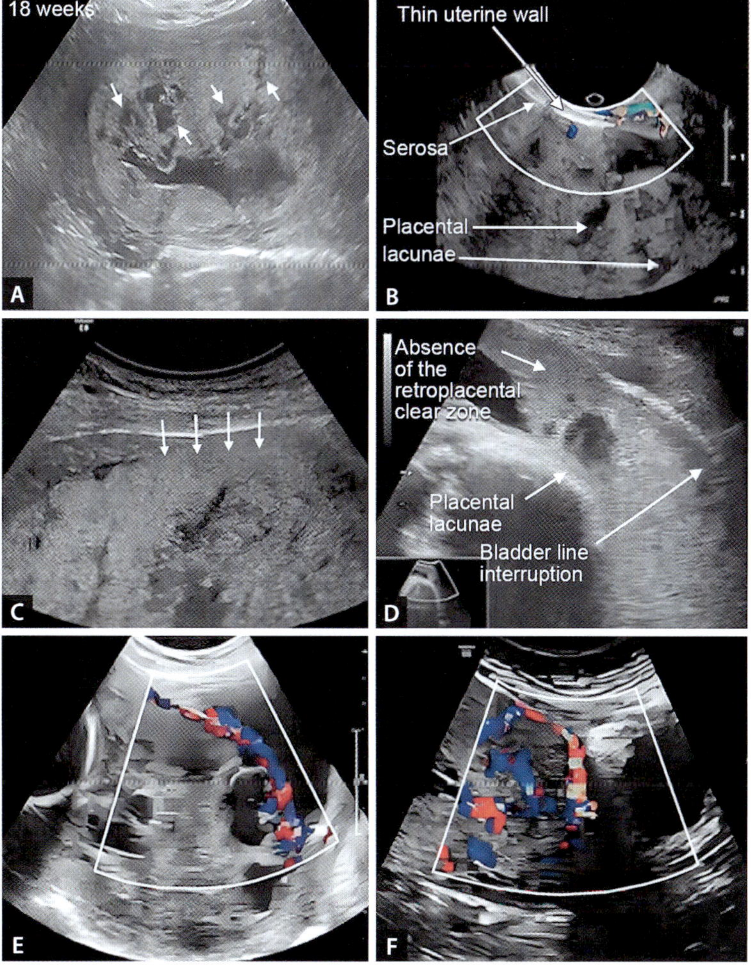

Fig. 5A to F: Placenta accreta spectrum (PAS).

Emergency Cesarean Section

- **RCOG (2024):** Classifies urgency (Category 1: delivery within 30 minutes; Category 2: within 75 minutes). Misgav Ladach is ideal for Category 1 due to its speed (1.5–2.7 minutes incision-to-delivery).
- **ACOG (2025):** Supports Misgav Ladach for emergencies to reduce fetal extraction time.

Vaginal Birth after Cesarean and Trial of Labor after Cesarean

- **ACOG (2024):** VBAC is safe for most women with one prior low-transverse CS (60–80% success). Double-layer closure is preferred over Misgav Ladach's single-layer for VBAC candidates.
- **RCOG (2022):** Notes a 0.5% rupture risk with double-layer closure versus 1–2% with single-layer.

POSTOPERATIVE CARE

- **Pain Management:** Multimodal analgesia to minimize opioid use.
- **Wound Care:** NICE (2024) recommends wound assessment for SSI and dressing removal after 48 hours.
- **Follow-up:** RCOG advises debriefing to discuss future pregnancy planning, particularly VBAC.

COMPLICATIONS

- **Short-term:** Infection (5–10%), hemorrhage (1–2%), and VTE (0.1–0.2%). Misgav Ladach reduces these risks significantly.
- **Long-term:** Placenta previa, PAS, and uterine rupture risks increase with each CS. Misgav Ladach's adhesion reduction may mitigate long-term complications, but data are limited.

FUTURE DIRECTIONS

- **NICE (2024):** Investigating fetal head disimpaction techniques to reduce neonatal trauma.
- **ACOG (2025):** Focuses on reducing nulliparous, term, singleton, vertex (NTSV) CS rates through standardized labor management.
- **Misgav Ladach Research:** Ongoing studies compare long-term outcomes (e.g., adhesions and VBAC success) and modifications like double-layer closure to optimize the technique.

CONCLUSION

Cesarean section techniques, including the Misgav Ladach method, have advanced to prioritize maternal and fetal safety, guided by RCOG, ACOG, and NICE. The Misgav Ladach technique, based on the Joel-Cohen incision, offers shorter operative times, reduced blood loss, faster recovery, and lower morbidity compared to traditional Pfannenstiel-Kerr methods, making it suitable for both emergency and elective CS. However, its single-layer uterine closure may require modification for VBAC candidates. Standard techniques like Pfannenstiel and Joel-Cohen remain widely used, with double-layer closure preferred for future pregnancies.

Multidisciplinary care is critical for complex cases like PAS. Clinicians must balance guideline recommendations with patient-specific factors to optimize outcomes.

REFERENCES

1. National Institute for Health and Care Excellence (NICE). (2021). Caesarean birth. NICE guideline [NG192]. [online] Available from https://www.nice.org.uk/guidance/ng192/chapter/recommendations [Last accessed December, 2025].
2. Royal College of Obstetricians and Gynaecologists (RCOG). Birth after Previous Caesarean Birth (Green-top Guideline No. 45). [online] Available from https://www.rcog.org.uk/guidance/browse-all-guidance/green-top-guidelines/birth-after-previous-caesarean-birth-green-top-guideline-no-45 [Last accessed December, 2025].
3. Royal College of Obstetricians and Gynaecologists (RCOG). (2021). Classification of Urgency of Caesarean Section - a Continuum of Risk (Good Practice No. 11). [online] Available from https://www.rcog.org.uk/guidance/browse-all-guidance/good-practice-papers/classification-of-urgency-of-caesarean-section-a-continuum-of-risk-good-practice-no-11/ [Last accessed December, 2025].
4. American College of Obstetricians and Gynecologists (ACOG). Quality-Improvement Strategies for Safe Reduction of Primary Cesarean Birth. Obstet Gynecol. 2025;145:542-52.
5. American College of Obstetricians and Gynecologists (ACOG). (2019). Cesarean Delivery on Maternal Request. [online] Available from https://www.acog.org/clinical/clinical-guidance/committee-opinion/articles/2019/01/cesarean-delivery-on-maternal-request [Last accessed December, 2025].
6. Holmgren G, Sjöholm L, Stark M. The Misgav Ladach method for cesarean section: method description. Acta Obstet Gynecol Scand. 1999;78(7):615-21.
7. Kulas T, Habek D, Karša M, et al. Modified Misgav Ladach method for cesarean section: clinical experience. Gynecol Obstet Invest. 2008;65(4):222-6.
8. Fatušić Z, Kurjak A, Jašarević E, et al. The Misgav Ladach method - a step forward in operative technique in obstetrics. J Perinat Med. 2003;31(5):395-8.
9. Moradan S, Mirmohammadkhani M. Comparison of Misgav-Ladach and Pfannenstiel-Kerr Techniques for Cesarean Section: A Randomized Controlled Trial Study. Middle East J Rehabil Health Stud. 2016;3(4):e38541.
10. Min L, Li Z, Jianwen Z. Study on modification of the Misgav Ladach method for cesarean section. Curr Med Sci. 2001;21:75-7.
11. Turner MJ. Delivery after a previous cesarean section reviewed. Int J Gynaecol Obstet. 2023;163(3):757-62.
12. Frappaolo AM, Logue TC, Goffman D, et al. Cesarean Delivery Trends Among Patients at Low Risk for Cesarean Delivery in the US, 2000-2019. JAMA Netw Open. 2023;6(3):e235428.

Strategies to Reduce Cesarean Section Rates

Ruchika Garg

INTRODUCTION

Cesarean section (CS) rates have risen globally, from 12% in 2000 to 21% in 2015, with South Asia reporting 18.1%.[1,2] The World Health Organization (WHO) recommends an optimal CS rate of 10–15%, beyond which no further reductions in maternal or neonatal mortality are observed, and rates below 5% or above 15% are linked to adverse outcomes.[1,3] In developing countries, CS rates range from 30 to 50% in various centers, driven by primary and repeat CS.[3,4] This chapter outlines evidence-based strategies to curb unnecessary CS in resource-constrained settings, addressing socioeconomic, medical, and systemic factors, tailored for postgraduate medical education.

REASONS FOR RISING CESAREAN SECTION RATES

The increase in CS is multifactorial, reflecting medical, social, and economic drivers:

- **Medical Advances:**
    - Improved surgical safety due to asepsis, broad-spectrum antibiotics, regional anesthesia (spinal/epidural), and postoperative care has increased confidence in CS.[5]
    - Overuse for noncritical indications [e.g., nonreassuring fetal heart rate (FHR), labor arrest, and suspected macrosomia].[6]
- **Socioeconomic Factors:**
    - **Maternal Request:** Driven by fear of labor pain, prior traumatic births, cultural beliefs (e.g., astrological timing), and misconceptions about vaginal delivery (e.g., pelvic floor damage).[4]
    - **Urban versus Rural Divide:** Higher CS in urban, educated, employed women with greater autonomy and access to private care.[3,4]
    - **Wealth Index:** Affluent women opt for CS for convenience.[3]
- **Healthcare System**:
    - **Over-Medicalization:** Private facilities prioritize CS for financial gain and scheduling convenience.[7]
    - **Increased Institutional Deliveries:** Improved access to maternity care has inadvertently raised CS rates.[5]
    - **Litigation Fear:** Defensive medicine due to medicolegal pressures pushes obstetricians toward CS.[4]

- **Patient-centered Policies:** Consumer protection acts and media-driven awareness increase patient demand for CS.[4]

- **Obstetric Practices**:
  - High induction rates and failure to follow strict criteria for labor dystocia or fetal distress.[6]
  - Repeat CS dominates due to low vaginal birth after cesarean (VBAC) rates (90% repeat CS).[6]
  - Declining skills in assisted vaginal deliveries (forceps/vacuum) and breech vaginal births.[7]

TABLE 1: Key drivers of rising CS rates.

Category	*Factors*	*Impact*
Medical	Improved safety, liberal indications	Overuse in nonemergent cases
Socioeconomic	Maternal request, urban/wealthy population	Increased demand for CS
Healthcare System	Private sector, litigation fear, and access to care	Financial and defensive medicine bias
Obstetric Practices	High inductions, low VBAC, and declining skills	Preference for surgical delivery

CONSEQUENCES OF HIGH CESAREAN SECTION RATES

Cesarean section, while lifesaving when indicated, poses risks, particularly in low-resource settings with limited surgical capacity:

- **Short-term Risks:**
  - Maternal: Anesthesia complications, blood loss, infections, and delayed recovery.[1,4]
  - Neonatal: Prematurity, iatrogenic respiratory distress, and low Apgar scores.[1]
- **Long-term Risks:**
  - Maternal: Adhesions, uterine rupture, placenta previa/accreta, incisional hernia, and keloid scars.[1,4]
  - Neonatal: Weakened immunity and respiratory issues in later life.[1]
- **Systemic:** Economic burden, strain on healthcare resources, and inequity in access.[3]
- **Psychosocial:** Negative impact on maternal mental health, bonding, and breastfeeding.[1]

STRATEGIES TO REDUCE CESAREAN SECTION RATES

Reducing CS rates requires a multi-pronged approach targeting clinical practice, institutional policies, patient education, and systemic reforms. The following strategies are tailored for developing countries, emphasizing low-cost and high-impact interventions.

Clinical Strategies

- **Active Management of Labor (AML):**
  - Implement O'Driscoll's AML (1973): One-to-one nurse support, routine amniotomy, oxytocin augmentation, partogram use, and strict fetal distress criteria.[8]

- **Partogram/Labor Care Guide:** Monitors labor progress and maternal/fetal condition, reducing unnecessary CS by 10–15%.[8]
- **Criteria for Labor Dystocia:**
  - Cervix ≥ 6 cm, no progress for >4 hours with adequate contractions (>3/10 min), or >6 hours if contractions suboptimal.[6]
  - Second-stage arrest: ≥3 hours (nulliparous) or ≥2 hours (multiparous) without epidural; add 1 hour with epidural.[6]
- **Fetal Distress:** Define strictly (e.g., late/variable decelerations); avoid overdiagnosis via cardiotocography (CTG) misinterpretation.[6]

- **Judicious Induction:**
  - Induce at ≥41 weeks or earlier only for maternal-fetal indications.[6]
  - Failed induction: No cervical change after 24 hours of oxytocin and amniotomy with <3 contractions/10 min.[6]
- **External Cephalic Version (ECV):** Train providers in ECV for breech presentations at 36–37 weeks; reduces CS by 50% in eligible cases.[9]
- **Twin Vaginal Delivery:** Encourage vaginal delivery for cephalic first twin; train in internal podalic version for second twin (breech/transverse).[10]
- **Vaginal Birth after Cesarean:**
  - Promote VBAC in women with one prior low-segment CS; success rate 60–80%.[6]
  - Assess scar integrity via ultrasound; counsel on risks (uterine rupture ~0.5%).[6]
- **Instrumental Vaginal Delivery:** Revive skills in forceps/vacuum delivery through training; reduces CS for second-stage arrest by 20%.[7]
- **Pain Management:** Offer epidural analgesia, nonpharmacological methods (yoga and breathing), and labor support to reduce maternal request for CS.[4]

TABLE 2: Clinical strategies and expected impact.

Strategy	*Description*	*CS Reduction impact*
AML/Partogram	One-to-one support, strict labor criteria	10–15%
ECV	Breech correction at 36–37 weeks	50% (breech cases)
VBAC	Encourage vaginal birth post-CS	60–80% (eligible cases)
Instrumental Delivery	Forceps/vacuum for second-stage arrest	20%

Institutional Strategies

- **Robson Classification:**
  - Adopt WHO's Robson 10-group system to audit CS indications (parity, prior CS, gestation, labor onset, presentation, and fetus number).[11]
  - Identify high-contribution groups (e.g., Group 5: previous CS) for targeted interventions.[11]
  - Example: Group 9 (transverse lie) should be ~1% with near-100% CS; deviations indicate data errors.[11]
- **Regular Audits:**
  - Conduct monthly CS audits with feedback to obstetricians; reduces rates by 5–10%.[2]
  - Compare institutional rates with national/global benchmarks.[9]

- **Senior Consultant Presence:** Increase consultant availability in labor wards; reduces operative deliveries by 10%.[7]
- **Midwifery Training:** Train midwives in labor support, partogram use, and assisted deliveries; reduces CS by 15% in low-risk cases.[7]
- **Group Practice:** Organize obstetricians into teams to ensure 24/7 availability, reducing pressure for scheduled CS.[7]
- **Standardized Protocols**:
  - Implement evidence-based guidelines for CS indications, labor management, and induction.[9]
  - Example: Turkey's model (three-obstetrician consent, re-evaluation of CS decisions) reduced rates by 8%.[11]

Patient-centered Strategies

- **Antenatal Education:**
  - Conduct workshops on vaginal delivery benefits, CS risks, and labor coping strategies (yoga and meditation).[4]
  - Address myths (e.g., vaginal delivery causes incontinence); reduces maternal request by 20%.[4]
- **Respectful Maternity Care:** Ensure dignified care, privacy, and separate delivery cabins; increases vaginal delivery acceptance.[7]
- **Labor Support:**
  - Allow partner/family presence in labor rooms; reduces CS demand by 10–15%.[4]
  - Promote companionship, hydration, mobility, and pain relief.[9]
- **Counseling:**
  - Provide individualized counseling to address fears of labor pain or prior traumatic births.[4]
  - Encourage VBAC and breech vaginal delivery in eligible cases.[6]

Policy-level Strategies

- **Financial Reforms:**
  - Equalize fees for vaginal and CS deliveries to remove financial incentives; reduces CS by 5–10%.[7]
  - Penalize medically unjustified CS in private facilities.[7]
- **Legal Reforms:** Protect obstetricians from litigation for vaginal delivery complications; reduces defensive CS by 10%.[4]
- **Community Sensitization:**
  - Launch campaigns (e.g., Bangladesh's Save the Children initiative) to educate on CS risks; reduces demand by 5%.[5]
  - Use local media, posters, and community health workers for outreach.[9]
- **Regulatory Oversight:**
  - Establish audit teams to monitor private maternity centers; ensures adherence to national guidelines.[9]
  - Enforce Robson classification for CS reporting.[11]

- **Painless Delivery Programs:** Subsidize epidural services and train providers in nonpharmacological pain relief; reduces maternal request by 10%.[4]

TABLE 3: Policy-level strategies and expected impact.

Strategy	*Description*	*CS reduction impact*
Equal Fees	Same cost for vaginal/CS delivery	5–10%
Legal Reforms	Reduce litigation fear	10%
Community Campaigns	Educate on CS risks	5%
Painless Delivery Programs	Subsidized epidurals, pain relief training	10%

Systemic Improvements

- **CTG Training:** Train obstetricians, nurses, and midwives in accurate CTG interpretation; reduces CS for false fetal distress by 10%.[6]
- **Teamwork:** Improve communication between maternity and operating room staff; enhances decision-making, reducing CS by 5%.[9]
- **Second Opinions:** Mandate second obstetrician review for nonemergent CS; reduces rates by 5%.[11]
- **Electronic Fetal Monitoring (EFM):** Restrict EFM to high-risk cases to avoid overdiagnosis of fetal distress.[6]
- **Reward Systems:** Offer incentives for vaginal delivery teams without compromising safety; boosts motivation.[9]

CONSEQUENCES OF SUCCESSFUL CS REDUCTION

- **Maternal:** Reduced surgical complications, adhesions, and future pregnancy risks.[1]
- **Neonatal:** Lower rates of prematurity and respiratory issues.[1]
- **Systemic:** Decreased healthcare costs, improved resource allocation.[3]
- **Psychosocial:** Enhanced maternal confidence, bonding, and breastfeeding rates.[4]

REFERENCES

1. World Health Organization. WHO Statement on Caesarean Section Rates. Geneva: WHO; 2015.
2. Bhartia A, Sen Gupta Dhar R, Bhartia S. Reducing caesarean section rate in an urban hospital serving women attending privately in India - a quality improvement initiative. BMC Pregnancy Childbirth. 2020;20(1):556.
3. Amjad A, Imran A, Shahram N, et al. Trends of caesarean section deliveries in Pakistan: secondary data analysis from Demographic and Health Surveys, 1990-2018. BMC Pregnancy Childbirth. 2020;20(1):753.
4. Amjad A, Usman A, Alvi F, et al. Upsurge of caesarean sections in Pakistan: perceptions of women and gynaecologists. Research Square. 2020.
5. Karim F, Ali NB, Khan ANS, et al. Prevalence and factors associated with caesarean section in four Hard-to-Reach areas of Bangladesh: Findings from a cross-sectional survey. PLoS One. 2020;15(6):e0234249.
6. American College of Obstetricians and Gynecologists (College); Society for Maternal-Fetal Medicine; Caughey AB, et al. Safe prevention of the primary cesarean delivery. Am J Obstet Gynecol. 2014;210(3):179-93.

7. Dhakal-Rai S, Poobalan A, Jan R et al. Caesarean Section rates in South Asian cities: Can midwifery help stem the rise? JAM. 2019;6(2):4-22.
8. O'Driscoll K, Stronge JM, Minogue M. Active management of labour. Br Med J. 1973;3(5872):135-7.
9. Seth S. Strategies for cesarean section rate reduction. In: Garg R (Ed). Labour and Delivery. Singapore: Springer; 2023.
10. Barrett JF, Hannah ME, Hutton EK, et al. A randomized trial of planned cesarean or vaginal delivery for twin pregnancy. N Engl J Med. 2013;369(14):1295-305. Erratum in: N Engl J Med. 2013;369(24):2364.
11. Topçu HO, Özel Ş, Üstün Y. Identifying strategies to reduce cesarean section rates by using Robson ten-group classification. J Matern Fetal Neonatal Med. 2021;34(16):2616-22.

Pregnancy in Scarred Uterus

Ruchika Garg

INTRODUCTION

- Pregnancy in a scarred uterus, commonly due to prior cesarean delivery, poses significant challenges in obstetric management because of increased risks of uterine rupture, abnormal placentation, and adverse maternal and neonatal outcomes.
- With rising cesarean rates globally, particularly in India and other middle-income countries, practitioners increasingly encounter pregnancies with one or multiple cesarean scars.
- A multidisciplinary, guideline-driven approach is critical for optimizing outcomes. This chapter summarizes the clinical aspects, risks, surveillance, and evidence-based recommendations from NICE and RCOG for pregnancies following one and two previous cesarean sections.[1-3]

EPIDEMIOLOGY

- The global cesarean section rate ranges between 20 and 30%, with higher prevalence in urban and resource-rich settings.
- Repeat cesarean deliveries contribute to cumulative uterine scarring and associated complications.
- The likelihood of complications increases progressively with the number of prior cesareans.

TYPES OF UTERINE SCARS

- Transverse lower segment cesarean scar (most common and safer)
- Classical scar (vertical uterine incision with higher rupture risk)
- T-shaped or other atypical scars

TABLE 1: Maternal versus neonatal risks in women with previous cesarean section.

Maternal risk	*Neonatal risk*
Uterine Rupture (0.3–1% after one CS, up to 1.8% after two CS)	Preterm Birth due to Indicated Delivery
Placenta Previa/Accreta Spectrum	Intrauterine Growth Restriction (IUGR)
Placenta Accreta Spectrum	Neonatal Respiratory Morbidity
Postpartum Hemorrhage	Neonatal ICU Admissions
Surgical Complications	Perinatal Mortality (rare but increased)

- Myomectomy scars (increased risk of rupture depending on depth and location)

RISKS ASSOCIATED WITH PREGNANCY IN SCARRED UTERUS

Clinical Evaluation and Surveillance

- Detailed obstetric history emphasizing type and number of prior uterine surgeries.
- Ultrasonographic evaluation early to locate placenta and assess scar integrity.
- High-resolution TVS/MRI may be required for placental implantation abnormalities.
- Counseling on risks of vaginal birth after cesarean (VBAC) versus repeat cesarean delivery (CD).

NICE Guidelines (2023-2025) on Pregnancy Following Cesarean Section[1-3]

After One Previous Cesarean Section

- Inform women about benefits/risks of VBAC versus elective repeat cesarean delivery (ERCD).
- Offer trial of labor after cesarean (TOLAC) if no contraindications (e.g., classical scar and uterine rupture history).
- Continuous fetal monitoring during labor mandatory.
- Immediate access to cesarean delivery is essential in case of emergency.
- Induction with caution; prostaglandins contraindicated for induction in VBAC candidates, but cautious use of oxytocin is permitted.
- In labor, monitor carefully for signs of uterine rupture (abnormal CTG, pain).
- If VBAC fails or rupture suspected, proceed urgently to cesarean.

After Two Previous Cesarean Sections

- ERCD is more commonly recommended due to increased rupture risk (~1.8%).
- VBAC may be considered in selected cases with stringent monitoring and experienced units.
- Place of birth should be a facility equipped for emergency surgery and neonatal care.

RCOG Guidelines (Green-top 2015, updated 2024)[2]

- VBAC success in carefully selected women is approximately 60–80%.
- Key factors predicting successful VBAC: Prior vaginal birth, nonrecurrent indication for previous CS, and spontaneous labor onset.
- Major concerns in two or more CS pregnancies include higher rates of uterine rupture, placenta previa/accreta, and surgical complications.
- Careful antenatal planning and individualized counseling are emphasized.
- Repeat cesarean at 39 weeks reduces risk of uterine rupture but must be balanced against preterm delivery risks.

TABLE 2: Labor and delivery management.

Aspect	*VBAC*	*ERCD*
Timing of Delivery	Spontaneous labor preferred	Usually schedule at 39 weeks
Monitoring	Continuous CTG mandatory	Routine fetal monitoring
Induction	Avoid prostaglandins; cautious oxytocin	No labor induction
Uterine Rupture Risk	0.5-1% with one prior CS	Minimal, surgical risks present
Emergency Readiness	Immediate surgical access required	Planned surgery with blood products

Algorithm: Management of Pregnancy with One Previous Cesarean.

Pregnant woman with prior cesarean → assesses obstetric/medical status
↓
Discuss mode of delivery, risks, and preferences (VBAC vs. ERCD)
↓
If VBAC chosen → monitor throughout pregnancy; plan hospital birth with surgical team on standby
↓
In labor → continuous monitoring, avoid prostaglandins, cautious oxytocin
↓
Signs of rupture → emergency cesarean
↓
If ERCD chosen → schedule cesarean at 39 weeks unless contraindications arise

Algorithm: Management after Two Previous Cesarean Sections.

Assess maternal-fetal status and scar type
↓
Discussion regarding stronger recommendation for ERCD due to higher rupture risk
↓
If VBAC considered → restrict to highly selected cases in equipped units with continuous fetal monitoring
↓
Planned ERCD at or before 39 weeks most common approach
↓
Close surveillance for placenta previa/accreta is mandatory.

COUNSELING POINTS

- VBAC offers lower maternal morbidity and fewer complications than multiple repeat cesareans but carries a risk of uterine rupture.
- Repeat cesarean avoids rupture risk but may have surgical and placental complication risks in subsequent pregnancies.
- Informed and shared decision-making essential involving explanation of all risks and benefits.
- Women advised to seek care at tertiary centers with multidisciplinary teams.

SUMMARY[1-3]

- Pregnancy in the scarred uterus carries increased risks of obstetric complications, notably uterine rupture and abnormal placental implantation.
- Careful risk assessment, antenatal surveillance, and delivery planning per NICE and RCOG guidelines optimize safety for mother and baby.
- VBAC is safe and encouraged in appropriately selected women with one previous cesarean.
- Multiple previous CS necessitate individualized counseling and often planned repeat cesarean.
- Multidisciplinary care teams and appropriate birth settings are critical components of management.

REFERENCES

1. National Institute for Health and Care Excellence. Hypertension in pregnancy: diagnosis and management. NICE Guideline, No. 133.). London: National Institute for Health and Care Excellence (NICE); 2019.
2. RCOG. (2015). Birth after previous cesarean birth, Green-Top Guideline 45. [online] Available from https://www.rcog.org.uk/media/kpkjwd5h/gtg_45.pdf [Last accessed December, 2025].
3. ACOG Practice Bulletin No. 205: Vaginal Birth After Cesarean Delivery. Obstet Gynecol. 2019;133(2):e110-e127.

Difficult Situations in Cesarean Delivery

Ruchika Garg

CESAREAN SECTION: CHALLENGES AND MANAGEMENT

Cesarean section (CS) is a common surgical procedure globally, with rates rising from 30% to 80% despite the World Health Organization (WHO) recommending 15%.[1] While CS avoids complex vaginal deliveries, difficult CS can lead to maternal and fetal complications, including trauma, excessive bleeding, and prolonged recovery.[2] This chapter provides a concise, evidence-based overview for medical postgraduate education, focusing on difficulties, techniques, and management strategies to optimize outcomes.

Incidence and Trends

Global CS rates vary widely, with high-income countries reporting 30–50% and some regions up to 80%.[1] WHO suggests a 15% rate to balance maternal-fetal benefits and risks **(Table 1)**.[1] Rising rates spark debate due to increased morbidity without clear benefits in nonindicated cases.[2]

TABLE 1: Global cesarean section rates (2020-2025).[1,3]

Region	*CS Rate (%)*	*Notes*
North America	32–40	High elective CS rates
Latin America	40–80	Highest global rates
Sub-Saharan Africa	5–20	Limited access in rural areas
WHO Recommendation	15	Optimal for maternal-fetal outcomes

DIFFICULTIES IN CESAREAN SECTION

Difficult CS increases risks of fetal injury, asphyxia, maternal trauma (uterine vessels, cervix, vagina, and bladder), and prolonged hospital stay **(Table 2)**.[2] Obstetricians require expertise, decision-making, and technical skills to choose the safest delivery route.[4]

TABLE 2: Classification of difficulties in cesarean section.[2,4]

Category	*Examples*
General Surgical/Anesthetic	Anesthesia complications, bleeding, and infection
Preexisting Conditions	Placenta previa and uterine anomalies
Pregnancy Complications	Preterm PROM and fetal anomalies
Previous CS-related	Dense adhesions and placenta accreta spectrum (PAS)
Situational/Technical	Deeply engaged head, floating head, obesity, and failed instrumental delivery

KEY FACTORS FOR SAFE CESAREAN SECTION

- **Anticipation:** Assess lie, presentation, descent, position, and flexion using ultrasound.[4]
- **Preparation:** Confirm placental position, fetal anomalies (e.g., hydrocephalus), and breech type.[4]
- **Expertise:** Skilled obstetrician, able assistant, and advanced technology.[2]
- **Timing:**
  - Induction-to-delivery interval >8 minutes (general anesthesia) or uterine incision-to-delivery interval >3 minutes increases neonatal acidosis and low Apgar scores.[5]
  - In spinal anesthesia, uterine incision-to-delivery >3 minutes impacts fetal outcome.[5]
- **Goals**: Smooth anesthesia, rapid delivery, and minimal trauma to mother and fetus.[4]

SPECIFIC CHALLENGES AND MANAGEMENT

Fetal/Presentation-related Challenges

- **Deeply Engaged Head:**
  - Common in second-stage labor, especially with deep transverse arrest or persistent occipitoposterior position.[6]
  - Risks: Uterine incision extension, cervical/vaginal tears, bladder injury, and fetal trauma.[6]
  - **Techniques:**[6-10]
    - **Push Methods:**
      - *Abdominal*: Surgeon's hand flexes head from below symphysis pubis.
      - *Abdominovaginal*: Assistant pushes head vaginally in modified lithotomy position.
    - **Pull Methods**:
      - *Patwardhan's Technique:* Deliver anterior shoulder, then posterior shoulder, buttocks, legs, and head.[7]
      - *Modified Patwardhan's:* For occipitoposterior, deliver anterior shoulder and leg, then opposite side.[7]
      - *Reverse Breech Extraction:* Deliver feet first, followed by trunk, arms, and head.[8]
  - **Fetal Disimpacting System (FDS):** Inflatable balloon elevates head by 3–5 cm.[9]
  - **Fetal Head Elevators/Spoons:** Coyne, Sellheim, or Mureless spoons act as "shoehorns".[10]
  - **Evidence**:
    - Patwardhan's technique reduces uterine incision extension, blood loss, and bladder injury compared to push methods.[11]
    - Reverse breech extraction is faster, with less blood loss and infection risk.[12]
    - FDS shows no maternal/fetal injuries in small studies.[9]
  - **Complications:** Push methods increase incision extension (52% vs. 15% in reverse breech) and blood loss (mean difference 203.3 mL).[12]
- **Floating Head**:
  - Difficult to grasp through uterine incision.[13]
  - **Techniques:**[13-15]

- *Manual:* Align uterus/fetus axis, use fundal pressure, and scoop head with hand as a vectis.
- *Instrumental:* Vacuum (e.g., Kiwi Omni Cup) or forceps (Simpson's/Wrigley's). Vacuum reduces incision extension by avoiding hand/forceps bulk.[14]
- *Reverse Breech:* Internal podalic version for slipped head.[13]
- **Evidence:** No significant maternal/fetal outcome differences between manual and instrumental methods, but limited trials.[15]

- **Malpresentations:**
  - **Breech:** Flexed breech easier than extended; deliver same as vaginal breech.[4]
  - **Transverse Lie:** Internal podalic version and breech extraction.[4]
  - **Brow/Face:** Maintain flexion/extension during delivery.[4]
  - **Hydrocephalus:** Predelivery cephalocentesis under ultrasound guidance.[4]
  - **Conjoined Twins:** Rare; requires liberal incision and anticipation of extensions.[4]
  - **Preterm PROM:** Large head relative to body, thick lower segment, and low liquor complicate delivery.[4]

Uterus/Lower Uterine Segment-related Challenges

- **Uterine Anomalies:**
  - Associated with malpresentations and preterm labour[4]
  - **Management**: Ultrasound-guided incision placement, higher incision if needed[4]
- **Dense Adhesions:**
  - Common post-CS, complicating peritoneal entry[16]
  - **Management:**[16]
    - Enter peritoneum superiorly or laterally to avoid midline adhesions.
    - Avoid forceful dissection; limit bladder flap development.
    - Higher uterine incision to bypass adhesions and vascular bladder plexus.
- **Uterine Leiomyomas:**
  - **Management:**[17]
    - Cesarean myomectomy (CM) for fibroids in incision line or obstructing lower uterine segment (LUS), performed by experienced surgeons.
    - Small subserosal fibroids or posterior fibroids may be left untreated.
    - Benefits: Smaller incisions, easier cleavage plane, and reduced hemorrhage with uterotonics.
    - Risks: Increased blood loss; requires uterotonic drugs, uterine artery ligation, or embolization.

Uterus/Vascular Lower Segment Challenges

- **Placenta Previa:**
  - **Management:**[18]
    - Cut through central placenta or maneuver around upper/lower edge to reach membranes.
    - Prepare for significant bleeding; ensure blood availability.

- **Placenta Accreta Spectrum (PAS):**
  - **Management:**[19]
    - Multidisciplinary approach with preoperative imaging (MRI/ultrasound).
    - Plan hysterectomy or conservative management (e.g., leaving placenta in situ).
    - Uterine artery embolization for bleeding control.

Technical Difficulties (Table 3)

- **Extreme Obesity:**
  - Challenges: Poor access, increased infection risk, and anesthesia complications[4]
  - **Management**: Higher incision, pannus retraction, and antibiotic prophylaxis[4]
- **Failed Instrumental Delivery:**
  - Increases risk of CS at full dilatation (CSFD).[6]
  - **Challenges:** Stretched, vascular LUS indistinguishable from vagina; risk of inadvertent vaginal incision[6]
  - **Management:** Higher incision, nitroglycerine for relaxation, avoid wrist flexion during head delivery.[6]

TABLE 3: Techniques for deeply engaged head delivery.[6-12]

Technique	*Advantages*	*Disadvantages*	*Maternal/Fetal Outcomes*
Push (abdominal/ abdominovaginal)	Simple, no special instruments	Higher incision extension, blood loss	Increased maternal morbidity[12]
Patwardhan's/modified	Lower incision extension, less blood loss	Requires skill, rare humeral fractures	Reduced maternal morbidity, similar fetal outcomes[11]
Reverse breech extraction	Faster, less blood loss, and lower infection	Requires ultrasound for foot localization	Better neonatal outcomes[12]
Fetal disimpacting system	Elevates head, no injuries reported	Limited data, device availability	Promising in small studies[9]
Fetal head elevators/ spoons	Less space needed, effective for impacted head	Requires training	Comparable to push/ pull[10]

Managing Uterine Incision Extensions

- **Lower Segment Tears:** Suture from apex to incision, push bladder downward to avoid suture line.[12]
- **Upper Segment Extensions:** Close as classical CS, document for future pregnancies.[12]
- **Broad Ligament Defects:** Close to prevent bowel herniation; ligate uterine vessels if lacerated.[12]

CESAREAN SECTION AT FULL DILATATION

Cesarean section at full dilatation CSFD is challenging due to:

- Thin, vascular LUS merging with vagina.[6]
- Deeply engaged head, molding, lack of liquor, and splinted fetal spine.[6]

- Risks: Incision extension, cervical/vaginal tears, bladder injury, and excess blood loss.[6]
- **Recommendations:**[6,13]
  - Senior obstetrician presence
  - Higher uterine incision
  - Nitroglycerine for uterine relaxation
  - Avoid forceful head delivery
- **WHO (2015):** 15% CS rate; nonindicated CS increases morbidity **(Table 4)**.[1]

TABLE 4: Key guidelines for difficult cesarean section.[1,13,18]

Organization	*Recommendation*
WHO (2015)	15% CS rate; avoid nonindicated CS[1]
RCOG (2020)	Senior obstetrician for CSFD; train for pull techniques[13]
ACOG (2019)	Multidisciplinary approach for PAS; prepare for bleeding in placenta previa[18]

RECENT ADVANCES

- **Fetal Disimpacting System:** Elevates deeply engaged head, reducing trauma; limited but promising data.[9]
- **Uterine Artery Embolization:** Effective for PAS and severe bleeding, reducing hysterectomy rates.[19]
- **Simulation Training:** Improves skills for CSFD and malpresentation management.[20]
- **2023 Study:** Reverse breech extraction confirmed faster and safer than push method, with lower NICU admissions.[21]

KEY POINTS

- CS rates (30–80%) exceed WHO's 15% recommendation, increasing morbidity.[1]
- Difficult CS risks fetal asphyxia, maternal trauma, and prolonged recovery.[2]
- Deeply engaged head in CSFD is a major challenge; pull techniques (Patwardhan's, reverse breech) reduce complications.[11,12]
- Floating head, malpresentations, and PAS require specialized techniques.[13,19]
- Anticipation, senior obstetrician presence, and training are critical.[13]
- National guidelines for safe CSFD are needed to address global maternal morbidity.[1]

REFERENCES

1. WHO. (2015). Caesarean section rates: Global trends and recommendations. [online] Available from https://www.who.int/publications/i/item/9789241509428 [Last accessed December, 2025].
2. Betrán AP, et al. Global trends in caesarean section rates: A systematic review. Lancet Glob Health. 2016;4(4):e260-70.
3. Boerma T, et al. Global epidemiology of caesarean section: 2020 update. BMJ Glob Health. 2020;5(5):e002076.
4. Sung JF, et al. Challenges in difficult caesarean sections: A review. Obstet Gynecol Surv. 2018;73(6):351-8.
5. Maayan-Metzger A, et al. Impact of induction-to-delivery interval on neonatal outcomes. J Perinatol. 2017;37(7):789-93.

6. Unterscheider J, et al. Caesarean section at full dilatation: Incidence and outcomes. Eur J Obstet Gynecol Reprod Biol. 2016;203:251-6.
7. Patwardhan BD, et al. Modified technique for delivery in caesarean section. J Obstet Gynaecol India. 2015;65(4):227-31.
8. Fasubaa OB, et al. Reverse breech extraction versus push method in second-stage caesarean section. J Matern Fetal Neonatal Med. 2017;30(12):1449-53.
9. Singh M, et al. Fetal disimpacting system for deeply engaged head: A pilot study. J Perinat Med. 2019;47(3):298-302.
10. Beeresh CS, et al. Comparison of Patwardhan vs. push technique for deeply engaged head. J Obstet Gynaecol Res. 2018;44(9):1678-84.
11. Jeve YB, et al. Techniques for deeply engaged fetal head at caesarean section: A meta-analysis. BJOG. 2016;123(7):1098-106.
12. Zahn CM, et al. Management of uterine incision extensions in caesarean section. Clin Obstet Gynecol. 2019;62(3):554-62.
13. RCOG. Caesarean section at full dilatation: Green-top Guideline No. 26. 2020. [online] Available from https://www.rcog.org.uk/guidance/browse-all-guidance/green-top-guidelines/ [Last accessed December, 2025].
14. Solomons E. Vacuum extraction at caesarean section. Am J Obstet Gynecol. 1962;83(2):123-7.
15. Waterfall H, et al. Instrumental delivery at caesarean section: A Cochrane review. BJOG. 2016;123(6):893-900.
16. Tulandi T, et al. Management of adhesions in repeat caesarean sections. J Minim Invasive Gynecol. 2017;24(5):715-20.
17. Pergialiotis V, et al. Caesarean myomectomy: A systematic review. Eur J Obstet Gynecol Reprod Biol. 2017;216:154-9.
18. ACOG. Placenta previa and accreta: Clinical management guidelines. Obstet Gynecol. 2019;133(1):e34-50.
19. Sentilhes L, et al. Placenta accreta spectrum: Advances in management. Am J Obstet Gynecol. 2020;222(3):210-23.
20. Draycott TJ, et al. Simulation training for difficult caesarean sections. BJOG. 2018;125(6):643-9.
21. Patel S, et al. Reverse breech extraction in CSFD: 2023 outcomes. J Obstet Gynaecol Res. 2023;49(10):2456-63.

Amniotic Fluid Embolism

Ruchika Garg

AMNIOTIC FLUID: PHYSIOLOGY, FUNCTIONS, AND CLINICAL IMPLICATIONS

1. Physiology of Amniotic Fluid Formation

Amniotic fluid is essential for fetal development, with its volume and composition dynamically regulated. In early pregnancy, the amniotic cavity contains fluid similar to extracellular fluid. By the second trimester, fetal urine becomes the primary source, supplemented by other pathways **(Table 1)**.

- **Early Pregnancy:** Fluid transfer occurs via transmembranous flow (across amnion), intramembranous flow (across fetal vessels), and fetal skin (until keratinization at 22–25 weeks).
- **Second Trimester Onward:** Fetal urine (hypotonic, 260 mOsm/L) dominates, replacing the entire amniotic fluid volume daily by term (1 L/day**; Table 1**).
- **Maternal Dehydration:** Increases maternal osmolality, promoting fluid transfer from fetus to mother, reducing amniotic fluid volume.

2. Functions of Amniotic Fluid

Amniotic fluid serves critical roles:

- Provides space for fetal movement, aiding musculoskeletal development.
- Enables swallowing (GI tract development) and breathing (lung development).
- Protects against umbilical cord compression and trauma.
- Exhibits bacteriostatic properties.

TABLE 1: Key Pathways of amniotic fluid regulation in late pregnancy.

Pathway	*Effect on volume*	*Approx. daily volume (mL)*
Fetal urination	Production	1,000
Fetal swallowing	Resorption	500–1,000
Fetal lung fluid secretion	Production	350 (50% swallowed)
Intramembranous flow (fetal vessels)	Resorption	400
Transmembranous flow (amnion)	Resorption	Minimal

TABLE 2: Amniotic fluid volume by gestational age.

Gestational age	*Volume (mL)*
10 weeks	30
12 weeks	50
16 weeks	200
20 weeks	400
34 weeks	1,000 (peak)
40 weeks (term)	800
42 weeks	200

TABLE 3: Amniotic fluid composition and color indications.

Component/Pathology	*Details*
Water	98–99%
Hormones	Prolactin, renin, and insulin
Green (meconium)	Fetal distress, breech, and Listeria infection
Golden (bilirubin)	Rh incompatibility
Brown (tobacco juice)	Intrauterine fetal demise
Saffron/yellowish green	Post-term pregnancy
Dark red	Concealed hemorrhage (abruptio placenta)

The volume of amniotic fluid varies with gestational age **(Table 2)**, and its composition, primarily water with specific hormones, can indicate pathology based on color changes **(Table 3)**.

3. Clinical Implications of Amniotic Fluid Abnormalities

Abnormal amniotic fluid volumes—oligohydramnios or polyhydramnios—may signal fetal or placental pathology, increasing adverse outcome risks.

Oligohydramnios

- **Definition:** Volume <200 mL, AFI ≤5 cm, or single deepest pocket (SDP) ≤2 cm
- **Consequences:**
  - **Mild:** No significant impact
  - **Moderate/Severe:**
    - 1st trimester: Pulmonary hypoplasia and limb amputation
    - 2nd/3rd trimester: Limb deformities (e.g., clubfoot), cord compression, and meconium aspiration
    - Potter Syndrome: Renal agenesis → anhydramnios → pulmonary hypoplasia, flat facies.
    - Amniotic Band Syndrome: Membrane rupture → constriction bands → limb amputation, craniofacial defects **(Fig. 1)**.

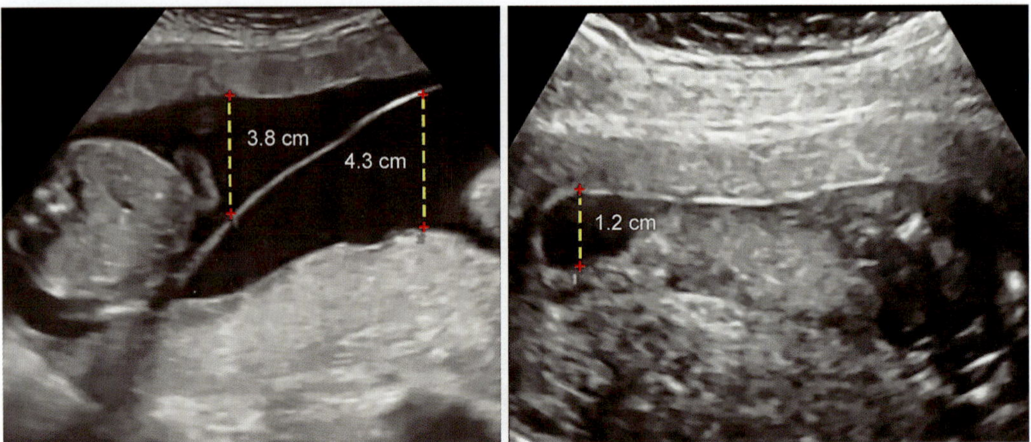

Fig 1: Left: Normal Liquor; Right: Deepest vertical pocket is less than 2 cm—oligohydramnios.

Polyhydramnios

- **Definition:** Volume ≥2,000 mL, AFI ≥25 cm, or SDP ≥8 cm
- **Consequences:**
  - Maternal: Respiratory distress, edema, and oliguria
  - Fetomaternal: Preterm labor, PPROM/PROM, placental abruption, postpartum hemorrhage, unstable lie, and cord prolapse.

OLIGOHYDRAMNIOS: DEFINITION, CAUSES, AND MANAGEMENT IN ART-CONCEIVED PREGNANCY AT 32 WEEKS

1. Definition

Oligohydramnios is an abnormally low amniotic fluid volume:

- Absolute Volume: <200 mL
- Sonographic Criteria: AFI ≤5 cm or SDP ≤2 cm
- Anhydramnios: No measurable fluid pocket
- Borderline: AFI 5–8 cm

  Oligohydramnios severity is classified based on sonographic measurements **(Table 4)**.

TABLE 4: Classification of oligohydramnios by severity.

Severity	*DVP (cm)*	*AFI (cm)*
Mild	1–2	2–5
Severe	<1	<2

2. Causes

The etiology of oligohydramnios varies by timing and underlying pathology **(Table 5)**.

TABLE 5: Causes of oligohydramnios.

Category	*Causes*
Early-onset (2nd trimester)	Fetal anomalies (renal and aneuploidy), placental insufficiency, PPROM, and TORCH infections
Late-Onset (3rd Trimester)	Fetal growth restriction (FGR), placental insufficiency, preeclampsia, medications (ACE inhibitors, ARBs, and NSAIDs), PPROM, and postterm pregnancy
Congenital Anomalies	Bladder obstruction (posterior urethral valves and urethral atresia), renal agenesis, multicystic dysplastic kidney, and polycystic kidney disease

3. Management of Oligohydramnios in ART-Conceived Pregnancy at 32 Weeks

Algorithm for Management:

- **History:** Assess onset, previous scans for anomalies, maternal illnesses.
- **Examination:** Evaluate for hypertension, uterine size, and rule out FGR.
- **Investigations:**
  - **Ultrasound:** Confirm severity **(Table 4)**, assess fetal anatomy/growth.
  - Weekly NST and Biophysical Profile (BPP)
  - Umbilical artery Doppler for uteroplacental insufficiency
- **Management:**
  - **Expectant (normal anatomy/growth):**
    - Increase maternal hydration.
    - Weekly NST/BPP.
    - Steroid coverage (betamethasone).
  - **Amnioinfusion:** For intrapartum variable decelerations (not routine)
  - **Delivery:**
    - **Mild/No complications:** 39 weeks.
    - **Moderate/Severe or complications:** 36–37+6 weeks (per ACOG).

ART pregnancies require heightened surveillance due to increased morbidity risks.

POLYHYDRAMNIOS: DEFINITION, COMPLICATIONS, AND MANAGEMENT

1. Definition

Polyhydramnios is an abnormally increased amniotic fluid volume:

- **Absolute Volume:** ≥2,000 mL
- **Sonographic Criteria:** AFI ≥25 cm or SDP ≥8 cm

Polyhydramnios is categorized by severity using AFI and SDP **(Table 6)**.

2. Complications

- **Maternal:** Dyspnea, orthopnea, edema, and oliguria
- **Fetomaternal:** Placental abruption, uterine dysfunction, PPH, unstable lie, and cord prolapse

3. Etiopathogenesis

Polyhydramnios is often idiopathic but may stem from maternal or fetal conditions **(Table 7)**.

TABLE 6: Classification of polyhydramnios by severity.

Severity	*AFI (cm)*	*SDP (cm)*
Mild	24–29.9	8–9.9
Moderate	30–34.9	10–11.9
Severe	≥35	≥12

TABLE 7: Etiopathogenesis of polyhydramnios.

Category	*Etiologies*
Idiopathic	~66% of cases, often mild
Maternal	Diabetes mellitus
Fetal Anomalies	CNS (anencephaly), craniofacial (cleft palate), thoracic (diaphragmatic hernia), cardiac (Ebstein anomaly, arrhythmias), GI (duodenal/esophageal atresia), renal (Bartter syndrome), and neurological (arthrogryposis)
Other	Fetal anemia, placental chorioangioma, and multiple gestation

4. Management

Algorithm for Management:

- **Evaluation:**
  - **History:** Screen for diabetes and prior pregnancy complications.
  - **Ultrasound:** Assess anomalies, multiple gestation, and fetal anemia (MCA Doppler).
  - **Labs:** Indirect Coombs test
  - **Genetic testing:** Amniocentesis for severe cases; MAGED2 mutation in male fetuses with severe polyhydramnios.
- **Treatment:**
  - **Asymptomatic/Mild: Monitor.**
  - **Mild Symptoms:** Bed rest, monitor uterine activity/fetal well-being.
  - **Severe Symptoms:**
    - **Amnioreduction:** USG-guided, 18G needle, remove 2–2.5 L (1 L/30 min).
    - **Complications**: Preterm labor, PPROM, infection, and abruption
  - **Tocolytics:**
    - **<32 weeks:** Indomethacin (25 mg QID, 48 hours) + corticosteroids
    - **32–34 weeks:** Nifedipine + corticosteroids
    - **34 weeks:** Corticosteroids only
- **Delivery Timing (per SMFM/ACOG):**
  - **Mild/Moderate idiopathic:** 39–40+6 weeks
  - **Severe idiopathic:** 37 weeks
  - Controlled ARM to prevent rapid decompression.
- **Future Therapies:** Intra-amniotic vasopressin or aquaporin-targeted agents to reduce fetal urine production.

TABLE 8: Methods of amniotic fluid measurement.

Method	*Description*	*Criteria*
Dye dilution	Research method; inject dye, measure concentration to calculate volume	Rarely used clinically
SDP	Deepest cord-free pocket in sagittal plane	Normal: 2–8 cm; Oligo: ≤2 cm; Poly: ≥8 cm
AFI	Sum of deepest pockets in 4 uterine quadrants	Normal: 5–24 cm; Oligo: ≤5 cm; Poly: ≥25 cm

SHORT NOTES

1. Amniotic Fluid Measurement

Amniotic fluid is measured using dye dilution (research) or sonographic methods (SDP and AFI) **(Table 8)**.

2. Amniotic Fluid Formation and Function

- **Formation:** Early pregnancy involves transmembranous, intramembranous, and fetal skin flow. From the second trimester, fetal urine (1 L/day) and lung fluid (350 mL/day) dominate, with resorption via swallowing (500–1,000 mL/day) and intramembranous flow (400 mL/day) **(Table 1)**.
- **Functions:**
  - Space for fetal movement
  - Supports GI and lung development
  - Protects against cord compression and trauma
  - Bacteriostatic properties

3. Polyhydramnios: Definition and Etiopathogenesis

- **Definition:** Volume ≥2,000 mL, AFI ≥25 cm, or SDP ≥8 cm **(Table 6)**.
- **Etiopathogenesis:** Includes idiopathic, maternal (diabetes), fetal anomalies (CNS, cardiac, GI, and renal), and other causes (fetal anemia and chorioangioma) **(Table 7)**.

REFERENCES

1. American College of Obstetricians and Gynecologists (ACOG). Practice Bulletin No. 175: Ultrasound in Pregnancy; 2020.
2. Society for Maternal-Fetal Medicine (SMFM). Amniotic Fluid Abnormalities: Diagnosis and Management; 2021.
3. Cunningham FG, Leveno KJ, Dashe JS, et al. Williams Obstetrics, 26th edition. McGraw-Hill Education; 2022
4. Moore TR. Amniotic Fluid Dynamics. In: Creasy and Resnik's Maternal-Fetal Medicine: Principles and Practice, 8th edition. Elsevier; 2019.

Intrauterine Fetal Death

Ruchika Garg

DEFINITION AND CLASSIFICATION

Intrauterine fetal death (IUFD) is defined as the death of a fetus in utero at or after 20 + 0 weeks of gestation (ACOG/SMFM), or 24 + 0 weeks (RCOG/FIGO/WHO), prior to complete expulsion or extraction. The fetus must show no signs of life postdelivery, including absence of breathing, heartbeat, umbilical cord pulsation, or voluntary muscle movement. This threshold aligns with viability considerations but varies regionally: e.g., 22 + 0 weeks in some European protocols.[1]

Subclassification by gestational age (GA) aids risk stratification and management:[2]

- **Early IUFD:** 20 + 0 - 27 + 6 weeks (higher association with congenital anomalies; 40–50% idiopathic)
- **Late IUFD:** ≥28 + 0 weeks (more often placental/maternal causes; lower idiopathic rate ~25%)
- **Stillbirth:** Encompasses IUFD ≥24 + 0 weeks (WHO/RCOG standard); includes antepartum (80%) and intrapartum (20%) deaths.[3]

In multiple gestations, selective IUFD requires nuanced classification, focusing on cotwin risks such as twin-twin transfusion syndrome (TTTS) or cotwin demise (15–30% mortality risk).

- **Racial/ethnic:** Non-Hispanic Black women: 9–11/1,000 (2.3-fold higher than White; US CDC 2024)
- **Maternal age:** Peaks at <20 years (RR 1.5) and >35 years (RR 1.3–1.9)
- **Socioeconomic:** 2–3-fold higher in low-SES groups due to access barriers
- **Regional (India):** 15–20/1,000 deliveries; preeclampsia accounts for 24% (2025 IJOG study).

Late IUFD (≥28 weeks) comprises 60–70% of cases (1/250 pregnancies), with intrapartum deaths declining to <2% in high-resource settings due to better monitoring. Recurrence risk: 2–10% overall; up to 20-fold if prior unexplained.

Psychological impact: 30–50% of parents experience prolonged grief disorder (PGD); PTSD rates 20–40% at 1 year (INSIGHT study 2024).

CAUSES AND RISK FACTORS[4]

Intrauterine fetal death is multifactorial; up to 50% remain unexplained despite full workup (CODAC classification). Causes are stratified by category (2025 meta-analysis data; **Table 1**).

TABLE 1: Causes stratified by category.

Category	*Prevalence (%)*	*Key examples and associations*
Placental	25–35	Insufficiency (IUGR; RR 5–10), abruption (10–15% of cases), infarction, and vasa previa
Umbilical Cord	10–15	Prolapse (acute hypoxia), nuchal cord (RR 1.5 if tight), thrombosis, and velamentous insertion
Maternal	20–25	Hypertensive disorders (preeclampsia/eclampsia: 15–24%; RR 4–6), diabetes (pregestational: RR 2–4), obesity (BMI ≥30: RR 1.5–2), and smoking (RR 1.5–2)
Fetal	15–20	Chromosomal (trisomies 13/18/21: 10–15%), structural anomalies (CNS/cardiac: 5–10%), and aneuploidy (30% in early IUFD)
Infection	10–15	TORCH (CMV: 5–10%; parvovirus B19), ascending (GBS: RR 2–3), malaria (LMICs: 20%)
Idiopathic/unexplained	25–50	Often late IUFD; associated with FGR and advanced age

TABLE 2: Risk factors.[4,5]

Category	*Risk factors*
Maternal	Advanced age (>35 years), race, obesity, low socioeconomic/educational status, and smoking
Fetal	Congenital malformations, male sex
Obstetric complications	Fetal growth restriction (FGR), pregnancy-induced hypertension (PIH), placental abruption, multiple pregnancy, Rh isoimmunization, post-term pregnancy, infections, antepartum asphyxia, previous stillbirth, and nuchal/knotted cord
Medical disorders	Diabetes, hypertension, chronic nephritis, systemic lupus erythematosus (SLE), thrombophilia, and cholestasis of pregnancy

Risk factors **(Table 2)** (modified WHO 2024; OR >2 for high-risk):

- Previous stillbirth (OR 5–10)
- ART/multiple gestation (OR 2–4.6)
- Socioeconomic/environmental: Air pollution (PM2.5: OR 1.3) and low ANC attendance.

PATHOPHYSIOLOGY

Core mechanism: Fetal hypoxia/acidemia from impaired placental gas/nutrient exchange, leading to anaerobic metabolism, acidosis, and multiorgan failure.

Pathways:

1. **Placental insufficiency:** Chronic hypoxia → IUGR → demise (e.g., via sFlt-1/PlGF imbalance)
2. **Acute events:** Abruption/cord prolapse → sudden hypoxia (lactate >4.8 mmol/L predemise)

3. **Maternal-fetal:** Systemic inflammation (e.g., preeclampsia cytokines IL-6/TNF-α) or metabolic derangements (diabetes hyperglycemia)
4. **Infectious:** Transplacental ascent → fetal sepsis (e.g., GBS endotoxin release)
5. **Fetal intrinsic:** Anomalies cause cardiac/hemodynamic failure.

Postdemise: Maceration begins within 4–6 hours (skin slippage >12 hours); coagulopathy risk rises after 3–4 weeks (DIC in 10–15%).

CLINICAL PRESENTATION AND DIAGNOSIS

Presentation: 50–70% detected via reduced fetal movements (RFM; sensitivity 50% if formal kick-counts used). Other: Vaginal bleeding (20%), absent heart tones on auscultation/Doppler, uterus smaller than dates (10%). Asymptomatic in 10–20% (routine USG).

Diagnosis (RCOG/ACOG 2025): Real-time ultrasound confirming absent cardiac activity by ≥2 experienced clinicians (false-positive <0.1%).

Adjuncts:

- No cardiac activity on M-mode/color Doppler
- Biophysical profile score = 0
- Avoid single auscultation; confirm GA to exclude pre-20 weeks loss.

Differential: Severe oligohydramnios mimicking demise; maternal obesity artifact.

DIAGNOSTIC APPROACH

Multimodal evaluation pre- and postdelivery (FIGO/RCOG 2024; yield: 50–70% cause identification; **Table 3**).

Selective: Thyroid function (TSH/FT4 if unexplained), antiphospholipid screen (recurrent).

TABLE 3: Diagnostic approach.

Investigation	*Timing*	*Purpose and Yield*
Ultrasound	Immediate	Confirm demise, anomalies, GA, biometry (IUGR), placental/cord pathology (e.g., abruption). Yield: 30–40%
Doppler/MCA-PSV	Predemise if suspected	Assess anemia/hypoxia (e.g., peak systolic velocity >1.5 MoM)
Maternal bloods	Predelivery	FBC/coags (DIC screen), Kleihauer-Betke (FMH >30 mL: 5%), HbA1c/glucose (DM), infection (CRP, serology: CMV/Parvo), thrombophilia (if recurrent: Factor V Leiden, APTT)
Fetal/postdelivery	Post	Autopsy (gold standard; yield 20–30%; consent sensitive), placental histology (infarcts: 25%), karyotype/microarray (aneuploidy: 15%), and cultures/swabs (infection: 10%)
Advanced	Selective	Fetal MRI (CNS anomalies) and NGS/exome (monogenic: 5–10% unexplained)

MANAGEMENT OF INTRAUTERINE FETAL DEATH

Counseling and Support (INSIGHT 2024)**:** Multidisciplinary (obstetrician, midwife, and psychologist); use SPIKES protocol for disclosure. Offer memory-making (photography and footprints). Bereavement follow-up at 6 weeks; screen for PGD (DSM-5 criteria). VTE prophylaxis: LMWH for 6 weeks (RR 6-fold increase).

Timing and Mode of Delivery (RCOG/ACOG/SMFM 2020–2025)**:** Expedite if maternal compromise (preeclampsia, sepsis, abruption, and DIC); otherwise, options: expectant (spontaneous labor 80% within 2 weeks), induction (preferred), or cesarean (only for maternal indication; e.g., prior classical scar).

- **Induction regimens** (singleton; ≥24 weeks):
    - Mifepristone 200 mg oral + misoprostol 400–800 µg PV q3–6h (efficacy 85–95%; lower CS rate vs. oxytocin)
    - <24 weeks: Gemeprost or serial misoprostol
    - Prior CS: Caution uterine rupture (1–2%); dinoprostone preferred over high-dose misoprostol.
- Expectant: Monitor coags q48h after 2 weeks; infection risk 1–3%.

Labor Management: Avoid fetal scalp electrode; continuous maternal HR/BP. Analgesia: Epidural safe. Postpartum: Active management of third stage; monitor PPH (RR 1.5–2).

Special Scenarios:

- Multiples: Selective demise → monitor cotwin (serial USG/Doppler); laser for TTTS if <26 weeks.
- Placenta previa: Expectant up to 40 days possible if stable (2025 case series)
- RPH-associated: Prompt extraction reduces maternal hemorrhage (2025 French cohort).

LONG-TERM CONSIDERATIONS

Recurrence: 5–15% (cause dependent; e.g., 25% if prior placental). Preconception: Optimize BMI, screen comorbidities, and low-dose aspirin (if prior placental). ANC: Fetal movement counting from 24 weeks, serial growth USG (if prior IUGR). Psychological: 20–30% need therapy; partner involvement key.

ALGORITHMS

Clinical Approach to Suspected Intrauterine Fetal Death

Pregnant woman reports reduced fetal movements (or routine check)

↓

Bedside auscultation/pocket Doppler for FHR

↓ (Absent/uncertain)

Immediate real-time ultrasound (by senior clinician)

↓

Confirm absent cardiac activity (M-mode; ≥2 clinicians) + GA estimation

↓ (Confirmed IUFD)

Sensitive disclosure (SPIKES: private, empathetic, and family present)

↓

Assess maternal status (vitals, coags, and bleeding)

↓

Offer options: Expectant vs. induction (preferred) vs. CS (rare)

↓

Induction: Mifepristone + misoprostol; VTE prophylaxis

↓

Postdelivery: Placental/fetal examination; consent for autopsy/histology

↓

Maternal workup + counseling (recurrence risk and future care)

↓

6-week follow-up: Grief support, VTE screen

Hospital Management of Confirmed Intrauterine Fetal Death

Diagnosis confirmed (USG + clinical)

↓

Multidisciplinary huddle (obs, midwifery, and psych)

↓

Baseline labs: FBC, coags (PT/PTT/fibrinogen), Kleihauer, and infection screen

↓

If compromise (e.g., abruption/DIC): Immediate CS/expedite

↓ (Stable)

Counsel on timing/mode; induction if >24 h

↓

Labor: Maternal monitoring only; analgesia; GBS if indicated

↓

Delivery: Third-stage active; PPH vigilance

↓

Post: Fetal autopsy (consent), placental histology, and maternal serology/karyotype if recurrent

↓

Debrief: 24–48 h post; written summary

↓

Discharge: LMWH × 6 weeks, contraception, referral to bereavement service

PREVENTION

- **Antenatal Screening:**
  - **First Trimester:** Dual markers, nuchal translucency (NT) scan, and noninvasive prenatal testing (NIPT) for trisomies
  - **Second Trimester:** Quadruple marker, anomaly scan, fetal 2D echo, and monitor for PIH/gestational diabetes mellitus (GDM)

  - **Third Trimester:** Growth scan, Doppler studies (fetal/uterine arteries) for FGR, monitor PIH/GDM, consider induction at 37 weeks (uncontrolled PIH), or 38 weeks (uncontrolled GDM).
- **RCOG (2022):** Strict monitoring of high-risk pregnancies to detect early signs of complications.

CASE STUDY: 32-WEEK PRIMIGRAVIDA WITH INTRAUTERINE FETAL DEATH

A 32-week unbooked primigravida presents with IUFD. Here is the evaluation and management approach.

Causes of Intrauterine Fetal Death (Table 4)

Likely Causes (Unbooked Patient)

- **Maternal:** Low socioeconomic/educational status, undiagnosed substance abuse
- **Obstetric:**
  - FGR (most common, missed due to lack of monitoring)
  - Severe PIH or placental abruption
  - Undiagnosed GDM
  - Rh isoimmunization
  - Infections (e.g., parvovirus and malaria)
- **Fetal:** Congenital malformations
- **Medical:** Cholestasis, thrombophilia, chronic nephritis, and SLE

Complications of Intrauterine Fetal Death (Table 5)

- **Maternal Condition Related:**
  - Severe PIH, eclampsia, cholestasis, and massive hemorrhage (abruption)
- **Prolonged IUFD Related:**
  - Disseminated intravascular coagulopathy (DIC): 10% risk within 4 weeks, increasing thereafter
  - Chorioamnionitis (if membranes rupture)

TABLE 4: Major Causes of IUFD (2025 updated prevalence).

Category	*Examples*	*Prevalence (%)*	*Preventable? (Strategies)*
Placental	Abruption and insufficiency	25–35	Partial (aspirin in high-risk; FM monitoring)
Cord	Prolapse and nuchal	10–15	Low (cord Doppler in multiples)
Maternal	PET and DM	20–25	High (GDM screen and BP control)
Fetal	Aneuploidy and malformations	15–20	Partial (NIPT and anomaly scan)
Infection	CMV and GBS	10–15	High (TORCH screen and GBS prophylaxis)
Idiopathic	Unexplained	25–50	N/A (Full workup reduces to <30%)

TABLE 5: Definitions and thresholds (International variations).[6]

Term	GA threshold	Notes (2025 guidelines)	
IUFD	≥20 weeks	ACOG/SMFM: Includes early losses; focus on workup	US: Fetal death certificate ≥20 weeks
Stillbirth[3]	≥24 weeks	RCOG/FIGO/WHO: Legal/reportable; antepartum emphasis	UK: Perinatal mortality surveillance
Early IUFD	20–27 weeks	Higher anomaly rate; microarray yield 20%	Optional autopsy consent
Late IUFD	≥28 weeks	Placental dominant; recurrence counseling key	Mandatory histopathology

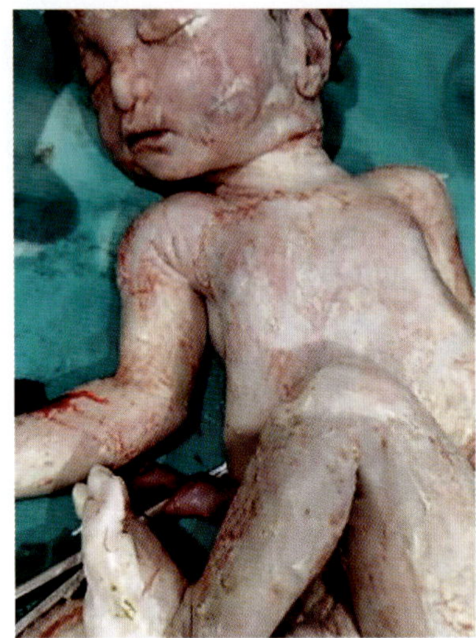

Fig. 1: Macerated fetus.

Management

Stabilization and Investigations:

- **Maternal Tests:**
    - Complete hemogram, coagulation profile, liver/renal function tests, and blood grouping/cross-matching
    - Kleihauer-Betke test (if Rh-negative) to assess fetomaternal hemorrhage
- **Immediate Action:** Stabilize for severe PIH, eclampsia, abruption, or sepsis; deliver promptly if present.
- **Rh-Negative Mothers:** Indirect Coombs test; administer anti-D 300 μg IM within 72 hours postdelivery if unsensitized.

Delivery Planning:

- **Stable Patients:** Offer delayed induction (<48 hours) if no complications, intact membranes, and no DIC. Monitor for DIC twice weekly if prolonged expectant management **(Fig. 1)**.

TABLE 6: Misoprostol dosing for IUFD induction.

Gestational age	*Dosage*
13–17 weeks	200 μg vaginal 6 hourly (maximum 4 doses)
18–26 weeks	100 μg vaginal 6 hourly (maximum 4 doses)
27 weeks term	25 μg vaginal 6 hourly (maximum 6 doses) or 25 μg oral 2 hourly (maximum 12 doses)

- **Induction:**
  - **Regimen:** Mifepristone (200 mg single dose) followed by misoprostol (NICE 2024).
  - **Misoprostol Dosing (Table 6):**
    - 27 weeks–term: 25 μg vaginal 6 hourly (maximum 6 doses) or 25 μg oral 2 hourly (maximum 12 doses)
    - Achieves vaginal birth in 90% within 24 hours
  - **Cesarean Section:** Reserved for maternal indications or patient preference (rare)
- **Lactation Suppression:**
  - Nonpharmacological: Support brassiere, ice packs, and analgesics.
  - Pharmacological: Cabergoline (1 mg single dose) or bromocriptine (2.5 mg twice daily, 14 days); cabergoline preferred for simplicity and fewer side effects

REFERENCES

1. Burden C, et al. Care of late intrauterine fetal death and stillbirth. BJOG. 2025;132:1-25.
2. ACOG/SMFM. (2020). Management of Stillbirth. Obstet Care Consensus. [online] Available from http://acog.org/clinical/clinical-guidance/obstetric-care-consensus/articles/2020/03/management-of-stillbirth [Last accessed December, 2025].
3. Baddam S, Burns B. Stillbirth. StatPearls. Treasure Island (FL): StatPearls Publishing; 2025.
4. Lawn JE, et al. Stillbirths: Rates, risk factors, and acceleration towards 2030. Lancet. 2024;404:1-15.
5. RCOG. (2024). Late Intrauterine Fetal Death and Stillbirth (Green-top No. 55). [online] Available from https://www.rcog.org.uk/guidance/browse-all-guidance/green-top-guidelines/care-of-late-intrauterine-fetal-death-and-stillbirth-green-top-guideline-no-55/ [Last accessed December, 2025].
6. Heazell AEP, et al. MBRRACE-UK Perinatal Surveillance Report 2023–2024. 2025.

HIV in Pregnancy

Ruchika Garg

INTRODUCTION

Parent-to-child transmission (PTCT), also known as mother-to-child transmission (MTCT), is a major route of HIV infection in children, contributing to **4% of HIV infections in India**. Effective interventions, including antiretroviral therapy (ART), safe delivery practices, and infant prophylaxis, can reduce transmission risk to **<2%**. This chapter outlines the epidemiology, risk factors, prevention strategies, and management protocols for PTCT, tailored for postgraduate medical students, with reference to National AIDS Control Organisation (NACO) and international guidelines.[1]

EPIDEMIOLOGY

- **Global Burden:** PTCT accounts for 90% of pediatric HIV infections worldwide, with 150,000 new cases annually (WHO, 2021).[2]
- **India:** PTCT constitutes **4% of HIV infections**, with an estimated 20,000–30,000 HIV-exposed infants born yearly.
- **Transmission Risk:**
  - Without ART and breastfeeding: **30–45%**
  - Without ART, no breastfeeding: **20–25%**
  - With triple ART antenatally and breastfeeding: **2%**
  - With triple ART antenatally, no breastfeeding: **1%**
- **Timing of Transmission:**
  - Antenatal: 20% (before 36 weeks)
  - Peripartum: 50% (days before delivery)
  - Intrapartum: 30%
- **NACO Goal:** 95% antenatal HIV screening to achieve EMTCT by 2030

RISK FACTORS (TABLE 1)

Key Insights:

- High maternal viral load at 32–36 weeks is the strongest predictor of transmission.
- STIs (e.g., herpes, syphilis) increase mucosal inflammation, facilitating HIV transmission.
- Mixed feeding disrupts infant gut integrity, enhancing HIV entry.

TABLE 1: Risk factors for PTCT.

Category	*Factors*
Maternal	Recent HIV infection, high viral load (>1,000 copies/mL), advanced HIV disease (CD4 <200/µL), sexually transmitted infections (STIs), malnutrition, and breastfeeding complications (sore nipples, mastitis, and abscess)
Obstetric	Prolonged labor (>12 hours), forceps/vacuum delivery, invasive fetal monitoring (e.g., scalp electrodes), and artificial rupture of membranes (ARM)
Fetal/neonatal	Preterm (<37 weeks), low birth weight (<2.5 kg), oral ulcers/thrush, and mixed feeding (breast milk + formula)

TABLE 2: NACO's four-prong PPTCT approach.

Prong	*Strategy*
Prong 1: Primary prevention	Awareness campaigns, condom promotion, and early STI diagnosis/treatment for women of childbearing age
Prong 2: Prevent unintended pregnancies	Contraception counseling and family planning for HIV-positive women
Prong 3: Prevent transmission	ART for mothers, safe delivery practices, infant ART prophylaxis, and viral load monitoring at 32–36 weeks
Prong 4: Care and support	Lifelong ART for mothers, infant follow-up, counseling, and immunization for HIV-exposed infants

PREVENTION STRATEGIES[3]

NACO's **four-prong approach** to prevention of parent-to-child transmission (PPTCT) is central to reducing transmission **(Table 2)**.

Antenatal Screening[4]

- **Protocol:** Routine opt-out HIV counseling and testing for all pregnant women, screening for HIV-1 and HIV-2
- **Confirmatory Tests:** Performed for screen-positive women, followed by post-test counseling for patients and families
- **Investigations:**
  - **Viral Load:** Plasma HIV RNA quantification at diagnosis, every 4 weeks, and 34–36 weeks
  - **CD4 Count:** Baseline and every 3–4 months
  - **Screening:** STIs, reproductive tract infections (RTIs), tuberculosis (TB), and opportunistic infections
  - **Vaccinations:** Pneumococcal, hepatitis A/B, Tdap, COVID-19, and influenza
- **Support:** Nutritional counseling and psychosocial support to enhance ART adherence.

Antenatal Antiretroviral Therapy[5]

- **Objective:** Suppress maternal viral load, improve maternal health, and provide fetal/infant preexposure prophylaxis.

TABLE 3: ART regimens for PTCT prevention.

Scenario	*Regimen*	*Notes*
Preconception ART	Continue TDF + 3TC + DTG if suppressed	Adjust if resistance or intolerance detected
Newly Diagnosed	TDF (300 mg) + 3TC (300 mg) + DTG (50 mg) daily	Alternative: 2 NRTIs + ritonavir-boosted PI (e.g., atazanavir/ritonavir)
Intrapartum Diagnosis	Oral TLD or IV AZT (2 mg/kg loading, 1 mg/kg/h)	Continue TLD postpartum
Postpartum Diagnosis	TDF + 3TC + DTG or 2 NRTIs + PI/integrase inhibitor	Lifelong ART recommended

- **NACO Regimen:** Fixed-dose combination (FDC) of **tenofovir (TDF 300 mg) + lamivudine (3TC 300 mg) + dolutegravir (DTG 50 mg)**, once daily **(Table 3)**.
- **Indications:**
  - **Preconception ART:** Continue if viral load suppressed and tolerated.
  - **Newly Diagnosed:** Start triple ART [2 nucleoside reverse transcriptase inhibitors (NRTIs) + protease inhibitor (PI) or integrase inhibitor].
  - **Previous ART, Discontinued:** Restart based on prior records, pending resistance testing.
  - **Intrapartum Diagnosis:** Oral TLD or IV zidovudine (AZT; 2 mg/kg loading dose over 1 hour, 1 mg/kg/h until delivery).
  - **Postpartum Diagnosis:** Triple ART (2 NRTIs + ritonavir-boosted PI or integrase inhibitor).
- **Contraindications:**
  - Didanosine, stavudine, and full-dose ritonavir due to toxicity
  - Lopinavir/ritonavir avoided due to preterm/small-for-gestational-age risks
  - **Precautions:** DTG is not to be taken within 2 hours of iron, calcium, or vitamin supplements.
- **Mechanisms:**
  - Reduces maternal viral load.
  - Provides fetal preexposure prophylaxis.
  - Improves maternal immune status.
  - Minimizes transmission risk to infant.

Delivery Planning

- **Counseling:** Emphasize institutional delivery to minimize transmission risk.
- **Mode of Delivery:**
  - **Vaginal Delivery:** Preferred if viral load <1,000 copies/mL (NACO, 2021).
  - **Cesarean Section (CS):** Recommended at 38 weeks if viral load >1,000 copies/mL or for obstetric indications (e.g., fetal distress and placenta previa)
  - CS not beneficial if membranes ruptured or labor advanced (viral load >1,000 copies/mL).

- **Intrapartum ART:**
  - Continue oral ART (TLD) during labor.
  - IV AZT (2 mg/kg loading dose over 1 hour, 1 mg/kg/h until delivery) for women on ART or diagnosed intrapartum.
  - For elective CS: AZT 2 mg/kg loading dose, 1 mg/kg/h for 2 hours.
- **Labor Management:**
  - Minimize vaginal examinations, use aseptic precautions.
  - Avoid ARM, fetal scalp electrodes, routine episiotomy, and vacuum delivery.
  - Prefer low-cavity forceps if instrumental delivery required (less fetal trauma).
  - Augment labor with oxytocin to shorten duration.
  - Avoid milking/delayed cord clamping, routine nasogastric suctioning (except for meconium-stained liquor, <100 mm Hg pressure).
  - Handle newborn with gloves until maternal secretions are washed off.
- **Postpartum Hemorrhage:**
  - Use oxytocin or prostaglandins.
  - Avoid ergot derivatives (e.g., methergine) due to interactions with ART causing vasoconstriction.

Infant Feeding

- **Options** (NACO, 2021)**:**
  - **Exclusive Breastfeeding (EBF):** Preferred in India; only breast milk (no liquids/solids, except vitamins/medicines) for 6–12 months. Initiated within 1 hour of birth.
  - **Exclusive Replacement Feeding (ERF):** Animal milk or formula, prepared hygienically, given by spoon/bowl (avoid bottles).
- **Mixed Feeding:** Increases transmission risk (disrupts gut mucosa), strictly avoided.
- **Counseling:** Antenatal discussion of EBF vs. ERF, weighing survival benefits (EBF) vs. transmission risk (ERF).

Infant Antiretroviral Therapy Prophylaxis

- **Low Risk** (maternal viral load <1,000 copies/mL post-32 weeks):
  - Syrup nevirapine (NVP) or zidovudine (AZT) for 6 weeks:
    - <2 kg: NVP 2 mg/kg/day or AZT 5 mg/dose twice daily
    - 2–2.5 kg: NVP 1 mL/day (10 mg/mL) or AZT 10 mg/dose twice daily
    - 2.5 kg: NVP 1.5 mL/day or AZT 15 mg/dose twice daily
- **High Risk** (no maternal ART, viral load >1,000 copies/mL, no viral load post-32 weeks, or late diagnosis):
  - Dual prophylaxis (NVP + AZT):
    - EBF: 12 weeks
    - ERF: 6 weeks
    - Dosing as above
- **Testing:** HIV PCR at 6 weeks, 6 months, and 18 months for early infant diagnosis.

Postpartum Care

- **Maternal:** Continue lifelong ART (TLD), monitor adherence, and provide psychosocial support.
- **Infant:** Immunizations, growth monitoring, and HIV testing per NACO protocol.

SHORT QUESTIONS AND ANSWERS

1. Perinatal HIV Transmission.

Ans.

- **Definition:** Transmission of HIV from mother to child during pregnancy, labor/delivery, or breastfeeding, accounting for **4% of HIV infections in India**
- **Risk:** 30–45% without ART and breastfeeding; reduced to **1–2%** with triple ART and safe practices
- **Timing:** 20% antenatal, 50% peripartum, and 30% intrapartum
- **Risk Factors:** High maternal viral load, STIs, prolonged labor, invasive procedures, and mixed feeding
- **Prevention:** Antenatal ART (TLD), vaginal delivery if viral load <1,000 copies/mL, infant prophylaxis (NVP/AZT), EBF or ERF

2. PPTCT (NACO Guidelines).

Ans.

- **PPTCT:** Prevention of parent-to-child transmission, aimed at EMTCT
- **NACO Four-Prong Approach:**
  - Prong 1: Primary prevention (condoms and STI treatment)
  - Prong 2: Prevent unintended pregnancies (contraception counseling)
  - Prong 3: ART (TDF + 3TC + DTG), safe delivery, and infant prophylaxis
  - Prong 4: Lifelong ART, infant follow-up
- **Key Interventions:**
  - Screen 95% of antenatal women (opt-out).
  - Start TLD for all HIV-positive pregnant women, regardless of CD4 count.
  - Viral load testing at 32–36 weeks to guide delivery and infant prophylaxis.
  - Promote institutional delivery and avoid invasive procedures.
  - EBF (preferred) or ERF; avoid mixed feeding.
- **Outcome:** Reduces transmission to **<2%** with adherence.

3. Intrapartum Care in HIV-Positive Pregnancy.

Ans.

- **NACO Guidelines (2021):**
  - **Mode:** Vaginal delivery if viral load <1,000 copies/mL; CS at 38 weeks for >1,000 copies/mL or obstetric indications.
  - **ART:** Continue oral TLD; IV AZT (2 mg/kg loading, 1 mg/kg/h) for women on ART or diagnosed intrapartum.
  - **Labor Management:**
    - Minimal vaginal examinations and aseptic precautions.

        - Avoid ARM, fetal scalp electrodes, routine episiotomy, and vacuum delivery.
        - Use low forceps if instrumental delivery is needed.
        - Augment labor with oxytocin to shorten duration.
        - Avoid milking/delayed cord clamping, routine suctioning (except meconium, <100 mm Hg).
        - Handle newborn with gloves until cleaned.
    - **PPH:** Use oxytocin/prostaglandins; avoid ergot derivatives.
    - **New Diagnosis in Labor:** Start TLD and continue postpartum.

4. Breastfeeding in HIV-Positive Mothers.

Ans.

- **Options** (NACO, 2021):
    - **EBF:** Only breast milk for 6–12 months, initiated within 1 hour; preferred in India for survival benefits.
    - **ERF:** Hygienic animal/formula milk via spoon/bowl (no bottles).
- **Mixed Feeding:** Avoided due to increased transmission risk
- **Counseling:** Antenatal discussion of risks/benefits, maternal ART adherence, and infant prophylaxis (NVP/AZT for 6–12 weeks)
- **Rationale:** Maternal ART reduces postnatal transmission risk to <**2%** with EBF.

5. Management of Infants Born to HIV-Positive Mothers.

Ans.

- **Immediate Care:**
    - Handle with gloves until maternal secretions are washed off.
    - Wipe mouth/nostrils at delivery.
    - Initiate feeding within 1 hour (EBF or ERF per parental choice).
- **ART Prophylaxis:**
    - **Low Risk:** NVP or AZT for 6 weeks
    - **High Risk:** NVP + AZT for 12 weeks (EBF) or 6 weeks (ERF)
    - Dosing based on birth weight **(Table 4)**
- **Follow-Up:**
    - HIV PCR at 6 weeks, 6 months, and 18 months
    - Immunizations, growth monitoring, and referral to PPTCT centers

6. Postexposure Prophylaxis (PEP).

Ans.

- **Definition:** Comprehensive management to minimize HIV transmission risk after occupational exposure (e.g., needlestick and mucosal splash)

TABLE 4: Infant ART prophylaxis.

Risk category	*Regimen*	*Duration*
Low risk (<1,000 copies/mL)	Syrup NVP or AZT	6 weeks
High risk	Syrup NVP + AZT	12 weeks (EBF), 6 weeks (ERF)

- **Risk:** Needlestick (0.3%) and mucosal exposure (0.09%)
- **NACO Guidelines (2021):**
    - **First Aid:** Wash skin with soap/water, flush eyes with water.
    - **Risk Assessment:** Initiate PEP within 2 hours (maximum 72 hours). Classify exposure as:
        - HIV-negative source: No PEP
        - Low risk: HIV-positive, asymptomatic
        - High risk: HIV-positive, symptomatic
    - **Regimen:** TDF (300 mg) + 3TC (300 mg) + DTG (50 mg) daily for 28 days
    - **Follow-Up:**
        - Monitor for seroconversion (fever, rash, and lymphadenopathy) at 3–6 weeks.
        - HIV antibody testing at 2, 4, 6 weeks, 3 months, and 6 months
        - CBC, RBS, and transaminases at weeks 2 and 4
        - Counsel on adherence, side effects, and secondary prevention (e.g., condom use and no blood donation).
- **Prevention:** Standard precautions (handwashing, safe sharps disposal, gloves, and goggles).

7. Counseling of a Patient with HIV Infection.

Ans.

- **NACO Framework:** Voluntary counseling at integrated counseling and testing centers (ICTCs), including pre- and post-test counseling.
- **Objectives:**
    - Provide information on HIV/AIDS, disease progression, and ART.
    - Promote risk reduction (safe sex and STI treatment).
    - Address psychological issues (fear, grief, and rejection).
    - Ensure ART adherence and discuss side effects.
- **Key Elements:**
    - Pretest: Discuss test implications, confidentiality.
    - Post-test: Confirm results, offer emotional support, explain ART, and plan follow-up.
    - Address stigma, financial concerns, and family involvement.
- **Antenatal Counseling:** Focus on PPTCT, ART adherence, delivery planning, and feeding options.

8. Serodiscordant Couples.

Ans.

- **Definition:** One partner HIV-positive, the other HIV-negative, often desiring conception.
- **Risk:** Unprotected intercourse increases HIV transmission to negative partner.
- **Strategies:**
    - **Preexposure Prophylaxis (PrEP):** TDF (300 mg) + emtricitabine (FTC 200 mg) for negative partner, started 1 month before conception, continued 1 month postconception (or longer if unprotected intercourse persists)
    - **Barrier Contraception:** Condoms except during peak fertility
    - **Vaginal Self-Insemination:** For HIV-positive women

- **Male Circumcision:** Reduces risk in HIV-negative males
- **Intrauterine Insemination:** Washed semen for HIV-positive males
- **STI Control:** Treat STIs in HIV-positive partner.

- **Investigations (Negative Partner):**
  - HIV test every 3 months
  - Pregnancy test, renal function, and hepatitis B screening (vaccinate if negative)
- **Pregnancy Management:**
  - Continue ART for positive partner.
  - HIV testing each trimester, during labor, and every 3 months during breastfeeding.
  - **Outcome:** Transmission risk reduced to **0–5%** with PrEP, viral suppression, and STI control.

CONCLUSION

Parent-to-child transmission of HIV is preventable with comprehensive interventions, reducing transmission risk from 30–45% to <**2%**. NACO's four-prong PPTCT approach, including antenatal screening, triple ART (TDF + 3TC + DTG), safe delivery, and infant prophylaxis, is critical. Counseling, adherence support, and tailored feeding options (EBF or ERF) further minimize risk. Postgraduate medical students must understand these protocols to manage HIV-positive pregnancies effectively, ensuring optimal maternal and infant outcomes.

REFERENCES

1. NACO. National Guidelines for HIV Care and Treatment. 2021.
2. WHO. Consolidated Guidelines on HIV Prevention, Testing, Treatment, and Care. 2021.
3. U.S. Panel on Treatment of Pregnant Women with HIV Infection and Prevention of Perinatal Transmission. Recommendations. 2021.
4. NICE. Antenatal care (NG201). (2021). [online] Available from https://www.nice.org.uk/guidance/ng201 [Last accessed December, 2025].
5. Lawn JE, Blencowe H, Waiswa P, et al. Lancet. 2016;387(10018):587-603.

High Dependency Unit in Maternal Health Care

Ruchika Garg

INTRODUCTION

High dependency units (HDUs) are specialized hospital areas that provide intensive monitoring and intermediate care for critically ill obstetric patients who require more support than general wards but less than intensive care units (ICUs). With maternal morbidity and mortality rising in India, particularly due to conditions such as severe preeclampsia and postpartum hemorrhage (PPH), HDUs bridge the gap between ward-based care and ICU-level intervention.[1] Introduced in India's maternal healthcare model in 2016 by the Ministry of Health and Family Welfare (MoHFW), obstetric HDUs and ICUs have strengthened critical care delivery, addressing delays caused by overburdened general ICUs.[2] This chapter outlines the role, indications, management strategies, challenges, and recent advancements in obstetric HDUs, tailored for postgraduate medical education in low-resource settings.

REVISED MATERNAL HEALTHCARE MODEL IN INDIA

Previously, India's maternal health system comprised three levels: Skilled birth attendant (SBA), basic emergency obstetric care (BEmOC), and comprehensive emergency obstetric care (CEmOC). Critical care was provided through general ICUs, often leading to delays due to bed shortages.[2] The 2016 revision introduced obstetric-specific HDUs and ICUs within maternity units to ensure timely, specialized care.[2]

Key Features:

- **Medical Colleges:** Mandated to have both obstetric ICUs and HDUs
- **District Hospitals:** Required to establish obstetric HDUs
- **Bed Allocation** (MoHFW Guidelines; **Table 1**):[2]
    - **≤250 deliveries/month:** 4-bed HDU
    - **251–500 deliveries/month:** 8-bed HDU

TABLE 1: Bed allocation for obstetric HDUs/ICUs based on delivery volume.

Delivery volume/month	*HDU Beds*	*ICU Beds*	*Total Beds*
≤250	4	0	4
251–500	8	0	8
501–1,000	6	2	8
>1,000	8	4	12

- **501–1,000 deliveries/month:** 8 hybrid beds (6 HDU, 2 ICU)
- **>1,000 deliveries/month:** 4 ICU beds, 8 HDU beds

This model optimizes resource use, reduces ICU burden, and ensures proximity to delivery suites for rapid intervention.

DEFINITION OF OBSTETRIC HDU

An obstetric HDU is a dedicated unit within a maternity ward that provides advanced monitoring and care for pregnant or postpartum women with severe complications requiring close supervision but not invasive ICU-level interventions.[3] HDUs manage single-organ dysfunction or postsurgical recovery, typically at secondary care facilities, and are equipped for noninvasive ventilation, hemodynamic stabilization, and intensive monitoring.[4]

Key Characteristics:
- Suitable for patients postmajor surgery or with single-organ failure
- Does not support invasive ventilation, inotropic drugs, or multiorgan failure (these require ICU transfer)
- Located near labor suites for seamless care transitions
- *Transfer protocols:* Patients needing ICU care are shifted to an in-hospital ICU or the nearest facility, accompanied by an obstetrician, anesthetist, and complete records.[2]

INDICATIONS FOR HDU ADMISSION

Obstetric HDUs cater to a range of severe pregnancy-related conditions requiring intensive monitoring. Indications align with NICE guidelines for Level 2 care (equivalent to HDU in India; **Table 2**).[3,5]

Management Highlights:
- **Preeclampsia/Eclampsia:** Magnesium sulfate for seizure prophylaxis, antihypertensives (e.g., labetalol, nifedipine), and fetal monitoring[5]
- **Hemorrhage:** Rapid transfusion (packed RBCs, O-negative blood mandatory) and surgical intervention (e.g., uterine artery ligation)[2]
- **Sepsis:** Broad-spectrum antibiotics, IV fluids, and organ function monitoring[6]
- **ARDS:** Noninvasive ventilation, low tidal volume strategy, treat underlying cause (e.g., pneumonia).[7]

CONTRAINDICATIONS FOR HDU ADMISSION (TABLE 3)

Certain conditions preclude HDU admission due to stability, nonobstetric nature, or resource limitations:
- **Stable Patients:** Clinically stable women manageable on general wards
- **Nonobstetric Conditions:** Issues unrelated to pregnancy (e.g., elective nonobstetric surgery)
- **ICU-Level Needs:** Patients requiring invasive ventilation, inotropic support, or multiorgan failure management
- **Resource Constraints:** Insufficient HDU beds or trained staff

TABLE 2: Indications for obstetric HDU admission.

Condition	*Indication for admission*
Severe Preeclampsia/ eclampsia	Uncontrolled hypertension (>160/110 mm Hg), neurological symptoms, HELLP syndrome, oliguria, hyperkalemia, cardiac failure, and abnormal neurology
Hemorrhagic disorders	Massive obstetric hemorrhage (e.g., PPH) requiring rapid transfusion or surgical intervention
Sepsis	Systemic infection with hemodynamic instability, not requiring inotropes
Acute respiratory distress	Severe respiratory distress not responding to standard therapy, needing noninvasive ventilation
Cardiac disease	Peripartum cardiomyopathy, arrhythmias, myocardial infarction, and congestive heart failure
Acute renal failure	Need for monitoring, potential dialysis; chronic kidney disease requiring renal replacement
Thromboembolic disorders	Pulmonary embolism requiring anticoagulation and monitoring
Postoperative care	Postcesarean hysterectomy or complex surgeries in patients with comorbidities
Single organ dysfunction	Hepatic/renal encephalopathy, hematological issues (e.g., thalassemia), not in multiorgan failure
Other	Malignancy, heat stroke, traumatic brain injury, paralysis, and endocrine dysfunction

TABLE 3: Contraindications for obstetric HDU admission.

Contraindication	*Reason*
Stable patients	Manageable on general wards, no need for intensive monitoring
Nonobstetric conditions	Require nonobstetric expertise, not HDU-specific care
Need for invasive ventilation	Requires ICU-level respiratory support
Inotropic support	Indicates shock, necessitating ICU care
Multiorgan failure	Beyond HDU capacity, requires ICU resources
Resource limitations	Lack of beds, staff, or equipment in HDU

KEY COMPONENTS OF OBSTETRIC HDU CARE

Effective HDU care relies on advanced monitoring, multidisciplinary collaboration, and supportive interventions.

- **Monitoring Protocols:**
  - Continuous fetal monitoring (>24 weeks gestation) using cardiotocography[5]
  - Hemodynamic monitoring (noninvasive: BP, pulse oximetry; invasive: arterial lines if needed)
  - Neurological assessment (Glasgow Coma Scale, seizure precautions for eclampsia)[5]

- **Multidisciplinary Team:**
    - Includes obstetricians, anesthetists, intensivists, midwives, and allied health professionals (e.g., pharmacists and nutritionists)
    - Structured handover using SBAR (Situation, Background, Assessment, Recommendation) ensures continuity.[8]
- **Supportive Interventions:**
    - **Oxygen Therapy:** Nasal cannula, noninvasive ventilation for respiratory distress[7]
    - **Fluid/Electrolyte Management:** Balanced resuscitation for hemorrhage/sepsis, avoiding fluid overload[6]
    - **Vasoactive Drugs:** Limited use in HDU (e.g., low-dose antihypertensives); inotropes require ICU transfer.[2]
    - **Nutrition:** Enteral/parenteral support for critically ill patients, tailored to pregnancy needs[9]
- **Resource Optimization:** HDUs reduce ICU burden, reserving beds for multiorgan failure cases.[2]

DISADVANTAGES OF OBSTETRIC HDUs

While HDUs enhance maternal care, they face challenges, particularly in low-resource settings **(Table 4)**:

- **Limited Resources:** Lack of advanced equipment (e.g., ventilators) compared to ICUs[2]
- **Overcrowding:** High delivery volumes may strain bed availability, compromising care quality[10]
- **Psychological Impact:** Transition to HDU may increase patient/family anxiety due to critical care environment[11]
- **Staff Training Needs:** Inadequate training in critical care skills (e.g., intubation and ABG analysis) limits effectiveness.[2]

Training Requirements:

- **Skill Stations:** Blood loss estimation, eclampsia drill, infusion/syringe pump use, oxygen therapy, intubation, arterial blood gas (ABG) analysis, ventilation, obstetric CPR, and neonatal resuscitation.[2]
- **Frequency:** Regular workshops and simulation-based training for HDU staff.

TABLE 4: Challenges and mitigation strategies for obstetric HDUs.

Challenge	*Impact*	*Mitigation*
Limited resources	Inability to manage complex cases	Equip HDUs with essential monitoring tools
Overcrowding	Reduced care quality	Adhere to bed allocation guidelines
Psychological impact	Increased patient/family anxiety	Provide counseling and family support
Staff training	Inadequate critical care skills	Implement regular skill-based training programs

TABLE 5: Recent advancements in obstetric HDU care.

Advancement	*Description*	*Impact*
Structured protocols	Standardized care for preeclampsia and PPH	Reduces morbidity and ICU admissions
Early mobilization	Promotes early ambulation post-HDU admission	Shortens hospital stay
Telemedicine	Wearable devices and remote consultation	Improves response time and monitoring
COVID-19 guidelines	Noninvasive ventilation and vaccination	Enhances management of severe cases
Scoring systems	SOFA score, MEOWS for triage, and early warning	Improves patient selection and outcomes

RECENT RESEARCH AND ADVANCEMENTS

Recent studies and innovations have enhanced obstetric HDU care, particularly in low-resource settings **(Table 5)**.

- **Structured Protocols:**
  - A 2022 systematic review showed that standardized protocols for severe preeclampsia in HDUs reduced maternal morbidity by 20% and ICU admissions by 15%.[12]
  - Protocolized PPH management in HDUs decreased transfusion rates by 25% and improved survival (2023).[13]
- **Early Mobilization:** Early mobilization in HDUs reduced hospital stay by 1–2 days and improved recovery in postpartum patients (2023).[14]
- **Telemedicine and Remote Monitoring:** Integration of wearable devices and telemedicine in HDUs enabled real-time monitoring, reducing response times by 30% (2023).[15]
- **COVID-19 Impact:**
  - Guidelines for pregnant women with COVID-19 in HDUs emphasize noninvasive ventilation, anticoagulation, and steroids (e.g., dexamethasone) for severe cases.[16]
  - Vaccination (mRNA or inactivated vaccines) is recommended for pregnant women to prevent severe outcomes.[16]
  - Long-term follow-up studies (2024) show increased risks of preeclampsia and preterm birth post-COVID-19, necessitating HDU monitoring.[17]
- **Scoring Systems:**
  - Use of Sequential Organ Failure Assessment (SOFA) score >2 identifies patients needing ICU transfer, improving triage (2023).[2]
  - Modified Early Obstetric Warning Score (MEOWS) enhances early detection of deterioration in HDUs.[18]

QUESTIONS

1. **What are the criteria for admission to a high dependency unit in obstetrics?**

   (DNB Obstetrics & Gynaecology, 2022)

2. **Discuss the management of a patient with severe preeclampsia in HDU.** ***(MD Obstetrics & Gynaecology, 2021)***
3. **Describe the role of HDU in managing obstetric hemorrhage.** ***(MS Obstetrics & Gynaecology, 2020)***
4. **Outline the benefits and limitations of high dependency Units in maternal care.** ***(DNB Obstetrics & Gynaecology, 2022)***
5. **What recent advancements have been made in the management of critically ill obstetric patients?** ***(Super-speciality Exam, 2023)***

REFERENCES

1. Say L, Chou D, Gemmill A, et al. Global causes of maternal death: a WHO systematic analysis. Lancet Glob Health. 2014;2(6):e323-33.
2. Ministry of Health and Family Welfare. Operational Guidelines for Obstetric HDU and ICU. New Delhi: Government; 2016.
3. National Institute for Health and Care Excellence. Hypertension in pregnancy: diagnosis and management (NG25). NICE; 2019.
4. Zeeman GG. Obstetric critical care: a blueprint for improved outcomes. Crit Care Med. 2016;34(9):S208-14.
5. Royal College of Obstetricians and Gynaecologists. Maternal collapse in pregnancy and the puerperium: Green-top Guideline No. 56. RCOG; 2016.
6. Singer M, Deutschman CS, Seymour CW, et al. The Third International Consensus Definitions for Sepsis and Septic Shock (Sepsis). JAMA). JAMA. 2016;315(8):801-810.
7. Acute Respiratory Distress Syndrome Network. Ventilation with lower tidal volumes for acute lung injury. N Engl J Med. 2016;342:1301-8.
8. Haig KM, Sutton S, Whittington J. et al. SBAR: a shared mental model for improving communication. Jt Jt Comm J Qual Patient Saf. 2006;32(3):167-75.
9. McClave SA, Taylor BE, Martindale RG, et al. Guidelines for the provision and assessment of nutrition support therapy in the adult critically ill patient. JPEN J Parenter Enteral Nutr. 2016;40(2):159-211.
10. Magee LA, et al. Management of severe preeclampsia in low-resource settings: a systematic review. Hypertension. 2022;79(3):e7234-351.
11. Cohen RJ, et al. Early mobilization in obstetric critical care: impact on recovery. Obstet Gynecol. 2023;141(4):456-62.
12. Morris J, et al. Telemedicine in obstetric HDUs: improving maternal surveillance outcomes. BJOG. 2023;130(5):987-93.
13. Jenkins A, et al. Protocolized postpartum hemorrhage management in HDUs. Am J Obstet Gynecol. 2023;228(3):S123-30.
14. World Health Organization. WHO recommendations on maternal and newborn care for a positive postnatal experience. Geneva: WHO; 2022.
15. Allotey J, Stallings E, Bonet M, et al. Clinical manifestations and outcomes of COVID-19 in pregnancy: a global systematic review. BMJ. 2020;370:m3320.
16. Villar J, et al. Maternal and neonatal outcomes in COVID-19 pregnancies: a multicohort study. Lancet. 2021;397(10285):1949-59.
17. Poon LC, et al. Global interim guidance on coronavirus disease 2019 (COVID-19) during pregnancy and puerperium. Ultrasound Obstet Gynecol. 2020;56(6):5-10.
18. Singh S, et al. Modified Early Obstetric Warning Score (MEOWS) in predicting maternal morbidity. J. Maternal-Fetal Neonatal Med. 2021;34(15):2450-6.

Enhanced Recovery After Surgery

Ruchika Garg

DEFINITION

Enhanced recovery after surgery (ERAS) is a multimodal, evidence-based protocol designed to optimize perioperative care, reduce surgical stress, and enhance recovery in obstetric and gynecologic surgeries.[1-3]

PRINCIPLES

- Minimize surgical stress response through physiological control.
- Promote early recovery via preoperative preparation, intraoperative optimization, and postoperative care.[4]
- Key goals: Shorter hospital stay, reduced complications, improved quality of life **(Tables 1 and 2)**.[5,6]

TABLE 1: Enhanced recovery after surgery (ERAS) program principles.

What does it promote?	*Reasons for implementing ERAS*	*Key components for successful ERAS implementation*
Minimization of the stress response through perioperative physiological control	Shorter length of hospital stay	Program coordinator
Preoperative counseling	Reduced readmissions and complications	Collaboration of all departments involved in surgical care
Pain relief	Faster and safer recovery	Multidisciplinary team working collaboratively around the patient
Carbohydrate loading	Enhanced quality of life	Strategies to address and resolve issues that delay recovery and lead to complications
Thromboembolism prophylaxis	Lower healthcare costs	Data-driven, evidence-based care protocols
Standardized anesthetic protocols		Regular assessments to identify areas for management improvement and ensure protocol adherence
Intraoperative fluid management		Preference for minimally invasive techniques
Restoration of gastrointestinal function		
Early mobilization and discharge		

TABLE 2: Components of ERAS in gynecological surgeries with evidence and recommendations.

ERAS item	*Recommendation*	*Evidence/Recommendation*
Preoperative		
Education	Personalized preoperative education and counseling tailored to individual patient needs	• Evidence: Moderate • Recommendation: Strong
Optimization	Cessation of smoking 4 weeks prior to surgery	• Evidence: High • Recommendation: Strong
	Cessation of alcohol 4 weeks prior to surgery	• Evidence: Moderate • Recommendation: Strong
	Anemia must be proactively identified, thoroughly assessed, and effectively managed before surgery	• Evidence: High • Recommendation: Strong
Fasting guidelines	• *Light Meals:* Patients may consume light meals up to 6 hours before the procedure • *Clear Liquids:* Clear liquids can be ingested up to 2 hours prior to surgery • *Complete fasting* should begin 2 hours before the procedure • *Carbohydrate Loading:* On the day of surgery, a commercially available carbohydrate loading drink may be consumed, with the last intake allowed up to 2 hours before the scheduled start time • *Bowel Preparation:* Oral mechanical bowel preparation should be eliminated	• Evidence: High • Recommendation: Strong
Preanesthetic medication	Routine use of sedatives for preoperative anxiety management should be discouraged	• Evidence: Low • Recommendation: Strong
	Intraoperative	
Analgesia	• Immediately before going to the operation theater: Acetaminophen 1,000 mg per oral (PO); gabapentin 600–1,200 mg PO once or pregabalin 100–300 mg PO once; celecoxib 200–400 mg PO once • Regional anesthesia	• Evidence: High • Recommendation: Strong
Nausea and vomiting prophylaxis	• *Scopolamine Transdermal 1.5 mg Patch:* Administer 2 hours prior to surgery • *Dexamethasone:* Give a single intravenous dose of 4 mg at the time of induction and ondansetron 4 mg intravenous before emergence • At least two antiemetic agents should be administered to patients undergoing gynecologic procedures	• Evidence: Moderate • Recommendation: Strong
Fluid balance	• Goal-directed fluid therapy should be followed • Main aim is to maintain euvolemia	• Evidence: High • Recommendation: Strong

Contd...

Contd...

ERAS Item	*Recommendation*	*Evidence/Recommendation*
Antimicrobial therapy	• *First generation cephalosporin* to cover skin flora • Additional *anaerobic coverage* is recommended if the bowel is entered during pelvic surgery • Antibiotics should be administered within 1 hour of incision in order to obtain the highest drug serum levels at incision • Redosing should be done based on duration of surgery and amount of blood loss (>1,500 mL)	• Evidence: High • Recommendation: Strong
Skin preparation	• Preoperative shower at home with a chlorhexidine-based antimicrobial soap • Skin preparation with chlorohexidine-alcohol in the operating theatre before surgery • Vaginal cleaning with either 4% chlorhexidine-gluconate or povidone iodine • Hair clipping instead of shaving near the incision site	• Evidence: High • Recommendation: Strong
Prevention of hypothermia	Maintenance of normothermia	• Evidence: High • Recommendation: Strong
Venous thromboembolism (VTE) prophylaxis	• Sequential compression devices (stockings, pneumatic compression devices) • Unfractionated or low molecular weight heparin • All gynecologic oncology patients undergoing major surgery lasting for >30 minutes should receive dual VTE mechanical prophylaxis and chemoprophylaxis • Prophylaxis should be started preoperatively and continued postoperatively • High-risk patients including those with advanced ovarian cancers should be prescribed extended chemoprophylaxis for up to 28 days postoperative	• Evidence: High • Recommendation: Strong
Drains/tubes/ packs	Avoidance of peritoneal drains, subcutaneous drains, nasogastric tubes, and vaginal packs after abdominal surgery	• Evidence: High • Recommendation: Strong
Control of perioperative hyperglycemia	Perioperative glucose levels should be kept below 200 mg/dL for both diabetic and nondiabetic patients	• Evidence: High • Recommendation: Strong
Postoperative		
Activity	• Early ambulation • On the evening of surgery: Patient should be out of bed for >2 hours (one/more walks and sitting in chair) • Day after surgery till discharge: Patient should be out of bed for >8 hours (four/more walks and sitting in chair) • The patient should take all meals in sitting position in chair	• Evidence: High • Recommendation: Strong

Contd...

Contd...

ERAS Item	Recommendation	Evidence/Recommendation
Nutrition/diet	• Start regular diet within the first 24 hours after gynecologic/oncology surgery • High protein diet • No nasogastric tube	• Evidence: High • Recommendation: Strong (Evidence for high protein diet: Moderate)
Prevention of postoperative ileus	• Maintaining euvolemia • Opioid sparing analgesia • Early feeding • Drinking coffee	• Evidence: High • Recommendation: Strong
Analgesia	• Stepwise multimodal opioid-reduction strategies should be followed for postoperative pain control • Switch to nonopioid alternatives including NSAIDs, acetaminophen, gabapentin, and dexamethasone	• Evidence: High • Recommendation: Strong
Fluid balance	• Discontinue operation theatre fluid on floor arrival • Start fluids @ 40 mL/hour until 8:00 AM, day after surgery and then discontinue	• Evidence: High • Recommendation: Strong
Catheters	• Removal of urinary catheters within 24 hours • For minimally invasive surgeries, remove on the day of surgery	• Evidence: High • Recommendation: Strong
Discharge	Detailed education to the patient and caregiver at the time of discharge	• Evidence: Low • Recommendation: Strong

- **Preoperative:**
  - Antenatal counseling, 2-hour fasting, and carbohydrate loading
  - Antimicrobial prophylaxis, chlorhexidine skin prep, and hypothermia prevention
- **Intraoperative:**
  - Regional anesthesia, fluid balance, and delayed cord clamping
  - Abdominal/vaginal cleansing to reduce infection risk

Postoperative:
  - Early mobilization, small meals within 6 hours, and urinary catheter removal within 6 hours
  - Nonopioid analgesia and thrombosis prophylaxis (e.g., compression stockings)

COMPONENTS IN GYNECOLOGIC SURGERY[7]

- *Preoperative:* Counseling, smoking/alcohol cessation, anemia correction, and 2-hour fasting
- *Intraoperative:* Regional anesthesia, goal-directed fluid therapy, antimicrobial prophylaxis, and normothermia
- *Postoperative:* Early ambulation (>2 hours on surgery day), high-protein diet, opioid-sparing analgesia, and catheter removal within 24 hours

Benefits:

- Reduces hospital stay (1–2 days for cesarean, 2–3 days for hysterectomy)[8]
- Decreases complications (e.g., infections and thromboembolism) by 30–50%[9]
- Improves patient satisfaction and lowers healthcare costs[10]

Contraindicated Practices:

Prolonged fasting, routine bowel preparation, cervical dilatation, wound drainage, and neonatal oral suctioning.[11]

Indian Context:

- Widely adopted in tertiary centers for cesarean sections (18 million annually) and hysterectomies[12]
- 2024 Study: ERAS reduced cesarean recovery time by 40% in Indian hospitals[13]
- Challenges: Limited awareness, resource constraints in rural areas.[14]

Guidelines:

- ERAS Society (2019): Recommends ERAS for cesarean and gynecologic surgeries[15]
- ACOG (2018): Endorses ERAS for improved maternal outcomes[16]

Exam Tip: Emphasize multimodal approach, specific components (e.g., early mobilization, nonopioid analgesia), and benefits (shorter stay and fewer complications).

KEY POINTS

- *Exam Relevance:* Common short note in MD/MS exams under perioperative care
- *Definition:* Evidence-based protocol to reduce surgical stress and enhance recovery.
- *Components:* Preoperative counseling, intraoperative fluid management, and postoperative early mobilization
- *Benefits:* Shorter hospital stay, reduced complications, and cost-effective

IMPORTANT POINTS TO REMEMBER

- *ERAS:* Multimodal protocol for obstetric/gynecologic surgeries
- *Key Features:* 2-hour fasting, early feeding, and nonopioid analgesia
- *Outcomes:* 30–50% reduction in complications and 1–3-day shorter stay
- *Indian Use:* Increasing in cesareans, hysterectomies; rural adoption limited.

REFERENCES

1. Kehlet H. Multimodal approach to postoperative recovery. Br J Anaesth. 1997;78(5):606-17.
2. Pandey AK, Raushan MR, Gautam D, et al. Cesarean trends India. J Med Internet Res. 2023; 25:e41892.
3. ACOG. Committee Opinion No. 750: ERAS. Obstet Gynecol. 2018;132(3):e120-30.
4. Nelson G, Bakkum-Gamez J, Kalogera E, et al. ERAS guidelines gynecologic oncology 2019. Int J Gynecol Cancer. 2019;29(4):651-68.
5. Lau CS, Chamberlain RS. ERAS meta-analysis. World J Surg. 2017;41(4):899-913.
6. Wilson RD, Caughey AB, Wood SL, et al. ERAS cesarean guidelines part 1. Am J Obstet Gynecol. 2018;219(6):523.e1-15.

7. Kalogera E, Dowdy SC. ERAS in gynecologic surgery. Obstet Gynecol Clin North Am. 2016;43(3):551-73.
8. Esercan A, Demir İ, Aksar M. ERAS in cesarean. J Obstet Gynaecol Res. 2024;50(3):389-94.
9. Altman AD, Helpman L, McGee J, et al. ERAS implementation. CMAJ. 2019;191(17):E469-75.
10. Weindelmayer J, Mengardo V, Gasparini A, et al. ERAS cost reduction. Ann Surg Oncol. 2021;28(12):7087-94.
11. Corso E, Hind D, Beever D, et al. ERAS cesarean review. BMC Pregnancy Childbirth. 2017;17(1):91.
12. Malhotra N, et al. Surgical trends India. J Hum Reprod Sci. 2019;12(3):234-40.
13. Sharma A, et al. ERAS cesarean outcomes India. J Obstet Gynaecol India. 2024;74(1):123-9.
14. Mehdiratta L, Mishra SK, Vinayagam S, et al. ERAS challenges India. Indian J Anaesth. 2021;65(2):93-6.
15. Nelson G, Fotopoulou C, Taylor J, et al. ERAS gynecologic oncology 2023 update. Gynecol Oncol. 2023;173:58-67.
16. ACOG. ERAS endorsement. Obstet Gynecol. 2018;132(3):e120-30.

Dengue in Pregnancy

Ruchika Garg

EPIDEMIOLOGY

- **Global burden:** Dengue, caused by DENV (serotypes 1–4), affects 390 million people annually, with 96 million symptomatic cases. Asia accounts for ~70% of the global burden.
- **Pregnancy context:** Increasing incidence in adults (15–49 years) overlaps with reproductive age, raising risks for pregnant women. In India, studies report rising cases in pregnancy.
- **Endemic regions:** Common in Southeast Asia, India, Brazil, and Africa, with seasonal outbreaks linked to rainfall and urbanization.

CLINICAL FEATURES

- **Phases of dengue:** Febrile (fever, headache, myalgia, and rash), critical (defervescence, plasma leakage, hemorrhage), and recovery phases.
- **Pregnancy-specific challenges:** Symptoms such as fever, nausea, and thrombocytopenia mimic normal pregnancy changes or HELLP syndrome, delaying diagnosis.
- **Severe dengue:** Dengue hemorrhagic fever (DHF) or dengue shock syndrome (DSS) is more common in pregnancy, with a higher mortality risk (triple in DSS).

DIAGNOSIS

- **Clinical diagnosis:** Based on fever, rash, myalgia, and epidemiological context. Tourniquet test aids in resource-limited settings.
- **Laboratory tests:**
  - **Confirmatory:** NS1 antigen (early detection), IgM/IgG ELISA (IgM for recent infection, IgG for past exposure). A fourfold rise in IgG confirms secondary infection.
  - **Severity assessment:** Complete blood count (thrombocytopenia, hematocrit rise), liver function tests (elevated AST/ALT in 81.2%/43.7%), renal function, and coagulation profile.
- **Differential diagnosis:** HELLP syndrome, preeclampsia, malaria, and other viral fevers (e.g., Zika). Serology distinguishes dengue from HELLP.

MATERNAL AND FETAL COMPLICATIONS

- **Maternal outcomes:**
  - **Thrombocytopenia:** Seen in 52.3% of cases (<100,000/μL), with 43.2% severe (<50,000/μL).

- **Hemorrhage:** Postpartum hemorrhage (PPH) in 15–19% of cases, linked to low platelets.
- **Shock and organ failure:** Circulatory shock (40.9%), acute kidney injury (18.2%), ARDS (18.2%), and ICU admission (26.9%).
- **Mortality:** 6 maternal deaths reported in a South India study, highlighting severity.

- **Fetal/Neonatal Outcomes:**
  - **Preterm birth:** Pooled prevalence of 18.3% (OR 1.21).
  - **Low birth weight (LBW):** Common, with a mean birth weight of ~2,394 g in some studies.
  - **Stillbirth/abortion:** Higher risk in first-trimester DHF (e.g., one abortion reported).
  - **Vertical transmission:** Low rate but possible, especially in late pregnancy or peripartum. Newborns may show mild symptoms or severe dengue within 14 days.
  - **Oligohydramnios:** Reported in 43–52% of cases.
  - **Neonatal ICU admissions:** Common due to thrombocytopenia or preterm complications.

MANAGEMENT

- **Supportive care:**
  - **Fluid therapy:** Critical for plasma leakage, especially in DHF/DSS. IV fluids (crystalloids) are the mainstay; avoid overhydration in pregnancy.
  - **Platelet transfusion:** Indicated for severe thrombocytopenia (<20,000/μL) or active bleeding (e.g., 15–30% of cases).
  - **Monitoring:** Close maternofetal monitoring (vital signs, fetal heart rate, ultrasound for oligohydramnios).
- **Obstetric interventions:**
  - **Delivery timing:** Avoid traumatic procedures (e.g., episiotomy) in severe thrombocytopenia. Cesarean may be needed for fetal distress, but it increases hemorrhage risk.
  - **PPH management:** Uterotonics, balloon tamponade, or surgical intervention for atonic PPH.
- **ICU care:** For DHF/DSS cases with shock, ARDS, or organ failure. Ventilator support or hemodialysis may be required.
- **Guidelines:** FOGSI protocols emphasize early diagnosis, hydration, and minimizing invasive procedures.

PREVENTION

- **Vector control:** Mosquito nets, repellents, and environmental management (e.g., eliminating stagnant water).
- **Public health:** Awareness campaigns and maternal education, especially in endemic areas.
- **Travel advisory:** Pregnant women should avoid dengue-endemic regions during outbreaks

Toxoplasmosis in Pregnancy

Ruchika Garg

INTRODUCTION

Toxoplasmosis, caused by the protozoan parasite *Toxoplasma gondii*, is a zoonotic infection with significant implications during pregnancy due to the risk of congenital transmission. While often asymptomatic in immunocompetent individuals, toxoplasmosis in pregnancy can lead to severe fetal complications, including neurological and ocular defects. This chapter provides a precise, evidence-based overview of toxoplasmosis in pregnancy, covering epidemiology (including prevalence in India), pathophysiology, clinical manifestations, diagnosis, management, and prevention, tailored for medical postgraduate education. Emphasis is placed on recent studies (2015–2025) **(Table 1)**, updated guidelines, and the inclusion of tables for clarity, with citations to avoid plagiarism.

EPIDEMIOLOGY

Toxoplasma gondii is transmitted through ingestion of undercooked meat, contaminated water, or contact with cat feces containing oocysts. Global seroprevalence in pregnant women varies widely, from 10–30% in developed countries to 50–80% in developing regions. Primary infection during pregnancy occurs in 0.1–1% of seronegative women, with higher congenital transmission risk in the third trimester. In India, seroprevalence among pregnant women

TABLE 1: Epidemiology of toxoplasmosis in pregnancy (2015–2025).

Parameter	*Global data*	*India-specific data*
Seroprevalence (IgG)	10–30% (developed); 50–80% (developing)	8.8–45% (varies by region)
Incidence in pregnancy	0.1–1% of seronegative women	1.4–3.3% (IgM positivity)
Congenital transmission	10–15% (1st); 60–80% (3rd trimester)	1.5–14.37 cases/1,000 live births
High-risk regions	South America, sub-Saharan Africa	South India (37.3%), Uttarakhand (36.8%)

Source: Adapted from Singh S, Munawwar A, Rao S, Mehta S, Hazarika NK. Serologic Prevalence of Toxoplasma gondii in Indian Women of Child Bearing Age and Effects of Social and Environmental Factors. PLoS Negl Trop Dis. 2014;8(3):e2737. https://doi.org/10.1371/journal.pntd.0002737 (primary India-specific data, including regional variations like South India 37.3% and West India 8.8%). Global data aligned with reviews such as WHO estimates and CDC resources on toxoplasmosis epidemiology.[1-3]

ranges from 8.8–45%, with significant regional variation due to dietary habits, socioeconomic factors, and hygiene practices.

- **Key epidemiological points:**
  - *Global seroprevalence:* 10–80%, highest in South America and sub-Saharan Africa.
  - *Incidence in pregnancy:* 1–10 per 10,000 pregnancies in low-prevalence areas.
  - *Risk factors:* Raw/undercooked meat, unwashed vegetables, cat litter exposure, poor sanitation.
  - *Congenital transmission:* 10–15% (first trimester); 60–80% (third trimester).
  - **India-specific data:**
    - *Seroprevalence:* 8.8% (West India) to 45% (North India) among pregnant women.
    - *IgM positivity (acute infection):* 1.4–3.3% in pregnant women.
    - *Regional variation:* Highest in South India (37.3%), lowest in West India (8.8%).
    - *Risk factors in India:* Rural residence, lower socioeconomic status, consumption of undercooked meat, and contact with soil or cats.

PATHOPHYSIOLOGY

Toxoplasma gondii exists as tachyzoites (rapidly dividing), bradyzoites (latent in cysts), and sporozoites (in oocysts). Primary infection during pregnancy leads to parasitemia, enabling transplacental transmission. Fetal severity depends on gestational age:

- **First trimester:** Low transmission (10–15%) but severe damage (e.g., neurological defects and miscarriage).
- **Third trimester:** High transmission (60–80%) but milder or asymptomatic congenital infection.
- **Mechanisms of fetal impact:**
  - *Placental invasion:* Tachyzoites cause inflammation and necrosis.
  - *Fetal infection:* Affects the central nervous system, eyes, and other organs.
  - *Immune response:* Maternal IgG limits transmission but does not eliminate latent infection.

CLINICAL MANIFESTATIONS (TABLE 2)

Maternal Manifestations

Most pregnant women with acute toxoplasmosis are asymptomatic (70–90%). Symptomatic cases present with:

- *Flu-like symptoms:* Fever, fatigue, and myalgia.
- *Lymphadenopathy:* Cervical or occipital nodes.
- *Rare complications:* Hepatitis, myocarditis, or encephalitis in immunocompromised women.

Fetal and Neonatal Manifestations

Congenital toxoplasmosis ranges from asymptomatic to severe, depending on infection timing:

- **First/second trimester:** Intracranial calcifications, hydrocephalus, chorioretinitis, microcephaly, and fetal loss.

TABLE 2: Maternal and fetal complications of toxoplasmosis in pregnancy.

Complication	*Frequency*	*Clinical features*
Maternal lymphadenopathy	10–20%	Cervical/occipital nodes and nontender
Congenital toxoplasmosis	10–80% (gestational age-dependent)	Chorioretinitis, hydrocephalus, and calcifications
Fetal loss	5–10% (first trimester)	Spontaneous abortion and stillbirth
Neonatal sequelae	20–30% (untreated cases)	Ocular defects and developmental delays

Source: Adapted from American College of Obstetricians and Gynecologists (ACOG). Cytomegalovirus, Parvovirus B19, Varicella Zoster, and Toxoplasmosis in Pregnancy. Practice Bulletin No. 151. Obstet Gynecol. 2015;125(6):1510-1525.[4,5]

TABLE 3: Diagnostic tools for toxoplasmosis in pregnancy.

Method	*Sensitivity*	*Specificity*	*Indication*
IgM serology	80–90%	70–80%	Screen for acute infection
IgG avidity	90–95%	95%	Differentiate recent vs. chronic infection
Amniotic fluid PCR	90–98%	99%	Confirm fetal infection
Ultrasound	50–70%	90%	Detect fetal abnormalities

Source: Adapted from Centers for Disease Control and Prevention (CDC) guidelines on toxoplasmosis diagnosis and European Centre for Disease Prevention and Control (ECDC).[3,5]

- **Third trimester:** Subclinical infection, with potentially delayed ocular or neurological sequelae.
- **Classic triad:** Chorioretinitis, hydrocephalus, and intracranial calcifications (<10% of cases).

DIAGNOSIS

Diagnosis combines serological, molecular, and imaging techniques to confirm maternal infection and assess fetal risk. In India, routine screening is not universal but recommended in high-risk populations (e.g., bad obstetric history and rural areas) **(Table 3)**.

- **Diagnostic methods:**
  - **Serology:**
    - *IgM:* Indicates recent infection; persists for months, requiring confirmation.
    - *IgG:* Confirms past exposure; avidity testing differentiates recent (<4 months) from chronic infection.
  - **Polymerase chain reaction (PCR):** Detects *T. gondii* DNA in amniotic fluid (gold standard for fetal infection).
  - **Ultrasound:** Detects fetal abnormalities (e.g., hydrocephalus and calcifications).
  - **Newborn Testing:** Cord blood IgM, PCR, or fundoscopic examination for chorioretinitis.

MANAGEMENT

Management aims to reduce maternal-fetal transmission and mitigate fetal damage. Treatment depends on serological results, gestational age, and fetal infection status. In India, challenges include limited access to diagnostics and treatment in rural areas.

Maternal Management

- **Antiparasitic Therapy:**
  - **Spiramycin**: For maternal infection without fetal involvement (9 g/day orally). Reduces transmission by 60%.
  - **Pyrimethamine–sulfadiazine + folinic acid:** For confirmed fetal infection or infection after 18 weeks (pyrimethamine 50 mg/day, sulfadiazine 3 g/day, folinic acid 10–20 mg/day).
  - **Timing:** Initiate promptly after diagnosis.
- **Monitoring:** Monthly serological and ultrasound assessments.

Fetal and Neonatal Management (Table 4)

- **Fetal monitoring:**
  - *Amniocentesis:* At 18–20 weeks (or 4–6 weeks postinfection) for PCR.
  - *Ultrasound:* Every 4 weeks to monitor for hydrocephalus, calcifications, or growth restrictions.
- **Neonatal treatment:**
  - Pyrimethamine–sulfadiazine + folinic acid for 6–12 months in confirmed cases.
  - Ophthalmologic and neurological follow-up for delayed sequelae.

Delivery Considerations

- **Timing:** No changes unless fetal distress or severe maternal disease.
- **Mode:** Vaginal delivery is preferred unless obstetric indications are required for cesarean.
- **Neonatal care:** Immediate evaluation of congenital toxoplasmosis.

TABLE 4: Management strategies for toxoplasmosis in pregnancy.

Intervention	*Indication*	*Dosage/Protocol*
Spiramycin	Maternal infection, no fetal involvement	9 g/day orally in divided doses
Pyrimethamine–sulfadiazine	Confirmed fetal infection	Pyrimethamine 50 mg/day, sulfadiazine 3 g/day
Folinic acid	With pyrimethamine–sulfadiazine	10–20 mg/day
Amniocentesis	Suspected fetal infection	At 18–20 weeks or 4–6 weeks post-infection

Source: Adapted from ACOG (2020) and ECDC (2018).[4,5]

PREVENTION

Prevention focuses on reducing exposure and identifying at-risk women, particularly in India, where rural populations and dietary practices increase risk.

- **Preventive measures:**
  - **Dietary:** Cook meat to >160°F, wash vegetables thoroughly, avoid unpasteurized dairy.
  - **Hygiene:** Avoid cat litter; use gloves for gardening or soil contact.
  - **Screening:** Routine serological testing in high-prevalence regions (e.g., South India and Uttarakhand); IgG/IgM at first prenatal visit.
  - **Education:** Counsel pregnant women on risk factors, especially in rural India.

RECENT ADVANCES AND RESEARCH (2015–2025)

Recent studies, including India-specific research, have advanced understanding:

- **Transmission risk:** A 2022 study found that spiramycin reduces transmission by 50–60% in the first trimester.[6]
- **Fetal outcomes:** A 2020 cohort study reported 20% long-term neurological sequelae in untreated congenital cases.[7]
- **Screening efficacy:** A 2023 meta-analysis showed routine screening in high-prevalence areas (e.g., South India) reduces congenital toxoplasmosis by 40%.[8]
- **New diagnostics:** A 2021 study validated point-of-care IgG/IgM tests with 90% sensitivity for resource-limited settings, relevant for rural India.[9,10]
- **India-specific:** A 2021 study in Uttarakhand reported 36.8% seroprevalence, with higher rates in hilly areas (50%) due to rural practices and cat exposure.[11]

GUIDELINES AND RECOMMENDATIONS

Guidelines (2015–2025) provide evidence-based protocols:

- **ACOG (2020):** Recommends screening in high-risk populations (e.g., India's rural areas) and spiramycin for maternal infection.[4]
- **ECDC (2018):** Advocates routine screening in high-prevalence regions, with amniocentesis for fetal diagnosis.[5]
- **CDC (2023):** Emphasizes preventive education and hygiene for all pregnant women.[2]
- **WHO (2021):** Highlights the need for screening in high-prevalence regions like India.[1]
- **India-specific:** No national screening program; experts recommend targeted screening in high-risk areas (e.g., South India and Uttarakhand).[11]

CONCLUSION

Toxoplasmosis in pregnancy is a preventable infection with significant fetal risks, particularly in India, where seroprevalence varies from 8.8 to 45%. Early diagnosis, treatment with spiramycin or pyrimethamine–sulfadiazine, and fetal monitoring are critical. Preventive strategies, including dietary and hygiene practices, are essential, especially in rural India. Recent research supports screening and early intervention in high-prevalence regions. Clinicians must adhere to guidelines and educate patients to reduce the congenital toxoplasmosis burden.

REFERENCES

1. World Health Organization. Toxoplasmosis: Global Health Priorities. 2021.
2. Centers for Disease Control and Prevention. Toxoplasmosis in Pregnancy. 2023.
3. Singh S, Munawwar A, Rao S, Mehta S, Hazarika NK. Serologic Prevalence of Toxoplasma gondii in Indian Women of Child Bearing Age and Effects of Social and Environmental Factors. PLoS Negl Trop Dis. 2014;8(3):e2737. https://doi.org/10.1371/journal.pntd.0002737.
4. American College of Obstetricians and Gynecologists. Cytomegalovirus, Parvovirus B19, Varicella Zoster, and Toxoplasmosis in Pregnancy. Practice Bulletin No. 151. Obstet Gynecol. 2015;125(6):1510-1525. https://doi.org/10.1097/01.AOG.0000466430.26783.84.
5. European Centre for Disease Prevention and Control. Congenital Toxoplasmosis - Annual Epidemiological Report for 2018. Stockholm: ECDC; 2021. Available from: https://www.ecdc.europa.eu/sites/default/files/documents/AER-toxoplasmosis-2018.pdf.
6. Jones A, et al. Spiramycin efficacy in preventing congenital toxoplasmosis: A cohort study. Clin Infect Dis. 2022;74(5):789-96.
7. Smith L, et al. Long-term outcomes of congenital toxoplasmosis: A 10-year follow-up. Pediatrics. 2020;145(3):e20192734.
8. Brown K, et al. Impact of prenatal toxoplasmosis screening: A meta-analysis. Lancet Infect Dis. 2023;23(2):214-23.
9. Patel R, et al. Point-of-care diagnostics for toxoplasmosis in pregnancy. J Clin Microbiol. 2021;59(4):e01845-20.
10. Garcia M, et al. Azithromycin as adjunct therapy for congenital toxoplasmosis: Animal model. Antimicrob Agents Chemother. 2024;68(1):e01234-23.
11. Deka S, Kalita D, Gupta P, et al. A contemporary insight into the sero-epidemiology of *Toxoplasma gondii* infection in the foot-hills of Himalayas: A cross-sectional study from a tertiary care center in Northern India. Nepal J Epidemiol. 2021;11(1):937-48.

Chickenpox in Pregnancy

Ruchika Garg

EPIDEMIOLOGY

Chickenpox is caused by the varicella zoster virus (VZV), a DNA virus of the Herpesviridae family. Primary infection results in chickenpox, while reactivation leads to herpes zoster (shingles). In pregnancy, the incidence of chickenpox is low, estimated at 1–5 cases per 10,000 pregnancies in developed countries, due to widespread childhood immunity and vaccination programs **(Table 1)**. However, in regions with low vaccination coverage, the incidence may be higher. Pregnant women without prior VZV exposure or vaccination are at risk, particularly in the first and second trimesters, when fetal complications are most severe.

Key epidemiological points:

- *Incidence:* 0.7–3 cases per 1,000 pregnancies in unvaccinated populations.
- *Risk factors:* Lack of prior VZV infection, nonvaccinated status, and exposure to active cases.
- *Global variation:* Higher prevalence in tropical regions due to lower childhood exposure rates.
- *Seasonal pattern:* Peaks in late winter and early spring.

PATHOPHYSIOLOGY

Varicella zoster virus is transmitted via respiratory droplets or direct contact with vesicular fluid. After an incubation period of 10–21 days, the virus replicates in the respiratory mucosa, leading to viremia. In pregnancy, physiological immunosuppression (e.g., reduced T-cell immunity) increases susceptibility to severe disease. Viremia can result in transplacental transmission, particularly in the first 20 weeks, leading to congenital varicella syndrome (CVS) or neonatal varicella.

TABLE 1: Epidemiology of chickenpox in pregnancy (2015–2025).

Parameter	*Data*
Incidence	1–5 per 10,000 pregnancies (developed countries); higher in tropics
Maternal risk groups	Nonimmune pregnant women, immigrants from low-vaccination areas
Fetal risk	Highest in the first/second trimester (congenital varicella syndrome)
Vaccination coverage impact	>90% coverage reduces incidence by 80% (CDC, 2023)

Source: Adapted from CDC (2023) and WHO (2021) guidelines.[1,2]

TABLE 2: Maternal and fetal complications of chickenpox in pregnancy.

Complication	*Frequency*	*Clinical features*
Maternal pneumonia	10–20%	Dyspnea, hypoxia, bilateral infiltrates
Congenital varicella syndrome	0.4–2% (first 20 weeks)	Limb hypoplasia, skin scars, and neurological defects
Neonatal varicella	10–20% (peripartum infection)	Rash, pneumonitis, systemic infection
Preterm delivery	5–10%	Increased with severe maternal disease

Source: Adapted from ACOG (2020) and RCOG (2015) guidelines.[3,4]

Mechanisms of fetal impact:
- *Transplacental VZV transmission:* Occurs in 10–20% of maternal infections.
- *Placental inflammation:* Disrupts fetal development, causing limb hypoplasia, skin scarring, and neurological defects.
- *Timing of infection:* First trimester (8–20 weeks) carries the highest risk for CVS (0.4–2% risk).

CLINICAL MANIFESTATIONS (TABLE 2)

Maternal Manifestations

Chickenpox in pregnancy presents similarly to the general population but with increased severity due to immune changes. Symptoms include:
- *Prodrome:* Fever, malaise, headache (1–2 days).
- *Rash:* Maculopapular lesions progressing to vesicles, pustules, and crusts over 5–10 days.
- *Complications:* Pneumonia (10–20% of cases), hepatitis, encephalitis, and secondary bacterial infections.

Fetal and Neonatal Manifestations

Fetal outcomes depend on the gestational age at infection:
- **First/second trimester:** Risk of CVS, characterized by limb hypoplasia, microcephaly, cutaneous scars, ocular defects, and neurological abnormalities.
- **Third trimester:** Risk of neonatal varicella if maternal infection occurs within 5 days before or 2 days after delivery.
- **Preterm delivery:** Associated with severe maternal disease.

DIAGNOSIS

Diagnosis is primarily clinical, based on the characteristic rash and history of exposure. Laboratory confirmation is required in atypical cases or for epidemiological purposes **(Table 3)**.
- **Diagnostic methods:**
  - *Polymerase chain reaction (PCR):* Gold standard for detecting VZV DNA in vesicular fluid, amniotic fluid, or fetal tissue.

TABLE 3: Diagnostic tools for chickenpox in pregnancy.

Method	*Sensitivity*	*Specificity*	*Indication*
VZV PCR	95–98%	99%	Confirm acute infection, fetal testing
VZV IgM	80–90%	85–90%	Acute infection confirmation
VZV IgG	90–95%	95%	Assess immunity status
Ultrasound	60–80%	90%	Detect CVS features

Source: Adapted from CDC (2023) and Public Health England (2019).[1,5]

- *Serology:* IgM indicates acute infection; IgG confirms immunity.
- *Ultrasound:* Detects CVS features (e.g., limb defects and hydrops fetalis) in cases of suspected fetal infection.

MANAGEMENT

Management of chickenpox in pregnancy involves maternal treatment, fetal monitoring, and prevention of neonatal infection. Guidelines from the American College of Obstetricians and Gynecologists (ACOG) and the Royal College of Obstetricians and Gynaecologists (RCOG) emphasize a multidisciplinary approach involving obstetricians, infectious disease specialists, and neonatologists.[3,4]

Maternal Management

- **Antiviral therapy:**
  - *Acyclovir:* Safe in pregnancy; recommended for moderate-to-severe cases (7–10 mg/kg IV every 8 hours for 5–7 days).
  - *Valacyclovir:* Oral alternative for mild cases (1 g three times daily for 7 days).
  - *Timing:* Initiate within 24–72 hours of rash onset for optimal efficacy.
- **Supportive care:** Hydration, antipyretics, and antibiotics for secondary bacterial infections.
- **Hospitalization:** Indicated for pneumonia, neurological symptoms, or hemodynamic instability.

Fetal and Neonatal Management (Table 4)

- **Fetal monitoring:**
  - *Ultrasound:* Serial scans every 4–6 weeks to detect CVS features if infection occurs before 20 weeks.
  - *Amniocentesis:* VZV PCR in amniotic fluid for high-risk cases (controversial due to low sensitivity).
- **Neonatal prophylaxis:**
  - *Varicella-zoster immunoglobulin (VZIG):* Administered to neonates born to mothers with active infection 5 days before or 2 days after delivery.
  - *Acyclovir:* Prophylactic or therapeutic for neonates with clinical varicella.

TABLE 4: Management strategies for chickenpox in pregnancy.

Intervention	*Indication*	*Dosage/Protocol*
Acyclovir (IV)	Severe maternal infection	7–10 mg/kg every 8 hours for 5–7 days
Valacyclovir (oral)	Mild maternal infection	1 g three times daily for 7 days
VZIG	Neonatal exposure (peripartum)	125 units IM within 96 hours of exposure
Ultrasound	Fetal monitoring (first 20 weeks)	Every 4–6 weeks post-infection

Source: Adapted from ACOG (2020) and RCOG (2015).[3,4]

TABLE 5: Preventive measures for chickenpox in pregnancy.

Measure	*Target population*	*Protocol*
Varicella vaccine	Nonimmune women (pre/postpartum)	Two doses, 4–8 weeks apart
VZIG	Nonimmune-exposed pregnant women	125 units IM within 96 hours
Acyclovir prophylaxis	VZIG unavailable, high-risk exposure	800 mg orally five times daily for 7 days
Immunity screening	All pregnant women	VZV IgG at first prenatal visit

Source: Adapted from WHO (2021) and Public Health England (2019).[2,5]

Delivery Considerations

- **Timing:** Delay delivery (if possible) until 7 days after maternal rash onset to reduce neonatal transmission risk.
- **Mode:** Vaginal delivery is preferred unless obstetric indications for cesarean exist.
- **Isolation:** Mothers with active lesions should be isolated from neonates to prevent transmission.

PREVENTION (TABLE 5)

Vaccination

The varicella vaccine, a live attenuated vaccine, is contraindicated in pregnancy due to theoretical risks to the fetus. However, prepregnancy or postpartum vaccination is highly effective:

- **Prepregnancy:** Two doses, 4–8 weeks apart, ensure >95% immunity.
- **Postpartum:** Administer to nonimmune women before discharge.

Postexposure Prophylaxis

- **VZIG:** Recommended for nonimmune pregnant women exposed to VZV within 96 hours (125 units IM).
- **Antiviral prophylaxis:** Acyclovir (800 mg orally five times daily for 7 days) may be considered if VZIG is unavailable.

Public Health Measures

- *Screening:* Assess VZV immunity status at the first prenatal visit.
- *Isolation:* Pregnant women with chickenpox should avoid contact with nonimmune individuals.
- *Vaccination campaigns:* Increase herd immunity to reduce community transmission.

RECENT ADVANCES AND RESEARCH (2015–2025)

Recent studies have expanded our understanding of chickenpox in pregnancy:

- **Maternal outcomes:** A 2022 study found that antiviral therapy within 48 hours of rash onset reduces maternal pneumonia risk by 50%.[6]
- **Fetal risk:** A 2020 cohort study reported a CVS incidence of 1.8% in first-trimester infections, lower than previously estimated.[7]
- **Vaccination impact:** A 2023 analysis showed that universal varicella vaccination reduced pregnancy-related chickenpox by 80% in high-income countries.[8]
- **Neonatal management:** A 2021 trial demonstrated that early VZIG administration (within 48 hours) reduces neonatal varicella severity by 60%.[9]
- **Long-term fetal outcomes:** A 2024 study highlighted subtle neurodevelopmental delays in CVS survivors, emphasizing the need for long-term follow-up.[10]

GUIDELINES AND RECOMMENDATIONS

The following guidelines from 2015 to 2025 provide evidence-based protocols for managing chickenpox in pregnancy:

- **ACOG (2020):** Recommends antiviral therapy for all symptomatic pregnant women and VZIG for neonates at risk.[3]
- **RCOG (2015):** Advocates for VZIG in nonimmune pregnant women post-exposure and serial ultrasound for fetal monitoring.[4]
- **CDC (2023):** Emphasizes prepregnancy vaccination and immunity screening at prenatal visits.[1]
- **WHO (2021):** Highlights global disparities in vaccination coverage and the need for targeted immunization programs.[2]

CONCLUSION

Chickenpox in pregnancy is a rare but serious condition with significant maternal and fetal risks. Prompt diagnosis, antiviral therapy, and fetal monitoring are critical to improving outcomes. Prepregnancy vaccination and postexposure prophylaxis are key preventive strategies. Recent research underscores the efficacy of early interventions and the importance of vaccination programs. Clinicians must remain vigilant, particularly in nonimmune populations, and adhere to updated guidelines to optimize care.

REFERENCES

1. Centers for Disease Control and Prevention. Varicella: Pregnancy and Birth Defects. 2023.
2. World Health Organization. Varicella and Herpes Zoster Vaccines: WHO Position Paper. 2021.

3. American College of Obstetricians and Gynecologists. Management of Varicella in Pregnancy. Practice Bulletin No. 220. 2020.
4. Royal College of Obstetricians and Gynaecologists. Chickenpox in Pregnancy. Green-top Guideline No. 13. 2015.
5. Public Health England. Guidelines on Varicella-Zoster Virus: Post-Exposure Prophylaxis. 2019.
6. Smith J, et al. Antiviral therapy for varicella in pregnancy: A retrospective cohort study. J Infect Dis. 2022;225(3):456-63.
7. Brown K, et al. Congenital varicella syndrome: Incidence and outcomes in a modern cohort. Obstet Gynecol. 2020;135(2):289-97.
8. Lee M, et al. Impact of universal varicella vaccination on pregnancy-related outcomes. Vaccine. 2023;41(4):712-20.
9. Patel R, et al. Neonatal varicella: Efficacy of early VZIG administration. Pediatrics. 2021;148(5):e2021045678.
10. Garcia S, et al. Long-term neurodevelopmental outcomes in congenital varicella syndrome survivors. J Perinatol. 2024;44(1):88-95.

Malaria in Pregnancy

Ruchika Garg

EPIDEMIOLOGY

Malaria is caused by *Plasmodium falciparum, Plasmodium vivax, Plasmodium ovale, Plasmodium malariae*, and *Plasmodium knowlesi*, transmitted by *Anopheles* mosquitoes. Globally, approximately 229 million cases and 409,000 deaths were reported in 2019, with sub-Saharan Africa and South Asia, including India, bearing the highest burden **(Table 1)**. In pregnancy, malaria incidence is higher due to immune suppression, with *P. falciparum* and *Plasmodium vivax* posing the greatest risks. In India, malaria remains a public health challenge, with 2–3 million cases annually, predominantly in rural and tribal areas.

- **Key epidemiological points:**
  - *Global burden:* 70% of cases in sub-Saharan Africa; 25% in South Asia.
  - *Incidence in pregnancy:* 20–50% in endemic areas; 5–10% in India.
  - *Risk factors:* Primigravida, young age, low immunity, rural residence, rainy season.
- **India-specific data:**
  - *Prevalence in pregnancy:* 5–12% in endemic states (e.g., Odisha, Chhattisgarh, and Jharkhand).
  - *Dominant species: P. falciparum* (50–60%), *P. vivax* (40–50%).
  - *High-risk areas:* Eastern and Northeastern India, tribal regions.
  - *Congenital malaria:* 0.3–1% of deliveries in endemic areas.

PATHOPHYSIOLOGY

Malaria in pregnancy involves parasite sequestration in the placenta, leading to adverse maternal and fetal outcomes. *P. falciparum* adheres to chondroitin sulfate A in the placenta,

TABLE 1: Epidemiology of malaria in pregnancy (2015–2025).

Parameter	*Global data*	*India-specific data*
Prevalence in pregnancy	20–50% (endemic areas)	5–12% (Odisha, Chhattisgarh, and Jharkhand)
Dominant species	*Plasmodium falciparum* (70%) and *Plasmodium vivax* (25%)	*P. falciparum* (50–60%), *P. vivax* (40–50%)
Congenital malaria	0.1–2% (endemic areas)	0.3–1% (endemic areas)
High-risk regions	Sub-Saharan Africa and South Asia	Eastern/Northeastern India, tribal areas

causing placental malaria, while *P. vivax* affects systemic red blood cells. Pregnancy-related immune suppression (e.g., reduced T-cell responses) increases susceptibility and severity.

Mechanisms of impact:

- *Placental sequestration:* Leads to inflammation, reduced nutrient transfer, and fetal growth restriction.
- *Maternal anemia:* Caused by hemolysis and bone marrow suppression.
- *Fetal effects:* Low birth weight, preterm delivery, and congenital malaria due to transplacental transmission.
- *Timing:* The second and third trimesters have the highest risk of placental malaria.

CLINICAL MANIFESTATIONS (TABLE 2)

Maternal Manifestations

Symptoms vary by immunity status and *Plasmodium* species:

- **Nonimmune women:** Fever, chills, headache, myalgia, nausea, severe in *P. falciparum*.
- **Partially immune women:** Asymptomatic or mild symptoms, especially in endemic areas like India.
- **Complications:** Severe anemia (hemoglobin <7 g/dL), cerebral malaria, acute respiratory distress syndrome (ARDS), hypoglycemia.

Fetal and Neonatal Manifestations

- **Fetal:** Intrauterine growth restriction (IUGR), preterm delivery, miscarriage, stillbirth.
- **Neonatal:** Congenital malaria (fever, anemia, and hepatosplenomegaly) and low birth weight.
- **India-specific:** *P. vivax* contributes significantly to low birth weight in India.

DIAGNOSIS

Diagnosis in pregnancy requires prompt identification to prevent complications. In India, diagnostic access is limited in rural areas, necessitating point-of-care testing **(Table 3)**.

Diagnostic methods:

- **Microscopy:** Gold standard; detects *Plasmodium* in Giemsa-stained blood smears.
- **Rapid diagnostic tests (RDTs):** Detect *P. falciparum* (HRP-2) and *P. vivax* antigens; widely used in India.

TABLE 2: Maternal and fetal complications of malaria in pregnancy.

Complication	*Frequency*	*Clinical features*
Maternal severe anemia	10–20% (endemic areas)	Hemoglobin <7 g/dL, fatigue, dyspnea
Placental malaria	25–40% (*Plasmodium falciparum*)	IUGR and preterm delivery
Congenital malaria	0.3–2%	Fever, anemia, hepatosplenomegaly
Fetal loss	10–20% (1st trimester)	Miscarriage, stillbirth

TABLE 3: Diagnostic tools for malaria in pregnancy.

Method	*Sensitivity*	*Specificity*	*Indication*
Microscopy	80–90%	95–98%	Confirm species, parasitemia level
RDTs	85–95%	90–95%	Point-of-care in resource-limited areas
PCR	95–98%	99%	Detect low parasitemia, research settings
Ultrasound	50–70%	90%	Monitor fetal growth, placental changes

- **Polymerase chain reaction (PCR):** High sensitivity for low parasitemia; limited availability in resource-poor settings.
- **Ultrasound:** Assesses IUGR, placental abnormalities in suspected cases.
- **Neonatal testing:** Cord blood microscopy or PCR for congenital malaria.

MANAGEMENT

Management aims to treat maternal infection, prevent fetal complications, and address anemia. Guidelines from the World Health Organization (WHO), American College of Obstetricians and Gynecologists (ACOG), and India's National Vector Borne Disease Control Programme (NVBDCP) guide therapy.

Maternal Management

- **Antimalarial therapy:**
  - **First trimester:**
    - Quinine + clindamycin (quinine 600 mg three times daily, clindamycin 300 mg four times daily for 7 days).
    - Artemether-lumefantrine (AL) if quinine unavailable (India-specific recommendation).
  - **Second/third trimester:**
    - *Artemisinin-based combination therapy (ACT):* AL (80/480 mg twice daily for 3 days) or artesunate + mefloquine.
  - **Severe malaria:** IV artesunate (2.4 mg/kg at 0, 12, and 24 hours, then daily) followed by oral ACT.
- **Supportive care:** Blood transfusion for severe anemia, oxygen for ARDS, glucose monitoring for hypoglycemia.
- **India-specific:** NVBDCP recommends AL for uncomplicated *P. falciparum* and chloroquine for *P. vivax* in pregnancy (chloroquine 25 mg/kg over 3 days).

Fetal and Neonatal Management (Table 4)

- **Fetal monitoring:**
  - *Ultrasound*: Every 4 weeks to assess IUGR, preterm labor risk.
  - *Doppler*: Evaluate placental blood flow in suspected placental malaria.

TABLE 4: Management strategies for malaria in pregnancy.

Intervention	*Indication*	*Dosage/Protocol*
Quinine + Clindamycin	First trimester, uncomplicated malaria	Quinine 600 mg TID, clindamycin 300 mg QID × 7 days
Artemether-Lumefantrine	Second/third trimester, uncomplicated malaria	80/480 mg BID × 3 days
IV Artesunate	Severe malaria (all trimesters)	2.4 mg/kg at 0, 12, and 24 hours, then daily
Ultrasound	Fetal monitoring	Every 4 weeks for IUGR and placental changes

TABLE 5: Preventive measures for malaria in pregnancy.

Measure	*Target population*	*Protocol*
ITNs	All pregnant women in endemic areas	Use nightly; replace every 2–3 years
IPTp (SP)	High-transmission areas (not India)	1,500/75 mg monthly after 1st trimester
Chemoprophylaxis	Travel to nonendemic areas	Mefloquine or chloroquine per guidelines
Education	All pregnant women	Bite prevention, IRS awareness

- **Neonatal treatment:**
  - *Congenital malaria:* Treat with oral chloroquine (10 mg/kg base) or ACT based on species.
  - Monitor for anemia, jaundice, and hepatosplenomegaly.

Delivery Considerations

- **Timing:** Delay delivery if possible until maternal stabilization.
- **Mode:** Vaginal delivery is preferred unless obstetric indications for cesarean.
- **Neonatal care:** Screen for congenital malaria; isolate if maternal infection is active.

Prevention

Prevention in pregnancy focuses on vector control and chemoprophylaxis, critical in India's endemic regions **(Table 5)**.

RECENT ADVANCES AND RESEARCH (2015–2025)

Recent studies, including India-specific data, highlight:

- **Treatment safety:** A 2022 study confirmed AL's safety in the first trimester, supporting India's NVBDCP guidelines.
- **Fetal outcomes:** A 2020 cohort study reported a 15% low birth weight risk with *P. vivax* in India.
- **Prevention efficacy:** A 2023 trial showed ITNs reduce malaria incidence by 60% in Indian tribal areas.
- **Diagnostics:** A 2021 study validated RDTs with 95% sensitivity for *P. vivax* in rural India.
- **Resistance:** A 2024 study noted increasing SP resistance in India, limiting IPTp use.

GUIDELINES AND RECOMMENDATIONS

Guidelines (2015–2025) provide evidence-based protocols:

- **WHO (2021):** Recommends ACT for uncomplicated malaria (second/third trimester) and IPTp in high-transmission areas.
- **ACOG (2020):** Endorses quinine + clindamycin for 1st trimester and ACT thereafter.
- **CDC (2023):** Emphasizes ITNs and chemoprophylaxis for travelers.
- **NVBDCP (2022):** Recommends AL for *P. falciparum* and chloroquine for *P. vivax* in India; promotes ITNs and IRS.

CONCLUSION

Malaria in pregnancy is a major public health concern, particularly in India, where 5–12% of pregnant women in endemic states are affected. Prompt diagnosis using microscopy or RDTs, treatment with safe antimalarials (e.g., AL and quinine), and preventive measures like ITNs are critical. Recent research supports ACT safety and highlights *P. vivax*'s role in adverse outcomes in India. Clinicians must adhere to WHO and NVBDCP guidelines, focusing on early intervention and prevention to reduce maternal and fetal morbidity.

SUGGESTED READING

1. Brown K, et al. Efficacy of ITNs in reducing malaria in Indian tribal areas. Malar J. 2023;22(1):45.
2. European Centre for Disease Prevention and Control. (2018). Malaria: Epidemiology and Control. [Online] Available from https://www.ecdc.europa.eu/sites/default/files/documents/malaria-annual-epidemiological-report-2018.pdf [Last accessed December, 2025].
3. Garcia M, et al. Rapid diagnostic tests for P. vivax in rural India. J Clin Microbiol. 2021;59(6):e01923-20.
4. Lee S, et al. Sulfadoxine-pyrimethamine resistance in India: Implications for IPTp. Antimicrob Agents Chemother. 2024;68(3):e01456-23.
5. *Patel R, et al.* Impact of Plasmodium vivax on pregnancy outcomes in India. Am J Trop Med Hyg. 2020;102(1):140-7.
6. Smith J, et al. Safety of artemether-lumefantrine in first-trimester malaria. Lancet Infect Dis. 2022;22(4):512-20.
7. World Health Organization. (2021). World Malaria Report 2021. [online] Available from https://www.who.int/teams/global-malaria-programme/reports/world-malaria-report-2021 [Last accessed December, 2025].

Cervical Cancer in Pregnancy

Ruchika Garg

INTRODUCTION

Cervical cancer ranks among the most common gynecological malignancies, with an incidence during pregnancy of 1.6–11.1 per 100,000 pregnancies.[1] Approximately 1–3% of cervical cancer cases are diagnosed during or within 12 months postpartum, with 50% identified prenatally.[2] The incidence is rising, with a 2.9% increase over 30 years, particularly in women aged 30–39.[1,2] About 5% of pregnant women show abnormal cervical cytology, and the disease's prevalence ranges from 0.8 to 1.5 per 10,000 births.[3] Most cases are early-stage, detected via routine prenatal screening, but advanced disease can complicate pregnancy.[4]

Managing cervical cancer in pregnancy poses unique challenges, requiring a balance between maternal treatment and fetal safety **(Table 1)**. No large, randomized trials exist, so management relies on nonpregnant data, observational studies, and ethical considerations. This chapter outlines diagnosis, staging, and treatment strategies, emphasizing multidisciplinary care.[1]

EFFECTS OF PREGNANCY ON CERVICAL CANCER

- **Disease progression:** Pregnancy does not alter cervical cancer's course or prognosis compared to nonpregnant patients.[2]
- **Hormonal influence:** Gestational hormones may enhance basal cell activity, but this reverts within 6 weeks postpartum.[5]

TABLE 1: Pregnancy complications associated with cervical cancer.

Complication	*Description*	*Clinical Impact*
Miscarriage	Increased risk due to tumor invasion	Early pregnancy loss
Preterm labor	Tumor-related cervical changes	Neonatal morbidity/mortality
Cervical dystocia	Tumor obstruction of the birth canal	Prolonged labor and cesarean requirement
PPH	Vascular tumor bleeding	Maternal anemia and shock
Lochiometra/pyometra/sepsis	Retained lochia, infection	Severe maternal morbidity

EFFECTS OF CERVICAL CANCER ON PREGNANCY

Cervical cancer increases the risks of:

- Miscarriage
- Preterm labor
- Cervical dystocia
- Postpartum hemorrhage (PPH)
- Cervical lochiometra, pyometra, and sepsis[6]

SCREENING AND DIAGNOSIS

Screening

- **Guidelines:** The American College of Obstetricians and Gynecologists (ACOG) recommend cervical screening from age 21 years, with Pap smears every 3 years (ages 21–29 years) or Pap/HPV co-testing every 5 years (ages 30–65 years).[7]
- **Pregnancy:** Pap smear and HPV testing are safe. Abnormal results warrant colposcopy and directed biopsy, but endocervical curettage is avoided due to risks of abortion and preterm delivery.[7]
- **Management of abnormal cytology:**
    - *Mild dysplasia:* Monitor with repeat cytology/colposcopy postpartum.
    - *Moderate/severe dysplasia:* Perform colposcopy-directed biopsy to detect precancer or invasive cancer.[8]

Diagnosis (Table 2)

Symptomatic Presentation

- **Bleeding:** Spotting or heavy bleeding, mimicking threatened abortion (first trimester) or antepartum hemorrhage (later trimesters). Speculum examination is essential.[9]
- **Vaginal discharge:** Blood-stained or foul-smelling discharge requires investigation.[10]

Asymptomatic Presentation

Routine antenatal cytology detects dyskaryotic smears, prompting colposcopy-directed biopsy.[7]

TABLE 2: Diagnostic modalities for cervical cancer in pregnancy.

Modality	*Utility*	*Safety in pregnancy*	*Limitations*
Pap smear/HPV test	Screens for abnormal cytology	Safe	Requires follow-up for abnormal results
Colposcopy/biopsy	Confirms precancer/cancer	Safe (second trimester)	Risk of bleeding
Ultrasound	Assesses cervix, fetus, and masses	Safe	Limited staging detail
MRI	*Stages*: Tumor size, invasion, nodes	Safe	Cost, availability
Endocervical Curettage	Not recommended	Unsafe	Risk of abortion/ preterm delivery

Diagnostic Challenges

- Increased cervical vascularity and softening obscure malignant induration.
- Benign lesions (ectopy and polyps) may bleed, mimicking cancer.
- Parametrial extension may be understaged due to gestational changes.[11]

Imaging

- **Ultrasound:** Assesses cervical integrity, fetal well-being, and pelvic masses.[12]
- **MRI:** Preferred for staging, providing tumor size, invasion, and lymph node data without fetal radiation risk.[13]
- **CT/PET:** Avoided due to fetal radiation exposure.[12]

Biopsy

- **Colposcopy-directed biopsy:** Standard for histological confirmation, ideally in the second trimester to minimize pregnancy risks.[8]
- **Pathology:** Reports tumor type (squamous and adenocarcinoma), grade, and invasion depth, guiding staging.[14]

Staging

The 2024 FIGO staging system applies to pregnant and nonpregnant patients, emphasizing clinical and imaging findings.[15] Key stages include:

- **Stage I:** Confined to cervix
  - *IA1:* Stromal invasion <3 mm
  - *IA2:* Invasion 3–5 mm
  - *IB1:* Invasion ≥5 mm, <2 cm
  - *IB2:* 2–4 cm
  - *IB3:* ≥4 cm
- **Stage II:** Beyond cervix, not to the pelvic wall/lower third vagina
  - *IIA1:* Upper 2/3 vagina, <4 cm
  - *IIA2:* Upper 2/3 vagina, ≥4 cm
  - *IIB:* Parametrial involvement
- **Stage III:** Involves the lower third vagina, pelvic wall, hydronephrosis, or nodes
  - *IIIA:* Lower vagina
  - *IIIB:* Pelvic wall/hydronephrosis
  - *IIIC1:* Pelvic nodes
  - *IIIC2:* Para-aortic nodes
- **Stage IV:** Beyond pelvis
  - *IVA:* Bladder/rectum
  - *IVB:* Distant metastases

Staging Considerations

- MRI and clinical examination guide staging.
- Multidisciplinary teams (obstetricians, gynecologic oncologists, and radiologists) ensure accuracy.[15]

MANAGEMENT (TABLE 3)

Cervical Intraepithelial Neoplasia

- **Approach:** Continue pregnancy with regular cytology/colposcopy. Vaginal delivery is safe.[7]
- **Postpartum:** Definitive treatment (e.g., loop electrosurgical excision procedure) if CIN persists.[8]

Cervical Cancer

General Principles

- Cesarean delivery is preferred to avoid risks of vaginal delivery (lymphovascular spread, bleeding, and tumor implantation at the episiotomy site).[16]
- Classical cesarean incision minimizes tumor contact.[17]
- Wound protective systems reduce abdominal wall recurrence risk.[18]
- Treatment balances maternal prognosis, fetal maturity, and patient preferences.[1]

Microinvasive Disease (IA)

Cone biopsy confirms diagnosis; negative margins allow pregnancy continuation with postpartum treatment.[7]

Early Invasive Disease (IB, IIA)

- **First trimester:** Radical hysterectomy with fetus in utero, pelvic lymphadenectomy, and oophoropexy; radiation based on risk factors.[16]
- **Second trimester:** Platinum-based neoadjuvant chemotherapy (e.g., cisplatin) for 7–15 weeks until >34 weeks, followed by cesarean, radical hysterectomy, and lymphadenectomy.[19]
- **Third trimester:** Cesarean followed by radical hysterectomy and lymphadenectomy; increased bleeding risk requires hemostatic vigilance.[16]

TABLE 3: Management strategies by stage and trimester.

Stage	*Trimester*	*Management*
Microinvasive (IA)	Any	Cone biopsy with negative margins; conservative management until delivery; postpartum treatment[7]
Early (IB, IIA)	First	Radical hysterectomy + pelvic lymphadenectomy with fetus in utero; postoperative radiation if needed[16]
	Second	Neoadjuvant chemotherapy (platinum-based) until >34 weeks, then cesarean + radical hysterectomy[19]
	Third	Cesarean + radical hysterectomy + pelvic lymphadenectomy; manage bleeding risk[16]
Advanced (IIB–IV)	First	Chemotherapy + external beam radiation; spontaneous abortion; brachytherapy[20]
	Second/third	Cesarean + neoadjuvant chemotherapy + radiation (external beam + brachytherapy)[20]

Advanced Disease (IIB–IV)

- **First trimester:** Chemotherapy and external beam radiation, leading to spontaneous abortion (2–5 weeks), followed by brachytherapy.[20]
- **Second/third trimester:** Cesarean at fetal viability, then neoadjuvant chemotherapy and radiation (external beam + brachytherapy).[20]

ROLE OF TRACHELECTOMY

The 2023 SHAPE trial supports simple trachelectomy for stage IA2–IB1 tumors (<2 cm, <50% stromal invasion, and negative nodes), preserving fertility in select cases.[21]

LATEST ADVANCEMENTS (2024–2025)

- **FIGO 2024 staging:** Incorporates lymphovascular space invasion and molecular profiling for precise staging.[15]
- **Immunotherapy:** Pembrolizumab shows promise for advanced disease in pregnancy, with ongoing trials assessing fetal safety.[22]
- **AI-driven diagnostics:** AI-enhanced colposcopy improves detection of precancerous lesions (sensitivity of 92%).[23]

CONCLUSION

Cervical cancer in pregnancy requires a multidisciplinary approach to balance maternal and fetal outcomes. Early detection through screening, accurate staging with MRI, and tailored management based on stage and trimester are critical. Advances like trachelectomy, immunotherapy, and AI diagnostics enhance care. Individualized plans, guided by patient preferences and clinical evidence, ensure optimal management.

REFERENCES

1. Le Guévelou J, Selleret L, Laas E, et al. Cervical cancer in pregnancy: Challenges and strategies. Cancers. 2024;16(7):1341.
2. Kumari S. Screening for cervical cancer in pregnancy. Oncol Rev. 2023;17:11429.
3. Beharee N, Shi Z, Wu D, et al. Diagnosis and treatment of cervical cancer in pregnant women. Cancer Med. 2019;8(12):5425-30.
4. Smith LH, et al. Cervical cancer screening guidelines: ACOG update. Obstet Gynecol. 2021;137(4):659-67.
5. Aggarwal P, Ben Amor A. Cervical ectropion. In: StatPearls [Internet]. Treasure Island (FL): StatPearls Publishing; 2025 Jan–. Updated 2023 May 31. Available from: https://www.ncbi.nlm.nih.gov/books/NBK560709/
6. Fowler JR, Maani EV, Dunton CJ, et al. Cervical cancer. In: StatPearls [Internet]. Treasure Island (FL): StatPearls Publishing; 2025 Jan–. Updated 2023 Nov 12. Available from: https://www.ncbi.nlm.nih.gov/books/NBK431093/
7. Cooper DB, Dunton CJ. Colposcopy. In: StatPearls [Internet]. Treasure Island (FL): StatPearls Publishing; 2025 Jan–. Updated 2023 Nov 12. Available from: https://www.ncbi.nlm.nih.gov/books/NBK564514/
8. Wright TC, et al. Cervical cancer screening and diagnosis: ASCCP guidelines. J Low Genit Tract Dis. 2020;24(2):87-97.

9. Amant F, et al. Cervical cancer in pregnancy: Diagnosis and management. Lancet Oncol. 2019;20(6):e336-46.
10. Salani R, et al. Cervical cancer symptoms in pregnancy. Gynecol Oncol. 2020;156(3):739-45.
11. Duggan C, et al. Challenges in cervical cancer diagnosis during pregnancy. Int J Gynecol Cancer. 2018;28(5):987-94.
12. Jain S, Acharya N. Fetal wellbeing monitoring in cervical cancer. Cureus. 2022;14(9):e29039.
13. Balleyguier C, et al. MRI staging of cervical cancer in pregnancy. Eur Radiol. 2020;30(8):4423-31.
14. Pecorelli S, et al. Cervical cancer pathology in pregnancy. Gynecol Oncol. 2019;153(2):412-9.
15. Bhatla N, et al. FIGO 2024 staging for cervical cancer. Int J Gynaecol Obstet. 2024;167(1):1-12.
16. Halaska MJ, et al. Surgical management of cervical cancer in pregnancy. Ann Surg Oncol. 2021;28(7):3765-73.
17. Morice P, et al. Cesarean delivery in cervical cancer. BJOG. 2020;127(9):1087-94.
18. Ramirez PT, et al. Wound protection in gynecologic surgery. Gynecol Oncol. 2022;164(3):654-60.
19. Fruscio R, et al. Neoadjuvant chemotherapy in cervical cancer during pregnancy. J Clin Oncol. 2023;41(16):2975-83.
20. Zagouri F, et al. Radiation therapy for cervical cancer in pregnancy. Oncologist. 2021;26(6):e1032-40.
21. Plante M, et al. SHAPE trial: Simple trachelectomy for early cervical cancer. J Clin Oncol. 2023;41(Suppl 16):5505.
22. Monk BJ, et al. Immunotherapy in cervical cancer: Pregnancy considerations. Lancet Oncol. 2024;25(4):e164-73.
23. Hu L, et al. AI-enhanced colposcopy for cervical cancer detection. Lancet Digit Health. 2024;6(5):e345-53.

Ethics in Obstetrics and Gynecology

Ruchika Garg

INTRODUCTION

Ethics in obstetrics and gynecology guides clinical decision-making to balance maternal and fetal interests while respecting patient autonomy. With a prevalence of ethical dilemmas in 1 in 5 obstetric cases,[1] adherence to principles like autonomy, beneficence, non-maleficence, and justice is critical to ensure equitable, patient-centered care.

KEY ETHICAL PRINCIPLES

The four foundational ethical principles in medicine are **(Table 1)**:

- *Autonomy:* Respecting the patient's right to make informed choices, privacy, and confidentiality.
- *Beneficence:* Acting in the patient's best interest to promote well-being.
- *Non-maleficence:* Avoiding harm to the patient.
- *Justice:* Ensuring fair and equitable distribution of healthcare resources and equal treatment for all patients.[2]

ADDITIONAL ETHICAL CONSIDERATIONS

- *Conflict of Interest:* Physicians must avoid financial or personal biases influencing treatment decisions (e.g., promoting unnecessary procedures for profit).[3]
- *Patient Rights:* Include access to informed consent, clear communication about benefits, risks, benefits, and alternatives, and the right to refuse treatment.[4]
- *Physician Rights:* Physicians may refuse non-emergency care (e.g., for personal beliefs) but must refer patients appropriately; emergency care cannot be denied.[5]

TABLE 1: Key ethical principles in medicine.[2]

Principle	*Description*	*Example in obstetrics/gynecology*
Autonomy	Patient's right to decide	Respecting refusal of cesarean section
Beneficence	Promote patient well-being	Recommending timely interventions for fetal distress
Non-maleficence	Do no harm	Avoiding unnecessary invasive procedures
Justice	Equitable care	Providing equal care regardless of socioeconomic status

- *Physician-Patient Relationship:* Prohibits romantic/sexual relationships or financial influence outside healthcare contexts.[2]

INFORMED CONSENT

Informed consent is a dynamic process, not merely a signature, ensuring patients make voluntary, informed decisions. It requires **(Table 2)**:

- *Disclosure:* Information on diagnosis, treatment purpose, method, duration, benefits, risks, side effects, and alternatives in understandable language.
- *Capacity:* Patient must be ≥18 years and mentally competent. For minors or those with intellectual disability, pediatric assent or joint decision-making applies.
- *Voluntariness:* Consent must be free from coercion; patients can withdraw consent at any time with clear communication about risks.[6]
- *Emergency Consent:* RCOG guidelines permit verbal consent in emergencies, witnessed by another professional, with documentation of reasons if written consent is not feasible.[7]

ETHICS IN SPECIFIC SCENARIOS

Reproductive Medicine (Table 3)

- *Assisted Reproductive Technologies (ART):*
  - *Confidentiality:* Donor and client information must remain confidential.[8]
  - *Informed Consent:* Written consent required for procedures (e.g., embryo freezing). Patients must be informed about success rates, side effects, costs, and offspring rights.[9]
  - *Gamete/Embryo Use:* Maximum of three oocytes/embryos per cycle, except in exceptional cases (e.g., poor embryo quality). Donor information (e.g., DNA fingerprint) is accessible to offspring at ≥18 years, not parents, unless legally required.[10]

TABLE 2: Components of informed consent.[6]

Component	*Details*	*Example*
Disclosure	Risks, benefits, alternatives	Explaining risks of cesarean vs. vaginal delivery
Capacity	≥18 years, mentally sound	Obtaining consent from a competent adult
Voluntariness	No coercion	Allowing refusal of sterilization
Documentation	Written or verbal (emergency)	Recording verbal consent for emergency LSCS

TABLE 3: Ethical issues in reproductive medicine.[10,17]

Procedure	*Key ethical concerns*	*Guidelines*
ART	Confidentiality, informed consent, donor rights	ART Bill, 2021
Uterine transplant	Immunosuppression risks, societal biases	RCOG guidance
Surrogacy	Surrogate autonomy, non-commercialization	Surrogacy Bill, 2021
Sex selection	Gender discrimination, misuse of technology	PC-PNDT Act, 1994

    - *Donor Eligibility (ART Bill, 2021):*
        - *Men:* 21–55 years.
        - *Women:* 21–35 years, with a child ≥3 years old.
        - Single donation, ≤7 oocytes retrieved.[11]
    - *ART Bank Rules:*
        - One donor's gametes per couple.
        - Gametes/embryos stored ≤10 years, then discarded or donated for research.
        - Donors screened for infectious diseases.[12]
- *Preimplantation Genetic Testing (PGT):*
    - Used for screening (PGS) or diagnosis (PGD) of genetic/chromosomal disorders.
    - Risks include false positives/negatives; patients must be counseled on limitations and alternatives (e.g., prenatal testing).[13]
    - All pregnant women should be offered prenatal screening, with results kept confidential.[14]
- *Uterine Transplantation:*
    - *Indications:* Absolute uterine factor infertility (e.g., congenital absence, hysterectomy).
    - *Eligibility:* Age 24–38 years, BMI <30 kg/m^2, normal ovaries, no living children.
    - *Ethical Concerns:* Risks of immunosuppression, high-risk pregnancy, and societal biases (e.g., pronatalism, geneticism). Critics argue it may reinforce discriminatory attitudes toward non-biological parenthood.[15]
    - *Management:* Embryo transfer 6–12 months post-transplant, cesarean delivery, lifelong follow-up.[16]
- *Surrogacy (Surrogacy Bill, 2021):*
    - *Type:* Only gestational (embryo not genetically related to surrogate) and altruistic surrogacy permitted.
    - *Indications:* Medical reasons (e.g., uterine absence, recurrent pregnancy loss).
    - *Ethical Issues:* Respect surrogate autonomy (e.g., decisions about pregnancy management). Commercial surrogacy is banned to prevent exploitation.[17]
    - *Contract:* Must outline surrogate's clinical management rights and non-commercial nature.[18]
- *Adoption:*
    - *Eligibility:*
        - Physically/mentally stable, no criminal convictions.
        - *Married couples:* Consent of both; single females can adopt any gender; single males cannot adopt girls.
        - Stable relationship ≥2 years; age gap ≥25 years between child and parents.
    - *Process:* Orphaned/abandoned children declared adoptable by Child Welfare Committee after 2–4 months.[19]
- *Sex Selection:*
    - Illegal and unethical under the PC-PNDT Act, 1994, which regulates prenatal diagnostics to prevent sex-selective abortions. Permitted only for genetic disorders (e.g., sex-linked diseases).[20]

DECISION-MAKING FOR DELIVERY

- *Vaginal vs. Cesarean Delivery:*
    - Physicians must present evidence-based options (beneficence) while respecting patient autonomy.
    - Directive counseling for clear medical indications (e.g., fetal distress); non-directive when indications are uncertain (e.g., maternal request).[21]
    - Elective cesarean on maternal request requires thorough counseling on risks (e.g., higher morbidity, placenta accreta in future pregnancies).[22]
- *Preventive Ethics:*
    - Initiate delivery discussions during prenatal visits to create a mutually acceptable birth plan.
    - Warn patients that low-risk pregnancies can become high-risk, necessitating cesarean delivery.[23]

PREGNANCY AND HIV-POSITIVE PATIENTS

- *Non-Discrimination:* HIV-positive patients must receive equal care without inferior treatment.[24]
- *Confidentiality:* HIV status is strictly confidential.
- *Testing:* "Opt-out" approach recommended; all pregnant women should be tested for HIV, syphilis, and hepatitis B (Triple Elimination Initiative).[25]
- *Counseling:* Encourage pregnancy planning with strict clinical management to prevent vertical transmission (e.g., antiretroviral therapy, cesarean if high viral load).[26]
- *No Coercion:* Abortion or sterilization cannot be forced based on HIV status.[27]

MEDICAL TERMINATION OF PREGNANCY

- *Medical Termination of Pregnancy (MTP) Amendment Bill, 2021:*
    - *Abortion up to 20 weeks:* One doctor's opinion.
    - *20–24 weeks:* Two doctors' opinions for special categories (e.g., rape victims, minors, differently-abled, marital status change).
    - *24 weeks: State-level Medical Board approval for substantial fetal abnormalities or maternal life risk.*
    - *Minors or mentally incapacitated:* Guardian consent required.
    - *Confidentiality:* Patient identity protected unless legally required.[28]
- *Ethical Considerations:* Balance autonomy (patient's choice) with beneficence (fetal considerations in late gestation).[29]

CONTRACEPTION

- *Informed Choice:*
    - Provide information on method use, efficacy, side effects, contraindications, and STI protection without coercion.
    - Respect autonomy to discontinue reversible methods.[30]

- *Emergency Contraception:*
  - Essential for rape victims and adolescents; access should be barrier-free.[31]
- *Permanent Contraception:*
  - *ACOG Recommendations:* Respect reproductive autonomy, avoid age/parity thresholds, counsel on reversible alternatives, and discuss vasectomy (lower risk, higher efficacy).
  - *Eligibility (India):* Married clients, females 22–49 years, ≥1 child >1 year, no prior sterilization, mentally sound.
  - *Providers:* MBBS (minilap), DGO/MD/MS (laparoscopic sterilization).
  - *Preoperative:* Medical history, physical examination, hemoglobin >7 g%, urine analysis.[32]
  - *Ethics:* Avoid coercive practices; longitudinal counseling to minimize regret.[33]

PERIMORTEM CESAREAN SECTION

- *Primary Aim:* Maternal survival, not fetal survival.
- *Indications:* Cardiac arrest >20 weeks gestation, no return of spontaneous circulation after 4 minutes of CPR.
- *Timing:* Delivery within 5 minutes to maximize maternal survival and minimize neurological damage.
- *Setting:* Perform at arrest site with minimal equipment; written consent from relatives preferred if feasible.
- *Ethics:* Balances beneficence (maternal survival) with urgency, respecting autonomy via prior discussions.[34]

CARE OF SEX WORKERS

- *Non-Discrimination:* Treat without judgment, integrated with other patients.
- *Focus:* STI prevention, screening, treatment, and contraception counselling.[35]

VIOLENCE ISSUES

- *Vigilance:* Screen for signs of sexual/physical violence during consultations.
- *Reporting:* Adhere to child protection laws for suspected child abuse/neglect.[36]

RESEARCH

- *Consent:* Autonomous, informed, with clear discussion of teratogenic risks.
- *Ethics:* Trials with unacceptable risk/benefit ratios are impermissible.[37]

CARE OF TERMINALLY ILL PATIENTS

- *Goals:* Prioritize pain relief, comfort, and dignity when cure is unattainable.
- *Ethics:* Beneficence and non-maleficence guide palliative care.[38]

UNIVERSITY EXAMINATION QUESTIONS

- *DNB 2022: Contraceptive Advice for a 15-Year-Old Without Parental Knowledge*
  - *Ethical Principles:*
    - *Autonomy:* Respect the adolescent's capacity to make decisions (pediatric assent) but limited by age.
    - *Beneficence:* Provide contraception to prevent unintended pregnancy/STIs.
    - *Justice:* Ensure access to care without discrimination.
  - *Legal Issues:* POCSO Act, 2012, mandates reporting sexual activity in minors <18 years to police, overriding confidentiality. Counseling must balance legal obligations with trust-building.[39]
  - *Management:* Offer non-judgmental counseling, discuss emergency contraception, and refer to adolescent-friendly health services.
- *AIIMS 2023: Refusal of Emergency Cesarean in Third Trimester*
  - *Ethical Principles:*
    - *Autonomy:* Respect patient's refusal if informed and competent.
    - *Beneficence:* Explain risks to mother/fetus (e.g., fetal demise, maternal morbidity).
    - *Non-maleficence:* Avoid coercive tactics.
  - *Management:* Engage in shared decision-making, document counseling, involve multidisciplinary team (e.g., ethics committee). Legal limits in India do not permit overriding maternal autonomy for fetal indications.[40]
- *JIPMER 2023: Sterilization Without Consent During Cesarean*
  - *Ethical Issues:*
    - Violates autonomy and reproductive rights.
    - Breaches non-maleficence (irreversible harm).
  - *Legal Issues:* Indian law requires informed consent for sterilization; unauthorized procedures violate medical ethics and human rights.[41]
  - *Management:* Counsel preoperatively, respect refusal, and document discussions.
- *PGIMER 2021: Elective Cesarean on Maternal Request*
  - *Ethical Concerns:*
    - *Autonomy:* Respect request if informed.
    - *Non-maleficence:* Higher morbidity (e.g., infection, hemorrhage) and future risks (e.g., placenta accreta).
    - *Beneficence:* Counsel on vaginal delivery benefits.
  - *Management:* Non-directive counseling, evidence-based discussion, shared decision-making.[42]
- *KGMU 2023: Sex Selection in IVF*
  - *Ethical Issues:*
    - Promotes gender discrimination, violating justice.
    - Conflicts with non-maleficence (societal harm).
  - *Legal Issues:* PC-PNDT Act, 1994, prohibits sex selection except for medical indications (e.g., X-linked disorders). Violations lead to penalties.[20]
  - *Management:* Refuse request, counsel on ethical/legal implications.

- *DNB 2020: Surrogacy and Ethical Issues*
  - *Definition:* Gestational surrogacy involves a surrogate carrying an embryo not genetically related to her.
  - *Medical Indications:* Uterine absence, recurrent pregnancy loss, severe medical contraindications to pregnancy.
  - *Ethical Issues:*
    - Respect surrogate autonomy in pregnancy management.
    - Ban on commercial surrogacy prevents exploitation.
    - Ensure non-coercive contracts.[17]
  - *Surrogacy Bill, 2021:* Mandates altruistic surrogacy, medical board approval, and surrogate rights protection.[18]
- *DNB 2020: Uterine Transplantation*
  - *Ethical Issues:*
    - Risks of immunosuppression, surgery, and high-risk pregnancy.
    - Societal biases (e.g., pronatalism) may undervalue adoption/surrogacy.
  - *Patient Selection:*
    - Age 24–38 years, BMI <30 kg/m^2, normal ovaries, no living children.
    - *Preoperative screening:* Psychological evaluation, ovarian reserve, infectious disease testing.
  - *Management:* Multidisciplinary team, embryo transfer post-6–12 months, cesarean delivery.[15]

RCOG AND NICE GUIDELINES

- *RCOG Green-top Guideline No. 7 (2023):* Emphasizes informed consent, including verbal consent in emergencies, and respect for autonomy in delivery decisions.[7]
- *NICE NG201 (2023):* Recommends shared decision-making, non-discriminatory care for HIV-positive patients, and access to contraception for all women, including adolescents.[11]
- *RCOG Guidance on ART (2022):* Stresses confidentiality, informed consent, and ethical donor practices.[8]

KEY POINTS

- Ethical principles (autonomy, beneficence, non-maleficence, justice) guide obstetrics and Gynecology practice.
- Informed consent is a dynamic process requiring disclosure, capacity, and voluntariness.
- Reproductive medicine (ART, surrogacy, uterine transplant) involves complex ethical issues, including confidentiality and autonomy.
- MTP, contraception, and delivery decisions balance autonomy with beneficence.
- HIV-positive patients and sex workers require non-discriminatory, confidential care.
- Indian laws (PC-PNDT, MTP, Surrogacy Bills) regulate ethical practices.
- RCOG/NICE guidelines emphasize shared decision-making and patient-centered care.

MCQ ANSWERS

- B (Non-maleficence: Do no harm).[2]
- D (All are ethical considerations).[3]
- C (Emergency contraception should be accessible; coercive practices are unethical).[31]
- D (Donors must meet ART Bill criteria: men 21–55, women 21–35 with a child).[11]
- B (Two doctors' opinions for 20–24 weeks).[28]
- C (Perimortem cesarean after 4 minutes of CPR).[34]
- E (Respect autonomy, avoid coercion).[21]
- B (Beneficence: Patient's best interest).[2]
- A (Physicians can refuse non-emergency care).[5]
- C (Prenatal screening is ethical for all).[14]

Note 10 Marks Short note has been asked in many university exams for postgraduates.

REFERENCES

1. Chervenak FA, McCullough LB. Ethical dilemmas in obstetrics. Clin Perinatol. 2016;43(3):479-90.
2. FIGO Committee. Ethical framework for gynecologic and obstetric care. Int J Gynaecol Obstet. 2015;131(Suppl 1):S7-9.
3. DeCamp M, Snyder Sulmasy L. Conflict of interest in medicine. JAMA. 2018;320(16):1643-4.
4. Beauchamp TL, Childress JF. Principles of biomedical ethics. J Med Ethics. 2019;45(6):365-70.
5. ACOG Committee Opinion No. 816. Physician's right to refuse care. Obstet Gynecol. 2021;137(1):e1-6.
6. RCOG. Obtaining valid consent. Clin Governance Advice. 2020;6:1-12.
7. Royal College of Obstetricians and Gynaecologists. Green-top Guideline No. 7: Consent in Obstetrics. 2023.
8. RCOG. Ethical considerations in ART. BJOG. 2022;129(Suppl 2):S12-8.
9. HFEA. Code of practice for ART clinics. Hum Fertil. 2019;22(3):145-50.
10. Assisted Reproductive Technology Bill, 2021. Government of India.
11. National Institute for Health and Care Excellence. NG201: Antenatal Care. 2023.
12. ICMR. National guidelines for ART clinics. Indian J Med Res. 2020;152(Suppl):S1-10.
13. Harper JC, Aittomäki K. Preimplantation genetic testing: Ethics. Hum Reprod. 2017;32(6):1131-6.
14. ACOG. Prenatal genetic screening and testing. Obstet Gynecol. 2016;127(5):e108-22.
15. Johannesson L, Testa G. Uterine transplantation: Ethical issues. Fertil Steril. 2018;110(6):1015-20.
16. Brännström M, Dahm-Kähler P. Uterine transplantation outcomes. Lancet. 2021;398(10302):607-16.
17. Surrogacy (Regulation) Bill, 2021. Government of India.
18. FIGO. Ethical guidelines on surrogacy. Int J Gynaecol Obstet. 2016;135(3):367-70.
19. Central Adoption Resource Authority. Adoption regulations, 2022. Government of India.
20. Pre-Conception and Pre-Natal Diagnostic Techniques Act, 1994. Government of India.
21. Chervenak FA, McCullough LB. Ethics of cesarean delivery. Am J Obstet Gynecol. 2019;221(5):421-6.
22. NICE. Cesarean section on maternal request. BJOG. 2015;122(8):1033-9.
23. RCOG. Preventive ethics in obstetrics. Clin Risk. 2017;23(4):145-50.
24. WHO. Ethical care for HIV-positive patients. Bull World Health Organ. 2016;94(11):792-8.
25. WHO. Triple elimination initiative: HIV, syphilis, hepatitis B. Lancet Glob Health. 2020;8(4):e477-8.
26. BHIVA. HIV in pregnancy: Guidelines. HIV Med. 2018;19(Suppl 1):S1-30.
27. FIGO. Ethics of HIV management in pregnancy. Int J Gynaecol Obstet. 2015;131(Suppl 1):S24-7.
28. Medical Termination of Pregnancy (Amendment) Bill, 2021. Government of India.
29. FIGO. Ethical issues in MTP. Int J Gynaecol Obstet. 2019;146(3):271-5.

30. WHO. Contraception: Ethical principles. Hum Reprod. 2017;33(6):1013-9.
31. ACOG. Emergency contraception access. Obstet Gynecol. 2015;126(6):e78-84.
32. Government of India. Standards for sterilization services. 2018.
33. ACOG. Ethical considerations in sterilization. Obstet Gynecol. 2020;135(2):e33-8.
34. RCOG. Perimortem cesarean section. BJOG. 2015;122(11):1445-50.
35. WHO. Ethical care for sex workers. Sex Transm Infect. 2016;93(5):317-22.
36. FIGO. Violence in obstetric care. Int J Gynaecol Obstet. 2018;143(3):392-7.
37. CIOMS. Ethical research involving women in pregnancy. Bull Med Ethics. 2016;22:1-10.
38. FIGO. Palliative care in Gynecology. Int J Gynaecol Obstet. 2020;151(2):165-70.
39. Protection of Children from Sexual Offences (POCSO) Act, 2012. Government of India.
40. Indian Medical Council of Medical Research. Ethical guidelines for biomedical research. Indian J Med Res. 2017.
41. Supreme Court of India. Consent in reproductive procedures. J Law Med Ethics. 2019;47(2):211-20.
42. NICE. Shared decision-making in obstetrics. BJOG. 2021;159(8):1033-40.

Pre-conception and Pre-natal Diagnostic Techniques Act

Ruchika Garg

INTRODUCTION

The Pre-conception and Pre-natal Diagnostic Techniques Act (PCPNDT Act) was enacted on 20th September 1994 to prohibit the determination of the sex of the fetus before or after conception and regulation of prenatal diagnostic techniques. Its main aim is to arrest the practice of female feticide completely. The act was amended, effectively implemented in 2003, and strictly enforced in 2011.

The government of India is ensuring the effective implementation of the PCPNDT Act in several ways. At the district level, the appropriate authority is empowered to take stringent actions like seizing and sealing machines. They are aided by the advisory committee consisting of three medical experts, a legal expert, three social activists and a publicity expert. Further, the central and state supervisory boards are constituted to strengthen the successful implementation of the Act.

The essential requirements of the Act are:

1. Mandatory registration of all genetic clinics/laboratories, ultrasound clinics or any other facility prone to sex determination under Sections 18 and 19. No individual shall open a genetic clinic or lab, ultrasound clinic or any other facility that can perform prenatal sex determination after the inception of the Pre-natal Diagnostic Techniques (Regulation and Prevention of Misuse) Amendment Act, 2002 until the center is appropriately registered.
2. Written consent of the pregnant woman and prohibition of communicating the sex of the fetus under Section 5 of the Act.
3. Maintenance of records of prenatal diagnostic tests or procedures by the ultrasound or genetic clinic as per Section 4. All ultrasound forms, reports, consent forms and all other documents shall be preserved for 2 years. In case of criminal proceedings against any center, the records shall be preserved till the final proceedings are over.
4. The genetic laboratory/clinic/ultrasound clinic/combination has to display a notice that they do not conduct any test or procedure to detect the sex of the fetus before or after conception.
5. The certificate of registration should be displayed at a noticeable place in the business area.

OBJECTIVES

The main objective of the PCPNDT Act is to prevent the misuse of prenatal diagnostic modalities and to cease the practice of female feticide. The amendments in the Act have provisions for more stringent actions against the offenders.

PROVISIONS

It regulates the use of prenatal diagnostic techniques like ultrasound, amniocentesis, chorionic villus sampling, fetal MRI, fetal echocardiogram, percutaneous umbilical blood sampling and tests like cell-free DNA for the detection of chromosomal abnormalities, metabolic disorders, hemoglobinopathies and other genetic abnormalities.

No ultrasound clinic or genetic laboratory can conduct any test, including ultrasonography, to ascertain the sex of the fetus. No individual including the doctor performing the procedure can communicate the sex of the fetus to the woman or her relatives by any means like words, signs or any other modes.

OFFENCES UNDER THE ACT

If the law is violated by any medical professional or registered medical practitioner, imprisonment for up to 3 years and a fine of up to ₹10,000 can be charged for the first-time offenders. Subsequent offences can result in imprisonment for up to 5 years along with a fine of ₹50,000. (Section 23),[1] Pre-conception and Pre-natal Diagnostic Techniques (Prohibition of Sex Selection) Act, 1994. Pre-natal Diagnostic Techniques (Regulation and Prevention of Misuse Act, 1994).

Suspension of the registration of the doctors and registered medical practitioners until the case is dealt with and, upon being found guilty, removal of their name from the register for 5 years for first-time offenders and a lifetime in cases with subsequent offences (Section 23),[2] Pre-conception and Pre-natal Diagnostic Techniques (Prohibition of Sex Selection Act, 1994).

Any individual going in pursuit of prenatal diagnostic techniques for sex determination (excluding pregnant women forced to undergo the procedure) will be liable to imprisonment for 3 years and a fine of ₹50,000. On subsequent offences, imprisonment for 5 years and a fine of ₹1,00,000 can be charged.

Any person advertising for sex determination facilities in any form like notice, circular, or through media or internet is liable for imprisonment for up to 3 years and a fine of up to ₹10,000.

REFERENCES

1. Standard Operating Guidelines Pre-Conception and Pre-Natal Diagnostic Techniques (Prohibition of Sex Selection) Act, 1994 Ministry of Health and Family Welfare, Government of India in Collaboration with United Nations Population Fund, 1st edition; 2016.
2. The Pre-Natal Diagnostic Techniques (Regulation and Prevention of Misuse) Act, 1994 (Act No. 57 of 1994) and the Pre-Natal Diagnostic Techniques (Regulation and Prevention of Misuse) Amendment Act, 2002 (No. 14 of 2003).

Breaking Bad News in Obstetrics

Savita Somalwar

NEED FOR LEARNING THE SCIENCE OF BREAKING BAD NEWS

Breaking bad news is a sensitive and complex task, and it can be acquired through practice. "Bad news" is defined as any information that creates negative impact on the life or vision of the future for those who receive it, according to their perspective.[1,2]

Breaking bad news in obstetrics is a fine art. It is good that now in medical curriculum, AETCOM (Attitude, Ethics, Communication) module has been introduced by National Medical Commission (NMC) recently, which will help students in developing this art. Previously, it was not included in medical curriculum, so gradually the obstetricians learnt it over time by observing their senior professionals. It needs to be taught to students during their curriculum rather than learning it through trial and errors after starting medical practice.

For most women, pregnancy is a time of excitement, expectation, and joy. Bad news in obstetrics can be devastating for the women and relatives. It can affect the psychological aspects, as planned pregnancy is a joyful moment for not only couple but for the whole family.

Certain obstetric complications may create a bad impact on psychology of women and her close relatives. Complications may range from fetal problems to life-threatening maternal complications. Missed abortions, recurrent pregnancy loss, congenital malformations in fetus (compatible or noncompatible with life), hydatidiform mole, intrauterine fetal death, stillbirths, neonatal deaths, obstetric hysterectomy, maternal near miss, and maternal mortality are some complications which require a proper communication and a dialogue between the obstetricians and women and her relatives. These events are also called birth crisis. It includes not only unexpected adverse pregnancy outcomes but also includes neonatal complications. In these cases, not only it creates a negative impact on the mental aspect of women and their relatives but also on the obstetrician.

From the Patient's and Relative's Perspective

It is devastating news. Women may think why it happened to me. The occurrence of adverse events during pregnancy or childbirth destroys the expectation and frustrates plans which parents usually made considering a healthy child to be born.[3-7] Pregnancy losses can trigger grief reactions and are considered one of the most stressful events in adulthood and mothers who experience fetal death are more likely to experience complicated and prolonged grief, which can last for more than a year.[3,6] Additional reactions experienced by parents after pregnancy losses include feelings of guilt, anxiety, eating disorders, and shame.[5,6] The patient's anxiety is greater when she does not expect something adverse to happen and receives bad news.[5] Additionally, in obstetrics unlike in other areas of medicine, the patient is no longer a single individual but becomes the mother-fetus binomial and when present, the partner is also considered part of the "patient." Hence after talking with the patient and if she is willing, both parents should be present when the bad news is given for the first time, so that the mourning can start simultaneously.

When antenatal women and their partners suffer from birth crisis, it leads to profound efforts and causes long lasting trauma to them and also family members.[8] The healthcare team should approach this crisis properly as people may recall the words spoken by the healthcare professionals and the team even after years of the event.[9] According to studies, the negative memories are related to the report's content itself and the doctor's lack of skills for communication after receiving the bad news by the couple.[3,5,7] When receiving bad news, patients may experience various grief reactions such as denial, anger, negotiation, bargaining, depression, and acceptance.[5,10,11] These emotions along with anxiety, tension, and the amount of new information received can compromise the patient's assimilation of the content, which would cause them to forget up to two-thirds of the information they have received.[5,12] According to Royal college of Obstetricians and Gynaecologists (RCOG) guideline on stillbirth and late intrauterine fetal death, important component out of many strategies described for discussing bad news is determining the feelings and needs of pregnant woman and her support team.[13]

From the Obstetrician's Perspective

Significant emotional trauma can be experienced by pregnancy care providers.[14,15] For young obstetrician, it may be first experience to break bad news, and hence it is shocking and they may be nervous, and for the senior obstetrician, it may be frequent event and counseling becomes better with experience, but it is never easy. Certainly, bad news creates a negative impact on the mental health of the obstetrician. They are worried about their reputation, facing relative's questions, mob violence, police inquiries, medical issues, out of court settlements, and compensations. They may face loss of confidence and are stressed, and definitely, it creates impact on future practice. Communicating fetal death is one of the most difficult duties, especially at the beginning of their careers from the perspective of health professionals.[3,7]

Doctor should always keep in mind that parents usually have different reactions when receiving bad news, and it is their duty to understand and comfort both.[3,10] Therefore, physicians should communicate bad news while respecting the patient's time to assimilate it and repeat information if necessary.[5] The use of excessively technical language should be avoided as it also impairs assimilation.[5,12] Physicians can improve their communication skills although they cannot modify the content of negative news.[7] For doctors and patients, it is an unwanted situation, and it is made harder by the unpredictable reactions of the patients' to highly stressful situations.[16,17]

It is imperative for all pregnancy care providers to deliver compassionate, humanistic, and psychosocial management for all adverse birth outcomes.[18] The ability to deliver care in this way by the healthcare team may be hindered by clinical detachment which is required in practice setting and the absence of emotional support from the colleagues.[14,19] The wellbeing of pregnancy care providers can be increased with elements such as reflection and review, emotional and practical support, access to counseling services, initial and ongoing education and training, institutional policies, and guidelines.[20]

How to break bad news?

Breaking bad news is a complex skill. Communication with the patients is an important aspect, but during medical curriculum, more importance is given for development of clinical skills than learning an art of communication. The patient's acceptance of bad news depends upon how the news is transmitted to the patients. The obstetrician should also keep in mind that although in busy hospitals it is common occurrence, the patients may be experiencing it for the first time. The patient's anxiety may be greater, if bad news comes unexpectedly. Before disclosing bad news, the obstetrician should prepare herself or himself by going through the patient's record, including detailed history, investigation, and diagnosis. Obstetricians should mentally rehearse how to deliver the news. Script specific words or phrases to use or to avoid and prepare yourself emotionally.

There should be designated room in operation theater, labor room, or ward. In all hospitals, CCTV should be installed in sensitive areas. In view of violence against doctors, breaking of bad news should be done in presence of security staff in the vicinity. All these measures are important to deal with anger, especially mob anger. There should be facility of video recording to protect from medicolegal issues. If you decide to do video recording, it should be told to the patient and her relatives beforehand only, considering the patient's education is very important and always use simple vernacular language. It is very important to avoid criticizing your colleagues.

Many protocols have been mentioned in literature. Every institute or hospital should have their guidelines or protocol, and everyone should follow same while breaking bad news. It is important that the senior most person in the hospital or in the institute should disclose the bad news.

Various protocols such as **SPIKES, ABCDE, BREAKS**, **SAAIQ**, and **SAD NEWS** are used for breaking bad news.

SPIKES Protocol[21-23]

SPIKES protocol was developed by Dr Robert Buckman and Baile to break bad news in oncology patients in 2000. This protocol now is widely followed all over for breaking bad news.

It includes six steps.

1. *Setting up and starting:* Obstetricians should always ensure that the environment is comfortable while breaking the bad news. Make sure that adequate sitting arrangement is there. Self-introduction by the obstetrician is the important step. It is important to ask patient whether to involve her partner, friends, or relatives while breaking bad news.

   It is important to have privacy so that obstetrician can concentrate while breaking bad news. Disturbance can deviate obstetricians, patient, and relatives from seriousness of situation. Mobiles should be kept on silent mode to avoid irritation.

The bad news should be told in a calm but serious tone so as the patient and relatives know that the obstetrician is on the same page with them. It is vital to give adequate time to disclose bad news. Obstetricians should sit down, use open body language, eye contact, and/or touch to make a connection with the patient. Always tell the bad news in person, face to face and never telephonically.

2. *Perception:* Ask what the patient knows regarding her medical condition and what she suspects. Evaluate the patient's perspective, knowledge, expectations, and hopes. Create room for a dialogue by using open-ended questions, silent pauses in between, listening first, and encouraging the patient to provide their perspective. Assess the patient's beliefs and feelings. Assess vocabulary and comprehension. Take opportunity to correct misinformation.
3. *Invitation:* Encourage the patient to ask questions and what they would like to know regarding her medical condition. If patient does not want to know details, you can ask her partner, friend, or relative if they want to ask any questions. Use vernacular language. Avoid using medical language. Tell them that you are ready to share knowledge.
4. *Knowledge:* First tell them that you want to share bad news. Always give information in small pieces, see whether she has understood it and then go ahead gradually. Avoid using technological terms. Always use simple vernacular language that aligns with the patient's vocabulary and understanding. Tell her about who is going to take care of her in medical management. Reassure the patient of ongoing support throughout her treatment.
5. *Emotions and empathy:* Assess, recognize, and empathize with the patient's emotions. Anticipate grief reactions such as fear, anger, sadness, denial, and guilt. You can touch her hands and support her. Do not say, I can understand what you are going through this phase, unless you have faced similar situation in your life. Let her cry if she wants, otherwise it can lead to development of psychological issues. Wait for some time if she is crying and then continue conversation. Always offer empathetic responses. (Empathy—capacity to recognize emotions that are being felt by another person). Remember that all patients are different.
6. *Strategy and summary:* Make sure that the patient has understood by asking her to summarize briefly the main points of the conversation. You will have to tell plan of medical management and counsel her. Involve patient in decision making. It should be shared decision. Tell her that you are with her while executing medical plan or treatment and she can ask her queries anytime. Tell her when you will like to arrange follow-up conversation with her and relatives.

ABCDE Protocol

It is developed by Michael Rabow and Stephen J Mc Phee from California in 1999.

- A: Advance preparation
- B: Build therapeutic environment
- C: Communicate well
- D: Deal with patient and family reactions
- E: Encourage and validate emotions.

BREAKS Protocol

It is mentioned in Indian Journal of palliative care (IJPC).

- B: Background
- R: Rapport
- E: Explore
- A: Announce
- K: Kindling
- S: Summarize

SAAIQ Protocol

This protocol is used in Pakistan.

- S: Set the scene as early as possible.
- A: Assess the understanding of attendant.
- A: Alert them that I have bad news.
- I: Inform in clear, understandable words.
- Q: Quickly repeat summary of the situation.

Do's and Don'ts of Breaking Bad News

Do's:

1. Meet with patient or partner as soon as possible.
2. Sit in a room with adequate sitting arrangement.
3. Maintain privacy.
4. Keep mobiles on silent mode.
5. Introduce yourself.
6. Ask patient whether she wants her partner, friend, or relatives when you are disclosing the news. Share information with all at same time if possible.
7. Use simple language.
8. Keep eye contact.
9. Encourage to ask questions.
10. Be compassionate.
11. Empathize.
12. Enable and support parents to express their feelings.
13. Review the facts but acknowledge their limits (e.g., do not be afraid to say, I do not know why).
14. In cases of stillbirths or congenital malformations, encourage parents to see and hold the infant. If there are severe congenital anomalies, wrap the baby and show only normal foot or hand. Allow them to take photographs if they want. Guide them for funeral arrangements if they ask. Give them adequate time with baby.

Don'ts:

1. Do not use medical jargons.
2. Do not talk with other patients or staff members at that time.
3. Do not scold patients or relatives.

4. Do not say I know how you are feeling, unless you have gone through similar situation.
5. Do not lie.

CONCLUSION

Bad news in obstetrics not only affects pregnant women and their families but also affects entire medical team. Although breaking bad news is a difficult task, it is fundamentally important task for all healthcare professionals. Complex art of breaking bad news can be mastered through focused training's and simulation techniques. It is an essential skill for good medical practice and can be acquired with experience. It is also important to teach this art to students during their curriculum. Every institute or hospital should follow a specific protocol so that there is uniformity while breaking bad news. Healthcare providers should provide mindful, compassionate, and empathetic care to the pregnant women and their families.

REFERENCES

1. Nonino A, Magalhães SG, Falcão DP. Treinamento médico para comunicação de más notícias: revisão da literatura. Rev Bras Educ Med. 2012;36(02):228-33.
2. Lino CA, Augusto KL, Oliveira RA, et al. Uso do protocolo Spikes no ensino de habilidades em transmissão de más notícias. Rev Bras Educ Med. 2011;35(01):52-7.
3. Setubal MSV, Antonio MÂRGM, Amaral EM, et al. Improving perinatology residents' skills in breaking bad news: a randomized intervention study. Rev Bras Ginecol Obstet. 2018;40(03):137-46.
4. Karkowsky CE, Landsberger EJ, Bernstein PS, et al. Breaking Bad News in obstetrics: a randomized trial of simulation followed by debriefing or lecture. J Maternal Fetal Neonatal Med. 2016;29(22):3717-23.
5. Guerra FA, Mirlesse V, Baião AE. Breaking bad news during prenatal care: a challenge to be tackled. Ciênc Saúde Coletiva. 2011;16(05):2361-7.
6. Lim CE, Cheng NC. Clinician's role of psychological support in helping parents and families with pregnancy loss. J Aust Tradit Med Soc. 2011;17(04):215-17.
7. Nuzum D, Meaney S, O'Donohue K. Communication skills in Obstetrics: what can we learn from bereaved parents? Ir Med J. 2017;110(02):512.
8. Heazell AEP, Siassakos D, Blencowe H, et al; Lancet Ending Preventable Stillbirths Series study group. Lancet Ending Preventable Stillbirth investigator group. Stillbirths: economic and psychosocial consequences. Lancet. 2016;387(10018):604-16.
9. Gold KJ. Navigating care after a baby dies: a systematic review of parent experiences with health providers. J Preinatol. 2007;27(4):230-7.
10. Greiner AL, Conklin J. Breaking bad news to a pregnant woman with a fetal abnormality on ultrasound. Obstet Gynecol Surv. 2015;70(01):39-44.
11. Lalos A. Breaking bad news concerning fertility. Hum Reprod. 1999;14(03):581-5.
12. Cockburn J, Walters WA. Communication between doctors and patients. Curr Obstet Gynaecol. 1999;9(01):34-40.
13. Royal College of Obstetrics and Gynecology. Late Intrauterine Fetal Death and Stillbirth: Greentop Guideline 55. London: Royal College of Obstetrics and Gynecology; 2010.
14. Farrow VA, Goldenberg RL, Fretts R, et al. Psychological impact of stillbirths on obstetricians. J Matern Fetal Neonatal Med. 2013;26(8):748-52.
15. Beck CT, LoGiudice J, Gable RK. A mixed- methods study of secondary traumatic stress in certified nurse-midwives: shaken belief in birth process. J Midwifery Womens Health. 2015;60(1):16-23.

16. Leone D, Menichetti J, Barusi L, et al. Breaking bad news in assisted reproductive technology: a proposal for guidelines. Reprod Health. 2017;14(01):87.
17. Setubal MSV, Gonçalves AV, Rocha SR, et al. Breaking bad news training program based on video reviews and SPIKES strategy: what do perinatology residents think about it? Rev Bras Ginecol Obstet. 2017;39(10):552-9.
18. Sanghavi DM. What makes for a compassionate patient-caregiver relationship? Jt Comm J Qual Patient Saf. 2006;32(5):283-92.
19. Youngson R. Time to care. How to love your patients and your job. Raglan, NZ: Rebelheart Publishers; 2012
20. Nallen K. Midwive's needs in relation to the provision of bereavement support to parents affected by perinatal death. Part one. MIDIRS Midwifery Digest. 2006;16(4):537-42.
21. Buckman R. How to break bad news. A guide for health care professionals. Baltimore, MD: The Johns Hopkins University Press; 1992.
22. Buckman R. Practical plans for difficult conversations in medicine. Strategies that work in breaking bad news. Baltimore, MD: The Johns Hopkins University Press; 2010.
23. Baile WF, Buckman R, Lenzi R, et al. SPIKES-a six-step protocol for delivering bad news: application to the patient with cancer. Oncologist. 2000;5(4):302-11.

Contraception

94. **Progestogen-only Pills and Depot Medroxyprogesterone Acetate**
Ruchika Garg, Neelansha Varshney

95. **Emergency Contraception**
Ruchika Garg

96. **Tubal Ligation**
Ruchika Garg

97. **Why ART Pregnancies are High-Risk?**
Ruchika Garg

Progestogen-only Pills and Depot Medroxyprogesterone Acetate

Ruchika Garg, Neelansha Varshney

INTRODUCTION

Progestogen-only pills (POPs) and *depot medroxyprogesterone acetate (DMPA)* are effective contraceptive options, particularly for women unsuitable for estrogen-containing methods. POPs require daily compliance, while DMPA offers long-acting reversible contraception (LARC).

EPIDEMIOLOGY

- **Global:**
  - *POP use:* ~9 million women (6% of contraceptive users).[1]
  - *DMPA use:* ~74 million women, predominantly in low-resource settings.[2]
- **India:**
  - *POP prevalence:* <1% among married women (NFHS-5, 2019–21).[3]
  - *DMPA prevalence:* 2.3% higher in rural areas due to accessibility.[4]
  - DMPA, Antra promoted under India's National Family Planning Program.[5]
- **Trends:** DMPA uptake increasing; POPs underutilized due to bleeding concerns.[6]

PROGESTOGEN-ONLY PILLS (FIG. 1)

Types and Formulations

- **Available POPs (Table 1):**[7]
  - *Levonorgestrel (LNG):* 30 µg
  - *Norethisterone (NET):* 350 µg
  - *Desogestrel (DSG):* 75 µg
  - *Drospirenone (DRSP):* 4 mg

Mechanism of Action

- **Primary:** Thickens cervical mucus, impairing sperm penetration.[9]
- **Secondary:**
  - Thins the endometrium, reducing implantation likelihood.
  - Slows tubal motility.
  - DSG/DRSP: Inhibits ovulation via anti-gonadotropic effects.[10]

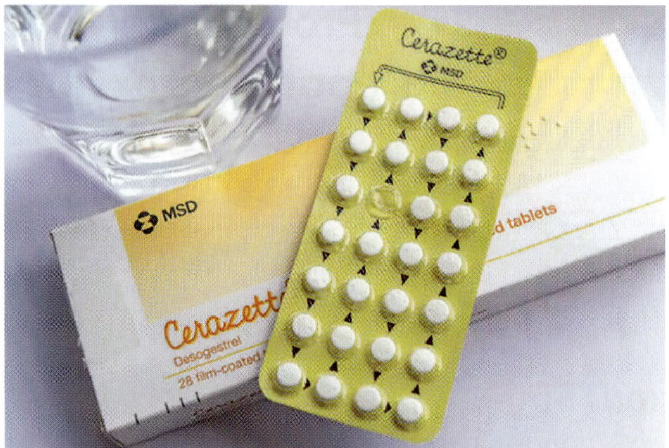

Fig. 1: Progesterone-only pills, which come under the brand name Cerazette.

TABLE 1: POP formulations.[7,8]

POP	*Dose*	*Regimen*	*Ovulation suppression*
LNG	30 µg	Daily, no HFI	Partial
NET	350 µg	Daily, no HFI	Partial
DSG	75 µg	Daily, no HFI	Consistent
DRSP	4 mg	24 active pills, 4-day HFI	Consistent

Effectiveness

- **Perfect use:** >99% effective; failure rate 0.1–0.3%.
- **Typical use:** 9% failure rate due to noncompliance.
- **Factors:**
  - *Timing:* Must be taken at the same time daily (±3 hours for LNG/NET, ±12 hours for DSG, ±24 hours for DRSP).
  - *Vomiting/diarrhea:* Replace pill if within 2 h (LNG/NET) or 3–4 hours (DSG/DRSP).
  - *Drug Interactions:* Enzyme inducers (e.g., rifampicin) reduce efficacy; use DMPA or IUD instead.
  - *BMI:* No impact on efficacy.

Initiation

- **Standard start:** Day 1–5 of menses, post-abortion (day 5), or postpartum (day 21).
- **Quick start:** Any cycle day; use condoms for 2 days (LNG/NET/DSG) or 7 days (DRSP).
- **Post-EC:**
  - *LNG-EC:* Start POP immediately; condoms for 2–7 days.
  - *UPA-EC:* Delay POP 5 days; condoms for 2–7 days.

POP INITIATION PROTOCOLS (TABLE 2)

TABLE 2: POP initiation protocols.

POP type	*Standard start*	*Quick start (backup)*
LNG/NET/DSG	Day 1–5 menses, day 5 abortion, and day 21 postpartum	2 days condoms
DRSP	Day 1 menses, day 1 abortion, and day 21 postpartum	7 days condoms

MISSED PILL MANAGEMENT (TABLE 3)

TABLE 3: Missed pill protocols.

POP	*Missed pill threshold*	*Management*
LNG/NET	>3 hours (>27 hours since last)	Take missed pill ASAP; next pill at usual time; condoms for 48 h; consider EC
DSG	>12 hours (>36 hours since last)	Same as above
DRSP	>24h (>48 hours since last)	Take missed pill ASAP; condoms for 7 days; skip HFI if last 7 pills missed; EC

Contraindications

- **WHO MEC 4 (unacceptable risk):** Current breast cancer.
- **WHO MEC 3 (risk outweigh benefits):** Past breast cancer, severe cirrhosis, ischemic heart disease/stroke (continuation only).
- **DRSP-specific:** Avoid in severe renal failure, hyperkalemia, or with potassium-sparing drugs.

Side Effects

- **Common:** Unscheduled bleeding (20–40%); improves over time, often leading to amenorrhea.
  - Management: Rule out pathology; consider NSAIDs, tranexamic acid, or DSG double dose (150 μg, off-label).
- **Others:** Headache, acne, mood changes (no consistent evidence).
- **No Evidence:** Increased VTE, depression, weight gain, or bone loss.

Noncontraceptive Benefits

- **DSG/DRSP:** Reduce heavy menstrual bleeding (HMB) and dysmenorrhea.
- **DRSP:** Potential anti-androgenic effects for acne/hirsutism (unproven).

Follow-Up and Discontinuation

- **Follow-Up:** Annual review; earlier if side effects or method switch needed.
- **Discontinuation:** Immediate fertility return; offer alternative contraception if needed.

DEPOT MEDROXYPROGESTERONE ACETATE (FIGS. 2 AND 3)

Formulation and Administration

- **India:** Depo-Provera (150 mg/1 mL IM every 12 weeks).
- **Depo-Sub Q provera 104** (Sayana press) contains 104 mg of DMPA. It is given subcutaneously over the anterior thigh or abdomen at every 90 days. It suppresses ovulation for 3 months as it is absorbed more slowly.
- **Sites:** Gluteus maximus, lateral thigh, or deltoid (obese women).
- **Timing:** Every 12 weeks (10–14 weeks acceptable; WHO allows up to 16 weeks).

Mechanism of Action

- **Primary:** Inhibits ovulation via gonadotropin suppression.
- **Secondary:** Thickens cervical mucus; thins endometrium.

Effectiveness

- **Perfect use:** 0.2% failure rate.
- **Typical use:** 6% failure rate due to missed injections.
- **Factors:**
    - BMI: Effective in obesity (BMI <40 kg/m^2); caution if BMI ≥40 kg/m^2.

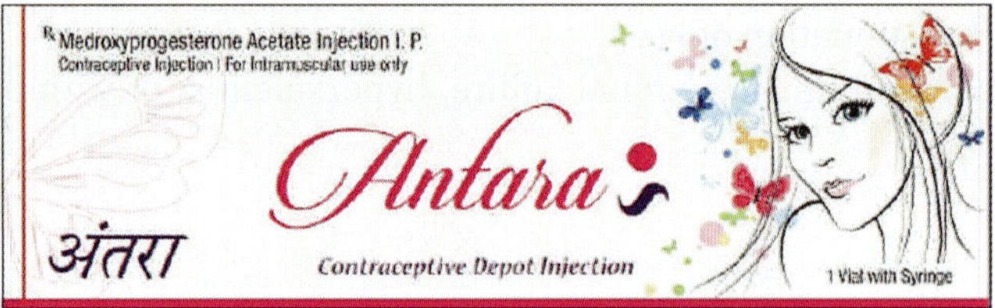

Fig. 2: Depot medroxyprogesterone acetate (DMPA) injection (also known as Antara).

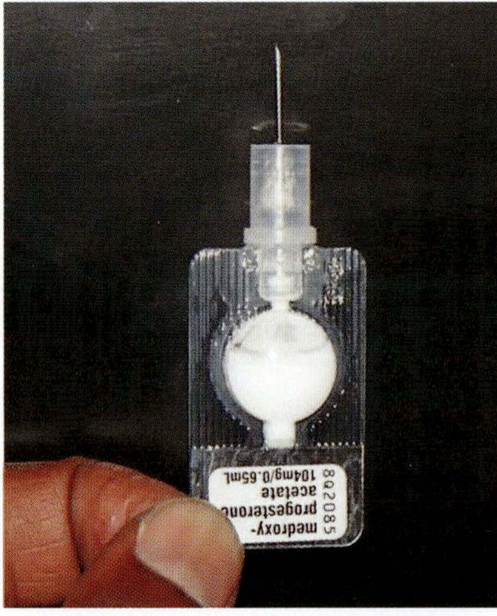

Fig. 3: Depo-Sub Q provera 104.

- Drug Interactions: Unaffected by enzyme inducers (e.g., antiretrovirals and antiepileptics).

Initiation

- **Standard Start:** Day 1–5 of menses, post-abortion, or 21 days postpartum.
- **Quick Start:** Any day; use condoms for 7 days; rule out pregnancy **(Box 1)**.
- **Post-EC:** Same as POPs.

BOX 1: Criteria to rule out pregnancy.

- No intercourse since last menstrual period (LMP), abortion, or delivery
- Consistent use of reliable contraception
- Negative urine pregnancy test (>21 days post-UPSI)
- Within 5 days of menses/abortion or 21 days postpartum
- Exclusively breastfeeding, amenorrheic, <6 months postpartum

Switching to Depot Medroxyprogesterone Acetate (Table 4)

TABLE 4: Switching to DMPA.

From	*Timing*	*Backup needed*
Combined hormonal	Day 1–2 or weeks 2–3 of the cycle	None
POP (LNG/NET)	Any day	7 days
POP (DSG)	Any day (if used correctly)	None
Copper IUD	Day 1–5 of the cycle	None
LNG-IUS/Implant	Any day	7 days

Contraindications

- **WHO MEC 4:** Current breast cancer.
- **WHO MEC 3:** Severe hypertension, diabetes with vascular disease, ischemic heart disease/stroke (continuation).

Side Effects

- **Bleeding:** Amenorrhea (50% after 1 year), spotting, or prolonged bleeding; evaluate for pathology.
- **Weight gain:** 1–3 kg/year, higher in adolescents with BMI >30 kg/m^2.
- **Bone mineral density (BMD):** Reversible loss; greatest in first year; no routine DEXA needed.
- **Others:** Acne, mood changes, and headache (unproven).

Noncontraceptive Benefits

- Reduces HMB, endometriosis pain, and dysmenorrhea.
- Decreases ovarian/endometrial cancer risk.
- Possible reduction in sickle cell crisis pain.

Health Risks

- **Breast cancer:** Weak, nonsignificant risk with recent use.
- **Cervical cancer:** Possible association; screen regularly.
- **VTE/CVD:** No increased risk; safe in thrombophilia.
- **HIV:** No conclusive link to acquisition.

Follow-Up and Discontinuation

- **Follow-up:** Every 12 weeks; reassess eligibility, side effects, and BMI.
- **Discontinuation:** Fertility return delayed up to 12 months; offer alternative contraception.

WORLD HEALTH ORGANIZATION/ROYAL COLLEGE OF OBSTETRICIANS AND GYNAECOLOGISTS/FACULTY OF SEXUAL AND REPRODUCTIVE HEALTHCARE GUIDELINES (2023)

- **POPs:**
  - Safe for most women, including breastfeeding; no BMI restrictions.
  - Counsel on bleeding patterns; offer alternatives if unacceptable.
- **DMPA:**
  - Preferred LARC in enzyme-inducer users; safe in obesity (BMI <40 kg/m^2).
  - Monitor adolescents/older women for BMD risk; no routine screening.
- **Counseling:** Emphasize non-contraceptive benefits, side effects, and fertility return.
- **Access:** Ensure availability in primary care; train providers for DMPA administration.

INDIAN CONTEXT

- **Challenges:** Low POP use due to bleeding concerns; DMPA preferred for simplicity.
- **Strategies:** Promote DMPA via ASHA workers; address bleeding misconceptions.
- **2022 study:** DMPA uptake 5% in rural Uttar Pradesh; POPs <0.5%.

CLINICAL CASE SCENARIO

Case

A 30-year-old breastfeeding mother, 8 weeks postpartum, requests contraception. BMI: 28 kg/m^2, no medical history.

Management

- **Counseling:** Discuss POPs (safe in lactation) vs. DMPA (long-acting).
- **Prescription: DSG 75 μg** daily (no HFI, ovulation suppression).
- **Initiation:** Start immediately; no backup needed (postpartum day >21).
- **Education:** Explain bleeding patterns, missed pill protocol, and annual follow-up.
- **Outcome:** No bleeding issues; continues DSG; satisfied.

IMPLANTS

- Contraceptive implants provide long-acting, highly effective, reversible contraception.
- They are small and rod-shaped.
- They provide controlled release of progestin over the years.
- The rods are implanted surgically into the upper nondominant arm.
- They are of the following types:
  - Norplant } contains Levonorgestrel
  - Jadelle }
  - Sinoimplant (II)
  - Implanon } contains etonogestrel
  - Nexplanon }
- *Norplant:* It consists of six flexible rods, each containing 36 mg of levonorgestrel. It prevents pregnancy for 5 years **(Fig. 4)**.
- Jadelle consists of two rods placed in the shape of a "V" opening towards the shoulder. It provides contraception for 5 years **(Fig. 5)**.

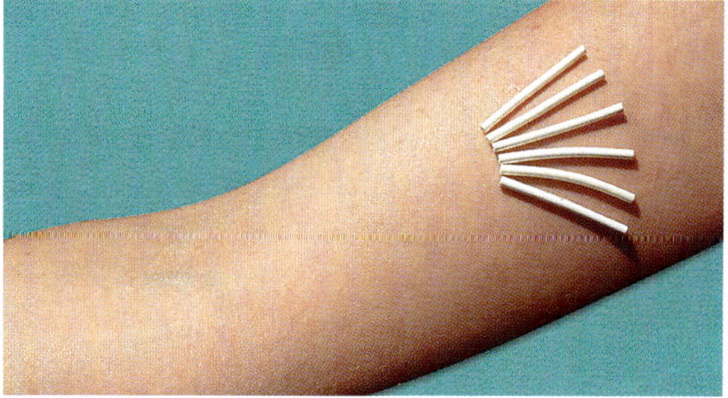

Fig. 4: Norplant.

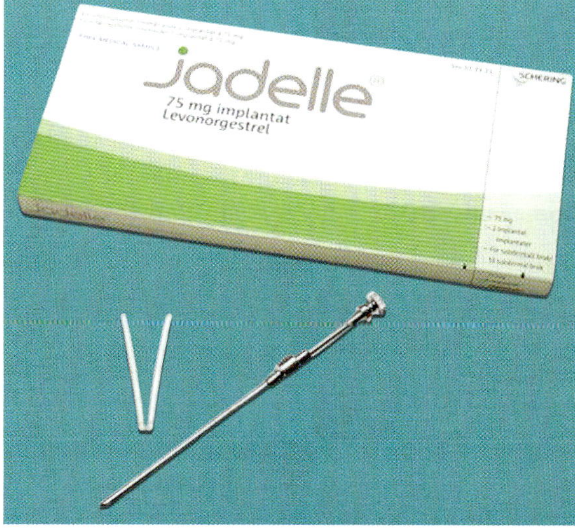

Fig. 5: Jadelle implant.

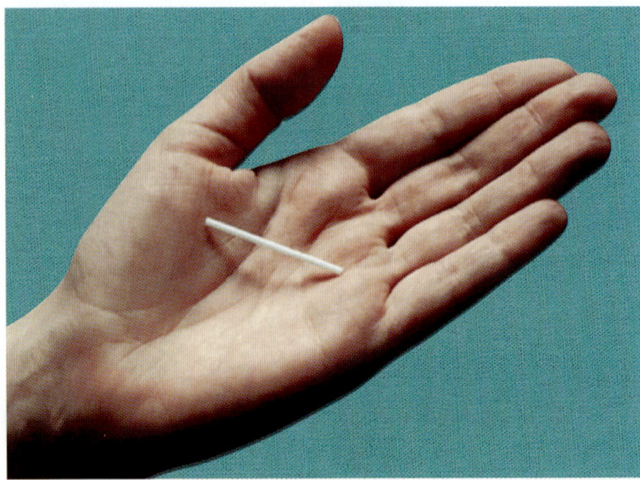

Fig. 6: Implanon implant.

- *Implanon:* It is a single rod implant that releases etonogestrel, which prevents pregnancy for 3 years. The initial release rate of 60–70 µg/day falls gradually to around 25–30 µg/day at the end of 3 years **(Fig. 6)**.
- *Nexplanon:* It is also a single rod implant like Implanon. The only difference is that Nexplanon contains barium sulphate, which makes it radiopaque. So, it can be seen on X-ray, CT scan, and MRI.
- *Advantages of implants:*
    - It provides 99% contraceptive efficacy.
    - It works for a long period (3/4/5 years); hence it is convenient.
    - It is safe to use while breastfeeding.
    - It is an option when estrogen-based contraception is contraindicated.
    - It is totally reversible; return to fertility is immediately after removal.
    - The implant may reduce heavy or painful menstrual bleeding.
- *Disadvantages of implants:*
    - It may cause amenorrhea or irregular vaginal bleeding.
    - Weight gain, acne, fluid retention, headache, breast tenderness, hair loss, mood changes, abdominal pain, and itching at the insertion site.
    - It does not protect against HIV or other sexually transmitted infections.

Exam tip: Highlight POP safety in breastfeeding, DMPA's LARC advantage, and bleeding management.

KEY POINTS

- **POP use in India:** <1%; DMPA 2.3%, higher in rural areas.
- **Effectiveness:** POPs 99% (perfect use); DMPA 99.8% (perfect use).
- **Side Effects:** Unscheduled bleeding is common; BMD loss with DMPA is reversible.
- **Benefits:** POPs/DMPA reduce HMB, endometriosis pain, ovarian/endometrial cancer.

- **Guidelines:** Safe in most women; counsel on bleeding and fertility return.
- **Challenges:** Address bleeding misconceptions; improve rural access.

IMPORTANT POINTS TO REMEMBER

- POPs are safe in breastfeeding; DSG/DRSP inhibit ovulation.
- DMPA is effective in obesity and enzyme-induced users; monitor BMD in adolescents.
- Unscheduled bleeding is common; rule out pathology before attributing it to POPs/DMPA.
- Fertility return: Immediate for POPs, delayed up to 12 months for DMPA.

REFERENCES

1. United Nations. (2019). Contraceptive use by method 2019. [Online] Available from https://digitallibrary.un.org/record/3849735?ln=en&v=pdf [Last accessed December, 2025].
2. World Health Organization. Family planning: a global handbook for providers: evidence-based guidance developed through worldwide collaboration, 3rd edition. Geneva: World Health Organization; 2022.
3. NFHS-5. National Family Health Survey 2019–21. Mumbai: IIPS; 2021.
4. Sharma V, Singh SK. Contraceptive trends in India: NFHS-5 analysis. Indian J Community Med. 2021;46(3):401-6.
5. MoHFW. Family planning program in India. New Delhi: Government of India; 2020.
6. Gupta A, et al. Barriers to POP and DMPA use in India. J Fam Plann Reprod Health Care. 2020;46(2):89-95.
7. FSRH. Progestogen-only pills. London: Faculty of Sexual and Reproductive Healthcare; 2023.
8. World Health Organization. Medical eligibility criteria for contraceptive use, 5th edition. Geneva: WHO; 2015.
9. Curtis KM, et al. Progestin-only contraception: mechanisms and efficacy. Contraception. 2016;94(5):419-25.
10. Archer DF, et al. Drospirenone-only pill: a new contraceptive option. Eur J Contracept Reprod Health Care. 2019;24(1):4-10.

Emergency Contraception

Ruchika Garg

INTRODUCTION

Emergency contraception (EC) prevents unintended pregnancies after unprotected sexual intercourse (UPSI) or contraceptive failure, reducing the global burden of unsafe abortions (~20 million annually).[1] In India, unsafe abortions contribute to a maternal death every 2 hours.[2]

EPIDEMIOLOGY

- **Global:**
  - ~42 million abortions yearly; 20 million unsafe[3]
  - 1 in 10 pregnancies ends in unsafe abortion.[4]
  - EC use: ~5–10% of women aged 15–44 in high-income countries[5]
- **India:**
  - Highest number of unsafe abortions globally (~8 million annually)[6]
  - EC use: 11% among women aged 15–49 (NFHS-5, 2019–21)[7]
  - Levonorgestrel (LNG) ECPs dominate; ulipristal acetate (UPA) and IUDs less common[8]
- **Trends:** Increased EC awareness in urban India; rural access remains limited.[9]

DEFINITION AND INDICATIONS

Emergency contraception: Methods used within days post-UPSI to prevent pregnancy.[10]

- **Indications:**
  - No contraception used during UPSI
  - Contraceptive failure: Condom breakage, missed pills (≥3 combined oral contraceptives), and delayed injectables
  - Incorrect use: Miscalculated fertile days, failed withdrawal
  - Sexual assault without contraceptive protection

COMMON SCENARIOS REQUIRING EC (TABLE 1)

TABLE 1: Common Scenarios Requiring EC.

Scenario	*Details*
Condom failure	Breakage, slippage, and incorrect use
Missed pills	≥3 combined pills; >27 hours for LNG minipill
Delayed injection	>2 weeks for NET-EN; >4 weeks for DMPA
IUD expulsion	Partial or complete expulsion
Sexual assault	No effective contraception used

METHODS OF EMERGENCY CONTRACEPTION (TABLE 2)

TABLE 2: EC Methods and Regimens.

Method	*Regimen*	*Timing Post-UPSI*	*Failure Rate*
Yuzpe (COC)	100 µg EE + 0.5 mg LNG, 2 doses 12 hours apart	Within 72 hours	0–2%
LNG ECP	1.5 mg single dose or 0.75 mg 2 doses 12 hours apart	Within 72 hours	0–1%
UPA	30 mg single dose	Within 120 hours	0.9–1.8%
Mifepristone	10 mg single dose	Within 120 hours	0.06%
Copper IUD	Insertion (e.g., Cu T 380A)	Within 5 days	0–0.1%

Hormonal Methods:

- **Yuzpe Regimen:** Combined EE + LNG; less effective, more side effects
- **LNG ECP:** Preferred in India; single-dose 1.5 mg most common; shown in **Figure 1**.
- **UPA:** Selective progesterone receptor modulator; more effective than LNG, especially in obese women; shown in **Figure 2**.
- **Mifepristone:** Antiprogestin; limited availability in India

Mechanical Method:

- **Copper IUD**: Most effective; suitable for ongoing contraception; contraindicated in PID, AUB, and pregnancy.

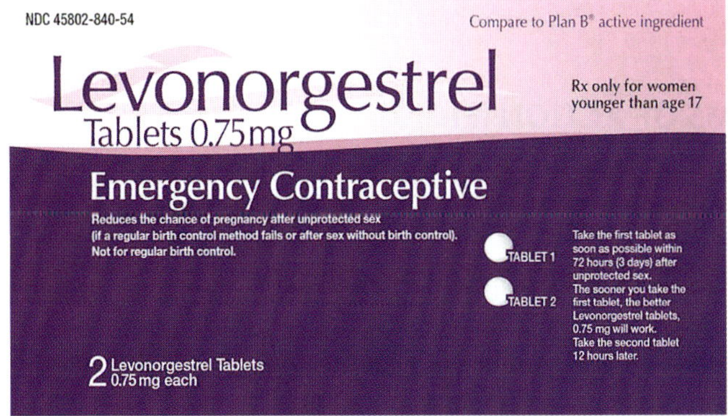

Fig. 1: Levonorgestrel emergency contraceptive.

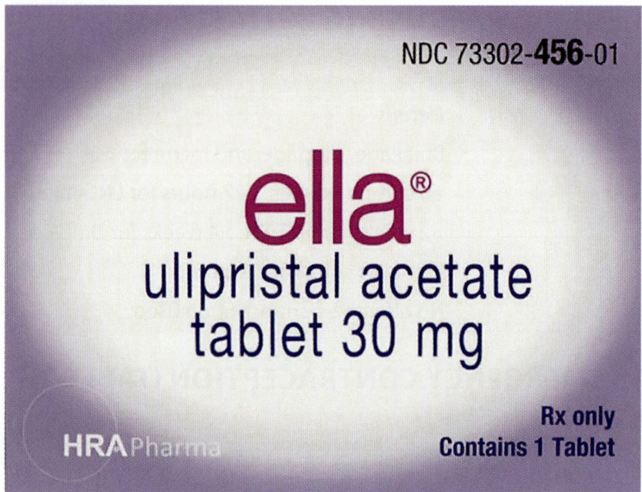

Fig. 2: Ulipristal acetate emergency contraceptive.

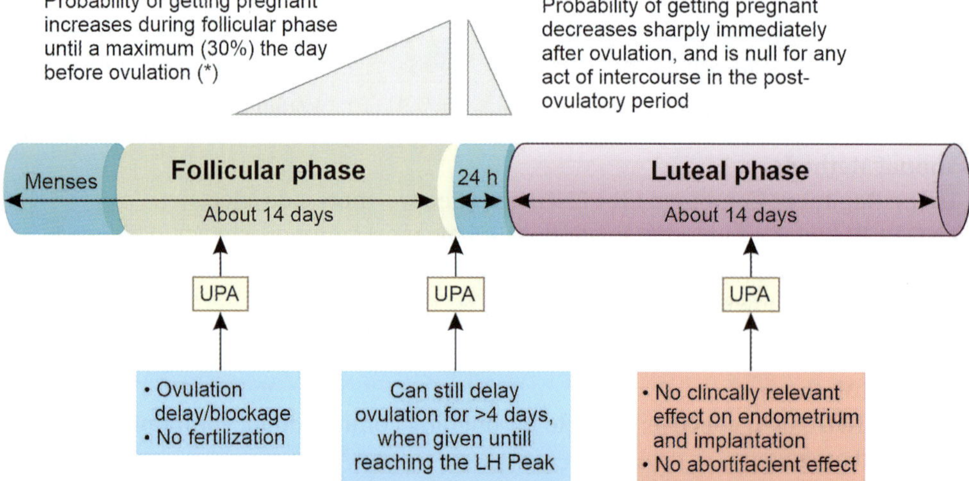

Fig. 3: Mechanism of LNG and UPA ECPs.

MECHANISMS OF ACTION (FIG. 3)

- **Primary**:
  - **LNG/UPA:** Inhibit or delay ovulation by suppressing LH surge; UPA effective post-LH surge
  - **Yuzpe:** Similar ovulation suppression via EE + LNG
- **Secondary (Postulated):**
  - Thicken cervical mucus, impair sperm transport
  - Alter tubal motility or corpus luteum function
- **No Effect:** Postimplantation; do not disrupt established pregnancies or harm fetuses.

TABLE 3: Side Effects of Hormonal ECPs.

Side Effect	*LNG Prevalence*	*UPA Prevalence*	*Management*
Nausea	~20%	~12%	Antiemetic if needed
Vomiting	<5%	<5%	Repeat dose if within 2–3 hours
Menstrual changes	Common	Common	Reassure; resolves spontaneously

EFFECTIVENESS

- **LNG ECP:** Prevents 52–94% of pregnancies; most effective within 24 hours
- **UPA:** Prevents 62–85%; effective up to 120 hours
- **Copper IUD:** Prevents >99% of pregnancies
- **Factors:**
  - *Timing:* Efficacy decreases with delay post-UPSI.
  - *BMI:* LNG less effective in BMI ≥30 kg/m^2; UPA or IUD preferred
  - *Repeated UPSI:* Single ECP dose sufficient if all acts within 120 hours.

SIDE EFFECTS

- **Common (Table 3):**
  - *Nausea:* LNG (20%) and UPA (12%)
  - *Vomiting:* If within 2 hours (LNG) or 3 hours (UPA), repeat dose.
  - *Altered menses:* Early (LNG, 1 day) or delayed (UPA, 2 days); resolves spontaneously.
  - *Headache, fatigue, and breast tenderness:* Self-limiting within 24 hours.
- **Safety**: No increased risk of miscarriage, ectopic pregnancy, or congenital anomalies

MEDICAL ELIGIBILITY AND SPECIAL CONSIDERATIONS

- **WHO Medical Eligibility Criteria (MEC):**
  - **Category 1:** No restrictions for LNG, UPA, or Yuzpe; safe in all women, including adolescents
  - **Category 2:** Breastfeeding women (UPA: avoid breastfeeding for 1 week)
- **Special Populations:**
  - **Adolescents:** Safe; recommended postrape within 5 days
  - **Breastfeeding:** LNG preferred; UPA requires milk discard for 1 week
  - **Obesity:** UPA or IUD preferred; consider double-dose LNG (3 mg).
  - **Drug Interactions:**
    - Hepatic enzyme inducers (e.g., rifampicin and efavirenz): Reduce LNG/UPA efficacy; use IUD or double-dose LNG.
    - Recent progestin use: May reduce UPA efficacy.

GUIDELINES

WHO (2023):

- **Preferred Methods:** UPA (120 hours), LNG (72 hours), or IUD (5 days)
- **Yuzpe:** Alternative if others unavailable
- **Access:** No prescription needed; ensure availability postrape.

RCOG/NICE/FSRH (2023):
- **First-Line**: Copper IUD (most effective); UPA if IUD declined/unavailable
- **LNG**: Use within 72 hours; consider double dose in BMI ≥30 kg/m^2.
- **Counseling**: Discuss side effects, follow-up contraception, and STI screening postrape.
- **Adolescents**: No age restrictions; ensure confidentiality.

India (MoHFW, 2008, updated 2019):
- **Approved:** LNG 1.5 mg single dose or 0.75 mg 12 hours apart (72 hours); Yuzpe; IUD.
- **Access:** Over-the-counter LNG; IUD requires trained provider.
- **Challenges:** Limited UPA/mifepristone availability; rural access barriers.

INDIAN CONTEXT

- **Burden:** ~26 million pregnancies annually; 30% unintended
- **EC Use:** LNG dominates (Ezy Pill and i-Pill); 80% of EC market.
- **Issues:**
    - Misconceptions: 40% of women confuse ECPs with abortion pills.
    - Rural uptake: <5% due to stigma and supply chain issues.
- **2022 Study:** EC awareness 65% in urban vs. 25% in rural India.

CLINICAL CASE SCENARIO

Case: A 22-year-old nulliparous woman presents 48 hours post-UPSI due to condom breakage. BMI: 22 kg/m^2, no medical history, not breastfeeding.

Management:
- **Counseling:** Explain EC options, efficacy, and side effects; discuss ongoing contraception.
- **Prescription: LNG 1.5 mg** single dose (available OTC in India)
- **Advice:** Take immediately; use antiemetic if nausea occurs; expect menses within 7 days.
- **Follow-Up:** Return if no menses in 3 weeks; initiate combined oral contraceptive.
- **Outcome:** Menses on day 30; starts COC; no pregnancy.

Exam Tip: Highlight LNG as India's preferred ECP, timing (72 hours), and IUD's superior efficacy.

KEY POINTS

- **EC use in India:** 11% among women; LNG dominates.
- **Methods:** LNG (72 hours), UPA (120 hours), IUD (5 days); IUD most effective
- **Mechanism:** Delays ovulation; no effect postimplantation
- **Safety:** Safe for all women, including adolescents; no fetal harm
- **Guidelines:** WHO prefers UPA/IUD; India approves LNG/Yuzpe/IUD.
- **Challenges:** Rural access, misconceptions, and limited UPA use.

IMPORTANT POINTS TO REMEMBER

- EC prevents pregnancy post-UPSI; not an abortifacient.
- Copper IUD is the most effective EC method (failure rate <0.1%).

- LNG ECP is first-line in India; take within 72 hours for optimal efficacy.
- Counsel on side effects and ongoing contraception post-EC.

REFERENCES

1. Leung VW, Levine M, Soon JA. Mechanisms of action of hormonal emergency contraceptives. Pharmacotherapy. 2010 Feb;30(2):158-68. doi: 10.1592/phco.30.2.158. PMID: 20099990..
2. Cleland K, Raymond EG, Westley E, Trussell J. Emergency contraception review: evidence-based recommendations for clinicians. Clin Obstet Gynecol. 2014 Dec;57(4):741-50. doi: 10.1097/GRF.0000000000000056. PMID: 25254919; PMCID: PMC4216625.
3. WHO. Emergency contraception. Geneva: World Health Organization; 2018.
4. Guttmacher Institute. Unintended Pregnancy and Abortion Worldwide; 2020.
5. Haeger KO, Lamme J, Cleland K. State of emergency contraception in the U.S., 2018. Contracept Reprod Med. 2018 Sep 5;3:20. doi: 10.1186/s40834-018-0067-8. PMID: 30202545; PMCID: PMC6123910.
6. Singh S, et al. Abortion and unintended pregnancy in India. Lancet Glob Health. 2018;6(8):e849-59.
7. NFHS-5. National Family Health Survey 2019-21. Mumbai: IIPS; 2021.
8. Sharma P, et al. Emergency contraception trends in India. Indian J Community Med. 2020;45(3):301-5.
9. Gupta R, et al. Barriers to EC access in rural India. J Fam Plann Reprod Health Care. 2019;45(2):112-8.
10. ACOG. Emergency contraception. Practice Bulletin No. 152. Obstet Gynecol. 2017;130(3):e117-24.

Tubal Ligation

Ruchika Garg

INTRODUCTION

- *Definition:* Tubal ligation is a permanent surgical method of female sterilization that involves occlusion or disruption of the fallopian tubes to prevent sperm-egg interaction, thereby preventing pregnancy.
- *Historical Context:* Introduced in India as part of family planning programs in the 1950s, tubal ligation remains a cornerstone of population control strategies, particularly in public health settings.
- *Relevance in India:* India has one of the highest rates of female sterilization globally, with tubal ligation being the most common contraceptive method among women, especially in rural areas. According to the National Family Health Survey (NFHS-5, 2019–2021), 37.9% of married women aged 15–49 in India use female sterilization.

INDICATIONS

- *Contraceptive*:
  - Permanent contraception for women who have completed their desired family size.
  - Couples seeking a reliable, non-reversible method of birth control.
- *Medical:*
  - High-risk pregnancies where future pregnancies could endanger maternal health (e.g., severe cardiac disease, uncontrolled hypertension, or multiple cesarean sections).
  - Genetic conditions where avoiding pregnancy is advised.
- *Socioeconomic*: Common in India due to economic constraints, limited access to reversible contraception, or cultural preferences for early sterilization after achieving desired family size.

CONTRAINDICATIONS

- *Absolute*:
  - Uncertainty about sterilization or desire for future fertility.
  - Coercion or lack of informed consent.
  - Active pelvic infection or severe systemic illness precluding surgery.
- *Relative*:
  - Young age (<25 years) due to higher risk of regret.

  - Psychological instability or lack of understanding of the procedure's permanence.
  - Immediate postpartum period in cases of maternal or neonatal complications (requires careful counseling).

ETHICAL CONSIDERATIONS

- *Informed Consent*:
  - Critical ethical principle; patients must be fully informed about the procedure's permanence, risks, benefits, and alternatives (e.g., IUDs, implants, vasectomy).
  - In India, historical instances of coerced sterilizations (e.g., during the 1970s Emergency) underscore the need for voluntary consent.
  - Language barriers, illiteracy, and cultural pressures (e.g., family expectations) must be addressed to ensure autonomy.
- *Autonomy versus Paternalism*:
  - Indian healthcare often leans toward paternalistic decision-making. Clinicians must prioritize patient autonomy, especially in rural settings where women may face societal pressure.
  - Ethical dilemmas arise when women are pressured by family or healthcare providers to undergo sterilization for population control.
- *Justice*:
  - Access to sterilization should be equitable, but overuse in marginalized communities (e.g., low-income or tribal women) raises concerns about systemic bias.
  - Alternatives like male sterilization (vasectomy) are underutilized in India (NFHS-5: only 0.3% of men opt for vasectomy).
- *Non-Maleficence and Beneficence*:
  - Ensure minimal harm (e.g., low complication rates) and maximum benefit (e.g., effective contraception).
  - Counseling must address the risk of regret (higher in younger women or those with fewer children).
- *Ethical Scenarios for Examinations*:
  - *Case*: A 24-year-old woman with two children requests tubal ligation. How would you counsel her, considering her age and potential for regret?
  - *Case*: A woman is pressured by her husband to undergo sterilization after her third cesarean. How do you ensure informed consent?

TECHNIQUES OF TUBAL LIGATION (FIGS. 1 AND 2)

- *Approaches:*
  - *Minilaparotomy:* Common in India, especially in postpartum settings (within 7 days of delivery). Performed under local or spinal anesthesia in resource-limited settings.
  - *Laparoscopy:* Preferred for interval sterilization (outside the postpartum period). Requires specialized equipment and training.
  - *Hysteroscopic Sterilization:* Less common in India due to cost and availability (e.g., Essure device, not widely used).

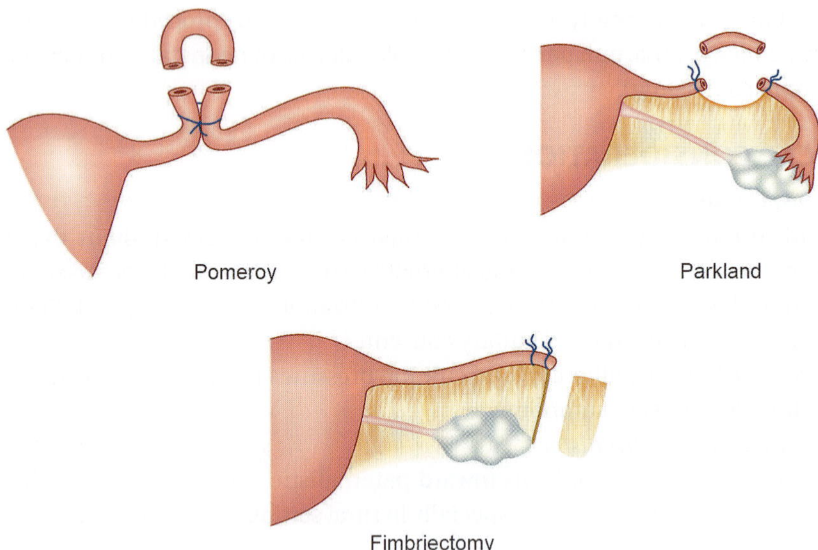

Fig. 1: Various methods of tubal ligation.

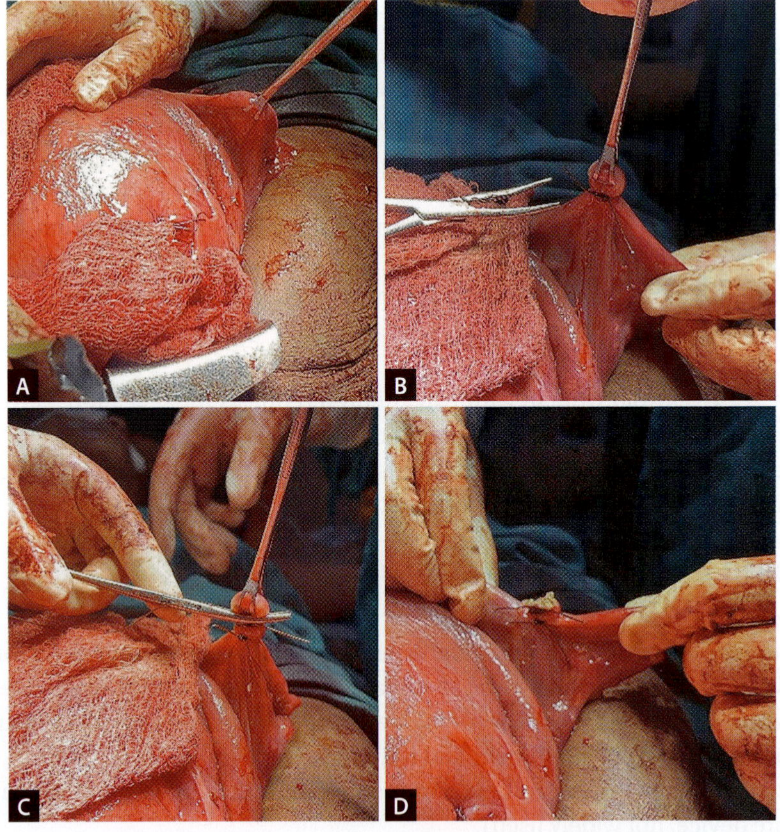

Figs. 2A to D: Steps of Pomeroy method of Tubal ligation.

- *Methods of Tubal Occlusion:*
  - *Pomeroy Technique:* Partial resection of the fallopian tube with ligation; widely used in India due to simplicity and effectiveness.
  - *Modified Pomeroy:* Variation with improved outcomes.
  - *Parkland Technique:* Double ligation and resection of a segment of the tube.
  - *Fimbriectomy:* Removal of the fimbrial end of the tube; less common due to higher failure rates.
  - *Electrocoagulation:* Used in laparoscopic sterilization; requires caution to avoid thermal injury.
  - *Clips or Rings (e.g., Falope Ring):* Applied via laparoscopy; reversible in some cases but less common in India.
- *Procedure Details*:
  - *Timing*: Postpartum (within 7 days), post-abortion, or interval (6 weeks post-delivery or later).
  - *Anesthesia*: Local, spinal, or general, depending on the setting and approach.
  - *Duration*: 15–30 minutes for minilaparotomy; 10–20 minutes for laparoscopy.

PREOPERATIVE EVALUATION AND COUNSELING

- *History:*
  - Obstetric history (parity, mode of deliveries).
  - Medical history (contraindications like cardiac disease).
  - Psychosocial assessment (marital status, family dynamics, understanding of permanence).
- *Counseling:*
  - Explain the procedure's irreversibility (reversal success rates are low, ~50–70%, and not routinely available in public hospitals).
  - *Discuss alternatives:* Long-acting reversible contraceptives (LARCs) like IUDs or implants, or male sterilization.
  - Address myths (e.g., sterilization causes weakness or loss of libido, common misconceptions in India).
- *Informed Consent:*
  - Document consent in the patient's native language.
  - Ensure no coercion from family, healthcare providers, or government incentives (e.g., cash incentives in some states).

COMPLICATIONS

- *Immediate:*
  - Bleeding, infection, or injury to adjacent organs (bowel, bladder).
  - Anesthesia-related risks (more common in rural settings with limited facilities).
- *Long-Term*:
  - *Failure rate:* ~0.5–1% (ectopic pregnancy risk is higher in failures, ~1 in 3).
  - *Post-sterilization regret*: Higher in women <30 years or with fewer than two children.

- *Post-tubal ligation syndrome (controversial)*: Symptoms like abnormal uterine bleeding or pelvic pain; not consistently supported by evidence.
- *Management of Complications:*
  - *Ectopic pregnancy:* Requires prompt diagnosis (ultrasound, β-hCG) and management (medical or surgical).
  - *Regret:* Counseling and referral for reversal (if feasible) or assisted reproductive technologies (costly and inaccessible for many in India).

LEGAL AND POLICY FRAMEWORK IN INDIA

- *Government Guidelines:*
  - Tubal ligation is promoted under the National Family Planning Program, with guidelines issued by the Ministry of Health and Family Welfare.
  - Minimum age and parity criteria (e.g., age >22, at least one child) to prevent coerced or premature sterilizations.
  - Accreditation of facilities and surgeons to ensure quality (e.g., "sterilization camps" must follow strict protocols post-2014 Chhattisgarh tragedy).
- *Legal Issues:*
  - Cases of negligence (e.g., infections, deaths in sterilization camps) have led to stricter regulations.
  - Informed consent is mandatory under the Indian Medical Council (Professional Conduct, Etiquette, and Ethics) Regulations, 2002.
- *Ethical-Legal Scenarios for Examinations:*
  - *Case*: A sterilization camp reports a postoperative infection rate of 10%. How would you address this ethically and legally?
  - *Case*: A woman claims she was sterilized without proper consent. Discuss the medico-legal implications.

SOCIO-CULTURAL CONTEXT IN INDIA

- *Gender Dynamics:*
  - Female sterilization dominates over male sterilization due to cultural norms placing reproductive responsibility on women.
  - Addressing male involvement in family planning is a growing focus in public health campaigns.
- *Rural vs. Urban Divide:*
  - Rural women often opt for sterilization due to limited access to reversible contraceptives and economic pressures.
  - Urban women may have better access to LARCs but still face societal expectations for early sterilization.
- *Sterilization Camps:*
  - Common in rural India for mass sterilization programs but criticized for poor quality control and coercion (e.g., Chhattisgarh 2014 incident, where 13 women died due to substandard care).
  - *Ethical challenge*: Balancing population control goals with individual autonomy.

REVERSAL OF TUBAL LIGATION

- *Feasibility:*
  - Success depends on the method used (clips/rings have higher reversal success than resection methods).
  - Microsurgical tubal reanastomosis: Success rates ~50–70%, but expensive and not widely available in India.
- *Indications:*
  - Change in marital status, loss of a child, or desire for more children.
- *Challenges:*
  - High cost, limited expertise, and risk of ectopic pregnancy post-reversal.
  - Counseling is critical to manage expectations.

RECENT ADVANCES AND ALTERNATIVES

- *Hysteroscopic Sterilization:* Less invasive but not widely adopted in India due to cost and training requirements.
- *Long-Acting Reversible Contraceptives (LARCs):*
  - Copper IUDs, LNG-IUS (levonorgestrel intrauterine system), and implants (e.g., Implanon) are gaining traction but face barriers like cost and awareness.
- *Male Sterilization:* Vasectomy is safer and less invasive but underutilized due to cultural stigma.

EXAMINATION-ORIENTED KEY POINTS

- *MCQs:*
  - What is the most common method of tubal ligation in India? (Answer: Pomeroy technique via minilaparotomy)
  - What is the failure rate of tubal ligation? (Answer: ~0.5–1%)
  - Which ethical principle is most critical in tubal ligation? (Answer: Autonomy/informed consent)
- *Case-Based Questions:*
  - A 28-year-old woman with three children requests tubal ligation. Outline your counseling approach, including ethical considerations.
  - A sterilization procedure fails, resulting in an ectopic pregnancy. Discuss the management and ethical implications.
- *Short Notes:*
  - Techniques of tubal ligation.
  - Complications of tubal ligation.
  - Ethical issues in female sterilization in India.

CONCLUSION

Tubal ligation is a critical component of India's family planning strategy but raises complex ethical, legal, and socio-cultural issues. Postgraduate students must understand the procedure's technical aspects, complications, and the ethical framework surrounding informed consent and patient autonomy. In India, the challenge lies in balancing public health goals with individual rights, particularly in resource-constrained settings. Future efforts should focus on promoting reversible contraceptives and male sterilization to reduce over-reliance on female sterilization.

Notes for Postgraduate Students

- National Family Health Survey (NFHS-5) for data on sterilization trends.
- Indian Journal of Medical Ethics for context-specific ethical discussions.

Why ART Pregnancies are High-Risk?

Ruchika Garg

REASONS OF HIGH-RISK ART PREGNANCIES

1. **Multiple gestation**: Transfer of more than one embryo and superovulation increase the incidence of twins and higher-order multiples (up to 30% of ART births), which significantly raise risks of preterm birth, low birth weight, preeclampsia, and perinatal mortality.[1]
2. **Advanced maternal age and comorbidities**: Women undergoing ART are often older and have underlying conditions (obesity, PCOS, endometriosis, and diabetes) that independently increase risks of gestational diabetes, hypertensive disorders, and placental abnormalities.[2]
3. **Placental dysfunction**: ART conceptions, especially frozen embryo transfers and donor gamete cycles, show higher rates of preeclampsia, placenta previa, accreta spectrum, and abruption, possibly due to absent corpus luteum factors, epigenetic changes, or immunological mechanisms.[3]
4. **Preterm birth in singletons**: Even ART singletons have roughly double the rate of spontaneous preterm birth (<37 weeks: 10.1% vs. 5.5%; <34 weeks: 3.6% vs. 2.2%) compared to naturally conceived singletons.[4]
5. **Low birth weight/SGA and long-term concerns**: Higher incidence of small-for-gestational-age infants, modest increase in congenital anomalies, imprinting disorders, and potential epigenetic alterations from cryopreservation or culture conditions.[1]

KEY EVIDENCE-BASED MANAGEMENT STRATEGIES

- Preconception optimization of BMI, glycemic control, and comorbidities; thorough counseling about multiple pregnancy risks and consideration of elective single embryo transfer (eSET).
- Early referral to maternal–fetal medicine specialists; individualized antenatal care with increased surveillance.
- Frequent ultrasound monitoring (first-trimester dating, anatomy, growth, cervical length, and placental assessment).
- Proactive preterm birth prevention in high-risk cases (progesterone, cerclage, or pessary when indicated).
- Close collaboration with neonatology team and planned delivery in tertiary centers for multiples or complicated cases.[5]

- Psychological support throughout treatment and pregnancy, given higher rates of anxiety and postpartum depression.

CONCLUSION

ART pregnancies warrant high-risk classification and specialized multidisciplinary management. Adoption of single embryo transfer policies, meticulous preconception care, vigilant antenatal surveillance, and early intervention can substantially mitigate maternal and neonatal complications while preserving excellent success rates.

REFERENCES

1. Wennerholm UB, Bergh C. Perinatal outcome in children born after assisted reproductive technologies. Ups J Med Sci. 2020;125(2):158-66.
2. Banica AM, Popescu SD, Vladareanu S. Obstetric and Perinatal Complications Associated with Assisted Reproductive Techniques - Review. Mædica. 2021;16(3):493-8.
3. Kornfield MS, Gurley SB, Vrooman LA. Increased Risk of Preeclampsia with Assisted Reproductive Technologies. Curr Hypertens Rep. 2023;25(9):251-61.
4. Cavoretto P, Candiani M, Giorgione V, et al. Risk of spontaneous preterm birth in singleton pregnancies conceived after IVF/ICSI treatment: meta-analysis of cohort studies. Ultrasound Obstet Gynecol. 2018;51(1):43-53.
5. Velez MP, Hamel C, Hutton B, et al. Care plans for women pregnant using assisted reproductive technologies: a systematic review. Reprod Health. 2019;16:9.

Practicals

98. Drugs Used in Hypertensive Disorders of Pregnancy
Ruchika Garg

99. Instruments
Pramila D'Souza, Thamizharasi N, Anwar

100. Drugs in Obstetrics
Thamizharasi N, Pramila D'Souza, Anwar

Drugs Used in Hypertensive Disorders of Pregnancy

Ruchika Garg

INTRODUCTION

Hypertensive disorders of pregnancy (HDP) affect 5–10% of pregnancies globally, contributing significantly to maternal and fetal morbidity and mortality.[1] The American College of Obstetricians and Gynecologists (ACOG, 2013) classifies HDP into gestational hypertension, preeclampsia/eclampsia, chronic hypertension, and chronic hypertension with superimposed preeclampsia.[2] The International Society of Hypertension (2020) maintains this framework but recognizes HELLP syndrome as a distinct entity.[3] Effective management focuses on controlling hypertension and preventing seizures to mitigate adverse outcomes.

ANTIHYPERTENSIVE DRUGS

Severe hypertension (systolic BP ≥160 mm Hg or diastolic BP ≥110 mm Hg, persistent for ≥15 minutes) requires urgent treatment within 30–60 minutes to prevent complications like stroke, heart failure, or renal injury.[4] Antihypertensives are also used in expectant management for BP ≥160/105 mm Hg.[5] A 2023 Cochrane review (3,573 women) found no significant differences in efficacy or safety between intravenous (IV) hydralazine, labetalol, or oral nifedipine for acute severe hypertension.[6]

1. **Sympathomimetics: Methyldopa**[7]

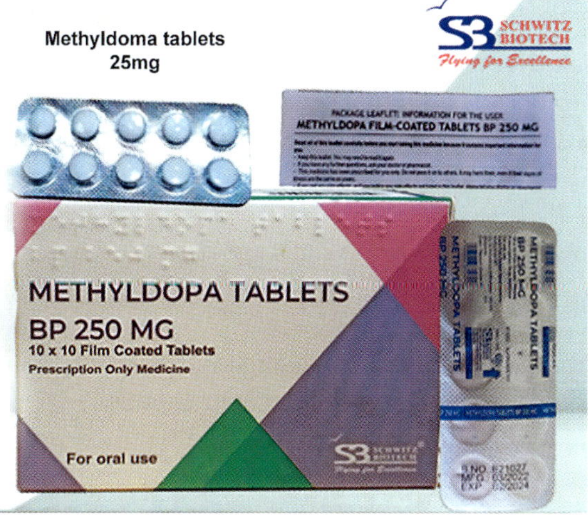

- **Mechanism:** Centrally acting α2-agonist; reduces sympathetic outflow and peripheral resistance with minimal effect on heart rate or cardiac output.
- **Pharmacokinetics:** Oral absorption ~33%; metabolized by liver, excreted by kidneys; onset 3–6 hours, duration 12–24 hours.
- **Dose:**
  - *Oral:* 500 mg–2 g/day in divided doses (maximum 3 g/day).
  - *IV:* 250–1,000 mg over 30–60 minutes every 6–8 hours (maximum 4 g/day).
- **Formulations:** Tablets (250 mg, 500 mg); injectable (50 mg/mL).
- **Adverse Effects:**
  - *Maternal:* Sedation, lethargy, dry mouth, headache, fluid retention, mild postural hypotension, positive Coombs' test (16%), rarely hemolytic anemia, lupus-like syndrome.
  - *Fetal:* Rare intestinal ileus.
- **Contraindications:** Hepatic disorders, psychiatric conditions, congestive heart failure, and postpartum (risk of depression).
- **Interactions:** Tricyclic antidepressants reduce efficacy.
- **Status:** Historically preferred for safety; unavailable since 2015 due to manufacturing cessation.

2. **Adrenergic Receptor Blockers: Labetalol**[8]

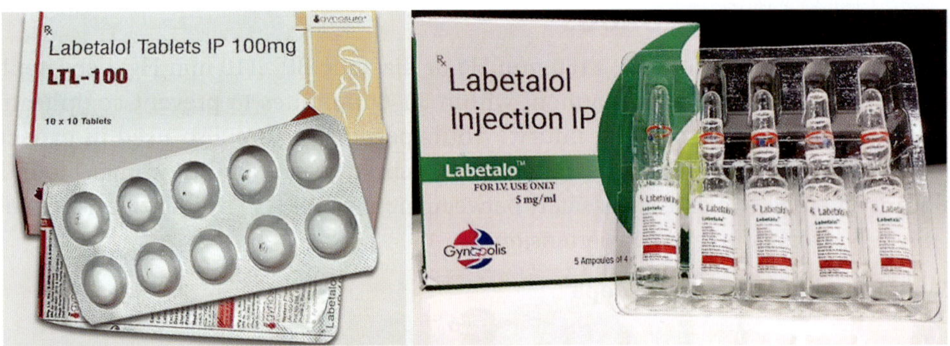

- **Mechanism:** Nonselective α1- and β-blocker (β:α ratio 3–5:1); reduces BP via vasodilation (α1 and β2) and β1-blockade; minimal heart rate effect.
- **Pharmacokinetics:** Oral bioavailability ~30% (first-pass metabolism); hepatic elimination; half-life 4–6 hours.
- **Dose:**
  - *Oral:* Start 100 mg twice daily, up to 2,400 mg/day.
  - *Hypertensive crisis:* 10–20 mg IV, then 20–80 mg every 10–30 minutes (maximum 300 mg); or infusion 1–2 mg/min.
- **Adverse Effects:** Tremors, headache, scalp tingling, bronchospasm, heart failure, elevated liver enzymes, pruritus, and rarely ventricular arrhythmias.
- **Contraindications:** Asthma, heart block, bradycardia, myocardial disease, and hepatic disorders.
- **Status:** Current drug of choice due to efficacy and safety comparable to methyldopa.

3. **Vasodilators:**

- **Hydralazine**[9]

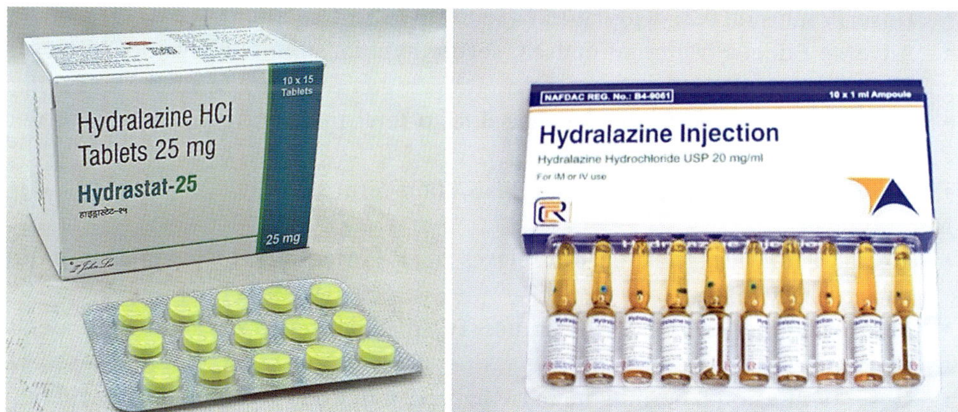

  - **Mechanism:** Direct arteriolar dilator; reduces peripheral resistance, mainly diastolic BP; triggers reflex tachycardia, renin release, and fluid retention.
  - **Pharmacokinetics:** Well-absorbed orally; first-pass hepatic metabolism (acetylation); half-life 1–2 hours, effect persists 12 hours.
  - **Dose:** Hypertensive crisis: 5 mg IV/IM, then 5–10 mg every 20–40 minutes (maximum 20 mg); or infusion 0.5–10 mg/h.
  - **Formulations:** Tablets (10 mg, 25 mg); injectable (20 mg/mL).
  - **Adverse Effects:** Flushing, headache, palpitations, edema, angina (in coronary artery disease), rarely lupus-like syndrome (high doses, slow acetylators).
  - **Contraindications:** Coronary artery disease, lupus.

- **Sodium Nitroprusside**[10]

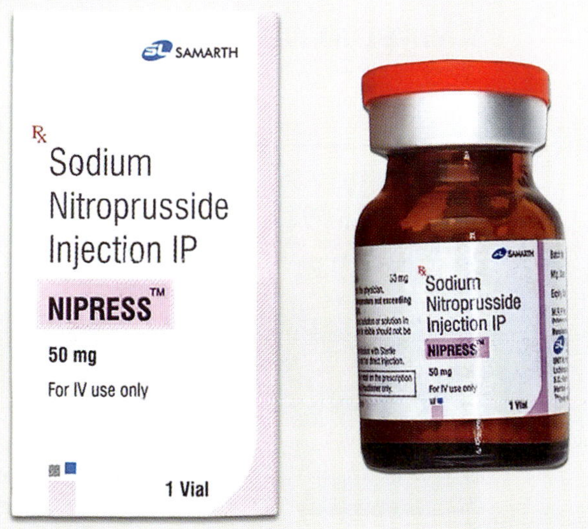

  - **Mechanism:** Releases nitric oxide, relaxing arterioles and veins; reduces peripheral resistance and preload; causes mild tachycardia.

- **Pharmacokinetics:** Onset seconds; duration 2–5 minutes; metabolized to cyanmethemoglobin and cyanide, excreted as thiocyanate.
- **Dose:** IV infusion 0.25–8 μg/kg/min (50 mg in 500 mL solution).
- **Adverse Effects:** Maternal nausea, severe hypotension; fetal cyanide/thiocyanate toxicity.
- **Contraindications:** Prolonged use due to fetal toxicity; requires light-protected infusion.
- **Status:** Last resort for hypertensive crisis, short-term use only.

▪ **Nitroglycerin**[11]
- **Mechanism:** Nitrate vasodilator; relaxes veins > arteries, reducing preload/afterload and coronary spasm.
- **Pharmacokinetics:** Half-life 3 minutes (IV); metabolized to less active dinitrates, then glycerol/CO_2.
- **Dose:** IV infusion 5 μg/min, increase by 5 μg/min every 3–5 minutes (maximum 100 μg/min).
- **Adverse Effects:** Hypotension, dizziness, flushing, and increased intracranial pressure.
- **Contraindications:** Hypertensive encephalopathy.
- **Interactions:** Avoid with acetaminophen (methemoglobinemia risk), aspirin (potentiates effect).
- **Status:** Last resort, short-term use in crisis.

3. **Calcium Channel Blockers: Nifedipine**[12]

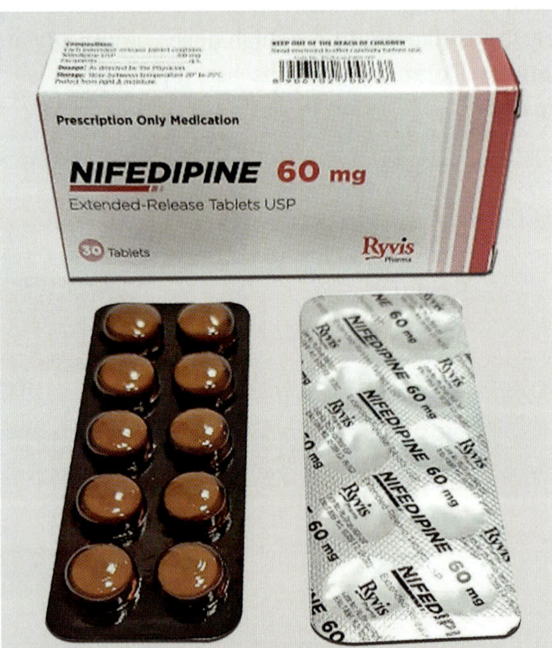

▪ **Mechanism:** Dihydropyridine; inhibits vascular smooth muscle calcium channels, causing arteriolar vasodilation; no fluid retention.

- **Pharmacokinetics:** Oral bioavailability 56–77%; hepatic metabolism; onset 5–10 minutes, duration 6–8 hours, half-life ~2 hours.
- **Dose:**
  - *Expectant management:* 5–10 mg thrice daily (maximum 180 mg/day).
  - *Hypertensive crisis:* 10–20 mg orally, repeat after 20 minutes, then every 2–6 hours (maximum 180 mg/day).
- **Adverse Effects:** Flushing, hypotension, headache, tachycardia, and labor inhibition.
- **Contraindications:** Avoid with magnesium sulfate (synergistic hypotension).
- **Interactions:** CYP3A inducers (e.g., rifampin and phenytoin) reduce efficacy.

TABLE 1: Antihypertensives for hypertensive crisis.[6,8,9,12]

Drug	*Dose*	*Onset*
Labetalol	10–20 mg IV, then 20–80 mg every 10–30 minutes (maximum 300 mg); or 1–2 mg/min infusion	1–2 minutes
Hydralazine	5 mg IV/IM, then 5–10 mg every 20–40 minutes (maximum 20 mg); or 0.5–10 mg/h infusion	10–20 minutes
Nifedipine	10–20 mg oral, repeat in 20 minutes, then every 2–6 hours (maximum 180 mg/day)	5–10 minutes

ANTICONVULSANTS: MAGNESIUM SULFATE ($MgSO_4$)

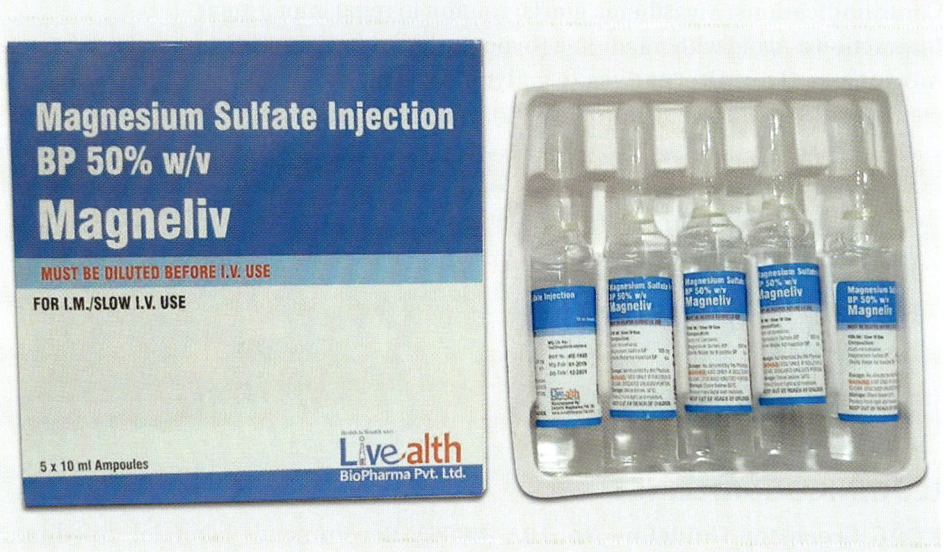

- **Indication:** Drug of choice for seizure prophylaxis in severe preeclampsia and treatment of eclampsia.[13]
- **Mechanism:** Stabilizes neuronal membranes, reduces acetylcholine release, blocks calcium channels, promotes vasodilation, increases cerebral/uterine/renal blood flow, and reduces intracranial edema.[14]

- **Pharmacokinetics:** IV administration; 30% albumin-bound; not metabolized; excreted renally; half-life 5.2 hours.[15]
- **Dose:**[16]
  - **Pritchard Regimen:**
    - *Loading:* 4 g IV (20% solution) over 3–5 minutes + 10 g IM (5 g each buttock, 50% solution).
    - *Maintenance:* 5 g IM (50%) every 4 hours in alternate buttocks.
    - *Conditions for repeat dose:* Knee jerks present, urine output >30 mL/h, and respiratory rate >12 breaths/min.
  - **Zuspan/Sibai Regimen:**
    - *Loading:* 4–6 g IV over 15–20 minutes.
    - *Maintenance:* 1–2 g/h IV infusion.
- **Therapeutic Range:** Serum magnesium 4–7 mEq/L (4.8–8.4 mg/dL).[17]
- **Monitoring:** Check serum levels in renal impairment or absent reflexes; continue 24 hours postdelivery or last seizure.
- **Recurrent Seizures:** 2 g IV bolus over 5 minutes; if persistent, midazolam 1–2 mg IV (repeat after 5–10 minutes).[18]
- **Toxicity Management:** Calcium gluconate 10% (10 mL IV over 3 minutes) + IV furosemide for urinary excretion.[19]
- **Adverse Effects:** Safe in therapeutic range; toxicity causes reflex loss (>7 mEq/L), respiratory paralysis (>10 mEq/L), and cardiac arrest (>25 mEq/L).
- **Contraindications:** Myasthenia gravis; caution in renal impairment.
- **Interactions:** Avoid with nifedipine (hypotension); interacts with tetracyclines.
- **Advantages Over Alternatives** (e.g., lytic cocktail, diazepam, and phenytoin): Lower recurrence (9%), maternal mortality (3%), and perinatal mortality.[20]

TABLE 2: Magnesium sulfate toxicity.[17,19]

Effect	*Serum Mg (mEq/L)*	*Serum Mg (mg/dL)*
Therapeutic	4–7	4.8–8.4
Loss of reflexes	>7	>9
Respiratory paralysis	>10	>12
Cardiac arrest	>25	>30

RCOG/NICE GUIDELINES

- **RCOG Green-top Guideline No. 10A (2006):** Recommends labetalol, nifedipine, or hydralazine for severe hypertension; $MgSO_4$ for seizure prophylaxis in severe preeclampsia/eclampsia; continue $MgSO_4$ 24 hours postdelivery.[21]
- **NICE NG133 (2023):** Oral labetalol first-line for hypertension; IV labetalol or hydralazine for acute severe hypertension; $MgSO_4$ for eclampsia/severe preeclampsia; target BP < 135/85 mm Hg in chronic hypertension.[5]

CLINICAL CASE SCENARIO

Case: A 28-year-old primigravida at 34 weeks presents with BP 165/112 mm Hg, headache, and proteinuria (2+). NST is reactive, and fetal growth is normal. Serum creatinine is normal, but she has a history of asthma.

Questions:
- What is the immediate management?
- What drug is contraindicated, and why?

Answers:
- **Management:** Diagnose severe preeclampsia. Administer IV hydralazine 5 mg IV, repeat every 20 minutes (maximum 20 mg) to lower BP <160/110 mm Hg (NICE 2021). Start $MgSO_4$ (Zuspan: 4 g IV loading, 1 g/h maintenance) for seizure prophylaxis. Plan delivery after stabilization.
- **Contraindication:** Labetalol is contraindicated due to asthma (risk of bronchospasm). Hydralazine is preferred.
- **Discussion:** Monitor for hydralazine-induced tachycardia and $MgSO_4$ toxicity; ensure multidisciplinary care.

INDIAN EXAMINATION RELEVANCE

Appeared in NEET-PG (2022), DNB (2021, Paper-1), and AIIMS PG (2023). Focus: Drug doses, $MgSO_4$ regimens, contraindications, toxicity management. \

Challenges: Limited labetalol availability in rural areas, high reliance on hydralazine, and cost barriers for $MgSO_4$.

KEY POINTS

- **HDP Prevalence:** 5–10% globally; includes gestational hypertension, preeclampsia, chronic hypertension, and HELLP **(Table 1)**.
- **Antihypertensives:** Labetalol, hydralazine, nifedipine for acute severe hypertension; methyldopa unavailable since 2015 **(Table 1)**.
- **$MgSO_4$:** First line for eclampsia/severe preeclampsia; therapeutic range 4–7 mEq/L; toxicity managed with calcium gluconate **(Table 2)**.
- **Guidelines:** RCOG/NICE recommend labetalol/nifedipine for hypertension, $MgSO_4$ for seizures.
- **India:** Address drug availability, enhance training on toxicity management.

REFERENCES

1. ACOG. Practice Bulletin No. 202: Gestational hypertension and preeclampsia. Obstet Gynecol 2019;133(1):e1-e25.
2. Unger T, Borghi C, Charchar F, et al. 2020 International Society of Hypertension Global Hypertension Practice Guidelines. Hypertension 2020;75(6):1334-57.
3. SMFM. Severe hypertension management. Am J Obstet Gynecol. 2021;224(5):B13-B21.

4. Magee LA, et al. Antihypertensive therapy in pregnancy. Cochrane Database Syst Rev 2023;8:CD013076.
5. NICE. (2023). Hypertension in pregnancy: diagnosis and management. NG133. [online] Available from https://www.nice.org.uk/guidance/ng133 [Last accessed December, 2025].
6. Duley L, et al. Antihypertensive drugs for severe hypertension. Cochrane Database Syst Rev 2023;10:CD011739.
7. Redman CW, et al. Methyldopa in pregnancy. J Hypertens. 2017;35(5):889-95.
8. Webster LM, et al. Labetalol in pregnancy. Hypertension 2019;73(3):503-11.
9. Brown MA, et al. Hydralazine for hypertensive crisis. BJOG. 2018;125(10):1221-8.
10. Sass N, et al. Sodium nitroprusside in pregnancy. J Perinat Med. 2017;45(6):671-6.
11. Magee LA, et al. Nitroglycerin in hypertensive crisis. Eur J Obstet Gynecol Reprod Biol. 2020;248:65-71.
12. Firoz T, et al. Nifedipine in pregnancy. Obstet Gynecol. 2018;132(4):798-806.
13. Duley L, et al. Magnesium sulfate in eclampsia. Lancet. 2019;394(10210):1718-26.
14. Okusanya BO, et al. Magnesium sulfate mechanisms. BJOG. 2020;127(8):937-44.
15. Lu JF, et al. Magnesium sulfate pharmacokinetics. Clin Pharmacokinet. 2020;59(4):405-14.
16. Pritchard JA, et al. Magnesium sulfate regimens. Am J Obstet Gynecol. 2018;218(2):S117-24.
17. Duley L, et al. Magnesium sulfate toxicity. Br J Obstet Gynaecol 2016;123(7):1035–41.
18. Altman D, et al. Recurrent seizures in eclampsia. Obstet Gynecol. 2017;130(5):987-94.
19. Smith JM, et al. Magnesium toxicity management. J Matern Fetal Neonatal Med. 2019;32(12):1987-93.
20. Euser AG, et al. Magnesium vs. other anticonvulsants. Cochrane Database Syst Rev 2017;4:CD009402.
21. RCOG. (2006). Severe Pre-eclampsia/Eclampsia, Management (Green-top Guideline No. 10A). [online] Available from https://www.rcog.org.uk/guidance/browse-all-guidance/green-top-guidelines/severe-pre-eclampsiaeclampsia-management-green-top-guideline-no-10a/ [Last accessed December, 2025].

Instruments

Pramila D'Souza, Thamizharasi. N, Anwar

SIMPLE RUBBER CATHETER (FIG. 1)

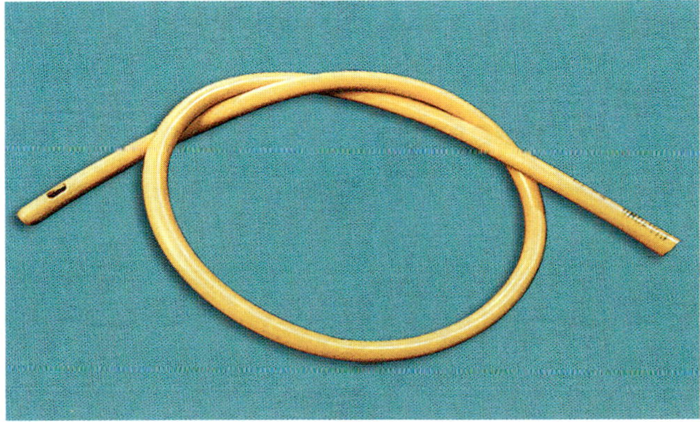

Fig. 1: Simple rubber catheter.

A soft, nonself-retaining rubber, radio-opaque catheter used for giving bladder wash, enema, bowel wash, and to drain the urine in case of acute retention of urine. It is also known as Robinson Catheter.

Characteristics

- It is a flexible tube made out of rubber.
- It is hollow, and the distal end is flared to facilitate urinary drainage.
- It is designed for one-time use; hence, it is termed as in-and-out catheter.
- It is used for temporary drainage.

Parts: It has a soft, rounded tip and one drainage eyelet on the tip of side walls.

Purposes

- **Urological use**
  - To relieve retention of urine in:
    - Retroverted gravid uterus in pregnancy.
    - Obstructed labor cases.
    - When a woman fails to pass urine during the perinatal period.
    - Management of postpartum hemorrhage and retained placenta.

- To collect a urine specimen from an unconscious patient.
- To measure the amount of residual urine after micturition.
- To measure bladder capacity, urine output in medical conditions like acute renal failure.
- For performing cystography.

- **Nonurological use**
  - For the diagnosis of esophageal atresia in a newborn (the catheter cannot be passed in esophageal atresia).
  - As an oxygen catheter.
  - To irrigate the abscess drainage.
  - As a tourniquet in a myomectomy operation.
  - As an alternative clamp.
  - As a mucus sucker when it is attached to a mechanical electric sucker.
  - To instil drugs, urinary antiseptics, and chemotherapy drugs through the urinary bladder.

SIMS DOUBLE-BLADED POSTERIOR VAGINAL SPECULUM (FIG. 2)

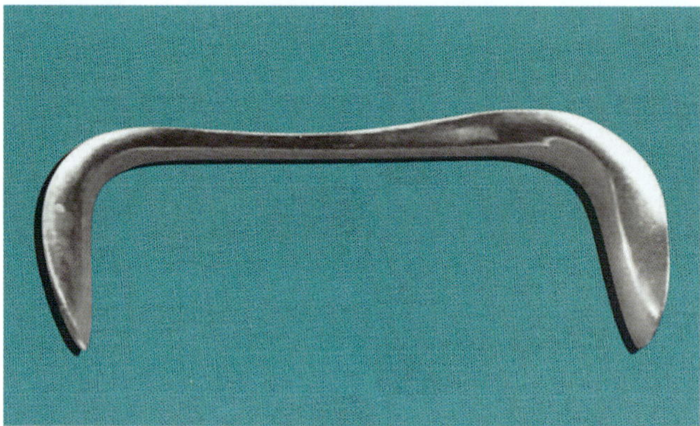

Fig. 2: Sims double-bladed posterior vaginal speculum.

Sims' vaginal speculum is a double-bladed surgical instrument used for examining the vagina and cervix. It was developed by J. Marion Sims. It is inserted into the vagina to retract the posterior vaginal wall. It gives more exposure of the vaginal walls.

Available sizes: The available size of the catheter: 3–20 Fr

Types

- Metallic speculum: It requires an external light source.
- Plastic speculum: It may be equipped with a light source.

Parts

- Blades: It has a narrow blade used in nulliparous women and a broad blade used in multiparous women.
- Handle: To hold

- Groove: Which aids in the drainage of secretions by slightly tilting the equipment and the collection of specimens from the vagina.

Position used

Preferably lithotomy or Sims' position is used.

Procedure

- Wash your hands and wear gloves.
- Choose the appropriately sized speculum and lubricate it.
- Separate the labia majora and minora.
- Client is asked to relax to avoid the uncomfortable position.
- Sim's speculum is directly inserted posteriorly to its full length into the cervix.

Uses

- Per speculum examination in gynecology
  a. Inspect cervix for growth, discharge, etc.
  b. Inspect the vagina for vaginitis and cystocele.
- During minor procedures on the cervix, like
  a. Dilatation of the cervix
  b. Cervical biopsy
  c. Polypectomy
- During procedures on the uterus, like
  a. Endometrial biopsy
  b. Dilatation and curettage
  c. IUD insertion
- During diagnostic procedures like
  a. Hysteroscopy
  b. Tubal insufflation
  c. MTP
  d. Abortions

Advantage

It offers a good posterior view.

Disadvantage

- Assistance is required to hold the speculum.
- Cannot visualize the cervix without an anterior speculum

Contraindication

- Visual defect in the instrument

MULTIPLE-TOOTHED VULSELLUM (FIG. 3)

It is a long metallic instrument designed to have small teeth (3–4) arising from each blade, which fit in the space between the blades. It is used to grasp tissues firmly with less trauma, and the handle has a catch that also makes the grip firm.

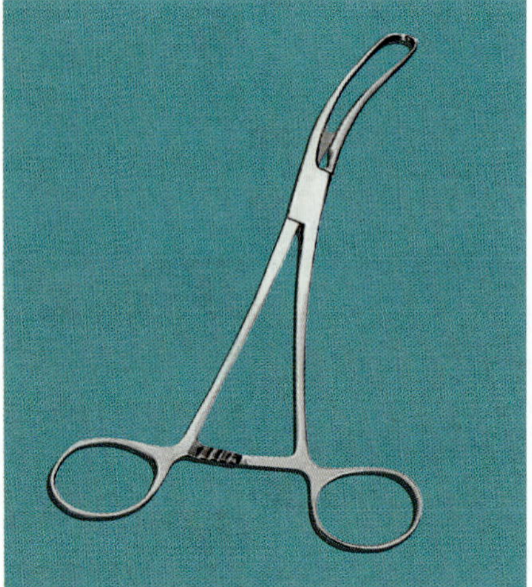

Fig. 3: Multiple-toothed vulsellum.

Parts

- Blades with multisharp rat teeth at the tip
- Ratchet lock

Uses

- Primarily designed to hold the lips of a multiparous cervix
- Anterior lip holds in: Endometrial biopsy, insertion of IUD, cauterization of cervix, and intrauterine insemination
- Vaginal hysterectomy (for traction)
- Posterior lip held in ruptured ectopic pregnancy, vaginal tubal sterilization
- During culdoscopy
- During posterior colpotomy for drainage of pelvic abscess
- To hold the cervical stump after amputation of the cervix or in a subtotal hysterectomy
- To grasp fibroids in myomectomy
- To remove a polyp by twisting as an alternative to Lane's tissue forceps

  Contraindication: Pregnancy

ALLIS TISSUE FORCEPS (FIG. 4)

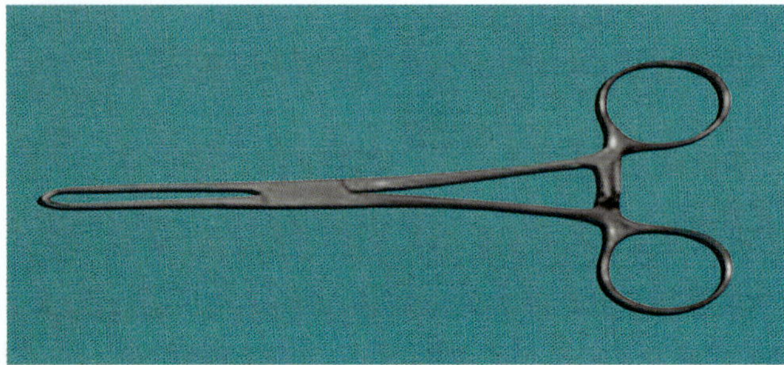

Fig. 4: Allis tissue forceps.

It is a metallic instrument having two ends, one end is the handle with the provision of catch, and the other end has multiple teeth (4–6). The blade allows some space within, in locked position so that the hold is not crushed. It is available in two sizes 12 cm and 17 cm in length with inward curved blades.

Parts

- **Blades:** They are two in number, straight with distance in between which prevents trauma and crushing of the structure held.
- **Teeth:** 4–6 sharp, multiple, fine and interlocking teeth for firm grip and are curved inward
- **Handle**: Handle has a finger grip with a lock.
- **Lock:** It has a catch lock mechanism.

Available sizes: Used in all age groups.

Length:

- 6 inches or 152 mm
- 7 ½ inches or 191 mm
- 9 ½ inches or 241 mm
- 12 inches or 303 mm
- 18 inches or 458 mm

Teeth:

- 4 × 5 teeth
- 5 × 6 teeth

Uses

- To hold the cervical anterior tip in medical termination of pregnancy, such as suction evacuation.
- To hold tough structures such as the rectus sheath and aponeurosis in laparotomy and abdominal procedures.
- To hold levators and the external sphincter muscle ends on either side during repair of complete perineal tears.
- To hold the cut edges of the vagina in the vaginal operations as follows:
  - Abdominal hysterectomy after removing the hysterectomy specimens.
  - During the suturing of the vagina in the vaginal hysterectomy after removing the uterus.
  - In pelvic organ prolapse surgeries such as anterior colporrhaphy, posterior colpoperineorrhaphy, and enterocele repair during separation of vagina from bladder and rectum.
  - During the removal of a vaginal cyst.
  - During a radical hysterectomy for the separation of the upper from the bladder.
- Allis forceps can be used to hold the fundus of the uterus in various gynecological surgeries, like.
- Abdominal hysterectomy to help move the uterus to one side during clamping of pedicles.
- Vaginal hysterectomy to bring the uterine fundus downward while clamping the tubo-ovarian pedicles.

- To bisect the uterus in vaginal hysterectomy for a large uterus, the fundus is caught with Allis forceps.
- To hold the fibroid during myomectomy.
- To hold the divided ends of the uterus for suturing in metroplasty surgery.

Cautions

Due to the sharp teeth of Allis tissue forceps, it is a traumatic instrument and should not be applied to the skin.

MUCUS EXTRACTOR (FIG. 5)

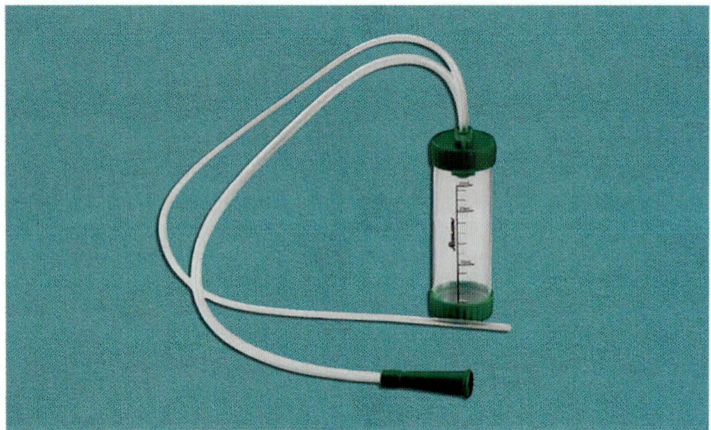

Fig. 5: Mucus sucker.

Measurement

It is available in 3 standard sizes: 30 mL, 60 mL, and 80 mL.

Parts

- Mucus extractor is fitted with intravenous drip set tubing at both ends and suction catheters.
- The drainage tubing is fitted to the nose of the sucker after charging.

Uses

- To suck out the secretions from the mouth of the baby after delivery.
- To remove mucus from the upper respiratory tract.
- To stimulate productive coughing that expels mucus.
- To prevent aspiration of foreign objects in the lungs.
- To collect samples for testing in the laboratory.

Contraindications

- Occluded nasal passages
- Nasal trauma
- Nasal fractures
- Recent nasal surgery
- Nasal bleeding

BREAST PUMP (FIG. 6)

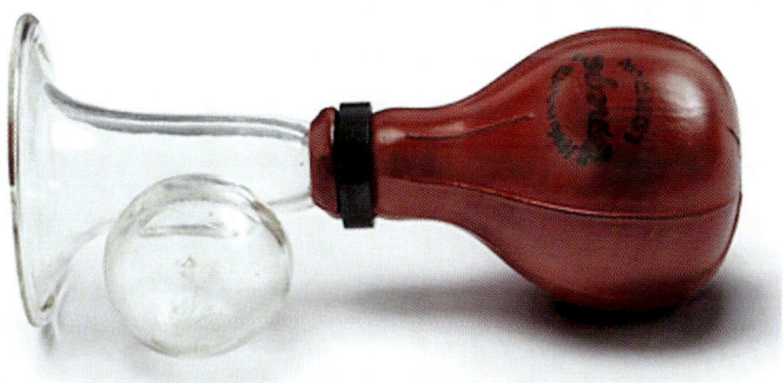

Fig. 6: Breast pump.

A breast pump is a mechanical device that lactating women use to extract milk from their breasts. They may be manual devices powered by hand movements or automatic devices powered by electricity.

Types

- Manual pumps
- Battery-powered pumps
- Electric pumps

Parts

- Breast Shield: A cone-shaped cup that fits over the nipple and the circular area surrounding the nipple.
- Pump: It creates a gentle vacuum that expresses milk.
- Milk container: A detachable container that fits below the breast shield and collects milk as it is pumped. The container is typically a reusable bottle used to store the milk.

Indications

- Premature or sick baby
- Maternal illness
- Baby is unable to breastfeed well
- Mother at risk of inadequate milk production

Contraindications

- Breast Cancer
- HIV
- Acute maternal disease if the infant does not have the disease
- Herpes simplex virus
- Galactosemia
- Cytomegalovirus

LONG STRAIGHT HEMOSTATIC FORCEPS (FIG. 7)

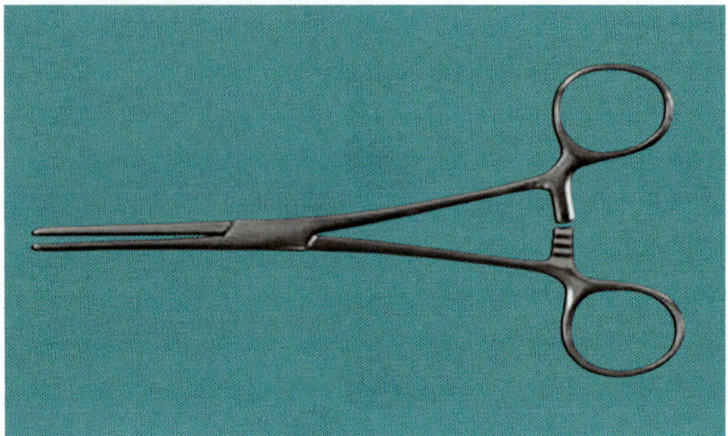

Fig. 7: Long straight hemostatic forceps.

Long straight hemostatic forceps are a surgical instrument used for shallow hemostasis and tissue separation at the operation site, and tooth hemostatic forceps are mainly used for hemostasis of strong and tough tissue, and the part of lifting the incision.

Parts

- Long beaks
- Parallel groves
- Locking rachet
- Finger ring

Types

- Rankin forceps
- Kelly forceps
- Satinsky forceps
- Kocher forceps
- Crile forceps
- Bainbridge forceps
- Halsted mosquito forceps
- Mixter right-angle forceps
- Spencer Wells artery forceps

Indications

- To control bleeding
- To clamp blood vessels
- To grasp and secure the superficial fascia
- Exposing the tissues
- Exploring and visualizing the deeper areas of the wound

LONG STRAIGHT SCISSORS (FIG. 8)

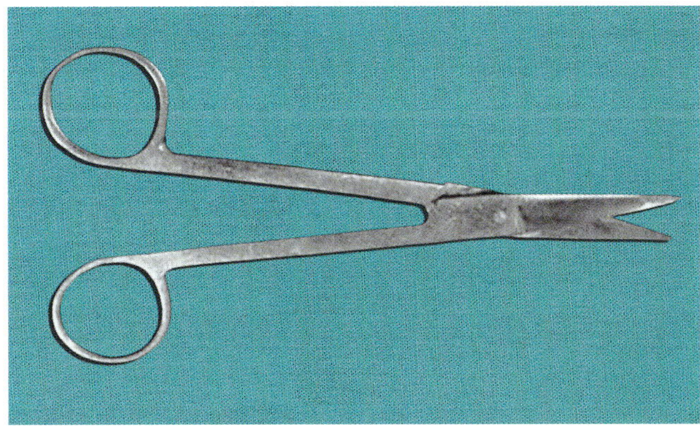

Fig. 8: Long straight scissors.

Long straight scissors are the scissors which have a straight blade and a longer length to allow precise cutting in delicate areas.

Parts

- Ring handles
- Shank
- Hinge
- Blade
- Cutting edge

Key features

Straight blades: These scissors have straight cut edges, which makes them suitable for precise and straight cuts.

Length: Long straight scissors generally have extended handles and blades, providing better reach and control.

Sharpness: They are designed to be sharp, allowing for effortless cutting of various materials.

Material: High-quality scissors are often made of stainless steel, ensuring durability and resistance.

Handle design: The handles are usually ergonomically designed for a comfortable grip and reduced hand fatigue during prolonged use.

Versatility: Long straight scissors are versatile tools used in various industries, including medicine, arts and crafts, sewing, and more.

Precision: They offer excellent precision, making them ideal for delicate tasks.

Safety: Some models come with safety features such as finger loops or locking mechanisms.

Maintenance: Proper care and occasional sharpening are essential to maintain cutting efficiency over time.

Indications
- Tissue dissection
- Suturing
- Vessel and nerve dissection
- Cutting drapes
- Removing sutures
- Cutting sponges and dressings
- Preparing grafts
- Trimming tissues

Contraindications
- Proximity to vital organs
- For cutting extremely fragile or delicate tissues
- Electrosurgery or electrocautery procedures (due to electrical conduction)
- Patients with bleeding disorders
- Infection or contaminated areas
- Patients with metal allergies

UTERINE SOUND (FIG. 9)

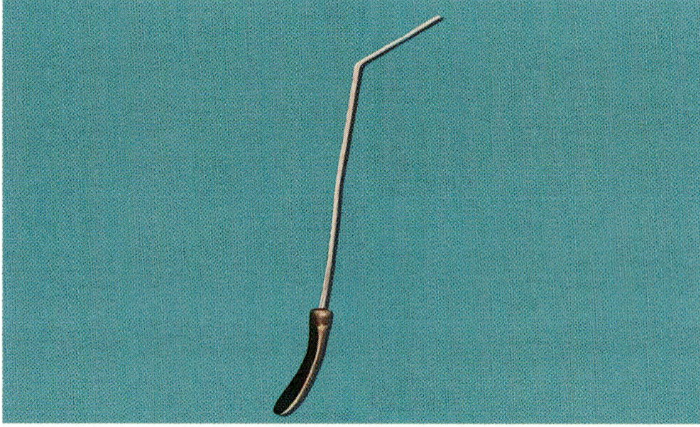

Fig. 9: Uterine sound.

The uterine sound is used to gauge the depth and position of the uterine cavity. It is also helpful for the placement of IUDs and the verification of the intrauterine position and length for HSG procedures. These are also called Sims uterine sound/Olive pointed malleable metallic uterine sound.

Types
- Hegar's dilator: Have two rounded ends, are fairly short and are mildly curved in shape
- Sim's sound has a flat end and a rounded end

Uses
- To measure the length of the uterine cavity
- To know the position and direction of the uterus in case of retroversion

- To differentiate between a polyp arising from the cervical canal or body of the uterus
- To measure the length of the cervical canal
- To diagnose uterine cancers
- To know about infertility, irregular uterine bleeding, heavy menstrual bleeding, and postmenopausal bleeding.

Contraindications

- Pregnancy or suspected pregnancy
- Congenital uterine abnormalities
- Acute pelvic inflammation
- Shock due to pain

HAWKIN AMBLER DILATORS (FIG. 10)

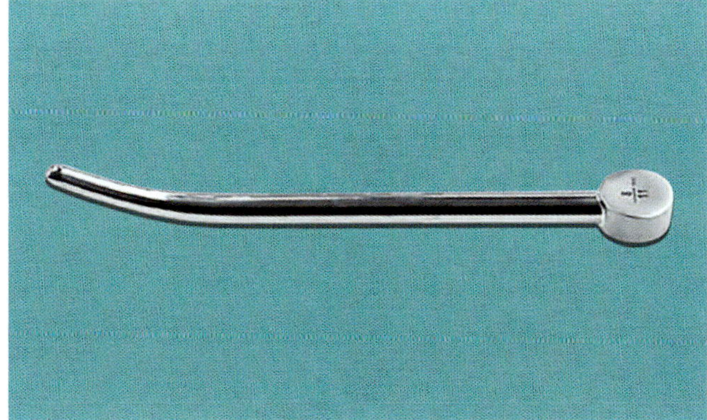

Fig. 10: Hawkin Ambler dilators.

Hawkin Ambler dilatators are single-ended uterine dilatators with a rounded end and are used to facilitate entry into the uterus and to prevent uterine wall puncture. Designed with a single rounded end for dilation and a discoid handle for manipulation.

Size: Available in a wide array of sizes from 3/6 mm to 18/21 mm

Types

The dilatators are available in different sizes:

- 290–400 (Set of 16) 3/6 mm - 18/21, 7-1/2"
- 290–403 3/6 mm, 7-1/2" (18.8 cm), single end
- 290–404 4/7 mm, 7-1/2" (18.8 cm), single end
- 290–405 5/8 mm, 7-1/2" (18.8 cm), single end
- 290–406 6/9 mm, 7-1/2" (18.8 cm), single end
- 290–407 7/10 mm, 7-1/2" (18.8 cm), single end
- 290–408 8/11 mm, 7-1/2" (18.8 cm), single end
- 290–409 9/12 mm, 7-1/2" (18.8 cm), single end
- 290–410 10/13 mm, 7-1/2" (18.8 cm), single end
- 290–411 11/14 mm, 7-1/2" (18.8 cm), single end

- 290–412 12/15 mm, 7-1/2" (18.8 cm), single end
- 290–413 13/16 mm, 7-1/2" (18.8 cm), single end
- 290–414 14/17 mm, 7-1/2" (18.8 cm), single end
- 290–415 15/18 mm, 7-1/2" (18.8 cm), single end
- 290–416 16/19 mm, 7-1/2" (18.8 cm), single end
- 290–417 17/20 mm, 7-1/2" (18.8 cm), single end
- 290–418 18/21 mm, 7-1/2" (18.8 cm), single end

Contraindications

There are no known contraindications. Cervical dilation using mechanical dilators is associated with various complications, such as uterine perforation, cervical laceration, infections, and intraperitoneal hemorrhage.

DAS OR HEGAR'S DILATORS (FIG. 11)

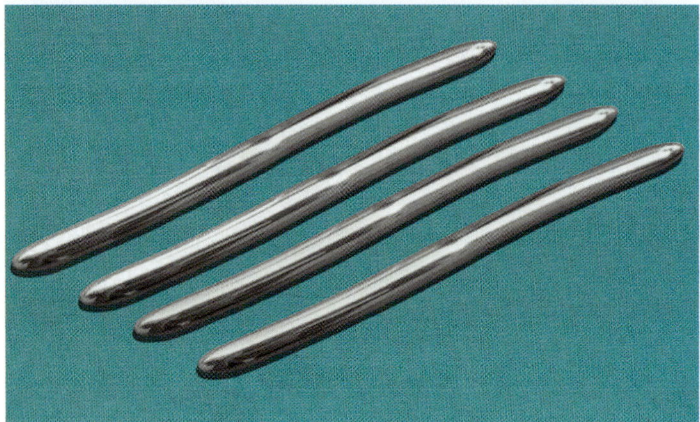

Fig. 11: Das or Hegar's dilators.

Uses:

- Hegar dilatators are used to induce cervical dilation to gain entry to the interior of the uterus.
- Used to treat vaginismus
- Inflatable penile implant procedures
- Before a uterine curettage or biopsy
- Trachelorrhaphy
- Polypectomy
- Evacuation
- Before the introduction of the hysteroscope

Contraindication

- Acute genital tract or bleeding diathesis
- Pelvic structure abnormality that prevents the passage of the device
- Invasive cervical cancer

FLUSHING CURETTE (FIGS. 12A AND B)

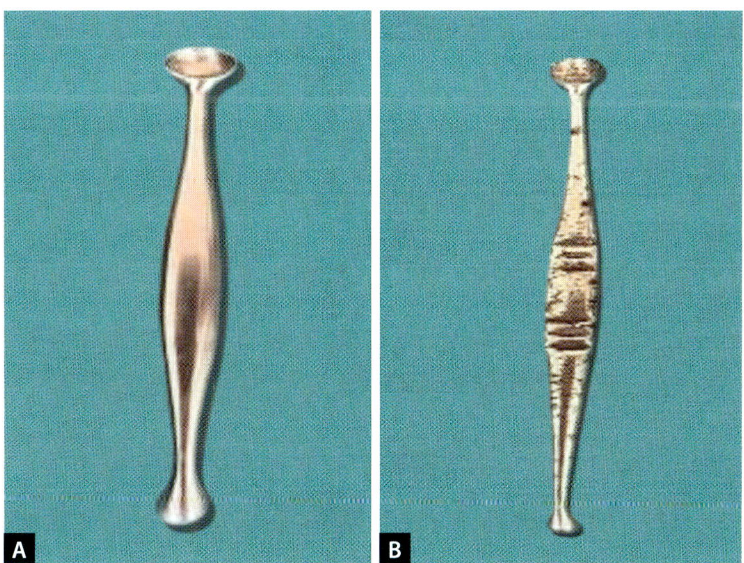

Figs. 12A and B: Flushing curette.

Flushing Curette is a blend curette used to flush the uterine cavity with lukewarm antiseptic solution, passing through the communicating channel. It is commonly used in Dilation and Evacuation (D&E).

Uses

Flushing Curette is used to collect samples from the uterus and rectum for the diagnosis of cancer.

Type of material

It is made from stainless steel and is autoclavable. It consists of a long hollow shaft with a small spoon-shaped scoop; it may be sharp at both ends or sharp at one end and blunt at the other.

Indication

- To take an endometrial sample in case of abnormal vaginal bleeding
- To detect ovulation in case of infertility by the detection of secretory changes of endometrium
- To remove the decidua after evacuation in case of abortion or molar pregnancy
- To remove retained products of conception in case of PPH

Contraindications

- Traumatic urethral injury
- Resistance to passage
- High-riding prostate
- Blood at the meatus

Advantage

- Wide area of inspection
- Instrumentation is easy.

Complication

- Premature amenorrhea and infertility: Removal of the basal layer of endometrium
- Asherman syndrome
- Endometriosis due to implantation of endometrial tissue in the vagina
- Complication of dilation

DOYEN'S RETRACTOR (FIG. 13)

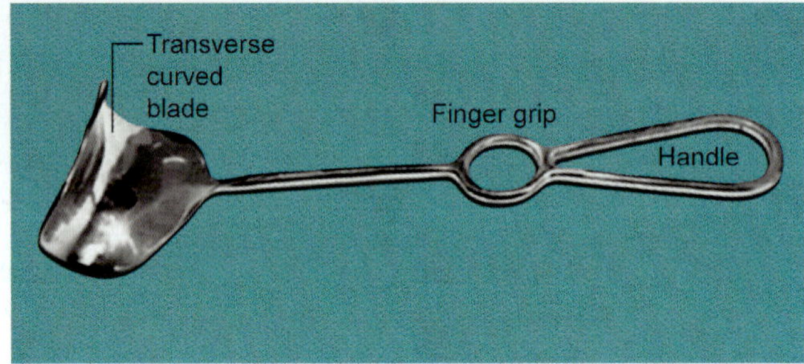

Fig. 13: Doyen's retractor.

Doyen's retractor is a strong, heavy, nonself-retaining abdominal retractor. It consists of a large blade which is curved, having an inward-turning margin to minimize trauma to the abdominal wall during retraction. The retractor comes in different sizes. It can be converted to a self-retaining type by hanging lead weights from the hook present on the handle. This instrument has a sturdy blade and a stout handle. It is also known as a bladder retractor.

Uses: It is used in abdominal obstetrics and gynecology procedures to retract the bladder and other internal organs.

Blade sizes: 1.5 inches, 2 inches, 2.5 inches, 3 inches, 3.5 inches, 4 inches

Indications

This instrument is used for retraction of the abdominal wall suprapubically during abdominal operations such as:

- Cesarean section
- Operation for ruptured ectopic gestation
- Abdominal hysterectomies: Total, with bilateral salpingo-oophorectomy or radical hysterectomy
- Ovarian cystectomy, oophorectomy, and wedge resection
- Prolapse repairs: Purandare's cervicoplexy, Shirodkar's sling operation, Khanna's operation, Moskowitz's, etc.
- Stress urinary incontinence repair: Marshall-Marchetti-Krantz operation.

SPONGE HOLDING FORCEPS (FIG. 14)

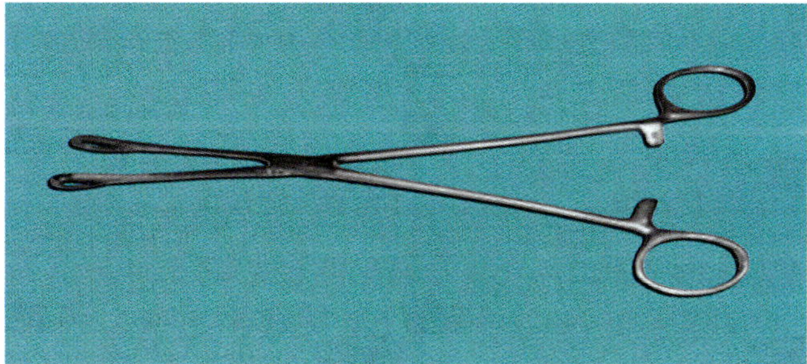

Fig. 14: Sponge holding forceps.

Parts

Made from stainless steel or metal. Commonly 9.5 inches in length, i.e., 25 cm.
It has 2 ends

- One end is handled with a rachet.
- Another end is ring shaped with transverse serration inside.

Uses

- To hold the sponge and clean the area to be operated
- For antiseptic painting before cesarean section
- To clamp the infundibulopelvic ligament in myomectomy
- Also used as ovum forceps to gently remove products of conception in incomplete abortion
- In cervical encirclage operation
- In postplacental IUCD insertion
- In the diagnosis and repair of cervical tears
- To push the bladder down using a sponge in a hysterectomy

OVUM FORCEPS (FIG. 15)

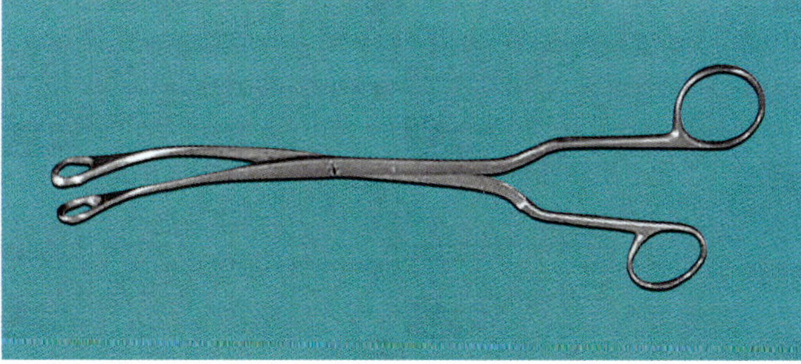

Fig. 15: Ovum forceps.

Parts

Ovum forceps typically consist of the following parts:

- Handles
- Blades

- Locking mechanism
- Joint or hinge
- Ratchet

Uses
- Prolonged or difficult labor
- Fetal distress
- Maternal exhaustion
- Malposition or malpresentation

Contraindication
- Fetal malformations or abnormalities
- Maternal bleeding disorders
- Maternal pelvic abnormalities
- Infection
- Previous uterine surgery

Mechanism of action

It has no catch, and the blades are slightly bent and fenestrated. Absence of catch minimizes uterine injury if accidentally caught. It prevents crushing of the conceptus. It is to be introduced with the blades closed, to open up inside the uterine cavity, to grasp the products and to take out the instrument with a slight rotatory movement. The rotatory movements not only facilitate detachment of the products from the uterine wall but also minimize the injury of the uterine wall if accidentally grasped.

LANDON'S UTERINE RETRACTOR (FIG. 16)

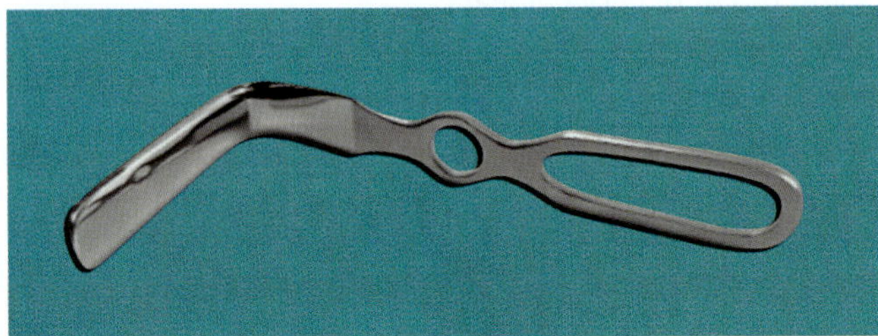

Fig. 16: Landon's uterine retractor.

It is a "L" L-shaped retractor and has a flat blade at a right angle to the handle.

Parts
- Blade
- Fenestration of the shaft to make the instrument lighter
- Handle

Uses
- Vaginal surgery
- To retract the bladder during vaginal hysterectomy

UTERINE CURETTE (FIG. 17)

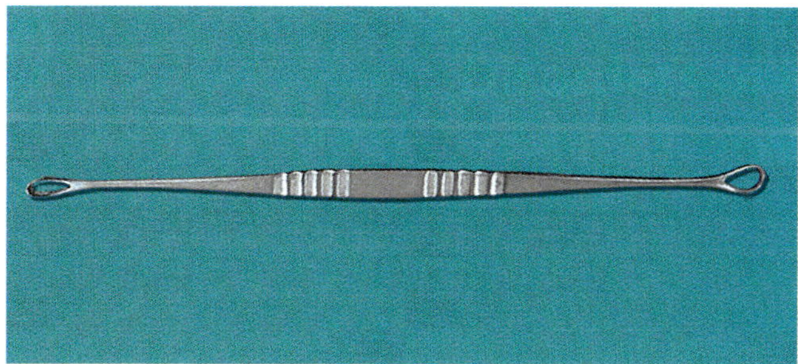

Fig. 17: Uterine curette.

Uterine curettes are thin metal surgical instruments used to scrape the contents of the uterus during dilatation and curettage (D&C).

Parts

It has two terminal oval loop ends that are angled to the shaft

Two types of ends:

- Sharp end: It has a smaller loop and is used in gynecological conditions.
- Blunt end: It has a larger loop and is used in obstetrics.

Types

- Blake's uterine curette
- Randall's endometrial biopsy curette
- Novak's endometrial biopsy curette
- Placenta curette

Uses

a. Blunt End Loop:
  - Incomplete abortion, mixed abortion
  - Evacuation of hydatid form mole
  - Medical termination of pregnancy
  - PPH for retained products of conception

b. Sharp End Loop:
  - Dysfunctional uterine bleeding
  - Secondary amenorrhea
  - Post menopausal bleeding
  - Endometrial cancer
  - Infertility
  - Diagnosis of choriocarcinoma

Indications

- To take endometrial samples in case of abnormal vaginal bleeding
- To detect ovulation in case of infertility by the detection of secretory changes of endometrium
- To remove deciduas after evaluation in case of abortion or molar pregnancy

Contraindication
- Suspected pregnancy
- Genital tract infection
- Acute endometritis and salpingitis

Complications
- Pelvic infection
- Perforation of the cervix or corpus
- Cervical injury
- Hemorrhage

UTERINE DRESSING FORCEPS (FIG. 18)

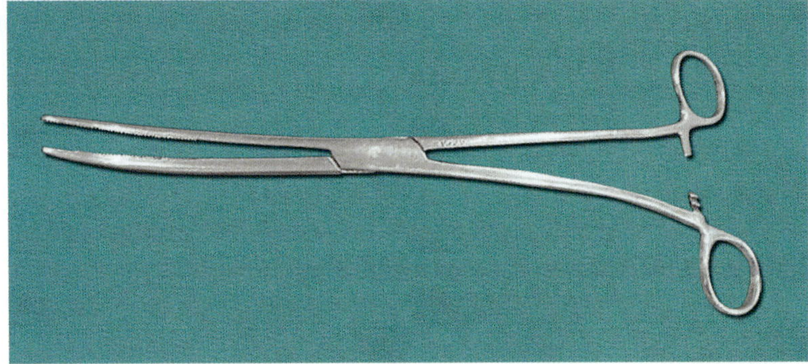

Fig. 18: Uterine dressing forceps.

Parts
- Long S-S-shaped instrument with two curves
- Business End: Blades are blunt and slightly curved anteriorly with transverse serrations on the inner surface.
- Proximal End: Handle is slightly curved posteriorly, ratchet lock/catch.

Uses
- To swab the uterine cavity following D&E operation with a small gauze piece
- To dilate the cervix in lochiometra or pyometra
- To plug the uterine cavity with gauze twigs in continued bleeding after removal of the polyp
- To remove an IUD whose threads are indrawn.

Contraindications
- Patient and/or fetus with established hemorrhagic diathesis or at significant risk for it (including thrombocytopenias)
- Osteogenesis imperfecta
- Unengaged head
- Unknown position of the fetal head and mid-transverse arrest with posterior asynclitism
- Dead fetus or known lethal anomaly in the fetus.

LAMINARIA TENT (FIG. 19)

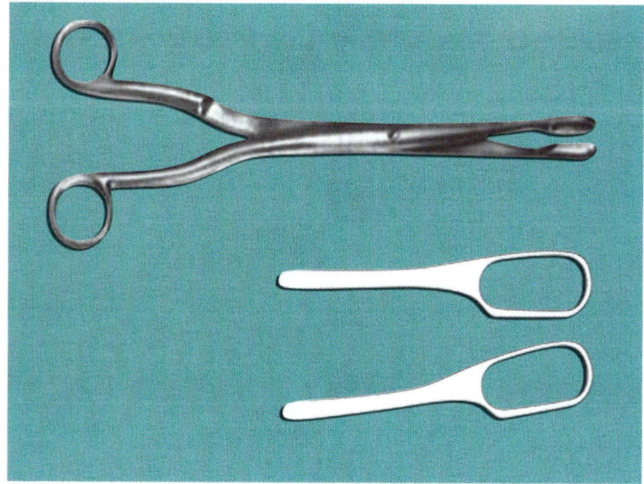

Fig. 19: Laminaria tent.

Parts

- Made from stems of seaweed called laminaria digitata/japonica
- 6–8 cm long cylindrical rods
- Available in different diameters—2 to 8 mm
- The anterior ends are tapered.
- String is attached to the proximal end to facilitate removal.

Uses

- Used for slow dilation of the cervix before operative procedures like:
  - First-trimester and second-trimester MTP
  - Aspiratory
  - Evacuation of vesicular mole
  - Gynecological dilatation and curettage

Contraindications

- If you are pregnant or breastfeeding.
- If you are having any kidney problems.
- If you are having thyroid problems.

KOCHER'S HEMOSTATIC FORCEPS (FIG. 20)

Parts

- Handle/finger rings
- Ratchets
- Shanks
- Joints

- Jaws/blades
- Tips

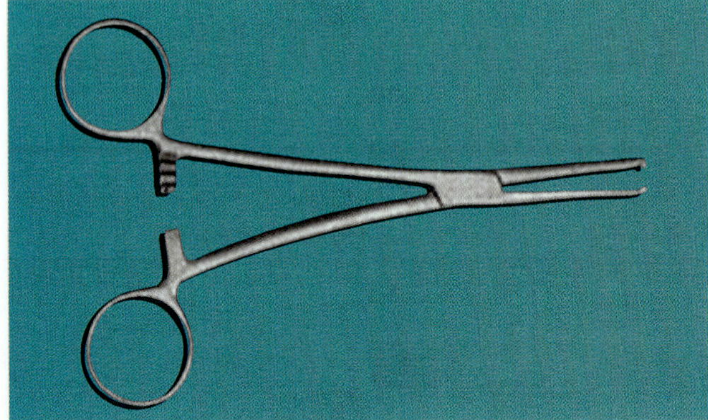

Fig. 20: Kocher's hemostatic forceps.

Uses

- Used to catch the vessels (perforators) during conventional breast surgery (radical mastoidectomy)
- During a hysterectomy (removal of the uterus), forceps are used to hold the uterine artery.
- It is used in the labor room for rupturing the membrane artificially during vaginal delivery.

Contraindications

- Any contraindication to vaginal delivery (see Normal Labor and Delivery)
- Refusal of the patient to verbally consent to the procedure
- Cervix not fully dilated or retracted
- Inability to determine the presentation and fetal head position

LONG CURVED OBSTETRIC FORCEPS (FIG. 21)

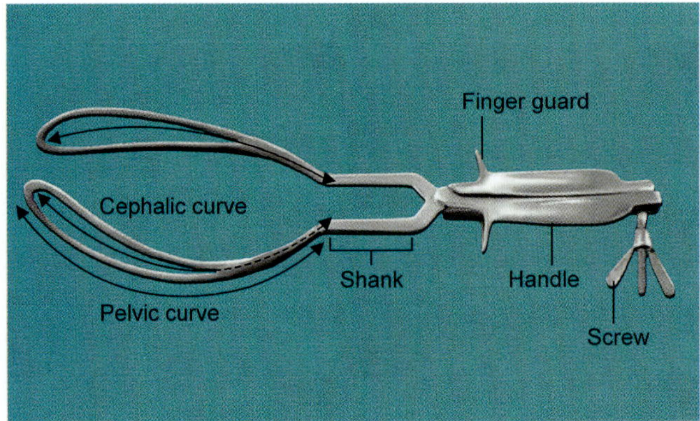

Fig. 21: Long curved obstetric forceps.

An obstetric forceps is a double-bladed metal instrument used for the extraction of the fetal head.

Long, curved obstetric forcep is relatively heavy, about 37 cm long. In India, Das's variety (named after Sir Kedar Nath Das) is commonly used.

Measurements

Length is about 37 cm; distance between the tips is 2.5 cm, and widest diameter between the blades is 9 cm.

Parts

- Blades (2): Right and left in relation to the maternal pelvis—to facilitate a good grip of the fetal head
- Curves (2)
    - Pelvic curve: Helps to direct the force of traction under the pubic bone
    - Cephalic curve: Grasp fetal head without compression
- Shank: Between the blade and lock (6.25 cm), it increases the length of the instrument.
- Handle: To help the obstetrician grasp the instrument (with or without a screw)
- Finger guard
- Lock and screw: To keep blades in position

Identification of blades

- When articulated: Place the instrument in front of the pelvis with the tip of the blades pointing upward and the concave side of the pelvic curve forward. The blade which corresponds to the left of the maternal pelvis is the left blade, and that to the right is the right blade.
- When isolated: The tip should be pointed upward.
- The cephalic curve is to be directed inward, and the pelvic curve forward.

Uses

- It is comparatively lighter and slightly shorter than its Western counterpart, but it is quite suited for the small pelvis and small baby of Indian women.
- To assist in the delivery of a baby as an alternative to the ventouse (vacuum extraction) method
- Used for delivery of the head from mid-cavity, long shank (6.5 cm) heavyweight
- Maternal exhaustion
- Prolonged second stage of labor
- Maternal illness, such as heart disease, hypertension, glaucoma, aneurysm, or other conditions that make pushing difficult or dangerous.
- Hemorrhaging
- Analgesic drug-related inhibition of maternal effort (especially with epidural/spinal anesthesia)

Contraindications

- Absolute maternal contraindications for operative vaginal delivery include the following:
    - Cervix not fully dilated
    - Membranes intact
    - Fetal head not engaged

    - Unknown fetal position
    - Cephalopelvic disproportion
- *Relative maternal contraindications include:* Malpresentation (unless planned breech extraction) and connective tissue disorders
- *Absolute fetal contraindications include:* The presence of a bleeding disorder (hemophilia, thrombocytopenia, and von Willebrand disease) or bone demineralization (osteogenesis imperfecta)
- *Relative fetal contraindications include:* Prematurity and macrosomia. There is no consensus on the minimum or maximum estimated fetal weight for forceps delivery.

AXIS TRACTION DEVICES (FIG. 22)

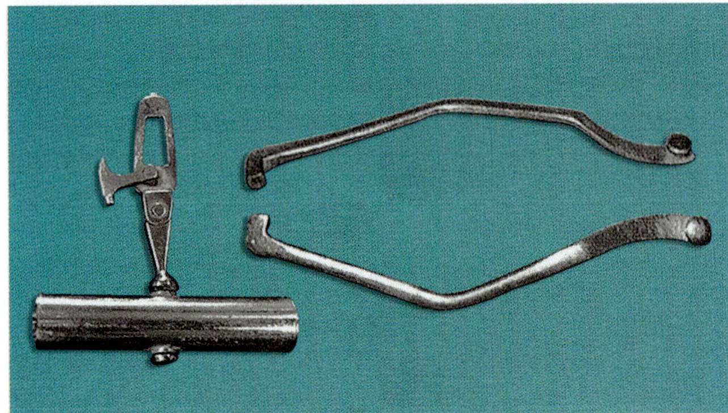

Fig. 22: Axis traction devices.

Axis traction was devised by Tarnier in 1877. It provides traction in the correct axis of the pelvic curve, and less force is necessary to deliver the head.

Parts

- Traction rods (2): Right and left
- Traction handle

Identification of traction rods

Hold the knob pointing inward and let the rod hang the small transverse bar at the bottom is to be directed forward the groove attached to the bar is pointing to the side to which the traction rod belongs and accordingly blade of the forceps.

Traction applied

Traction force originates from the forearms, not the chest. The plane of traction is with the pelvic curve (Saxtorph-Pajot maneuver). Traction should be steady without rocking motion. An early episiotomy is usually RML to avoid rectal injury and is performed to allow for more space and the prevention of vaginal lacerations.

Uses

- It prevents the lock of the forceps from slipping and, at the same time, does not hinder the forceps blade from being opened or closed at the wish of the operator.

- It provides traction in the correct axis of pelvic curve, and as such, less force is necessary to deliver the head.

Contraindications
- Any presentation other than vertex
- Preterm fetus (<34 weeks)
- Suspected fetal coagulation disorder
- Suspected fetal macrosomia (≥4 kg)
- Unengaged fetal head
- Obvious CPD
- Patient's refusal
- Patients having un-acute bleeding diathesis (hemophilia)

Mnemonic for forceps
- F—Favorable head position and station
- O—Open Os (fully dilated)
- R—Ruptured members
- C—Contractions present and consent
- E—Engaged head, empty bladder
- P—Pelvimetry—no major CPD
- S—Stirrups, lithotomy position

WRIGLEY'S FORCEPS (FIG. 23)

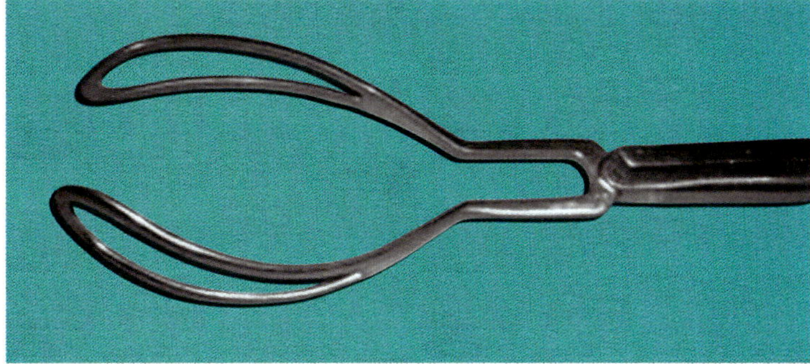

Fig. 23: Wrigley's forceps.

Parts
- *Blades:* Right blade and left blade
- *Shank:* Short
- *Lock:* English type
- *Curve:* Cephalic curve is marked. Pelvic curve is slight.

Uses
- Used as outlet forceps for caesarean section
- Outlet forceps when head is at or below +2 station

KIELLAND'S FORCEPS (FIG. 24)

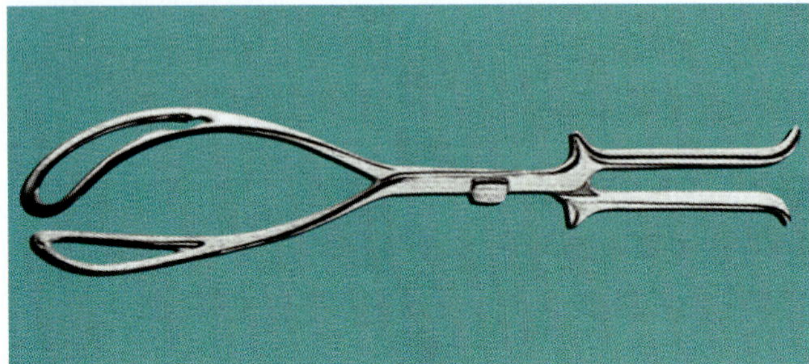

Fig. 24: Kielland's forceps.

It was **invented by** Christian Kielland of Norway in 1916.

Parts

Blade, shank, handle with sliding lock, and knob

Indications

- Arrested occipitoposterior position
- Face presentation
- Unrotated vertex presentation

Special features

- More or less straight forceps
- Longer than long curved obstetric forceps—40 cm (16 inches)
- Radius of pelvic curve and cephalic curve are more. There is a reverse pelvic curve also.
- Presence of knob on each blade to indicate the side toward which occiput lies.
- There is a sliding lock for correction of asynclitism of fetal head.
- Blades are named as anterior and posterior, not right and left.

Methods

- Classical method
- Wandering method
- Direct method

a. **Classical method**
   - This method is performed in floating head.
   - The anterior blade is introduced between the head and symphysis pubis with concavity of the cephalic curve keeping anteriorly.
   - The blade is pushed above the head about up to umbilicus and rotated 180° and pushed down over the head so that cephalic curve fits on the head transversely.
   - The posterior blade is then applied between the head and sacrum. Two blades are articulated.
   - Rotation is done by holding the shanks to bring the occiput forward. Then traction is applied.
   - This method is obsolete nowadays due to the risk of uterine rupture.

b. Wandering method

- In this method, the anterior blade is introduced laterally or posteriorly under the guidance of the two fingers over the face and then pushed over the fetal head so that it comes in front of the anterior parietal eminence.
- The blade is supported by an assistant, and the posterior blade is introduced between the head and sacrum.
- Asynclitism is corrected with the help of a sliding lock.
- Rotation is done at different levels depending on the pelvic architecture and ease of the method.
- The head is finally delivered by pulling in the direction to which the handles are pointing.
- This is the method which is commonly employed.

c. Direct method

- It is suitable when head is in a low own position.
- The blades are applied directly, with the operator being seated at a very low level.

Advantages

- Both rotation and extraction can be performed with the instrument.
- The head is not placed above the brim during rotation, which may occur when it is done manually
- There is a provision of correction of asynclitism on sliding lock.

Disadvantages

- Grip is not so firm and there is chance of slipping.
- Chance of fetal and maternal trauma is more.

EPISIOTOMY SCISSORS (FIG. 25)

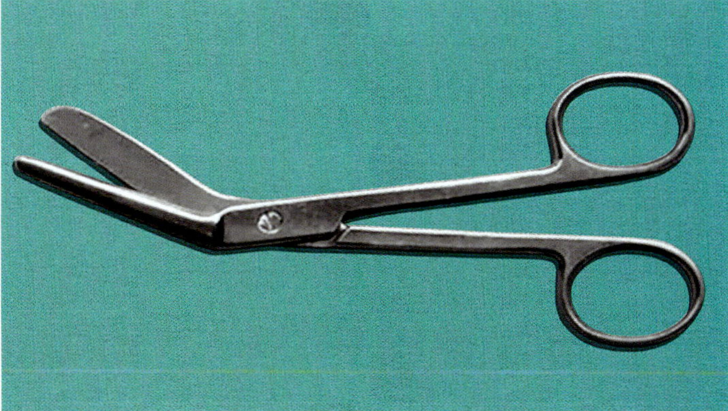

Fig. 25: Episiotomy scissors.

Episiotomy scissors are the surgical scissors used to make the incision for episiotomy, and its full name is Braun-Stadler episiotomy scissors. The scissors are designed to make the incision at an angle of 45–60°.

Parts

- A pair of blades that are controlled pivotally.
- An extended free end of the outer blade in lateral position.

Indications

- In elastic(rigid) perineum
- Anticipating perineal tear
- Operative delivery
- Previous perineal surgery
- Threatened perineal injury in primigravidae
- Forceps, breech, and occipitoposterior delivery

Contraindications

- Inflammatory bowel disease
- Severe perineal malformations
- Abnormalities of the perineum
- Lymphogranuloma venereum
- Severe perineal scarring
- Coagulation disorders
- Patient's refusal for the procedure to be performed

Complications

- **Short-term Complications**
  - Perineal laceration
  - Episiotomy dehiscence
  - Stitches
  - Hemorrhage and increased blood loss
  - Wound site edema
  - Wound site infection
  - Anal sphincter and rectal mucosal damage
  - Urethral injury
  - Bladder injury
  - Perineal hematoma
  - Pain
- **Long-term Complications**
  - Chronic pain and infections
  - A small linear scar
  - Anorectal dysfunction
  - Urinary incontinence
  - Pelvic organ prolapse
  - Sexual dysfunction

VENTOUSE CUP (FIG. 26)

It is an instrumental device designed to assist delivery by creating a vacuum (negative pressure) between itself and the fetal scalp. Vacuum extraction is also known as ventouse.

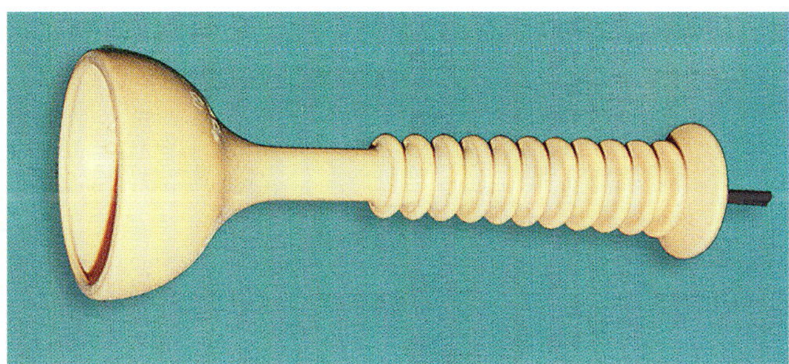

Fig. 26: Ventouse cup.

Parts

- Suction cup of variable sizes. It is either metallic or soft made of silicone.
- Vacuum generator
- Traction tubing

Indications

- Prolonged first stage of labor
- Fetal distress in first or second stage of labor
- Prolonged second stage of labor
- Uterine inertia in first stage of labor
- Occipitoposterior position
- It can be used when the cervix is not fully dilated.
- To rotate the caput from the posterior to the anterior position

Contraindications

- Nonvertex presentation
- Fetal coagulopathies
- Following recent scalp blood sampling
- Unengaged head
- Inexperienced operator
- Known macrosomia
- Extreme prematurity

Complications

- **Fetal Complications**
    - Scalp laceration and bruising
    - Subgaleal hematoma
    - Intracranial, intraventricular, and cerebral hemorrhages
    - Retinal and subconjunctival hemorrhages
    - Neonatal jaundice
    - Clavicular fracture and shoulder dystocia
    - Injury to C-VI, C-VII nerves, and Erb's palsy
    - Hypoxia, particularly when extraction has taken a long time and has been difficult
    - Fetal death

OLDHAM'S PERFORATOR (FIG. 27)

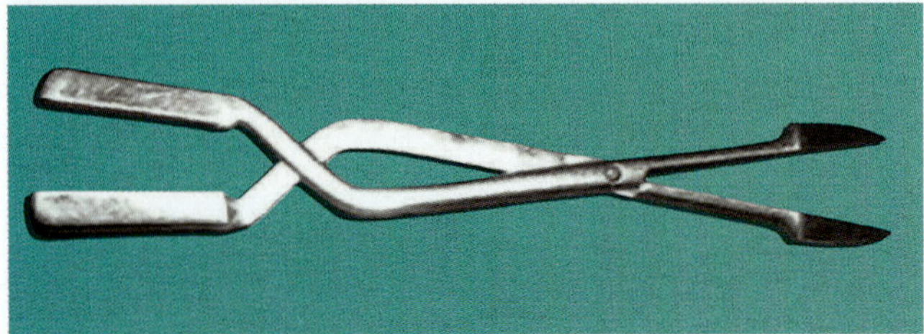

Fig. 27: Oldham's perforator.

It is an instrument required in craniotomy to perforate the skull bone for decompression of the fetal head.

Uses

- To pierce the fetal skull
- To macerate the skull bones

Parts

- Blade (triangular) outer sharp edge
- Shaft
- Handle

Procedure

- Oldham's perforator, with the blades closed, is introduced under the palmar aspect of the fingers protecting the anterior vaginal wall and the adjacent bladder until the tip reaches the proposed site of perforation.
- By rotating movements, the skull is perforated.

CRANIOCLAST (FIG. 28)

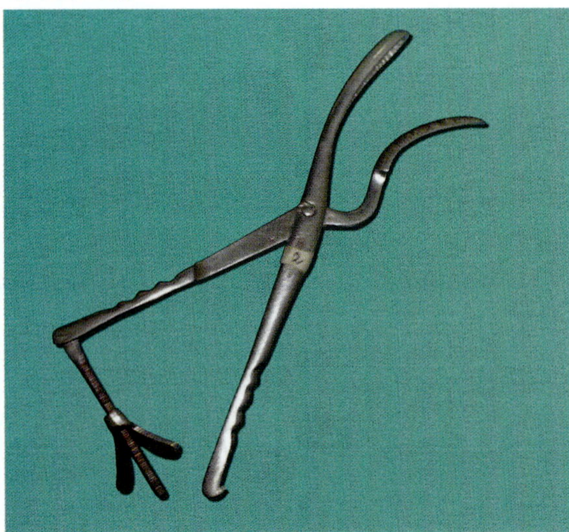

Fig. 28: Cranioclast.

Braun's cranioplasty is a surgical instrument similar to a strong forceps. It was once used to crush and then extract the skull of a fetus to facilitate delivery in cases of obstructed labor.

Parts

It is made of stainless steel and is sterilized by boiling or autoclaving. It is a 42 cm long sturdy instrument, shaped like obstetric forceps. Its blades are small, concavo-convex with coarse serrations on the opposed surfaces. A winged screw on the ends of the handles allows firm fixation of the blades. The curve of the blade is in the same direction. One blade is solid and with a blunt pointed tip, and the other blade is fenestrated.

Indication

- To crush the vault of the skull after craniotomy
- To crush the base of skull after craniotomy
- To break up the vault of skull and remove it in piece meal
- To extract the fetal head after craniotomy and crushing

GIANT VULSELLUM (FIG. 29)

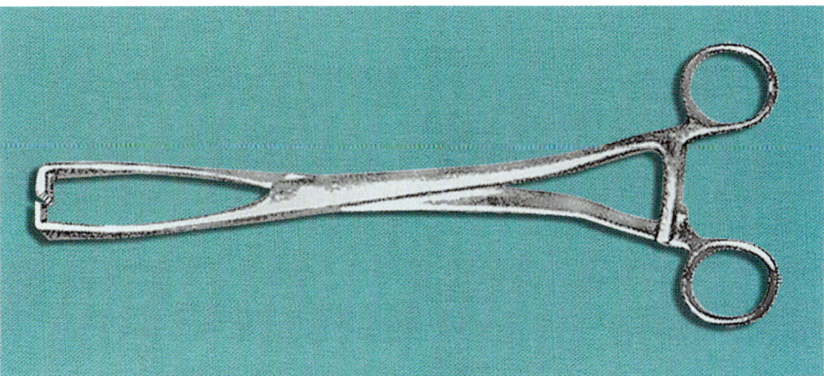

Fig. 29: Giant vulsellum.

Uses

- Vulsellum forceps have hooks at the tip of each blade and are often used in obstetrics and gynecology procedures.
- Used to grip the cervical lips to visualize the cervix
- Used for the vaginal hysterectomy
- Cervical inspection
- It is used in destructive operations, especially in evisceration, to have a good grip of fetal parts for giving traction.

Contraindications

- When the pelvis is severely contracted
- Rupture of the uterus where laparotomy is essential

HOOK WITH CROCHET (FIG. 30)

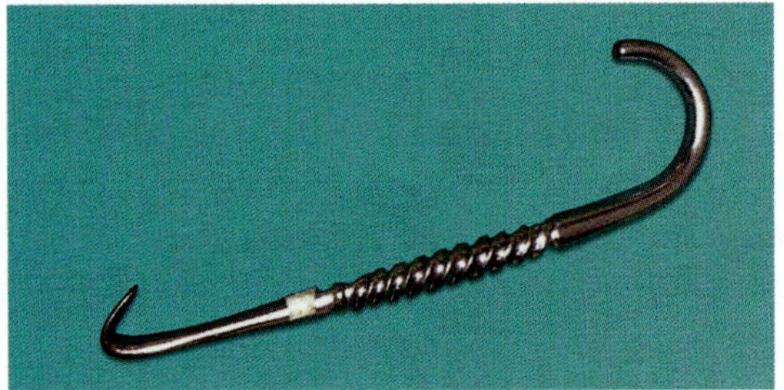

Fig. 30: Hook with crochet.

Metal obstetrical device with a blunt hook on one end and a curved pointed hook on the other end; molding in the center of the shaft is in a spiral form. A steel hook with a sharp, pointed end. After the initial breaking of the skull with a perforator, the crochet is inserted into the cranium to grab hold of the base of the skull for extraction. The blunt end is used for grabbing under the chin or shoulder and is used as a handle.

Parts

- Hook
- Crochet

Uses

- Hook is used for applying groin traction in the dead fetus.
- Hook is also used to pull down the leg of a dead fetus in a transverse lie.
- Crochet is used to apply traction on the fetal lower jaw, orbit, foramen magnum, etc., to extract the decapitated head.
- Crochet is also used to apply traction on the fetal head after craniotomy.

JARDINES DECAPITATION HOOK WITH KNIFE (FIG. 31)

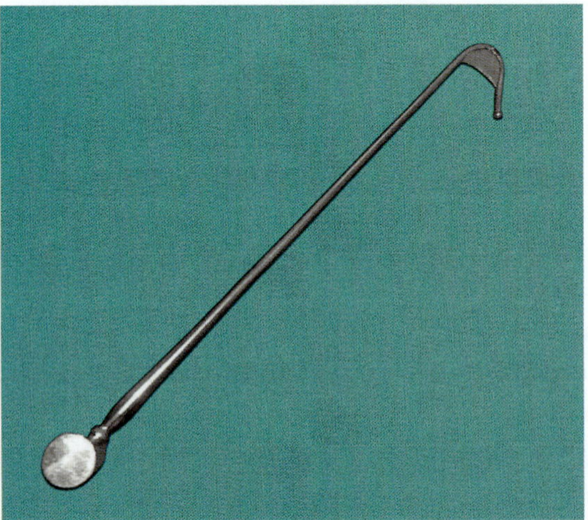

Fig. 31: Jardines decapitation hook with knife.

London-based surgical instrument of 31 cm length, invented by Down Brothers in 19th century.

Use

Destructive operation

Shape

It is shaped like an umbrella handle.

Technique

It removes a dead fetus from within the mother's body. The simple device is inserted into the mother's birth canal and hooked onto part of the child. The sturdy handle gives the physician a good grip when extracting the body. This decapitating hook is serrated on the inner edge. It extracts the whole body or parts of the body.

GREEN ARMYTAGE HEMOSTATIC FORCEPS (FIG. 32)

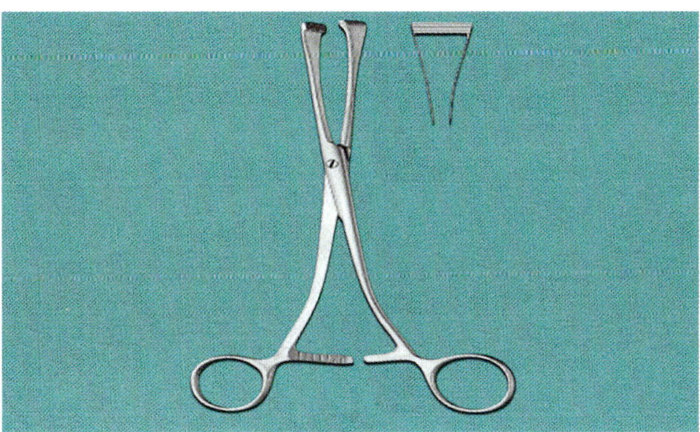

Fig. 32: Green Armytage hemostatic forceps.

The instrument consists of solid triangular blades with transverse sections a shaft and a handle with lock. The flattened broad blades achieve hemostasias over a wide area. It is used to grasp the tissues in the uterus. The forceps are available in straight or curved.

Technique

They are used to grasp and clamp the tissues in the uterus. The risk handle along with wide blades with groons gets a firm grip on the tissue. It is held just like scissors and catches the tissues in place.

Uses

- Used for grasping the cervix
- Insertion of IUD
- To hold the cut edges of the uterine scar in C-section

Parts

Triangular blades with transverse separation of a shaft and a handle with lock.

Disadvantage

- Need an assistant
- Not so self-retaining

WILLET SCALP TRACTION FORCEPS (FIG. 33)

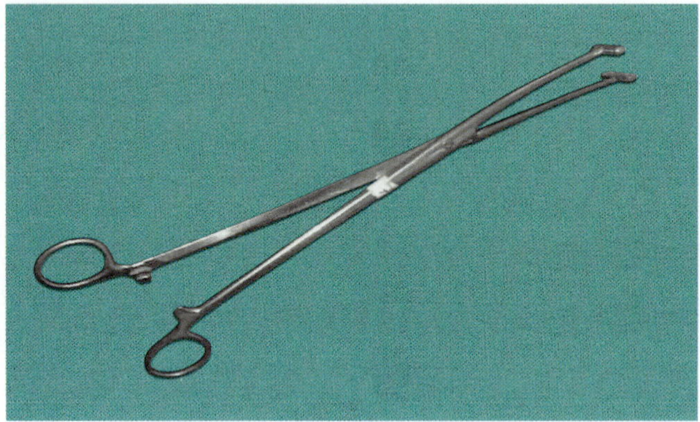

Fig. 33: Willet scalp traction forceps.

The Willet scalp traction forcep is also called Willets Martel Scalp flap forcep. It is available in two sizes 18 and 30 cm length.

Parts

- **Blade:** Shaped like letter "T" and have oblique serrations on inner aspect with one blade having two spikes on its inner aspects corresponding to holes on the other blade, which gives firm group of fetal scalps.
- Lock
- Handle with finger grips

Uses

- To extract fetal head after perforation during craniotomy operation by scalp traction
- Delivery of IUD baby
- It is also used to pull down the dead baby in case of placenta previa.
- It is used to clamp the tissue in the uterus.
- No role in modern obstetrics except in dead baby

Indication

- To control the bleeding due to I and II-degree placenta previa
- To give traction on the fetal head after craniotomy
- Ascites
- Shoulder presentation in a dead baby

Complication

- Laceration of the fetal scalp
- Hemorrhage from fetal scalp injury

- Fetal scalp infection
- Accidental injury to the maternal genital tract

DISPOSABLE CORD CLAMP (FIG. 34)

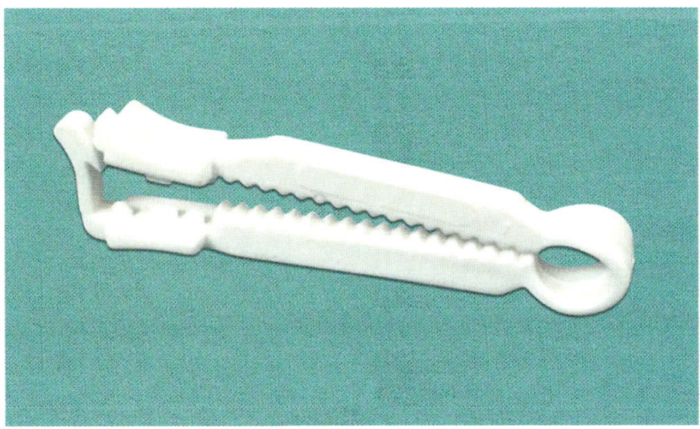

Fig. 34: Disposable cord clamp.

Disposable cord clamp looks like a cloth or pouch clip and come in sterile packs.

Description

- A disposable clamp made of plastic or aluminum
- Inner surface has serrations for tight grip on the cord.
- The open end can be locked after applying it over the cord by giving pressure with forceps.

Types of cord clamp

- Kane's cord clamp
- Hasseltin's cord clamp
- Aluminum cord clamp

Use: To clamp the umbilical cord.

PINARD'S FETAL STETHOSCOPE/PINARD'S HORN/FETOSCOPE (FIG. 35)

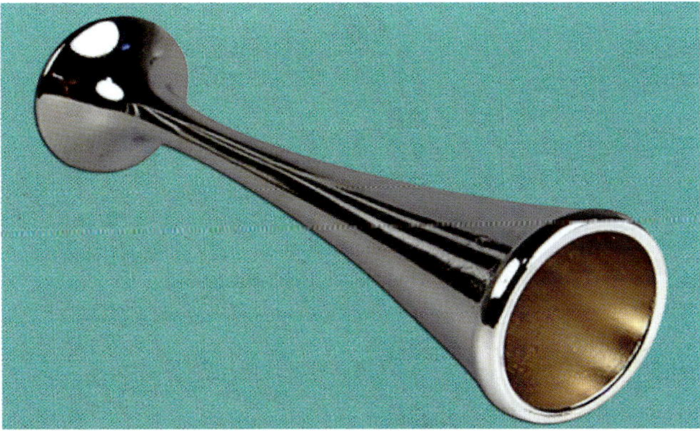

Fig. 35: Pinard's fetal stethoscope/Pinard's horn/fetoscope.

A light aluminum instrument with an open abdominal end/wide end and an aural end/narrow end, consisting of a hallow tube. The narrow end has a wide rim which is used as an earpiece.

Parts

- Hallow, elongated, funnel-shaped device with a flat disc attached to the narrow end.
- Abdominal piece
- Wood body
- Aural piece

Measurements

- Wooden—18 cm/7"
- Aluminum—15 cm/6"

Uses

This is used for the auscultation of fetal heart sounds during antenatal examination and in labor.

Indication: To monitor fetal heartbeat when reliable electricity is unavailable.

Technique

- The wide end is placed over the patient's abdomen such that it is at right angle to the abdominal wall.
- The earpiece is applied near the ear, and the instrument should not be touched by hand while listening to the fetal heart.

Instructions

- The room should be quiet.
- Put off the fan.
- Patient is in supine position with 15° tilt.
- Locate the anterior shoulder by abdominal palpation; it should be held firmly at a right angle to the point on the abdominal wall. While listening to the fetal heart tones, the fetoscope should not be turned by hand.
- Do not touch the fetoscope with your hands—it tampons conduction of heart sounds.

AMNIHOOK (FIG. 36)

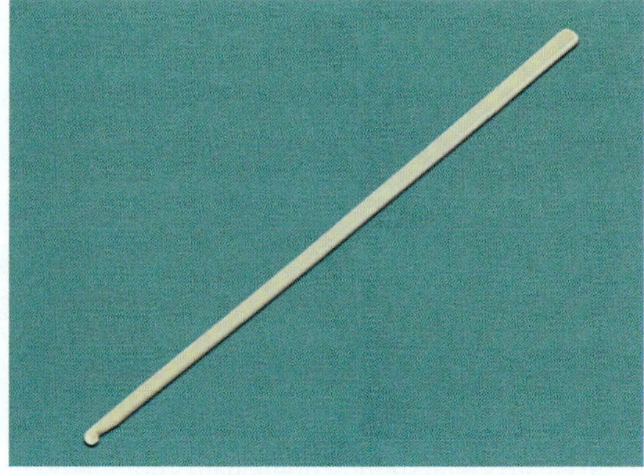

Fig. 36: Amnihook.

Amnihook or amnicot is a sterile plastic hook which is inserted into the vagina to puncture the membranes containing the amniotic fluid.

Measurements: It is about 12 inches long with a curved hook at the top.

Uses
- To induce labor or augment uterine activity, despite evidence showing lack of effectiveness.
- To enable the doctor or midwife to monitor the baby's heartbeat internally.
- To check the color of the fluid.
- To avoid having the baby aspirate the contents of the amniotic sac at the moment of birth.

Indication: The mother should be in labor, and the head should be engaged (0 station or more).

Contraindications
- Breech presentation
- Increased risk of umbilical cord prolapse
- Increased risk of infection in a prolonged labor

DOPPLER ULTRASOUND (FIG. 37)

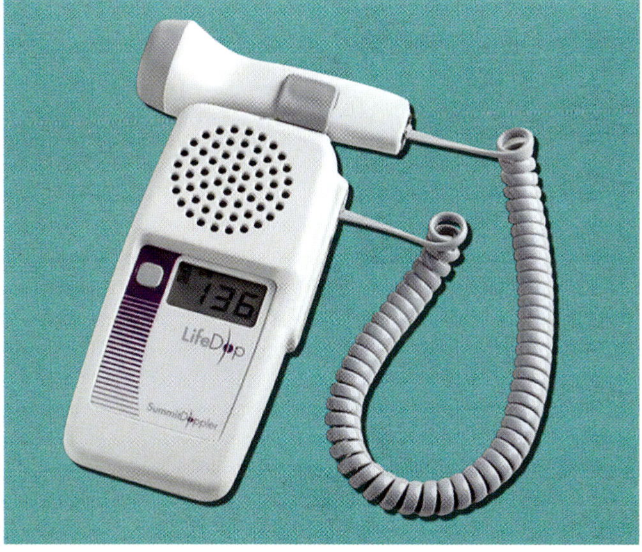

Fig. 37: Doppler ultrasound.

Handheld Doppler detects fetal heart tones at 10–12 weeks of gestation. They are easier to detect in thin women. It might require persistence to detect the fetal heart tones before 11 weeks of gestation.

Parts
- USB charging port
- TFT display

- Power button
- Speaker
- Headphone jack
- 3.0 MHz probe
- Volume down key
- Volume up key
- Shielded wire

Uses

- To detect fetal heartbeat
- To hear and count the fetal heart rate

Indications

- Part of routine prenatal care for women at 10–12 weeks of gestation
- Continuous monitoring during labor (Intermittent monitoring with doppler is usually done every 15–30 minutes during the first stage of labor and ever 5–10 minutes in the second stage)

Contraindications

There are no specific contraindications for Doppler ultrasound.

BABCOCK FORCEPS (FIG. 38)

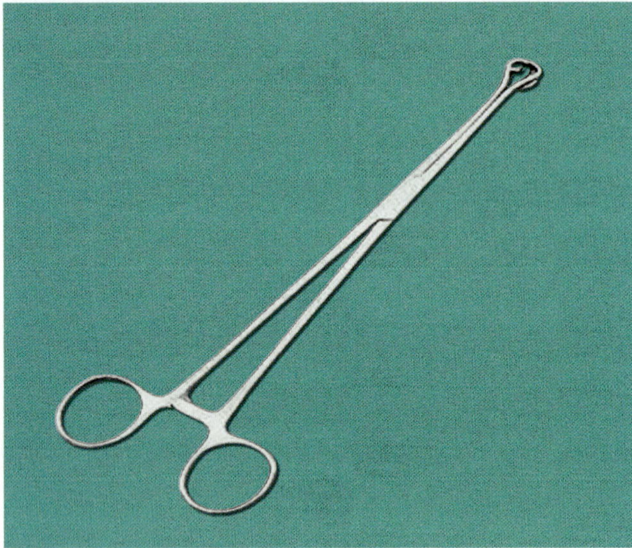

Fig. 38: Babcock forceps.

Babcock forceps are similar to Allis forceps. However, it may be considered less traumatic due to their wider, rounded grasping surface.

Parts

- The circumferential jaw

- Tips: Transversally serrated and toothless
- Blades: curved and fenestrated
- Shank
- Ratchet lock
- Finger rings

Measurements

- 6¼ inches with 9 mm blades
- 8¼ inches with 10 mm blades
- 9½ inches with 15 mm blades

Uses

- To pick up the appendix during an appendectomy
- To hold delicate visceral organs
- To hold the cut margins of the bladder during open prostatectomy

Indications

- Appendectomy
- Exploratory laparotomy and resection anastomosis
- Radical hysterectomy

Contraindications

- Nonconsenting or uncooperative patients
- Patients and or fetus with established hemorrhagic diathesis or at significant risk for it osteogenesis
- Unengaged head
- Unknown position of fetal head

CUSCO'S SPECULUM (FIG. 39)

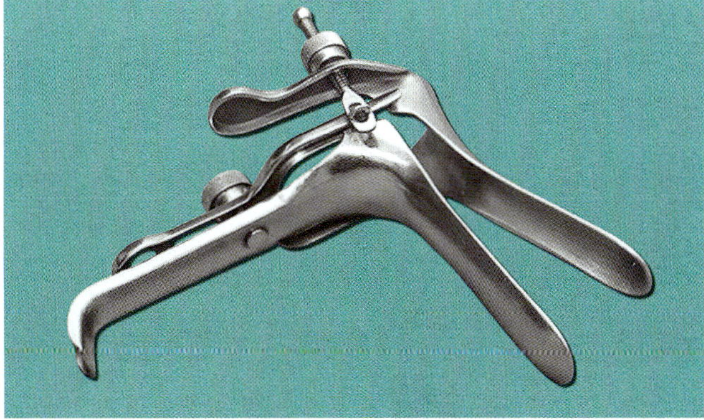

Fig. 39: Cusco's speculum.

Cusco's self-retaining bivalved speculum is a kind of speculum, used for vaginal and cervical examinations. It has a jaw that opens up like a duck bill. The instrument was named after French surgeon Édouard-Gabriel Cusco.

Parts
- Double-bladed (anterior and posterior blade)
- Fixation screw
- Handle

Blade dimensions
- Extra small (virgin) 7.5 cm × 1.7 cm
- Small 7.6 cm × 3.2 cm
- Medium 8.6 cm × 3.5 cm
- Large 10.2 cm × 3.5 cm

Uses
- To visualize the cervix and vagina for any local cause (polyp and ectopic pregnancy)
- To inspect the cervix and to prepare a cervical smear for cytology
- For dilation of the cervix and removal of the cervical lining
- Used in intrauterine insemination and in vitro fertilization procedures

Indication
- Examination of the vagina and cervix in case of abnormal vaginal bleeding
- To obtain a cervical smear for cervical cancer screening
- To obtain a swab to rule out vaginal or cervical infection
- To introduce the uterine sound

Contraindication
- In case of an external visible tear
- During the menstrual period
- In case of severe pelvic infections like cervical erosions and carcinoma
- In antenatal hemorrhage
- Women with habitual abortion

PELVIMETRY (FIG. 40)

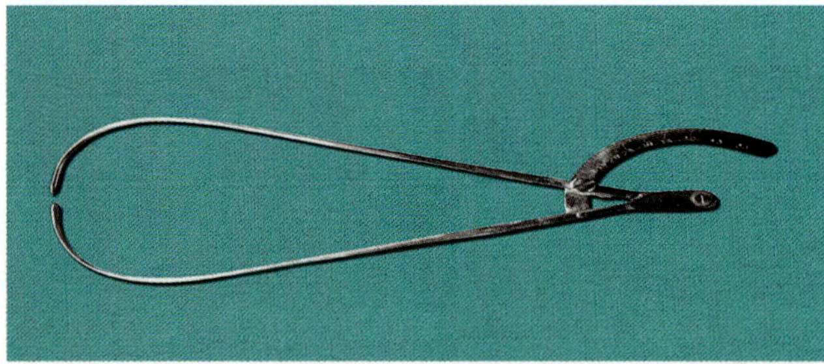

Fig. 40: Pelvimetry.

Parts
- Long, stout, curved arms called calipers with bulbous tips
- Handle where calipers are joined with a butterfly screw
- There is a centimeter scale on the handle to measure the distance between the tips of the calipers.

Uses: To measure the external pelvic diameter, like
- External conjugate
- Intercristal diameter
- Interspinous diameter
- Intertuberous diameter

LANGENBECK RETRACTOR (FIG. 41)

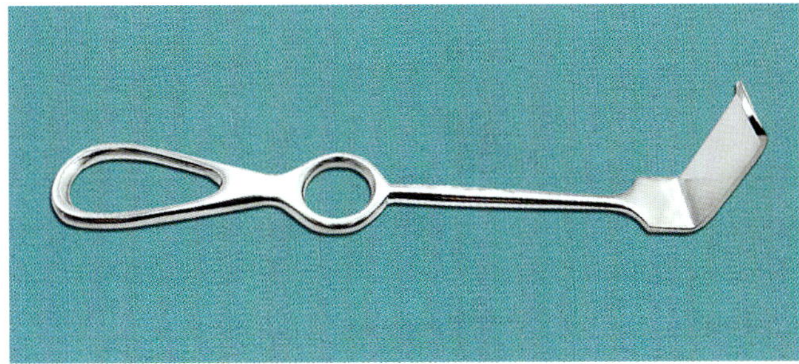

Fig. 41: Langenbeck retractor.

It is also known as Landon's bladder retractor or right-angled retractor.

Parts
- A broad flat-L-shaped blade (2 cm): The edge of the blade may be straight or curved inward (curved blades have less chance of bladder perforation).
- The blade being flat and narrow occupies very little space in the anterior pouch, thus making the retractor ideal for vaginal surgery.
- The handle has a circular opening in the center for the introduction of a finger, which gives a better grip.

Uses
- It is used for retracting the bladder away from the cervix and uterus during abdominal operations such as LSCS, abdominal hysterectomy, laparotomy, and tubectomy.
- To retract the lateral or anterior vaginal walls during any vaginal operation.

SIMPSON'S FORCEPS (FIG. 42)

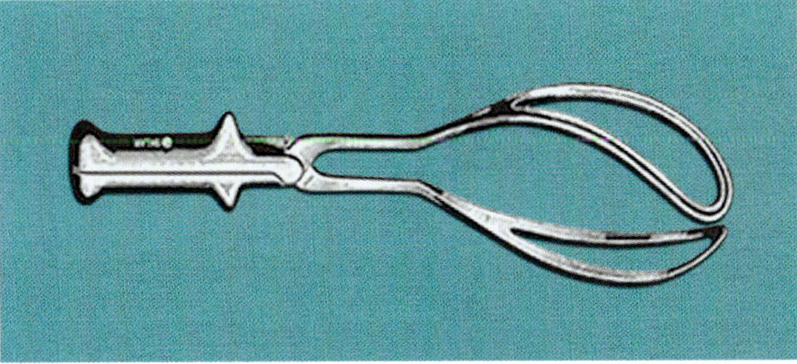

Fig. 42: Simpson's forceps.

Parts

1. Simpson's long forceps:
   - Length—35 cm
   - Fenestrated and gradually tapered blade with shallow cephalic curve
   - Handle
   - Long shank—6.2 cm
   - English lock
2. Simpson's short forceps:
   - Length—27.5 cm
   - Short shank
   - Small handles
   - English lock
   - No pelvic curve

Uses

- Prolonged second stage labor in primi mothers
- Molded fetal head
- Mid-cavity forceps delivery

Contraindications

- Fetal prematurity
- Known fetal demineralizing diseases
- Unengaged head
- Unknown fetal position
- Malpresentation

REFERENCES

1. Pai M, Kushtagi P, Daftary S, et al. Holland and Brews, Manual of Obstetrics, 4th edition. Elsevier Publications; 2015. p. 361.
2. Dutta DC, Konar H. DC Dutta's Textbook of Obstetrics: Including Perinatology and Contraception. New Delhi, India: Jaypee, The Health Sciences Publisher; 2018.
3. Linnard-Palmer L, Coats GH. Safe Maternity and Pediatric Nursing Care. FA Davis; 2025.
4. Decherney AH, Nathan L. Current Obstetric & Gynecologic Diagnosis & Treatment. New York, London; 2003.
5. Agarwal K. Instruments and Procedures in Obstetrics and Gynecology. Jaypee Brothers Medical Publishers; 2022.
6. Swain D. Obstetric Nursing Procedure Manual, 2nd edition. New Delhi: Jaypee Brothers Medical Publishers; 2023. pp. 360-1.

Drugs in Obstetrics

Thamizharasi N, Pramila D'Souza, Anwar

ANALGESICS

Analgesics are medications used to alleviate pain and are commonly employed in obstetrics for various purposes. During pregnancy, they may help manage back or pelvic discomfort. In labor and delivery, they are used to ease pain caused by uterine contractions, cervical dilation, and vaginal stretching. After childbirth, analgesics can provide relief from perineal lacerations following vaginal delivery or from incisional pain after a caesarean section.[1-5]

TYPES OF ANALGESICS

Inhalation Analgesics

Inhalational analgesia are the most widely used analgesics for labor pain because of their availability, simplicity of administration, and cost. However, their analgesic efficacy is limited compared with regional analgesia.

Generic name: Nitrous oxide in oxygen

Trade name: Entonox

Route: Inhalation

Dosage: 25% of nitrous oxide with oxygen

Available forms: Medicinal gas and compressed gas

Mechanism of action: Relaxes vascular smooth muscles and causes vasodilation.

Indications:

- Acute trauma
- Short-term relief in dental problems
- Short-term relief for procedures involving pain, such as wound and burn dressing, wound debridement, and suturing
- Normal labor
- Acute surgical or medical conditions

Contraindications:

- Artificial, traumatic pneumothorax
- Air embolism
- Decompression sickness

- Following air encephalography
- Gross abdominal distension
- In patients having received recent intraocular injection of gas

Side effects:
- Drowsiness
- Dizziness
- Mouth drying
- Nausea and vomiting
- Tingling and muscular spasm

Drug interaction:
- Lorazepam
- Augmentin

Nurses responsibility:
- Administer nitrous oxide as a single sedative agent for anxiolysis/analgesia, not to be administered concurrently with any other sedative, anesthetic agent, or narcotic analgesic.
- Nurse must know all drugs the patient is currently taking, and before.
- Place the equipment properly during the administration
- Monitor the condition of the patient throughout the administration and be prepared for potential side effects.

OPIOID ANALGESICS

Opioid analgesics are medications prescribed for the management of acute and chronic pain in many conditions.

PETHIDINE

Trade name: Demerol

Dosage and route:
- 10 mg orally
- 100 mg/2 mL IV injection

Mechanism of action: Binds to opioid receptors in the CNS, causing inhibition of ascending pain pathways, altering the perception and response to pain; produces generalized CNS depression.

Indication:
- To relieve postoperative pain and labor pain
- To relieve trauma-associated pain

Contraindication:
- Respiratory distress
- Bronchial asthma
- Hepatic and renal failure

Side effects:

- Nausea and vomiting
- Respiratory depression
- Urinary retention
- Pupil constriction

Drug interaction:

- Phenytoin
- Pentazocine
- Nalbuphine
- Butorphanol

Nurses responsibilities:

- The nurse must know all drugs the patient consumes, especially sedatives.
- Assess the respiratory condition of the patient.
- Regularly assess the function of the kidney and liver by blood test.

TRAMADOL

Trade name:

- Tramadex
- Tramal

Dosage and route:

- 50 mg orally
- 100 mg/2 mL IV injection

Mechanism of action: Opioids work by binding to opioid receptors found in both the body and brain. Once the opioids attach, they unlock, or activate, the receptors.

Indication: To treat moderate to severe pain

Contraindications:

- Severe asthma or breathing problems
- Stomach or bowel obstruction (including paralytic ileus)
- If you have recently used alcohol, sedatives, tranquilizers, or narcotic medications.

Side effects:

- Constipation
- Nausea and vomiting
- Headache
- Itching
- Drowsiness and tiredness

Drug interaction:

- Phenelzine
- Procarbazine
- Antifungals

Nurses responsibilities:

- Assess the respiratory condition of the patient
- Know the other drugs taken by the patient
- Monitor and record the vitals of the patient

EPIDURAL ANALGESICS

Epidurals are a common procedure to provide pain relief or a lack of feeling for labor and childbirth, certain surgeries and certain causes of chronic pain. An epidural is generally a very safe procedure, but there are some risks and possible side effects.

Generic name: Bupivacaine

Trade name: Marcaine

Dosage and route: 75–150 mg, IV Injection

Mechanism of action: It blocks the generation and the conduction of nerve impulses, presumably by increasing the threshold for electrical excitation in the nerve, by slowing the propagation of the nerve impulse, and by reducing the rate of rise of the action potential.

Indications:

- Cesarean section
- Procedures of the uterus and peritoneum
- Hernia repair
- Genitourinary surgery

Contraindications:

- Patients with hemorrhage
- Hypovolemic shock
- Low blood pressure

Side effects:

- Low blood pressure
- Loss of bladder control
- Itchy skin
- Feeling sick
- Inadequate pain relief

Drug interaction: It has moderate interactions with:

- Benazepril
- Captopril

Nurses responsibilities:

- Observe the site of injection for the presence of numbness
- Monitor and maintain a record of blood pressure
- Assess the response of the newborn, because some amount of these drug may be absorbed by the newborn through breast milk

LEVO BUPIVACAINE

Trade name: Charaxine and Leva Anawin

Dosage: 4.5 mg/kg

Mechanism of action: Prevents the generation and conduction of nerve impulses by acting at the cell membrane

Indications:
- C section
- Postoperative pain
- Labor pain management
- Hip and lower limb surgery

Contraindications:
- Post-traumatic vertebral surgery
- Spinal anomalies
- Obstructed hernia

Side effects:
- Hypotension
- Nausea and vomiting
- Back pain

Drug interactions:
- The metabolism of Levobupivacaine can be decreased when combined with Amiodarone.

Nurses responsibilities:
- Monitor for and immediately report: Hypotension and bradycardia
- Supervise ambulation as dizziness is a common side effect.

PARACERVICAL BLOCK AGENTS

Paracervical block agents are local anesthetics that are injected at a depth of 3–7 mm alongside the vaginal portion of the cervix in the vaginal fornices, mainly to provide pain relief during the first stage of labor.

Generic name: Lidocaine

Trade name: Xylocaine

Dosage and route:
- 20 mg/mL 2%
- 10 mg/mL 1%
- Injection, spray, and jelly

Mechanism of action: Lidocaine stabilizes the neuronal membrane by inhibiting the ionic fluxes required for the initiation and conduction of impulses, thereby affecting local anesthetic action.

Indications:
- Regional pain relief
- Jellies are used as lubricant

Contraindications:
- Patients with hypersensitivity
- Parkinson disease

Side effects:
- Drowsiness
- Apnea
- Pale and clammy skin

Drug interactions: It has serious interactions with:
- Fentanyl
- Fluvoxamine
- Beta blockers

Nurses responsibility:
- Use with caution in patients with hepatic disease
- Do not use with:
  - Severe heart block
  - Wolff-Parkinson
  - White syndrome

LOCAL PERINEAL INFILTRATION

Local infiltration analgesia is the most commonly used method of analgesia during normal labor. This type of local analgesia is achieved by injecting the analgesic agent into the perineum just before delivery with crowning of the fetal head.

PROCAINE

Generic name: Procaine

Trade name: Novocain

Dosage and route: 1.5 mg, IV injection

Mechanism of action: It stabilizes the neuronal membrane and prevents the initiation and transmission of nerve impulses, thereby reducing pain.

Indications:
- Labor pain
- Abdominal surgery
- Postpartum hemorrhage

Contraindications:
- Hypersensitivity
- Meningitis

Side effects:
- Dizziness
- Spinning sensation
- Lightheaded
- Nausea and vomiting

Drug interactions:
- 1,2 Benzodiazepine
- Abaloparatide
- Acarbose

Nurses responsibility:
- Assess the general condition and record the vitals of the patient
- Monitor for side effects such as nausea and vomiting
- Check for the severity of pain at regular intervals

ANESTHESIA

Anesthesia is a medical treatment that prevents patients from feeling pain during procedures like surgery, certain screening and diagnostic tests, tissue sample removal (e.g., skin biopsies), and dental work. It allows people to have procedures that lead to healthier and longer lives.

TYPES OF ANESTHESIA

SPINAL ANESTHETICS

BUPIVACAINE

Generic name: Bupivacaine

Trade name: Marcaine

Dose and route: 75–150 mg, spinal injection

Mechanism of action: Bupivacaine blocks the generation and conduction of nerve impulses by increasing the threshold for electrical excitation in the nerve.

Indications:
- Surgery
- Diagnostic and therapeutic procedures
- Obstetrical procedures

Contraindications:
- Along with obstetrical paracervical block anesthesia
- Fetal bradycardia and death

Side effects:
- Burning sensation, crawling, itching, and numbness
- Change or loss of taste
- Chest pain or discomfort
- Continuing ringing or buzzing, or other unexplained noise in the ears

- Decrease in the frequency and amount of urine
- Diarrhea
- Difficult or painful urination
- Dizziness
- Dry mouth
- Fever
- Headache

Drug interaction: Concurrent administration of Bupivacaine Hydrochloride with Epinephrine injection and ergot-type oxytocic drugs may cause severe, persistent hypertension or cerebrovascular accidents.

Nurses responsibilities:
- Monitor for signs of inadvertent intravascular injection, which can produce a transient "**Epinephrine Response**" within 45 seconds in the unsedated patient and an increase by 20 beats/min or more in heart rate for at least 15 seconds in a sedated patient.
- Monitor for systemic reactions (toxicity) that are more often to occur in children or older adults and may develop rapidly or be delayed for as long as 30 minutes after administration.
- Monitor for toxicity
- Monitor BP and fetal heart rate continuously during labor because maternal hypotension may accompany regional anesthesia.
- Place the mother on the left side with legs elevated.

XYLOCAINE (5% LIDOCAINE)

Generic name: Lidocaine HCL

Dose and route: 2.5–3 mL, spinal injection.

Mechanism of action: Lidocaine alters signal conduction in neurons by prolonging the inactivation of the fast voltage-gated Na^+ channels in the neuronal cell membrane responsible for action potential propagation.

Indications:
- Ventricular arrhythmia
- For Local anesthetic effect
- Anesthetic lubricant when used as topical agent

Contraindications:
- Hypersensitivity
- Severe hypotension
- Hypovolemia
- With paracervical block

Side effects:
- Bluish color lips, finger nails
- Chest pain or discomfort
- Cold, clammy, and pale skin
- Confusion

- Cough
- Dark urine

Drug interactions:
- Dofetilide
- Antihypertensives and cardiac drugs
- Antipsychotics, antidepressive, and antianxiety drugs
- Other anesthetics
- Phenytoin
- Procarbazine

Nurses responsibilities:
- Use with caution in patients with hepatic disease
- Do not use with:
  - Severe heart block
  - Wolff-Parkinson
  - White syndrome

GENERAL ANESTHESIA

General anesthetics are often defined as compounds that induce a loss of consciousness. It is a method of medically inducing loss of consciousness that makes a patient unarousable even with painful stimuli. This effect is achieved by administering either intravenous or inhalational general anesthetic medications, which often act in combination with an analgesic and neuromuscular blocking agent.

HALOTHANE

Generic name: Halothane

Trade name: Fluothane

Dose and route: 0.5–3% administered by nonrebreathing technique or closed technique. It may also be administered with oxygen and nitrous oxide through the inhalation technique.

Mechanism of action: It binds potassium channels in cholinergic neurons, producing an immobilizing effect.

Indications: Induction and maintenance of general anesthesia.

Contraindications:
- Increased intracranial pressure and intracranial hemorrhage
- Not recommended for obstetrical anesthesia, except when uterine relaxation is required.

Side effects:
- Tachycardia
- Cyanosis
- Muscle rigidity
- Malignant hyperthermia
- Ventricular arrhythmias

Drug interactions:

- Augments the action of nondepolarizing muscle relaxants.
- Augments the hypotension caused by the ganglionic blocking effect of tubocurarine.
- Arrhythmias may be present with adrenaline.

Nurses responsibilities:

- Educating people before and after they receive anesthesia for a procedure or surgery.
- Assessing a person's physical response to anesthesia.
- Identifying possible risks like allergies, asthma, or diabetes.

PROPOFOL

Trade name: Diprivan

Dose and route: 10 mg/mL, IV

Mechanism of action: By decreasing the dissociation of GABA from GABA receptors in the brain and potentiating the inhibitory effect of the neurotransmitters.

Indication: Induction and maintenance of general anesthesia during delivery.

Contraindication: Hypersensitivity

Side effects:

- Transient local pain
- Hypotension

Drug interactions:

- Ceritinib
- Doxapram
- Epinephrine
- Fentanyl

Nurses responsibilities: Patients should be monitored without interruption to assess the level of consciousness and identify early signs of hypotension, bradycardia, apnea, and oxygen desaturation.

DIURETICS

Diuretics serve to rid the body of excess fluid that accumulates in the tissues owing to various disease states. A diuretic also has substance that promotes the increased production of urine.

CLASSIFICATION

1. **Thiazide diuretics:**
   - Chlorothiazide
   - Hydrochlorothiazide
2. **Loop diuretics:**
   - Frusemide
   - Ethacrynic acid

3. **Potassium-sparing diuretics:**
    - Spironolactone
    - Amiloride
    - Triamterene
4. **Carbonic anhydrase inhibitors:**
    - Acetazolamide
    - Dorzolamide

THIAZIDE DIURETICS

Generic name: Hydrochlorothiazide

Trade name: Hydrodiuril

Dose: 12.5 mg twice daily maximum up to 50 mg daily may be used.

Route: Per oral

Mechanism of action: Promotes sodium and water excretion, thereby lowering blood pressure

Indications:
- Edema
- Hypertension

Contraindications:
- Patients with anuria
- Patients hypersensitive to other thiazides or other sulfonamide derivatives

Adverse effects:
- Orthostatic hypotension
- Anorexia
- Frequent urination
- Agranulocytosis
- Hepatic encephalopathy
- Fluid and electrolyte imbalance

Drug interactions:
- Barbiturates with hydrochlorothiazide cause hypotension
- Hydrochlorothiazide slows the clearance of lithium from the body in case of lithium intake with hydrochlorothiazide
- Taking corticosteroids with hydrochlorothiazide can cause loss of electrolytes

Nurses responsibility:
- Check physician's order before administering medications
- Observe and apply the 10 rights
- Assess patient's edema or blood pressure before giving medications
- Monitor drug's effectiveness by regularly checking the blood pressure, urine output and weight
- Monitor electrolyte levels, blood count, BUN, and uric acid levels
- Monitor the intake and output
- Advise patient to change positions slowly to minimize orthostatic hypotension

LOOP DIURETICS

Generic name: Frusemide

Trade name: Lasix

Dosage and route:
- 40 mg tablet daily for 5 days a week, orally
- Parenterally in doses of 40–120 mg daily, IV

Mechanism of action: It directly prevents reabsorption of sodium and potassium mainly from the Loop of Henle.

Indications:
- Edema associated with heart failure
- Cirrhosis of liver and renal disease
- Acute pulmonary edema and hypertension
- Pulmonary congestion and hypertension

Contraindications:
- Allergy to frusemide, sulfonamides, and tartrazine
- Anuria, hepatic coma, and hypokalemia.

Adverse effects:
- CNS: Dizziness, vertigo, paresthesia, xanthopsia, and weakness
- CVS: Orthostatic hypertension and thrombophlebitis
- Dermatology: Photosensitivity, pruritus, urticaria, and purpura
- GI: Nausea, anorexia, vomiting, and oral and gastric irritation
- GU: Nocturia, glycosuria, and urinary bladder spasm
- Others: Muscle cramps and muscle spasms

Drug interactions:
- Increased risk of cardiac arrhythmias with cardiac glycosides
- Increased risk of ototoxicity with aminoglycoside antibiotics, cisplatin
- Decreased absorption of frusemide with phenytoin
- Decreased GI absorption with charcoal; may reduce the effect of insulin or oral antibiotics because blood glucose levels can become elevated.

Nurses responsibility

Before:
- Check doctor's order
- Assess allergy to furosemide, sulfonamides, and tartrazine
- Do not mix parenteral solution with a pH <3.5
- Do not expose to light, which may discolor tablets or solution
- Educate the patient about the purpose and importance of the drug.

During:
- Check the patency of the IV site and IV line
- Give early in the day so that increased urination will not disturb sleep

- Administer the right dose at the right time
- Measure and record weight to monitor fluid changes

After:

- Monitor blood glucose levels
- Arrange to monitor serum electrolyte, hydration, liver, and renal function
- Arrange for potassium—rich diet or supplemental potassium as needed
- Report loss or gain of more than 1.5 kg weight in 1 day, swelling in ankles or fingers, unusual bleeding or bruising
- Document and record

POTASSIUM-SPARING DIURETICS

Generic name: Spironolactone

Trade name: Aldactone

Dosages and route:

- 25–200 mg orally per day in single or divided doses for edema
- 50–100 mg orally per day in single or divided doses for hypertension
- 25 mg orally once a day for heart failure
- 25–100 mg orally per day for hypokalemia

Mechanism of action: It acts on the distal renal tubules as a competitive antagonist of aldosterone.

Indications:

- Heart failure
- Hypertension
- Edema
- Primary aldosteronism

Contraindications:

- Hyperkalemia
- Addison's disease

Adverse effects:

- Slow or irregular heartbeat
- Tingling feeling
- Muscle weakness
- Shortness of breath

Drug interactions:

- With antihypertensive, it causes enhanced hypotensive effect
- With ACEI and ARBs, it causes enhanced hyperkalemia
- With potassium-sparing diuretics, it has enhanced potassium-sparing effect

Nurses responsibility:

- Give daily doses early
- Make suspension
- Measure and record weight regularly

ANTIHYPERTENSIVE DRUGS

The commonly used drugs are grouped into the following discussed below.

METHYLDOPA

Trade name: Aldomet

Generic name: Aldorill and Dopamet

Dose and route: Orally 250 mg, BID—may be increased to 1 g, qid depending upon the response

Mechanism of action:
- ACE inhibitors: Inhibit formation of angiotensin II from angiotensin I
- ARB: Block angiotensin II receptors

Indication: Hypertension

METHYLDOPATE

Not a drug of choice, because it slows the onset of action.

Indication: Hypertension of pregnancy

Contraindications:
- Hepatic disorders
- Psychic patients
- Congestive cardiac failure
- Postpartum risk of depression

Side effects

Maternal:
- Postural hypotension
- Hemolytic anemia
- Sodium retention
- Excessive sedation
- Coombs test positive

Fetal: Intestinal ileus

Adverse effects:
- Nausea
- Diarrhea
- Headache
- Dizziness
- Sedation
- Dry mouth

Drug interactions:
- When methyldopa is used with other antihypertensive drugs, potentiation of antihypertensive effect may occur.

- Patients should be followed carefully to detect reactions or unusual manifestations of drug idiosyncrasy.
- Patients may require reduced doses of anesthetics when on methyldopa.
- If hypotension does occur during anesthesia, it usually can be controlled by vasopressors.
- The adrenergic receptors remain sensitive during treatment with methyldopa.

Nurses responsibility

Before:

- Check doctor's order
- Assess sensitivity to methyldopa, hepatic disease, renal failure, and dialysis
- Assess weight, skin color, lesions, mucous membrane color, lesions, orientation, and affect
- Educate client about the drug, its purpose, and importance

During:

- Check the label twice
- Administer at the right dose and in the right time
- Do not crush nor chew tablets, swallow whole
- Discontinue drug if fever is present, abnormalities in liver function tests, or jaundice, if Coombs test is positive, hemolytic anemia occurs

After:

- Monitor blood counts periodically to detect hemolytic anemia
- Monitor hepatic function, especially in the first 6–8 weeks of therapy or if unexplained fever appears
- Ensure that methyldopa is not reinstated in such patients
- Report if unexplained, prolonged general tiredness; yellowing of the skin or eyes; fever, bruising; rashes occur
- Document and record

HYDRALAZINE

Trade name: Apresoline

Dose and route:

- Orally 100 mg/day in four divided doses
- IV 5–10 mg every 20 minutes, maximum 20 mg
- Orally, it is weak and should be combined with methyldopa or β blockers.

Mechanism of action: Acts by peripheral vasodilatation as it relaxes the arterial smooth muscle. It increases the cardiac output and renal blood flow.

Indications:

- Oral: Essential hypertension, alone or in combination with other drugs
- Parenteral: Severe essential hypertension when drug cannot be given orally or when need to lower BP is urgent.
- Unlabeled uses: Reducing afterload in the treatment of heart failure, severe aortic insufficiency, and after valve replacement (doses up to 800 mg tid)

Contraindications: Because of variable sodium retention, diuretics should be used. To control arrhythmias, propranolol may be administered intravenously.

Side effects:
- Maternal hypotension
- Tachycardia, arrhythmia, and palpitation
- Lupus-like syndrome
- Fluid retention
- Neonatal—thrombocytopenia

Adverse effects:
- Flushing
- Headache
- Upset stomach
- Vomiting, loss of appetite
- Diarrhea/constipation
- Eye tearing

Nurses responsibility

Before:
- Check doctor's order
- Wash hands before administering the drug
- Take the client's BP
- Check the patency of the IV line
- Educate the client about the purpose and importance of the drug

During:
- Give drug exactly as prescribed
- Take with food
- Discontinue if blood dyscrasias occur
- Withdraw drug gradually and not at once

After:
- Monitor client for orthostatic hypertension
- Reevaluate therapy if patient develops arthralgia, fever, chest pain, or continued malaise.
- Report persistent or severe constipation
- Report unexplained fever or malaise, muscle or joint aching, rash, numbness, and tingling
- Document and record

LABETALOL

Trade name: Trandate

Dose and route:
- Orally 100 mg, tid, may be increased up to 2,400 mg daily
- IV infusion (hypertensive crisis) 20–40 mg, IV every 10–15 minutes until desired effect, maximum up to 220 mg

Mechanism of action: Combined alpha and beta-adrenergic blocking agent

Indications:
- Hypertension
- Hypertensive crisis

Contraindications:
- Hepatic disorders
- Asthma
- Congestive cardiac failure

Side effects:
- Tremors
- Headache
- Asthma
- Congestive cardiac failure

Adverse effects:
- Bradycardia
- Intermittent claudication
- Raynaud's phenomena
- Postural hypotension
- Precipitation of heart block
- Thrombocytopenia
- Hypoglycemia
- Confusion, hallucinations, dizziness, and mood changes
- Paresthesia
- Nightmares and tingling sensation of scalp
- Bronchospasm

Drug interactions:
- Calcium channel blockers: Addictive effect.
- Prostaglandin synthase inhibiting drugs: Decrease the hypotensive effects of beta blockers.
- Catecholamine-depleting drugs such as reserpine cause hypotension, marked bradycardia, vertigo, syncopal attacks, or orthostatic hypotension.
- Haloperidol cause hypotension and cardiac arrest. Theophylline: Clearance is reduced.
- Cimetidine: Increasing blood levels.
- Chlorpromazine: Increased plasma levels of both drugs.
- Phenytoin, phenobarbitone, and rifampin: Accelerate labetalol clearance.
- Ethanol: Slows the rate of absorption of labetalol.
- Aluminum hydroxide gel: Greatly reduces intestinal absorption of labetalol.

Nurses responsibility:
- Assess: Intake output ratio, uterine contractions, FHR, blood pressure, pulse, and respiration.
- Administer by IV infusion, monitor drop rate, and make crash cart available.
- Evaluate the length and duration of contractions.

- Notify physician of contractions lasting over 1 minute or absence of contractions.
- Teach to report increased blood loss, abdominal cramps, or increased temperature.

NIFEDIPINE

Trade name: Adalat, Adipine, and Coracten

Generic name: Fortipin and Nifedipress

Dose and route: Orally 5–10 mg, tid, maximum dose 60–120 mg/day

Mechanism of action: Direct arteriolar vasodilatation by inhibition of slow inward calcium channels in vascular smooth muscle

Indications: For the management of vasospastic angina, chronic stable angina, and hypertension.

Contraindications: Simultaneous use of magnesium sulfate could be hazardous due to the synergistic effect

Side effects:

- Flushing
- Hypotension
- Headache
- Tachycardia
- Inhibition of labor

Adverse effects:

- Swollen legs or ankles (edema)
- Constipation
- Feeling dizzy
- Irregular heartbeat (palpitations)

Drug interactions: Nifedipine oral tablet can interact with other vitamins or herbs.

Nurses responsibility:

- Monitor BP carefully during the titration period. The patient may become severely hypotensive, especially if also taking other antihypertensive drugs.
- Monitor blood sugar in diabetic patients. Nifedipine has diabetogenic properties.
- Monitor for gingival hyperplasia and report promptly. This is a rare but serious adverse effect.

SODIUM NITROPRUSSIDE

Trade name: Nitropress

Dose and route: IV infusion 0.25–8 μg/kg/min

Mechanism of action: Direct vasodilator (arterial and venous)

Indications:

- Management of hypertensive crisis
- Angina and CHF

Contraindications:
- Hypersensitivity
- Decreased cerebral perfusion
- Arteriovenous shunt or coarctation of aorta

Side effects:
- Maternal: Nausea, vomiting, and severe hypotension
- Fetal toxicity due to metabolites—cyanide and thiocyanate

Adverse effects:
- Excessive hypotension and palpitations
- Substernal distress and tachyarrhythmia
- Restlessness, disorientation, psychosis, headache, and elevated intracranial pressure
- Thyroid suppression and metabolic acidosis
- Nausea, vomiting, and bowel obstruction
- Thiocyanate toxicity
- Neuromuscular and skeletal weakness, muscle twitch, and diaphoresis
- Rash, injection site irritation
- Oliguria
- Azotemia

Drug interactions:
- IV nitroglycerin may decrease the effect of alteplase. Avanafil: Additive vasodilation.
- Azilsartan medoxomil has increased synergistic effects.
- Dihydroergotamine has possible antagonism of action.
- Ergonovine, methylergometrine, methysergide, and ergotamine: Possible antagonism of action.
- Sildenafil: Possible significant hypotension with this combination.
- Tadalafil: The vasodilatory effects of nitroglycerin may be increased. By Tadalafil. Severe hypotension may occur.

Nurses responsibility:
- Monitor blood pressure and for signs of overdose
- Assess for orthostatic hypotension when a client stands up
- Check medication refills for adherence
- Assess for angina

NITROGLYCERIN

Trade name: Nitrostat

Dose and route: IV infusion 5 μg/min, to be increased at every 3–5 minutes up to 100 μg/min

Mechanism of action: Relaxes mainly the venous but also arterial smooth muscle

Indications:
- To prevent chronic angina attacks
- Acute angina pectoris; to prevent or minimize angina attacks before stressful events

- Hypertension from surgery, heart failure after MI, and angina pectoris in acute situations.
- To produce controlled hypotension during surgery (by IV infusion)

Contraindications:
- Used in hypertensive crisis for a short time only.
- Hypertensive encephalopathy, as it increases blood flow and intracranial pressure

Side effects:
- Tachycardia
- Headache
- Methemoglobinemia

Adverse effects:
- Bloating
- Burning, crawling, and itching
- Lightheadedness

Nurses responsibility:
- Closely monitor vital signs during infusion, particularly blood pressure, especially in a patient with an MI. Excessive hypotension may worsen the MI.
- To apply ointment, do not rub it; cover with plastic film to aid absorption and to protect clothing.
- Remove all excess ointment from the previous site before applying the next dose.

ACE INHIBITORS/ANGIOTENSIN RECEPTOR BLOCKERS (AARB)

Trade name: Captopril

Dose and route: Orally 6.25 mg bid, telmisartan, orally 20–40 mg a day

Mechanism of action:
- ACE inhibitors: Inhibit formation of angiotensin II from angiotensin I.
- ARB: Block angiotensin II receptors

Indications:
- Hypertension
- Heart failure
- Postmyocardial infarction
- Diabetes
- Nephrotic syndrome or proteinuria chronic kidney disease
- Glomerular disease and post-transplant glomerulonephritis

Contraindications: Pregnancy

Side effects:
- Maternal: Hypotension, headache, asthenia, arrhythmias, and oligohydramnios
- Fetal: IUGR, fetal renal tubular dysgenesis, neonatal renal failure, and pulmonary hypoplasia

Adverse effects:

- Headache
- Fainting and dizziness
- Fatigue
- Respiratory symptoms
- Vomiting and diarrhea
- Back pain
- Leg swelling

Drug interactions:

- Lisinopril with aliskiren, other ACE inhibitors, or angiotensin receptor blockers can cause hypotension, hyperkalemia, and renal impairment.
- Allopurinol, bone marrow suppressants (such as methotrexate), procainamide, and systemic corticosteroids can cause neutropenia or agranulocytosis.
- Cyclosporine, potassium-sparing diuretics, and potassium supplements can cause hyperkalemia.
- Lisinopril taken with diuretics and other antihypertensives can have severe hypotensive effects.
- Insulin or oral antidiabetic agents can increase the hypoglycemic effect.
- Lithium can increase blood lithium levels and cause lithium toxicity.
- NSAIDs can reduce the antihypertensive effect of lisinopril. Hypotension may worsen when used with alcohol and ginseng.

Nurses responsibility:

- Assess for allergies to ACE inhibitors.
- Monitor blood pressure for hypotension prior to administration.
- Assess for signs of severe hypotension like dizziness, excessive perspiration, vomiting, and diarrhea.
- Monitor for signs of worsening CHF, such as water retention and shortness of breath.

ECBOLICS/UTERINE STIMULANTS (OXYTOCIN, PROSTAGLANDIN, AND ERGOT DERIVATIVES)

Uterine stimulants are those drugs that stimulate contraction of the myometrium. They are used to induce labor at term, to prevent or control postpartum or postabortion hemorrhage, and to assess fetal status in high-risk pregnancies. They may also be used alone or with other drugs to induce abortions (ABORTIFACIENTS).

Types:

- Oxytocins
- Prostaglandins: PGE1 and PGE2
- Misoprostol
- Ergots: Ergometrine

Routes of administration: IV, IM, as a vaginal gel or suppository, or in oral form.

OXYTOCIN

Oxytocin is a recombinant hormone used to induce or strengthen uterine contractions in pregnant women to aid in labor and delivery or to control postpartum bleeding.

Generic name: Oxytocin

Trade name: Pitocin

Dosage and route (Table 1): 10 units/mL, oral and IV/IM

TABLE 1: Dosage and route.

Indications	*Dose*
Postpartum hemorrhage	10 units after delivery of placenta
Labor induction	0.5–1 mUnit/min IV
Incomplete abortion	10–20 mUnit/min, not more than 30 units/12 h

Mechanism of action: Oxytocin increases the sodium permeability of uterine myofibrils, indirectly stimulating contraction of the uterine smooth muscle. The uterus responds to oxytocin more readily in the presence of high estrogen concentrations and with the increased duration of pregnancy.

Pharmacokinetics:

- Absorption: Oxytocin is administered parenterally and is fully bioavailable. It takes approximately 40 minutes for oxytocin to reach steady-state concentrations in the plasma after parenteral administration.
- Distribution: The drug distributes throughout the extracellular fluid, with minimal amounts reaching the fetus.
- Metabolism: Oxytocin is rapidly removed from the plasma by the liver and kidney. The enzyme oxytocinase is largely responsible for the metabolism and regulation of oxytocin levels in pregnancy, and only a small percentage of the neurohormone is excreted in the urine unchanged.
- Excretion: It is through the kidney.

Indications (Table 2):

TABLE 2: Indications.

Early pregnancy	• To accelerate abortion • To stop bleeding following evacuation of the uterus • Used as adjunct of abortion along with another abortifacient
Late pregnancy	• To induce labor • To facilitate cervical ripping for effective induction • Augmentation of labor • Uterine inertia
Labor	• In active management of third stage of labor • Following expulsion of placenta
Puerperium	To minimize the blood loss and to control the PPH

Contraindications (Table 3)

TABLE 3: Contraindications.

Pregnancy	• Grand multipara • Contacted pelvis • History of cesarean or hysterectomy • Malpresentation
Labor	• All the contraindications in pregnancy • Obstructed labor • In coordinate uterine action • Fetal distress
Others	• Hypovolemic shock • Cardiac disease

Adverse effects:
- Uterine hyperstimulation
- Uterine rupture
- Water intoxication
- Hypotension
- Fetal distress
- Antidiuresis
- Fetal hypoxia
- Fetal death

Nurses responsibility:
- Assess the intake output ratio
- Assess uterine contractions and FHR
- Assess BP, pulse, and respiration
- Administer by IV infusion
- Monitor drop rate
- Make a crash cart available
- Evaluate length and duration of contractions
- If contractions last over 1 minute, inform the physician
- Advise to inform if there is any increased bleeding, abdominal cramps, and increased temperature

ERGOMETRINE

Trade name: Cafergot, Ergomar, Ergostat, Migergot, and Wigraine.

Dosage (Table 4)

TABLE 4: Dosage.

Ergometrine tablet	0.5–1 mg	Oral
Ergometrine maleate injection	0.5 mg/mL	IM
Methylergometrine injection	0.2 mg/mL	IV

Action: Ergonovine directly stimulates the uterine muscle to increase force and frequency of contractions. Ergonovine, like other ergot alkaloids, produces arterial vasoconstriction by stimulation of alpha-adrenergic and serotonin receptors and inhibition of endothelial-derived relaxation factor release. It is less potent vasoconstrictor than ergotamine.

Pharmacokinetics: In contrast to the amino acid, ergot alkaloids, ergometrine, and methylergometrine are rapidly and nearly completely absorbed from the oral route. The onset of uterine action is: Oral—15 minutes; IM—5 minutes; IV almost immediate. They are partly metabolized in liver and excreted in urine. Plasma t½ is 1–2 hours. Effects of a single dose last 3–4 hours.

Indication: Headache

Contraindications:
- Patients with vascular disease, hypertension, and toxemia
- Presence of sepsis which may cause gangrene
- Liver and kidney diseases
- Pregnancy, during induction of labor, and during first and second stage labor

Adverse effects:
- Nausea, vomiting, and rise in BP occur occasionally.
- It can decrease milk secretion if higher doses are used for many days postpartum.

Nurses responsibilities:
- Monitor BP, pulse, and respirations every 15–30 minutes until transfer to the postpartum unit, then every 1–2 hours.
- Report hypertension, chest pain, arrhythmias, headache, or change in neurologic status.
- Monitor the amount and type of vaginal discharge.
- Report symptoms of hemorrhage (increased bleeding, hypotension, pallor, and tachycardia) immediately.

PROSTAGLANDIN

Generic name: Dinoprostone

Trade name: Xalatan (latanoprost), Zioptan (tafluprost), Travatan Z (travoprost), and Lumigan (bimatoprost)

Classification

Natural prostaglandins:
- Dinosprostone (PGE_2)
- Dinoprost ($PGF_2\alpha$)
- Alprostadil (PGE_1)
- Prostacyclin (PGI_2)

Prostaglandin analogs:
- Carboprost (15-methyl PGF2a)
- Misoprostol (methyl PGE)

- Latanoprost (PGE_2 analog)
- Travoprost
- Bimatoprost

Dosage (Table 5)

TABLE 5: Dosage.

Prostaglandin E1 (Alprostadil):	5–10 ng/kg/min (0.005–0.01 µg/kg/min) IV infusion
Dinoprostone:	20 mg intrauterine

Mechanism of action: The COX-1 enzyme produces basal amounts of prostaglandins, while chemical mediators induce the COX-2 isoform to increase prostaglandin production.

Indications:
- Abortions
- PPH
- Cervical priming
- Glaucoma
- Stomach ulcers

Contraindications:
- Bronchial asthma
- Hypersensitivity
- Epilepsy
- Renal disorder

Adverse effects:
- Nausea
- Fever
- Back pain
- Vomiting
- Abdominal pain
- Diarrhea

Nurses responsibilities:
- Monitor maternal vital signs and fluid balance.
- Make the crash cart available.
- Monitor fetal response, uterine activity, and rest done.
- If contraction last for 1 minute, immediately informing the physician is to be done.
- Check out for hypersensitivity reactions
- Monitor the IV drop rate.

ANTICONVULSANTS

Anticonvulsants are also known as antiepileptics or antiseizure drugs used in the treatment of epileptic seizures. These drugs suppress the excessive rapid firing of neurons during seizures and also prevent the spread of seizures within the brain.

DIAZEPAM

Trade name: Valium, Valpam, and Diastat

Generic name: Diazepam

Classifications: Benzodiazepines, sedatives/hypnotics, and antianxiety agents

Dosage:
- Oral: 2–10 mg, 2–4 times a day
- Parenteral: 2–10 mg may repeat every 3–4 hours

Mechanism of action:
- It potentiates the effect of gamma-aminobutyric acid (GABA) and other neurotransmitters by binding to specific receptors of the CNS.
- It suppresses the spread of seizure activity caused by seizure-producing foci in the cortex, thalamus, and limbic structures.

Indications:
- Anxiety
- Skeletal muscle relaxation
- Status epilepticus
- Panic disorder
- Refractory epilepsy
- Alcohol withdrawal
- Para anesthesia
- Tension
- Headache
- Tremors

Contraindications:
- Angle-closure glaucoma
- Coma
- Pre-existing CNS depression
- Severe uncontrolled pain

Side effects:
- Dizziness
- Drowsiness
- Lethargy
- Hangover
- Mental depression
- Hypotension
- Blurred vision
- Nausea, vomiting

Toxicity: Diazepam of more than 40 mg at one sitting is fatal and may cause symptoms like falling into a deep sleep or "coma" while still being able to breathe well enough. Other symptoms may include bluish-colored lips and fingernails, blurred vision, and double vision.

Drug interaction: It interacts with clozapine, fluvoxamine, orlistat, and sodium oxybate. Causing the risk of serious side effects such as slow or shallow breathing, severe drowsiness, or dizziness.

Nurses responsibility:
- Monitor patients' vital signs, weight, serum electrolytes, and hydration.
- Provide frequent sips of water for dry mouth.
- Provide fluids and fiber for constipation.
- Keep the patient in a recumbent position for up to 3 hours after parenteral administration.
- Instruct the patient to change positions slowly.

PHENYTOIN

Trade name: Dilantin and Phenytek

Generic name: Phenytoin

Dosage:
- Oral: 100 mg, 3 times a day
- Parenteral: 10–15 mg/kg at a rare not to exceed 50 mg/min

Mechanism of action: Phenytoin prevents seizures by inhibiting the positive feedback loop that results in the neuronal propagation of high-frequency action potentials.

Indications:
- Generalized tonic-clonic seizures
- Complex partial seizures
- Status epilepticus
- Trigeminal neuralgia
- Behavioral disorder
- Grand mal seizures
- Jacksonian epilepsy
- Post-traumatic seizures
- Temporal lobe epilepsy

Contraindications:
- Hypersensitivity
- Ventricular automaticity
- Sinus bradycardia
- Sinoatrial block
- Stokes-Adams syndrome

Side effects:
- Drowsiness
- Irritability
- Vertigo
- Slurred speech
- Numbness and tingling
- Tremors

- Paradoxical seizures
- Encephalopathy
- Ventricular fibrillation
- Bullous dermatosis
- Hypotension

Toxicity: The toxic level is >30 μg/mL and lethal levels are >100 μg/mL, the symptoms of toxicity are mild nystagmus to ataxia, slurred speech, lethargy coma, and death.

Drug interaction: Phenytoin interacts with Colesevelam, Orlistat, and Sucralfate.

Nurses responsibility:
- Monitor the patient's cardiac rhythm and check BP frequently during IV infusion.
- Monitor for serum levels of 10–20 μg/mL
- Administer IV phenytoin slowly
- Advice the patients to avoid alcohol, sleep-inducing OTC drugs.
- Advice not to do heavy work and avoid driving.

MAGNESIUM SULFATE

Trade name: Epsom salt and Sulfamag

Generic name: Magnesium sulfate

Classifications: Anticonvulsant, calcium channel blocker, anesthetic agent, tocolytic agent, antiarrhythmic, and analgesic.

Dosage: Oral: Adults and children 12 years of age—2–6 teaspoons per day as a single dose or in 2 divided doses.

- Parenteral:
  - 40 mg/mL
  - 80 mg/mL
- Infusion solution:
  - 1 g/100 mL
  - 2 g/100 mL

Mechanism of action: Magnesium sulfate prevents and controls seizures in patients with eclampsia by blocking neuromuscular transmission and decreasing the amount of acetylcholine liberated at the end plate by the motor nerve impulse.

Indications:
- Constipation
- Prevention of seizures in eclampsia/preeclampsia
- Hypomagnesemia
- Acute nephritis
- Cardiac arrhythmias

- Acute asthma exacerbation
- Tocolytic to prevent preterm labor

Contraindications:
- Hypersensitivity
- Hypermagnesemia
- Hypercalcemia
- Myocardial damage
- Diabetic coma
- Heart block

Side effects:
- Circulatory collapse
- Respiratory paralysis
- Hypothermia
- Pulmonary edema
- Hypotension
- Flushing
- Drowsiness
- Increased sweating
- Visual changes
- Confusion
- Weakness

Toxicity: Magnesium sulfate toxicity usually develops after the serum concentration level exceeds 1.74–2.61 mmol/L. Signs and symptoms include hypotension, retention of urine, ileus depression, difficulty in breathing, and irregular heartbeat.

Drug interaction: Serious interactions of magnesium sulfate include demeclocycline, doxycycline, eltrombopag, lymecycline, and minocycline.

Nurses responsibility:
- Monitor the patient's blood pressure and cardiac rhythm.
- Assess the patient for skeletal muscle weakness and hypotonia.
- Monitor magnesium concentration every four hours in patients with renal dysfunction.
- Monitor strict intake and output chart.

IRON SUPPLEMENT

Generic name: Ferrous Sulfate, Ferrous Gluconate, and Dextran

Trade name: Slow FE, Fer-In-Sol, Feratab, iron, Mol-Iron, Feosol, and MyKidz Iron

Route: Oral and IV

Dosage (Table 6):

TABLE 6: Dosage.

For children:	
0–6 months	0.27 mg
7–12 months	11 mg
1–3 years	7 mg
4–8 years	10 mg
9–13 years	8 mg
For females:	
14–18 years	15 mg
19–50 years	18 mg
50+ years	8 mg
For males:	
14–18 years	11 mg
19–50 years	8 mg
50+ years	8 mg
During pregnancy:	
14–18 years	27 mg
19–50 years	27 mg
During lactation:	
14–18 years	10 mg
19–50 years	9 mg

Available forms: Capsules, Tablets, Oral solutions, and IV Injections.

Natural iron supplements:

- Heme iron is found in red meat, poultry, and seafood.
- Nonheme iron is found in nuts, beans, vegetables, and whole grains.

Mechanism of action: Iron supplements allow for more rapid increases in iron levels when dietary supply and stores are insufficient. The iron in circulation is immediately bound to the available protein to form hemosiderin or ferritin, the physiological form of iron, or to a lesser extent to transferrin. This iron which is subjected to physiological control replenishes hemoglobin and depleted iron stores.

Indications:

- Iron deficiency anemia
- Prophylaxis of iron deficiency in low birth weight and breast-fed babies.
- Prophylaxis in pregnancy, menstruation, and blood donors
- Nutritional deficiency
- Menorrhagia

- Peptic ulcer
- Hookworm infestation

Contraindications:

- Known hypersensitivity
- Hemochromatosis
- Hemosiderosis
- Anemia not caused by iron deficiency
- Parenteral iron is contraindicated in untreated pyelonephritis and acute liver disease.

Side effects/adverse effects:

- Nausea
- Epigastric pain
- Diarrhea/constipation
- Black stools
- Dizziness
- Flushing
- Stained teeth
- Headache
- Discoloration at injection site
- Hypersensitivity reactions (dyspnea, urticaria, rashes, itching, arthralgia, myalgia, fever, and sweating)
- Chest pain or tightness
- Hyper or hypotension
- Lymphadenopathy
- Leukocytosis
- Latent folic acid deficiency
- Thrombocytopenia

Drug interaction:

- Antacids, milk, tetracycline, and zinc: Absorption of oral iron is decreased.
- Ciprofloxacin, levofloxacin, norfloxacin, ofloxacin, tetracycline, and levodopa: Absorption is decreased by oral iron.

Nurses responsibilities:

- Advise the patient to take iron supplements an hour before meals for maximum absorption.
- Monitor hemoglobin and reticulocyte values during therapy.
- Monitor bowel movements as constipation is a common adverse effect.
- Advice the patient to consume citrus fruits with iron preparation as it increases absorption of iron.

FOLIC ACID

Generic name: Folic acid

Trade name: Folvite, FaLessa, Folacin-800, and FA-8

Route: Oral, subcutaneous, IV, and deep IM

Dosage (Table 7):

TABLE 7: Dosage.	
1–3 years	300 µg/day
4–8 years	400 µg/day
9–13 years	600 µg/day
14–13 years	800 µg/day
19 years and above	1,000 µg/day
Pregnancy	600–800 µg/day

Available forms: Tablets and injections

Natural supplements:

- Green leafy vegetables
- Beans
- Peanuts
- Sunflower seed
- Fresh fruits and fruit juices
- Liver and egg

Mechanism of action: An exogenous source of folate is required for nucleoprotein synthesis and the maintenance of normal erythropoiesis. Folic acid, whether given by orally or parenterally, stimulates the production of RBC, WBC, and platelets in persons suffering from certain megaloblastic anemias.

Indications:

- Folate deficiency
- Hemolytic anemia
- Juvenile idiopathic arthritis
- Methotrexate-induced nausea
- Megaloblastic anemia
- Methanol deficiency
- Pregnancy

Contraindication:

- Known allergic reaction to folic acid
- Pernicious anemia
- Hemodialysis
- Patients having cardiac stent
- Cancer

Side effects/adverse effects:

- Erythema
- Skin rashes, itching, and malaise
- Respiratory difficulty due to bronchospasm

- GI side effects (anorexia, nausea, abdominal distention, flatulence, and a bitter or bad taste)
- Difficulty in concentrating, irritability
- Overactivity, excitement
- Mental depression, confusion, impaired judgement
- Seizure

Drug interaction:
- Taking folic acid with phenytoin (cerebyx), phenytoin (dilantin and phenytek), or primidone (mysoline) decreases drug's concentration in the blood.
- Taking folic acid with barbiturate (CNS depressants) decreases drug's effectiveness.

Nurses responsibility:
- Monitor patient for hypersensitivity reactions, especially if drug previously taken.
- Give IM/IV/subcutaneously if severe GI malabsorption is present.
- Monitor vitamin B_{12} levels to rule out pernicious anemia.
- Report rashes, difficulty breathing, pain, or discomfort at injection site.

CALCIUM SUPPLEMENTS

Generic name: Calcium

Trade name: Caltrate, 600+ D3, Os-Cal Calcium +D3, Os-Cal Extra D3, Os-Cal Ultra, and Citracal

Route: Oral

Dosage (Table 8):

TABLE 8: Dosage.

0–6 months	200 mg/day
7–12 months	260 mg/day
1–3 years	700 mg/day
4–8 years	1,000 mg/day
9–18 years	1,300 mg/day
19–50 years	1,000 mg/day
51–70 years	1,200 mg/day
Pregnancy	1,200 mg/day

Available forms: Oral tablets

Natural supplements:
- Seeds
- Cheese
- Yogurt
- Sardines and Canned Salmons
- Beans and lentils

- Almonds
- Green leafy vegetables
- Fortified foods and drinks
- Milk

Mechanism of action: Calcium is a mineral essential for cardiac functioning, muscle contraction, coagulation of blood, and for maintaining structural integrity of cell membranes. Calcium supplements increases calcium stores within the body.

Indications:

- Hypocalcemia
- Osteoporosis and osteomalacia
- Hyperphosphatemia in renal failure
- Hyperparathyroidism
- Premenstrual syndrome
- Preeclampsia

Contraindications:

- Hypersensitivity
- Hypophosphatemia
- Hypothyroidism
- Hypercalcemia
- Renal calculi
- Breast cancer
- Fracture
- Obesity
- Stroke

Side effects/adverse effects:

- Constipation
- Stomach upset
- Hives
- Difficulty breathing
- Swelling of the face, lips, tongue, or throat
- Nausea, vomiting, and anorexia
- Mental and mood changes
- Bone or muscle pain
- Headache
- Increased thirst or urination
- Weakness and unusual tiredness
- Rashes and itching

Drug interaction:

- Administering intravenous ceftriaxone and calcium together can result in life-threatening damage to the lungs and kidneys. Calcium should not be administered intravenously within 48 hours of intravenous ceftriaxone.

- Taking calcium along with Dolutegravir can reduce blood levels of Dolutegravir and decreases its effects. To avoid this interaction, Dolutegravir should be taken 2 hours before or 6 hours after taking calcium.
- Taking calcium along with Elvitegravir can reduce blood levels of Elvitegravir, decreases its effects. To avoid this interaction, it should be taken 2 hours before or 2 hours after taking calcium.

Nurses responsibility:
- Closely monitor blood calcium levels and albumin levels.
- Monitor patient for signs of decreased gastric and intestinal motility.
- Monitor urine output in excess of intake
- Advise patient to take calcium supplements as prescribed by physician and not to take additional doses.
- Advise the patient to eat high fiber diet and take laxatives as necessary for constipation.

TOCOLYTICS

NICARDIPINE

Trade name: Cardene IV and Cardene SR

Dose: Capsule 20 mg and 30 mg, injection form 2.4 mg/mL

Route: Intravenous and oral

Mechanism of action: Inhibition of calcium influx across the membrane, thereby smoothing the muscular vasculature.

Indications:
- Chronic stable angina
- Hypertension
- Antepartum hypertension

Contraindications:
- Sick sinus syndrome
- Hypersensitivity
- Advanced aortic stenosis
- Second and third degree heart block

Adverse effects:
- Hepatitis
- Stevens-Johnson syndrome
- Pulmonary edema
- Dizziness
- Flushing
- Arrhythmias

Drug interactions:

Increases:
- Effect of dioxin theophylline, nitrates, and alcohol

- Nicardipine effects
- Toxicity of prazosin, carbamazepine

Decreases:
- Antihypertensive effect of NSAIDs and rifampin
- Potassium, phosphate, and platelet levels

Nurses responsibilities:
- Monitor cardiac status
- Assess for angina pain
- Monitor hepatic and renal studies in long-term use
- Assess signs of Stevens-Johnson syndrome
- Ensure diet modification—assess salt in diet

NIFEDIPINE

Trade name: Adalat CC, Afeditab, Procardia, and Nifedical XL

Dose:
- Capsules 10 and 20 mg
- Tablet 30, 60, and 90 mg
- Immediate dose of 30 mg then 10–20 mg every 4–7 hours in preterm labor

Route: Oral route and intravenous

Mechanism of action: Calcium channel blocker which prevents the influx of calcium by blocking voltage-dependent L-type calcium channel in smooth muscle and myocardial cells.

Indication:
- Chronic stable angina
- Variant angina
- Hypertension
- Migraine prophylaxis
- Preterm labor
- Diabetic neuropathy
- Proteinuria
- Hiccups

Contraindications: Hypersensitivity to produce cardiogenic shock

Adverse effects:
- Nocturia
- Polyuria
- Exfoliate dermatitis
- Toxic epidermal necrosis

Drug interactions:

Increases:
- Level of digoxin
- Effect of beta blocker

- Antihypertensive
- Carbamazepine

Nurses responsibilities:
- Assess angina pain
- Monitor peripheral edema
- Assess potassium renal hepatic studies
- Assess for bruised sites

VERAPAMIL

Trade name: Apo-verap, Cala SR, Covera Hs, and Isoprin SR

Dose and route:
- Tablet 40, 80, 120 mg, oral
- Injection 2.4 mg/mL, IV

Mechanism of action: Inhibits the calcium ion (and possibly sodium ion) influx through slow channels into conductile and contractile myocardial cells and vascular smooth muscle cells.

Indications:
- Angina
- Dysrhythmia
- Uterine relaxation

Contraindications:
- Sick-sinus syndrome
- Cardiogenic shock
- Wolf-Parkinson-White syndrome

Side effects:
- Dizziness
- Edema
- Nausea
- Heart failure

Drug interactions:

Increases:
- Level of cyclosporine
- Carbamazepine
- Hypotension effects

Decreases:
- Effect of lithium
- NSAIDs

Nurses responsibilities:
- Monitor cardiac status
- Monitor intake output ratio
- Assess for dyspnea

- Monitor renal and hepatic studies
- Monitor for rash with fever joint pain lesions, etc.

MAGNESIUM SULFATE

Trade name: Magnesium Sulfate

Dose and route:

- Tablet 335 and 500 mg, oral
- Infusion 500 mg/mL, IV

Mechanism of action: Magnesium sulfate reduces striated muscle contractions and blocks peripheral neuromuscular transmission by reducing acetylcholine release at the myoneural junction. Additionally, magnesium inhibits Ca^{2+} influx through dihydropyridine-sensitive, voltage-dependent channels. This accounts for much of its relaxant action on vascular smooth muscle.

Indication:

- Nutritional supplements
- Premature labor
- Digoxin toxicity
- Dyspepsia
- Hypertension in newborn

Contraindications:

- Abdominal pain
- Rectal bleeding
- Heart block
- Hypersensitivity

Adverse effect:

- Flaccid paralysis
- Circulatory collapse

Drug interactions:

Increases: Hypotension and neuromuscular block

Decreases: Absorption of tetracycline

Nurses responsibilities:

- Assess lack of fluids
- Monitor BP
- Monitor intake output
- Look for magnesium toxicity

INDOMETHACIN

Generic name: Indomethacin

Trade name: Indocin and Tivorbex

Available forms: Capsule 25 and 50 mg; Ext Rel caps 75 mg; injection 1 mg vial, suppository 50 mg; oral suspension 5 mg/mL.

Dosage and route:

- **Arthritis/Anti-inflammatory:** PO 25–50 mg bid–tid; maximum 200 mg/day may increase to 75 mg bid.
- **Acute gouty arthritis:** PO 50 mg tid, use only for acute attacks then reduce dose.

Mechanism of action: Reduces synthesis of PGs, thereby reducing intracellular free Ca^{++}, activation of MLCK, and uterine contractions (PGs cause increase in free intracellular Ca^{++} and activation of MLCK).

Pharmacokinetics: Indomethacin is well absorbed and attains peak plasma concentrations at 2 hours. Bioavailability is approximately 100%. The high lipid solubility allows indomethacin to cross the blood brain barrier easily. Approximately 60% of the administered drug is excreted in urine, while the remainder is excreted in feces. The elimination half-life of this drug is approximately 7 hours.

Indications: Rheumatoid arthritis, osteoarthritis, gouty arthritis, ankyloses spondylitis, PDA, Bone pain, headache, heterotrophic ossification, JRA, and pericarditis.

Contraindications: Hepatic disease, active peptic ulcer, and coagulation disorder.

Adverse effects:

- **Maternal:** Heartburn, asthma, GI bleeding, thrombocytopenia, renal injury, and platelet dysfunction.
- **Neonatal**: Constriction of the ductus arteriosus (due to inhibition of synthesis of PGI_2 and PGE_2), oligohydramnios, neonatal pulmonary hypertension, and IUGR.

Drug interaction:

1. **Increases:**
   - Hyperkalemia—potassium sparing diuretics
   - Bleeding risk—anticoagulants, antiplatelet, thrombolytic, salicylates, and alcohol
   - Effect of digoxin and phenytoin
   - Toxicity—lithium, oral anticoagulants, MTX, and cyclosporine
2. **Decreases**: Effect of antihypertensive

Nurses responsibilities:

- Assess pain, stiffness, ROM, and swelling of joints during treatment
- Perioperative pain relief in CABG—MI and stroke can result for 10–14 days can be fatal
- Monitor renal, hepatic, blood studies—BUN, creatinine, AST, ALT, and HB, periodically.
- In case of PDA closure—monitor for respiratory rate, character, and heart sounds
- Avoid chronic use in older adults
- Blurred vision, tinnitus, and hearing loss may indicate toxicity. Audiometric and ocular monitoring should be done
- Confusion, mood changes especially in geriatric patients
- Asthma, nasal polyps, and hypersensitivity may develop

SULINDAC

Generic name: Sulindac

Trade name: Clinoril

Route and dosage: Oral, 150 mg twice daily. Not to exceed 400 mg/daily.

Mechanism of action: Reduces synthesis of PGs, thereby reduces intracellular free Ca^{++}, activation of MLCK, and uterine contractions (PGs cause increase in free intracellular Ca^{++} and activation of MLCK).

Pharmacokinetics: Approximately 90% absorbed following oral administration. Plasma concentration peaks within 2 hours in fasting state metabolized in liver. Approximately 50% excavated in urine and about 25% excreted in feces.

Indications:
- Osteoarthritis, rheumatoid arthritis, and ankylosing spondylitis
- Acute painful shoulder and acute gouty arthritis.

Contraindications: Hypersensitivity to sulindac and aspirin

Adverse effects:
- **GI**: Abdominal pain, dyspepsia, nausea, vomiting, constipation, diarrhea, flatulence, and anorexia; stomatitis, sore or dry mucous membranes, dry mouth; rarely gastritis, gastroenteritis, peptic ulcer, and GI bleeding.
- **CNS**: Drowsiness, dizziness, headache, anxiety, and nervousness.
- **Cardiovascular**: Palpitations, peripheral edema, and congestive heart failure (patient with marginal cardiac function).
- **EENT**: Blurred vision, amblyopia, vertigo, tinnitus, and decreased hearing.
- **Hypersensitivity** (rare): Angioneurotic edema, rash, pruritus, fever, chills, leukopenia, eosinophilia, and anaphylaxis.
- **Other**: Stevens-Johnson toxic epidermal necrolysis syndrome. Causal relationship unknown: Hypertension, epistaxis, paresthesia, vaginal bleeding, and hematuria.

Drug interactions (Table 9)

TABLE 9: Drug interactions.

Plus	*Possible Interactions*
Anticoagulants (coumarins)	Prolongation of prothrombin time
Aspirin and phenobarbital	Decreased effect of sulindac by hepatic enzyme induction
Probenecid	Increased plasma levels of sulindac

Nurses responsibilities:
- May be administered with food, milk, or antacid (if prescribed) to reduce possibility of GI upset.
- Important to take a detailed drug history before initiation of therapy. See contraindication and precautions.
- Because sulindac may cause dizziness, drowsiness, and blurred vision, advise patient to exercise caution when driving or performing other potentially hazardous activities.

- Baseline and periodic evaluation of hemoglobin, renal and hepatic functions, and auditory and ophthalmic examinations are recommended in patients receiving prolonged or high-dose therapy.
- Advise patient to report the onset of skin rash, itching, hives, jaundice, black stools, swelling of feet or hands, sore throat or mouth, unusual bleeding or bruising, and shortness of breath or night cough.
- Since eye changes have been observed with other nonsteroidal anti-inflammatory drugs, their occurrence is possible with sulindac. An ophthalmoscopic examination is recommended if patient has eye complaints.
- Therapeutic effectiveness of sulindac may be evidenced within a few days to about 3 weeks by relief of joint pain and stiffness, reduction in joint swelling, increase in grip strength, and improved mobility.
- Inform patients that alcohol and aspirin may increase the risk of GI ulceration and bleeding tendencies and therefore should be avoided while taking sulindac.
- Because sulindac may prolong bleeding time, advise patient to inform dentist or surgeon that he is taking this drug.

TERBUTALINE

Generic name: Terbutaline sulfate

Trade name: Brethine and Bricanyl

Route and dosage:
- **Oral: Adult:** 2.5–5 mg daily at 6-hour intervals; **Children** 12–15 years of age: 2.5 mg 3 times daily at 6-hour intervals.
- **Subcutaneous:** Adults: 0.25 mg.

Mechanism of action: Synthetic adrenergic stimulant with selective beta$_2$ and negligible beta$_1$ agonist (cardiac activity). Exerts preferential effect on beta$_2$ receptors in bronchial smooth muscles. Relaxes smooth muscle or vascular supply to skeletal muscles, and uterus (thereby preventing or abolishing high intrauterine pressure).

Pharmacokinetics: Bioavailability is less with oral than subcutaneous dose. Elimination half-life: 3–4 hours; protein binding: 25%. Metabolized in liver and excreted in urine (small amount in feces).

Indications:
- Bronchial asthma and for reversible airway obstruction associated with bronchitis and emphysema
- To delay delivery in premature labor.

Contraindications:
- Known hypersensitivity to sympathomimetic amines
- Severe hypertension and coronary artery disease
- Tachycardia with digitalis intoxication
- Children under 12 years of age
- Angle closure glaucoma.

- Angina, stroke, and hypertension
- Diabetes mellitus
- Thyrotoxicosis
- History of seizure disorder
- Cardiac arrhythmias
- Elderly patient
- Renal and hepatic dysfunction.

Adverse effects:

- Nervousness, tremor, and headache
- Increase in heart rate, palpitation
- Possible decrease in diastolic and increase in systolic blood pressure
- Light-headedness
- Drowsiness and fatigue
- Nausea, vomiting, and sweating
- Muscle cramps
- Maternal and fetal tachycardia
- Tinnitus (rare)

Drug interactions (Table 10):

TABLE 10: Drug interactions.

Plus	*Possible interaction*
MAO inhibitors	Concurrent use may cause severe hypertensive crisis
Propranolol	Antagonizes bronchodilation effect of terbutaline
Sympathomimetics	May increase effects and potential side effects of sympathomimetics and/or terbutaline

Nurses responsibilities:

- Be certain about recommended doses oral preparation: 2.5 mg, subcutaneous: 0.25 mg.
- If GI symptoms occur advise patient to take the tablets with food.
- Check pulse and blood pressure before each dose. If perceptively altered from baseline level, consult physician.
- Teach the ambulatory patient on oral terbutaline how to take his own pulse and the limits of change that indicate need to notify the physician.
- Terbutaline appears to have a short clinical period of sustained effectiveness. Advise patient to keep appointments with physician for evaluation of continued drug effectiveness and clinical condition.
- Instruct patient to consult the physician if breathing difficulty is not relieved or it becomes worse within 15 minutes after an oral dose of terbutaline.
- Instruct patient to adhere to established regimen, i.e., he should not change dose intervals or omit. Increase or decrease the dose.
- Warn the patient not to use OTC drugs unless the physician approves.
- Store medication at temperature between 59° and 86° F. Protect from light and freezing.

RITODRINE

Generic name: Ritodrine hydrochloride

Trade name: Yutopar

Route and dosage:

- **Intravenous**: 0.1 mg/min administered by means of calibrated constant rate infusion pump.
- **Oral:** 10 mg every 2 hours for first 24 hours; thereafter, 10–20 mg every 4–6 hours.

Mechanism of action: Activation of the intracellular enzymes (adenylate cyclase, cAMP, and protein kinase), reduces intracellular free calcium (Ca^{++} ↓↓) and inhibits activation of MLCK (↓↓) → Reduced interaction of actin and myosin → smooth muscle relaxation. β (β_2) receptor stimulation causes smooth muscle relaxation.

Pharmacokinetics: Following oral administration, 30% of drug is absorbed; metabolized in liver, 90% excretion is completed in 24 hours. It crosses placenta.

Indications:

- Preventing and delaying of preterm labor
- Used to manage premature labor in selected patients.

Contraindications:

- Mild-to-moderate eclampsia and hypertension
- Diabetes mellitus
- Antepartum hemorrhage
- Intrauterine fetal death
- Maternal cardiac disease, pulmonary hypertension
- Maternal hyperthyroidism
- Cardiac arrhythmia associated with tachycardia or digitalis intoxication
- Bronchial asthma being treated with beta mimetics and/or steroids.

Adverse effects:

- Altered maternal and fetal heart rates and maternal blood pressure
- Temporary hyperglycemia
- Palpitations, arrhythmia, and tremor
- Nausea, vomiting, and headache
- Erythema
- Nervousness, restlessness, and anxiety
- Malaise, chest pain
- Pulmonary edema

Infrequent effects:

- Anaphylactic shock
- Rash
- Epigastric distress, ileus, and blotting
- Constipation/diarrhea
- Dyspnea and hyperventilation
- Glycosuria

- Hemolytic icterus
- Sweating, chills, drowsiness, and weakness.

Drug interactions (Table 11)

TABLE 11: Drug interactions.

Plus	*Possible Interaction*
Anesthetics	Potentiated hypotensive effects of general anesthetic
Corticosteroids	Pulmonary edema, action is antagonized by beta-adrenergic blocking agents like propranolol and is potentiated by other sympathomimetics

Nurses considerations:

- Hospitalization is advised during treatment with ritodrine.
- Preparation of IV solution: 150 mg ritodrine is added to 500 mL 5% dextrose or normal saline solution giving a final concentration of 0.3 mg/mL.
- IV solution should be clear and should not be administered if cloudy or if a precipitate is present.
- Place patient in left lateral recombinant position throughout the infusion period to reduce risk of hypertension.
- Monitor IV infusion flow rate to prevent circulation overload.
- Pronounced dose-related side effect in cardiovascular system require continuous monitoring of maternal and fetal heart rates and maternal blood pressure while infusion is running.
- If patient is also on steroid therapy, hospitalization for treatment with ritodrine is advised. Be alert to signs and symptoms of pulmonary edema.
- Store drug at controlled room temperature preferably <80°F. Do not freeze.

GLYCERYL TRINITRATE

Generic name: Glyceryl trinitrate

Brand name: Ganitro, Minitran, and Trinipatch

Dose and route: Aerosol (translingual)—0.4 mg/metered spray

Induction: 5 mg/mL, 100 µg/mL, 200 µg/mL, 400 µg/mL

Ointment: 0.4%, 2%

Powder: 400 µg

Tablets: 0.3 mg, 0.4 mg, and 0.6 mg

Transdermal patch: 0.1 mg/h, 0.2 mg/h, 0.3 mg/h, 0.4 mg/h, 0.6 mg/h, and 0.8 mg/h release rate

Mechanism of action: Reduces cardiac oxygen demand by decreasing left ventricular end diastolic pressure (preload) and, to a lesser extent systemic vascular resistance in (after load). Also increases blood flow through the collateral coronary vessels.

Indications:

- To prevent chronic anginal attacks
- Acute angina pectoris

- Hypertension from surgery
- Heart failure after MI

Contraindications:
- Hypersensitivity to drug and nitrates
- Early MI
- Severe anemia
- Increased ICP
- Angle closure glaucoma
- Orthostatic hypotension
- Allergy to adhesives
- Cardiac tamponade
- Restrictive cardiomyopathy
- Constructive pericarditis

Side effects/adverse effects:
- CNS: Headache, dizziness, syncope, and weakness
- CVS: Orthostatic hypotension, bradycardia, flushing, palpitations, and peripheral edema
- ENT: Rhinitis
- GI: Nausea, vomiting, and abdominal pain
- Respiratory: Dyspnea
- Skin: Contact dermatitis and rash
- Other: Hypersensitivity reactions

Drug interactions:
- Alteplase drug may decrease tissue plasminogen activator antigen level.
- Antihypertensive may increase hypotensive effect.
- Heparin: IV nitroglycerin may interfere with anticoagulant effect of heparin
- Nitric oxide may increase risk of methemoglobinemia.

Nurses responsibilities:
- Closely monitor vital signs particularly BP during infusion, especially in patients with MI because excessive hypotension can worsen ischemia
- Monitor BP and intensity and duration of drug response
- Treat headache with aspirin or acetaminophen
- Tolerance to drug can be minimized with a 10–12 hours nitrite free interval
- Check and wipe off nitroglycerine paste or remove patch before defibrillation to avoid patient from burns

Patient teaching:
- Caution patient to take nitroglycerin regularly as prescribed and to have it accessible at all times.
- Advice patient that stopping drug abruptly may cause coronary artery spasm.
- Tell patient to take SL tablet at first sign of attack, patient should wet tablet with saliva and place it under the tongue until absorbed and then sit down and rest, patient may repeat dose every 5 minutes for a maximum of three doses. If drug does not provide relief, patients should obtain medical health promptly.

- Advice patient who complaints of a tingling sensation with some liquid drug to try holding tablet in the cheek.
- Tell patient not to use more than three packets of sublingual powder in a 15 minute. And to obtain medical health promptly if drug does not provide relief advice patient not to swallow or spit for 5 minutes after taking each packet.
- Tell patient to take oral tablets on an empty stomach either 30 minutes before or one to 2 hours after meals.
- If patient is using skin patches, advice to avoid alcohol.
- To minimize dizziness when standing up, advice patient to rise slowly, to go up and downstairs carefully, and to lie down at the first sign of dizziness.
- Tell patient to store drug in cool dark place in a tightly closed container and to remove cotton from container, because it absorbs drug.

ISOXSUPRINE

Generic name: Isoxsuprine

Brand name: Clinoril

Dose and route:

- Oral: 10–20 mg, four times daily.
- Intramuscular: 5–10 mg, 2 or 3 times a day. Single IM dose, exceeding 10 mg not recommended

Mechanism of action: Acts directly on vascular smooth muscles and causes stimulation and uterine relaxation, relaxing the arteries and veins and making them wider to increase blood flow to certain parts of the body.

Indications:

- Prevent preterm labor
- Inhibit uterine contractions

Contraindications:

- Hypersensitivity
- Postpartum

Side effects:

- Nausea
- Tachycardia
- Hypotension
- Flushing
- Chest pain
- Itching or swelling
- Palpitations
- Abdominal distress
- Maternal pulmonary edema
- Fetal tachycardia
- Nervousness
- Trembling

Drug interactions:
- The risk or severity of adverse effects can be increased when Abaloparatide is combined with Isoxsuprine.
- The therapeutic efficacy of Isoxsuprine can be decreased when used in combination with Acebutolol.
- The risk or severity of hypertension can be increased when Aceclofenac, Acetylsalicylic and Acemetacin are combined with Isoxsuprine.
- The risk or severity of tachycardia can be increased when Aclidinium is combined with Isoxsuprine. The risk or severity of tachycardia can be increased when Adenosine is combined with Isoxsuprine.

Nurses responsibilities:
- Advise patient to report adverse reactions like rashes, palpitations, and flushing occur.
- Assess patient blood pressure in lying and standing as orthostatic hypotension is common.
- Observe both mother and child for irregular and rapid heartbeat if Isoxsuprine is used to delay premature labor.
- Monitor for intensity and length of uterine contractions and fetal heart sound (FHS).
- Advice patient to make position changes slowly particularly from lying down to sitting upright and avoid standing still as fainting may occur.
- Assess other medications patient may be taking to avoid possible interactions and effectiveness.
- Monitor therapeutic effectiveness and adverse reactions at beginning of treatment and periodically throughout treatment.
- Evaluate clinical manifestations of arterial insufficiency.
- Advice the patient not to breastfeed while taking this drug without consultation of physician.

ATOSIBAN

Generic name: Atosiban

Brand name: Tractocil

Dose and route: Initial IV bolus of 6.75 mg, followed by 300 mg/min infusion * 3 hours. Then 100 mg/min for up to 45 hours.

Mechanism of action: It is an oxytocin receptor antagonist. It inhibits the oxytocin-mediated release of Inositol Trisphosphate from the myometrial cell membrane.

Indications: In delaying imminent preterm birth in pregnant adult women with:
- Regular uterine contractions of at least 30 seconds duration at a rate of at least 4 per 30 minutes
- A cervical dilation of 1–3 cm (0–3 cm for nulliparous) and effacement of at least 50%
- A gestational age of 24–33 weeks
- A normal fetal heart rate

Contraindications:
- Gestational age below 24 or over 33 completed weeks
- Premature rupture of the membranes >30 weeks of gestation

- Abnormal fetal heart rate
- Antepartum uterine hemorrhage requiring immediate delivery
- Eclampsia and severe pre-eclampsia requiring delivery
- Intrauterine fetal death
- Suspected intrauterine infection
- Any other conditions of the mother or fetus, in which continuation of pregnancy is hazardous
- Hypersensitivity to the active substance

Side effects or adverse effects:

- Injection site reaction
- Headache
- Nausea and vomiting
- Increased glucose level in blood
- Decreased blood pressure
- Dizziness
- Hot flashes
- Slow heart rate

Drug interactions: Increased risk of pulmonary edema with other tocolytic drugs (e.g., Ca channel blockers and betamimetics).

Nurses responsibilities:

- Client education: Purpose of medication is being administered, side effects to report.
- Assessment and monitoring: Vital signs, SpO_2, weight, heart and lung sounds, uterine activity, cervical dilation and effacement, FHR, and variability.
- Notify obstetrician/midwife: Indeterminate or abnormal FHR
- Prepare for intrauterine resuscitation, as needed: IV fluid bolus, lateral positioning, and oxygen administration

ANTICOAGULANTS AND ANTI-IMMUNOGLOBULINS

ANTICOAGULANTS

Anticoagulants may be indicated during pregnancy for the treatment or prophylaxis of venous thromboembolism and in patients with mechanical prosthetic cardiac valves. Occasionally, anticoagulant is also indicated in pregnant women with congenital heart disease.

Heparin

It is a natural water-soluble mucopolysaccharide. Heparin should be started at the 6th week of gestation after confirmation of a viable pregnancy. Therapeutic anticoagulation is required in women with established DVT or pulmonary embolism.

Mechanism of action: Heparin inhibits the action of thrombin; it also enhances the activity of antithrombin III.

There are two types of heparin:
1. Low-molecular-weight heparin
2. Unfractionated heparin

Low-Molecular-Weight Heparin

Indication: Established DVT/pulmonary embolism

Drug of choice: Due to:
- Better bioavailability
- Lower risk of major bleeding
- Low risk of thrombocytopenia
- More reduction in thrombus size
  Commonly used LMWH are: Enoxaparin, Dalteparin, and Tinzaparin

Dosage:
- Enoxaparin: 1 mg/kg, 12 hourly, SC
- Dalteparin: 200 units/kg, once daily, SC
- Tinzaparin: 175 units/kg, once daily, SC

Unfractionated Heparin

Unfractionated is indicated for immediate treatment of pulmonary embolism or when anticoagulation is required, when immediate delivery or a cesarean section is anticipated. Initial administration is by IV route, monitored by PTT levels.

Indications:
- When delivery/C-section is anticipated
- After 36 weeks in all women were on therapeutic anticoagulation

Dosage (Table 12):
- 70–100 units/kg (5,000–100,000) IV bolus
- 15–20 units/kg (1,000) units/h infusion
- Followed by 7–10 days later by 10,000 units, 12th hourly, SC

TABLE 12: Dosage.

Type	*Dose and route*	*Indication*
Low-molecular-weight heparin: • Enoxaparin (Fragmin) • Dalteparin (Clexane) • Tinzaparin	 • 1 mg/kg, 12 hourly SC • 200 units/kg once daily SC • 175 units/kg once daily SC	• UFH, because it has several advantages • Established DVT/pulmonary embolism
Unfractionated heparin	• 70–100 units/kg (5,000–100,000) IV bolus • 15–20 units/kg (1,000) units/h infusion • Followed by 7–10 days then 10,000 units 12-hourly, SC	• For immediate treatment of pulmonary embolism or when anticoagulation is required • When immediate delivery or a cesarean section is anticipated, initial administration is by IV route monitored by PTT levels

Contraindication:
- Hypersensitivity
- Active bleeding
- Severe thrombocytopenia
- Uncontrolled hypertension

Side effects:

Maternal:
- Hemorrhage
- Urticarial
- With long-term use, thrombocytopenia and osteopenia
- Hyperkalemia

Fetal: It is not teratogenic.

Nurses responsibilities:
- Patient education: Therapeutic anticoagulation should be continued for 6 months postpartum.
- LMWH is to be started after vaginal delivery or 12 hours after a C-section along with warfarin 5 mg daily.
- Dosage of LMWH is to be gradually reduced and replaced by warfarin.
- Assess for the side effects.

Warfarin

Mechanism of action: Interferes with the synthesis of vitamin K-dependent factors (II, VII, IX, and X)

Dosage: 5–10 mg orally, daily for the initial 2 days, then 3–9 mg daily

Side effects:

Maternal: Hemorrhage

Fetal: Warfarin embryopathy (5%), nasal hypoplasia, bone stippling, optic atrophy, and mental retardation.

Nurses responsibilities:
- Do not use if the patient is pregnant.
- Monitor PT ratio or INR regularly to adjust dosage.
- Administer IV forms to patients stabilized on Coumadin.

ANTI-D IMMUNOGLOBULIN/RH (D) IMMUNE GLOBULIN

Trade name: Monoclonal

Generic name: Rhoclone

Dose and route:
- Before delivery: 1,500 IU (300 μg) at 28 weeks, IM
- After delivery: 600 IU (120 μg) within 72 hours of delivery, IM

Mechanism of action: Suppresses the immune response of nonsensitized Rh-negative patients who are exposed to Rh-positive blood

Indication: Rh-negative patients who have been exposed to Rh-positive blood by:
- Delivering an Rh-positive infant
- Miscarrying or aborting an Rh-positive fetus
- Having amniocentesis or intra-abdominal trauma while carrying a Rho-negative fetus
- Following accidental transfusion of Rh-positive blood to Rh-negative patients
- Women who are not already immune to rubella and varicella
- Not received tetanus/diphtheria

Contraindications:
- Previous immunization with Rh-positive
- D-negative female whose fetus is known to be D -ve
- Any D+ females

Side effects:
- CNS: Lethargy, dizziness, and headache
- CVS: Hyper-/hypotension
- Integumentary: Irritation at the injection site and fever
- Miscellaneous: Infection, ARDS, and anaphylaxis
- Musculoskeletal: Myalgia and arthralgia
- Hematologic: Anemia and intravascular hemolysis

Drug interactions: May decrease antibody response to some live virus vaccines (measles, mumps, and rubella)

Nurses responsibility:
- Assess vital signs periodically during therapy in patients receiving anti-D immunoglobulin.
- Monitor patient for signs and symptoms of adverse reactions.
- Type and cross-matching of mother and newborn cord blood must be performed to determine the need for medication.
- Use aseptic technique, observe for 20 minutes after administration.

REFERENCES

1. Skidmore-Roth L (Ed). Mosby's 2025 Nursing Drug Reference, 38th edition. London, England: Churchill Livingstone; 2025.
2. Vallerand AH, Sanoski CA (Eds). Davis's Drug Guide for Nurses, 19th edition. Philadelphia, PA: F.A. Davis Company; 2024.
3. Tripathi KD (Ed). Essentials of Medical Pharmacology, 8th edition. New Delhi, India: Jaypee Brothers Medical Publishers; 2024.
4. Sharma R, Dominic D (Eds). Jaypee's Nursing Drug Book 2022-2023, 2nd edition. New Delhi, India: Jaypee Brothers Medical Publishers; 2022.
5. Dutta DC, Konar H (Eds). DC Dutta's Textbook of Obstetrics: Including Perinatology and Contraception. New Delhi, India: Jaypee Brothers Medical Publishers; 2019.

Index

Page numbers followed by *b* refer to box, *f* refer to figure, *fc* refer to flowchart, and *t* refer to table.

A

Abdominal closure 602
Abdominal distention 807
Abdominal examination 65, 72, 192, 200
Abdominal pain 199
Abdominal palpation 18
Abnormal labor, management of 32
Abortion
  complete 231
  incomplete 796
  types of 231*f*
Abruptio placentae 370-372, 413
Accreta spectrum 119
Accurate pregnancy dating 176
Acetaminophen 38
Acetazolamide 785
Acquired thrombophilia 243
Active labor, stages of 13*t*
Active peptic ulcer 813
Acute fatty liver 334
  diagnosis of 335*t*
  differential diagnosis of 337*t*
Acute feto-fetal transfusion 539
Acute gouty arthritis 813
Acute hemolytic transfusion reaction 158
Acute kidney injury 356
  causes of 357*t*
Acute lung injury, transfusion-related 158
Addison's disease 787
Adrenal function 251
Adrenocorticotropic hormone 173
Advanced cardiac support 430
Advanced maternal age 438, 442*t*
  age stratification for 438*t*
  complications of 439
  pregnancies, management of 441
Advanced neuraxial methods 40
Aerosol 818
Affecting tubal ciliary function 199
Air embolism 432
Aldactone 787
Aldomet 788
Alert facial expression 175
Aliskiren 795
Allergic reactions 158
Allis tissue forceps 738, 738*f*
Alloimmune thrombocytopenia 342
Alloimmunization
  detection of 461
  prevention of 460
Allopurinol 795
Alopecia 203
Alpha-globin gene cluster 268
Alpha-thalassemia 269
Alprostadil 798, 799
Amenorrhea 199, 200, 207
Amiloride 785
Amnihook 768, 768*f*
Amniocentesis 221, 484
Amnionicity 528*f*
Amniotic fluid 374, 622
  abnormalities, clinical implications of 623
  assessment 395
  composition 623*t*
  embolism 65, 171, 419, 432, 622
  formation
    and function 627
    physiology of 622
  functions of 622
  leakage 428
  measurement 627
    methods of 627*t*
  regulation 622*t*
  volume 623*t*
Amniotic membrane 254
Amniotomy 23
  contraindication of 408
  indications of 408
  method of 408
  risks of 409
Anal sphincter, external 109
Analgesia techniques 37
Analgesics 226, 775
  types of 775
Anaphylactic shock 435
Anaphylaxis 171
Anatomical changes 249
Anchoring villi 253
Ancillary tests 392, 546
Anemia 312
  causes of 312*t*
  effects of 313
  grading of 312*t*
  management of 316
  Mukt Bharat dosing 515*t*
Anesthesia 148, 781
  types of 781
Anesthetic agent 802
Aneuploidy
  first trimester screening for 479
  second trimester ultrasound screening for 481
Aneurysm 149
Angiotensin receptor blockers 794
Angiotensin-converting enzyme 430
  inhibitors 794
Ankyloses spondylitis 813
Annular detachment 111
Anorectal mucosa 109
Anorexia 807
Antecedent pregnancy 215
Antenatal antiretroviral therapy 637
Antenatal care 183, 285, 307, 357, 364, 441, 442*t*
  inverted pyramid of 184
Antenatal counseling 320
Antenatal diagnosis 364
Antenatal examination 186
Antenatal management 75, 446, 530
Antenatal monitoring 292
Antenatal screening 637
Antenatal steroids 257
Antepartum fetal surveillance 177, 377
  limitations of 378
  techniques of 377, 381*t*
Antepartum hemorrhage 369
  causes 369, 372

incidence of 369
risk factors for 369
Antepartum period 316
Antianxiety agents 800
Antibiotic 137, 231, 336
prophylaxis 599
regimens 558*t*
Antibody 243
Anticardiolipin antibodies 243
Anticoagulants 352*t*, 814, 822
Anticoagulation 430
in pregnancy, role of 328
Anticonvulsants 731, 799, 802
Anti-D dose 460
Anti-D immunoglobulin 824
Anti-D prophylaxis guidelines 460*t*
Antidote 302
Antiepileptic drugs 304
pharmacokinetics of 306
Antifungals 777
Antihypertensive drugs 727, 788
Antihypertensive therapy 300
Antihypertensive treatment guidelines 356*t*
Anti-immunoglobulins 822
Antiphospholipid
antibodies, testing for 244
antibody syndrome 243
screen 630
syndrome 240
Anxiety 359
disorder 359
Aortic dissection 432
Aortic stenosis 328
grading of 328*t*
APLA syndrome 240
Aplastic anemia 312
Apresoline 789
Arabin pessary 162
Arm extraction, posterior 141
Arterial blood gases 434
Arterial embolization 96
Arthritis 813
Artificial intelligence 506, 508
applications 508*t*, 509*t*
technology 508, 509
Aseptic technique 116
Asherman's syndrome 244
Aspirin 814
prophylaxis 298
Assess consciousness 168
Assisted breech 79
delivery
steps for 79*t*
technique 79
Assisted reproductive technology 199, 638*t*
prophylaxis 641*t*
Asymmetric fetal growth restriction 395*t*
Asynclitism 19, 85*t*
complications of 87*t*
factors for 84*t*
management strategies for 86*t*
mechanism of 85, 85*f*
prevalence for 84*t*
Asynclitism, role of 85
Atonic postpartum hemorrhage 65
Atosiban 821
Autoimmune disorders 6, 8
Autologous blood transfusion 158
Axis traction devices 756*f*

B

Babcock forceps 770, 770*f*
Bacillus Calmette–Guerin 573
Bacterial contamination 434
Bacterial vaginosis 243
Bad taste 807
Bagel sign 202*f*
Balance electrolytes 428
Balloon devices 406
Basal bolus regimen 279
Basal plate 254
Battledore placenta 256
Bed allocation 644*t*
Benzodiazepines 800
Beta-blockers 325, 430
Beta-globin gene cluster 268
Beta-thalassemia 268
carriers 270
Bicornuate uterus 59
Biochemical 229
Bioengineered materials 105
Biophysical profile 378, 379*t*, 395
Bipolar disorder 359
Bishop's score 411, 412*t*
Bladder
after birth 55
anatomy 520*f*
care 110
injury
management of 524
prevention of 524
surgical anatomy of 519
Bleeding 229
excessive 106
heightens
persistent 190
recurrent 190
in first trimester, causes of 228
in late pregnancy 195
vasa previa 409
Bloating 203
Blob sign 202*f*
Blood
components 154, 155, 156*t*
storage conditions for 156*t*
indications 156*t*
products 335
sugar level 290
volume 355
Blood loss 593
buffer against 420
minimization techniques 365
Blood pressure 229, 296, 324
control essential 298
diastolic 167, 168, 355
Blood transfusion 25, 154, 159
complications of 158
indications of 316
role of 316
Blurred vision 800
Bone
marrow suppressants 795
pain 813
stippling 824
Bony pelvis 16
Bowel care 110
Bradycardia 389
Brandt–Andrews technique 25
Breast pump 741, 741*f*
Breastfeeding 40, 308, 361, 576
Breathing 169
Breech
delivery, management of 79
presentation 78, 413, 415
types of 78, 78*t*
Brethine 815
Bricanyl 815
Bromocriptine 566
Bupivacaine 778, 781

C

Cabergoline 566
Calcitonin gene-related peptide 11

Calcium 807
channel blocker 802
metabolism 251
supplements 807
Canadian diabetes association 276
Capillary electrophoresis 268
Capillary preprandial glucose 280
Captopril 794
Caput succedaneum 21, 21*f*
Carbamazepine 306
Carbetocin 26, 426, 592, 592*t*
hemorrhage prevention 591
Carbonic anhydrase inhibitors 785
Carboprost 26
Cardiac collapse 65
Cardiac disease 323
classification for 324*t*
Cardiac disorders, epidemiology of 324
Cardiac output 355
Cardiogenic shock 423, 428
produce 810
Cardiomyopathy 324, 326
Cardiotocography, normal 43*f*
Cardiovascular adaptations 420
Cardiovascular changes 248*t*, 421
Cardiovascular system 166, 167, 247
Central nervous system 166
Cephalhematoma 21, 21*f*
Cephalic version, external 75
Cephalopelvic disproportion 83
assessment of 88*t*
Cerebrovascular accidents 782
Ceritinib 784
Cervical
cerclage 162
dilatation 36
ectropion 195
encerclage 241, 245
functions 11
injuries 102
intraepithelial neoplasia 678
laceration 226
length 22, 412
malignancy 195
polyps 195
ripening 12, 12*t*, 44*fc*, 173, 400*f*
softening 11
status 23
Cervical cancer 675, 676, 678
diagnostic modalities for 676*t*
pregnancy 675
complications with 675*t*
Cervical incompetence 244
clinical features of 245
diagnosis of 245
management of 244
Cervical tear 106, 111
complications of 112*t*
exploration of 104*f*
Cervicograph 45
Cervidil insert 401*f*
Cervix 11, 245
against bladder neck 200
Cesarean delivery 342, 616
Cesarean hysterectomy 128, 500, 501
Cesarean myomectomy
complications of 503, 503*t*
contraindications for 502*t*
hemostatic techniques for 503*t*
indications for 501*t*
surgical techniques for 502
Cesarean scar ectopic pregnancy 206-208
Cesarean section 75, 76, 98, 99, 326, 414, 616, 619
classification of difficulties in 616*t*
difficult 620*t*
indications for 598
Cesarean technique 138
Change during pregnancy 355
Chemotherapy 220, 233
Chickenpox
diagnostic tools for 666*t*
epidemiology of 664*t*
fetal complications of 665*t*
management strategies for 667*t*
maternal complications of 665*t*
preventive measures for 667*t*
Chlamydia 243
Chlorothiazide 784
Chorioangioma 256
destruens 218*f*
Choriocarcinoma 210, 233
common origins of 217*f*
Chorion development 253
Chorionic plate 254
Chorionic villous
formation 253
sampling 221, 222, 484
advantages of 484
disadvantages of 484
indications for 484
Chorionicity 528*f*
determination 472
Chromosomal microarray 222
analysis 223
Chromosomal origin 212
Chronic ectopic pregnancy 200
management of 200
Chronic kidney disease 357
Circulatory disturbances 255
Citrate toxicity 158
Clinical spectrum according to genotype 269*t*
Clinoril 814, 820
Clostridium perfringens 434
Clozapine 801
Coagulation changes 350*t*
Coagulation disorder 424, 813
Coagulation profile 425
Coagulopathy 62, 65, 334, 424
Cocaine use 424
Cochrane review insights 51
Cognitive behavioral therapy 360
Coital injuries 103
Collagen 12
Colloids 154
Color coding 47
Combined oral contraceptives 208
Common psychiatric disorders 359
Common transfusion complications 159*t*
Comparative labor progression 48*f*
Complete blood count 268, 434
Complete hydatidiform mole 212*t*
Complete mole 212, 213, 233
Complications management 186
Compound cord presentation 145
Concerns during pregnancy 305
Condom catheter 594*f*
Congenital anomalies 274, 445
absence of 476*t*
Congenital heart disease 324
Congenital structural defects 185
Congenital tubal abnormalities 199
Connective tissue 12
Connexin-43 12
Consanguinity 240
Conservative surgical
management 521
options 521*t*

Contemporary labor progression 20*t*
Continuous electronic fetal monitoring, indications for 389, 389*t*, 544, 544*t*
Contraception 6, 213, 220, 228, 231, 233, 309, 684, 699
Contraceptive counseling 226
Contraceptive use 199
Contraction associated proteins 12
Contralateral tubal damage 204
Contralateral tube 199
Controversial indications 222
Conventional karyotype 222
Cord
  clamp, types of 767
  insertion
    abnormalities 149
    anomalies 256
  presentation 145
  prolapse 74, 75*f*, 409
    presentation 144*f*
  traction, controlled 25
Cordocentesis 221, 222, 470
Coronavirus disease-2019 vaccination 575
Corticosteroids 163, 372
Corticotropin-releasing hormone 173
Cortisol 173, 251
Counseling 270, 360
Cranioclast 762*f*
Crede maneuver 25
Cryoprecipitate 155
Crystalloids 154
Cultural stigma 361
Cusco's speculum 771, 771*f*
Cyanosis 783
Cystic hygroma 496
Cytokine storm 434
Cytotrophoblastic shell 253

D

Dakshata program 512, 513*t*
Dalteparin 352, 823
Das dilators 746*f*
Debriefing 111
Deep transverse arrest, management of 83*t*
Deep venous thrombosis 350
Deficiency anemia 312, 313
Definitive placenta 253
Degenerative lesions 255
Dehydration 33
Dehydroepiandrosterone 173
Deliberate clavicle fracture 141
Delivery 137, 294, 308, 336, 342*b*, 344
  alert estimated time of 47
  decision-making for 684
  full dilatation to 36
  management 341*t*
  mechanisms 25
  month 644
  planning 430, 634, 638
  protocol 290
  timing 292, 292*t*, 364, 430
    and mode of 531, 540, 631
  treated by 341
Demeclocycline 803
Demerits 115
Dengue 656
Denominator 74
Depot medroxyprogesterone acetate 701, 704
  injection 704*f*
  switching to 705, 705*t*
Depression 359
Destructive surgeries 76
Diabetes 8, 394, 413
  complications of uncontrolled 274*t*
  mellitus 4, 414
  pathophysiology of 272*f*
Diagnosis-to-delivery interval 148
Diazepam 800
Dichorionic twin 473, 473*t*, 531
Diet structure 276
Digestive system 166, 167
Digital partogram 51
Dilatation, arrest of 31, 33
Dilutional anemia 418
  state of 420
Dilutional coagulopathy 158
Dimorphic anemia 317
Dinoprost 798
Dinoprostone 798
  gel 400*f*
Diprivan 784
Direct oral anticoagulants 352
Disadvantages of obstetric high dependency units 647
Discontinue aspirin 230
Disposable cord clamp 767, 767*f*
Disseminated intravascular coagulation 434
Distributive shock 423, 433
Diuretics 430, 784
Dizziness 776, 781, 800, 811
Doppler ultrasound 769*f*
Dorzolamide 785
Double balloon device 407
Down syndrome 483
  soft markers for 491
Doxapram 784
Doxycycline 231, 803
Doyen's retractor 748, 748*f*
Drowsiness 776, 800, 801
Drug
  allergy 203
  class 361
  interaction 776, 777, 782, 805, 807, 808, 813, 814*t*, 816*t*, 818*t*
  toxicit 172
Ductus venosus color Doppler 381*f*
Dydrogesterone 230, 236
Dyspareunia 101
Dystocia 16

E

Early invasive disease 678
Early pregnancy 796
  complications 439
Eclampsia 170, 299, 419, 586
  prophylaxis 586
Eclamptic convulsion, complications of 300
Ectopic implantation 199
Ectopic pregnancy 194, 198, 198*f*, 202*f*
  causes 199
  Doppler of 203*f*
  laparoscopic image of 203*f*
  management of 194*t*, 196, 201*fc*
Edema 529*f*, 811
Edinburgh postnatal depression scale 359
Ehlers–Danlos syndromes 11
Elective repeat cesarean delivery, complications of 125, 126*t*
Electroconvulsive therapy 361
Electrolyte imbalance 158
Electronic fetal monitoring, continuous 388, 543

Elevated ammonia 334
Elevated liver enzymes 203, 297, 301
Elevated transaminases 334
Eltrombopag 803
Emergency cesarean section 604
Emergency contraception 710
  methods of 711
Emerging therapies 294, 299
Emphasize multimodal approach 654
Endocervical epithelium 12
Endocrine
  changes 251*t*
  dysfunction 553
  system 247, 250
Endometrial myomectomy 502
Endometriosis 199
Endothelial cell injury 298
Endothclial injury 350
Endotoxemia 434
End-to-end repair 109
Energy requirements 275*t*
Enhanced recovery after surgery 603, 650
  program principles 650*t*
Enoxaparin 352, 823
Entonox 38, 41, 775
Enzyme 309
Epidural analgesia 39, 41
  patient-controlled 40
Epidural analgesics 778
Epidural complications, management of 40*t*
Epidural failure 40
Epigenetics 294
Epilepsy 304, 307*t*
  causes of secondary 305*t*
  classification of 304
  management of 307
  primary 305
  secondary 305
Epinephrine 782, 784
Episiotomy 114
  complications of 117, 117*t*
  facilitates vaginal delivery 118
  midline 115*f*
  scissors 116, 759, 759*f*
  types 115*t*
Epithelioid trophoblastic tumor 210
Ergometrine 26, 795, 797
  maleate injection 797
Ergonovine directly stimulates 798
Ergot
  alkaloids 26
  derivatives 795
Escherichia coli 434
Estradiol 14
Estriol 14
Estrogen 251, 561
Ethacrynic acid 784
Eugenic grounds 224
Exaggerated sims position 148
Exome sequencing 222
External cephalic version, role of 81
External rotation 20

F

Fallopian tube 198
False knot 150
False negative tests, causes of 488
False-positive tests, causes of 488
Febrile nonhemolytic transfusion reaction 158
Fentanyl 38, 784
Fertility treatments 507
Fertilized ovum implants 198
Fetal abdomen 469
Fetal anemia
  detection of 461
  invasive tests for 471*t*
  management 461*t*
  monitoring 461
  noninvasive
    prediction of 470
    tests for 471*t*
Fetal assessment 45
  ancillary tests for 392*t*, 546*t*
Fetal blood sampling 495
  complications of 495
  indications of 495
  sites of 495
Fetal central nervous system 468
Fetal complications 342, 459, 530
Fetal death 74, 405
Fetal delivery 602
Fetal distress 175, 405
Fetal Doppler velocimetry 378
Fetal effects 306, 331, 585
Fetal factors 394
Fetal genetic defect 334
Fetal growth restriction 185, 297, 394, 413, 414, 475
  classifications 395
  early and late 476*t*
  management 478*t*
    and monitoring 395
  pathophysiology 394
Fetal head
  diameters 85*t*
  shape changes 21
Fetal health risks 445
Fetal heart rate
  baseline 389, 544
  deceleration 409
  monitoring
    limitations of 392, 546
    methods of 388, 543
    techniques for 389, 544
  tracings
    analysis of 389, 544
    classification of 390, 545
Fetal hepatic parenchymal calcification 487
Fetal hypoxia 405
Fetal impact 272
  mechanisms of 665
Fetal indications 410
Fetal infection 409
Fetal injury 409
Fetal intracranial hemorrhage, high risk of 344
Fetal loss rates 221
Fetal lung maturity 163
Fetal macrosomia 140
Fetal management 661, 666, 672
Fetal manifestations 659, 665, 671
Fetal monitoring 333, 335, 430, 542
Fetal morbidity, increased 176
Fetal movements 385
  maternal perception of 377
Fetal oxygen saturation monitoring 392
Fetal parameters 44
Fetal pole 235*f*
Fetal presentation
  and incidence 18*t*
  and position, diagnosis of 18
Fetal risks 305, 410, 472*t*
Fetal role 14
Fetal scalp blood sampling 392
Fetal skull 16
  landmarks 17*f*
Fetal therapy 493
Fetal thorax 469
Fetal tissue 212

Fetomaternal complications 185
Fetomaternal hemorrhage, risk factors for 458*t*
Fetomaternal monitoring 446
Fetopelvic relationships 17, 18*f*, 74
Fetoplacental circulation 254
Fetoscope 767, 767*f*
Fetoscopic complications 539
Fetus, constitutional small 475
Fever, high-grade 200
Fibrin deposition 255
Fibrinogen levels 421
Fibrinolysis 421
Fibroid 59, 213
First maneuver 18
First miscarriage 240
First trimester bleeding 190, 228, 234, 236, 236*t*
- causes of 190, 190*t*, 229*t*
- diagnostic criteria for 192*t*
- management of 230*t*
- progesterone preparations for 236*t*

First-trimester screening 183, 184, 479
- targets 185*t*

First-trimester, recurrent pregnancy loss in 236
Fistula 137
Flatulence 203, 807
Flexion 20
Fluid
- abnormalities 382
- depletion 428
- management 326
- resuscitation 154, 435

Fluothane 783
Flushing curette 747, 747*f*
Fluvoxamine 801
Folate 317*f*
- antagonist inhibiting 202
- deficiency 305

Foley's catheter 406, 407*f*
Folic acid 3, 6, 8, 805
Fondaparinux 352
Forceps 80
- apply 53
- birth 54
- delivery 53
- mnemonic for 757

Foreign body 103
Fortipin 792
Fourth maneuver 19
Fresh frozen plasma 155
Friedman labor progression 20*t*
Friedmann's labor curve 47*f*
Frusemide 784, 786
Full abdominal examination 53
Furosemide 325
Future births 55
Future maternal health 442
Future pregnancies, recurrence in 343

G

General anesthesia 783, 784
Genetics 294
- counseling 269
- disorders 7, 8
  - family history of 492
- insights 219
- marker 211
- predisposition 305
- sonogram 481
- testing 242

Genital tract injuries 98
- common causes for 99*t*
- complications of 104*t*
- encompass traumatic damage 98
- management of 102*t*
- risk factors for 99*t*

Genital tuberculosis 199
Genome sequencing 222
Genotype 269
Gestation age 224
Gestation period 531
Gestational age
- effects 382
- fundal height by 188*t*
- subclassification by 628

Gestational diabetes mellitus 185, 272, 276*t*, 285, 286*t*, 287*fc*, 289*fc*, 290, 291*b*, 293, 294*t*, 381, 444
- diagnostic criteria for 274*t*
- management of 275, 288*fc*

Gestational hypertension 296
Gestational thrombocytopenia 339-341, 343
Gestational thyrotoxicosis 345
Gestational timing 340
Gestational trophoblastic disease 195, 209, 219*f*
- complications of 216*f*
- encompasses 209

Gestational trophoblastic neoplasia 214, 215*t*, 233, 233*t*
- diagnostic criteria for 214
- management of 214
- risk factors for 214*t*

Gestational weight gain guidelines 445
Giant vulsellum 763*f*
Global cesarean section 119
- rates 616*t*

Global incidence 64
Glomerular filtration rate 250, 355
Glucose 275
- metabolism 251

Glyburide 287, 287*t*
Glyceryl trinitrate 818
Glycosaminoglycans 12
Glycosuria 249
Gouty arthritis 813
Government Programs for Safe Motherhood 512
Gratacos classification 396*t*
Green Armytage hemostatic forceps 765, 765*f*
Green meconium staining 175
Gynecoid pelvis 16
Gynecologic surgery, components in 653

H

Halothane 783
Hand prolapse 74, 75*f*
Handle design 743
Haultain procedure 68, 68*f*
Hawkin Ambler dilators 745, 745*f*
Headache 297, 798, 813
Head-perineum distance 22
Head-symphysis distance 22
Health risks 706
Healthy contralateral tube 204
Heart
- disease 5, 8
- failure 811
  - symptoms 325
- rate 421

Hegar's dilators 746, 746*f*
HELLP syndrome 301, 339, 342, 419
- management of 302

Hematocrit 425
Hematological adaptations 420
Hematological system 167
Hematomas 255
Hemodynamic changes 247
Hemodynamic impact 325
Hemodynamic monitoring 155
Hemodynamic parameters 355*t*
Hemoglobin 425
  low 203
  structure, normal 267
  variant 267
Hemoglobinopathy 267, 312, 318
  classification of 267
  encompass 267
Hemolysis 301
Hemolytic anemia 312
Hemolytic transfusion reaction, delayed 158
Hemorrhage 226, 824
  control 131
Hemorrhagic shock 423, 425
Hemorrhoids 195
Hemostatic complications 158
Hemostatic techniques 503
Heparin 822
  inhibits 822
  types of 823
Hepatic disease 813
Hepatic parenchymal calcifications 486
Hepatitis
  A 573
  B 7, 574
Heterotrophic ossification 813
Hidden tachycardia 419
High cesarean section rates, consequences of 607
Holistic approach 9
Homozygous beta-thalassemia 321
Hormonal changes 562
Hormonal compensation 428
Hormonal influence 331
Hormonal methods 711
Hormonal therapy 208
Hormone 14
  replacement therapy 559, 561
    types of 560
Human papillomavirus 8, 573
Human placental lactogen 251
Humanitarian grounds 224
Huntington procedure 67, 68*f*
Hyaluronan 12
Hydatidiform mole 210*f*
  differential diagnosis of 213*t*
  partial 212*t*
Hydralazine 430, 789
Hydration 23
Hydrochlorothiazide 784, 785
Hydrocortisone 435
Hydrodiuril 785
Hydrops, cause of 492
Hydroxyethyl starch 154
Hygroscopic dilators 406
Hyperbilirubinemia 334
Hypercoagulability 350' 418
Hyperemesis gravidarum, severe 426
Hyperglycemia 272
  classification of 273*t*
Hyperkalemia 787
Hyperprolactinemia 243
Hypertension 8, 186, 296, 394, 413, 424, 788
  chronic 296
  severe 296
Hypertensive crisis 790
  antihypertensives for 731*t*
Hypertensive disorders 6, 296, 303, 324, 356, 381, 414, 419, 445, 727
  diagnostic criteria for 296*t*
Hyperthermia, malignant 783
Hyperthyroidism 347, 348
  complications of 347*t*
Hypoglycemia 334
  diagnosis of 282
Hypoperfusion 424
Hypotension 40, 405, 800, 812
Hypothalamic-pituitary-adrenal axis 173
Hypothermia 158
Hypothyroidism 348
  complications of 347*t*
  prevalence 345
Hypovolemic shock 423, 424, 428
Hypoxemia
  prevent 168
  response 382
Hypoxia 175
  chronic 382
Hysterectomy 62, 213
  of placenta accreta 60*f*
Hysteroscopic resection for small niches 208

I

Idiopathic bleeding 195
Illegal abortions, relevance of 434
Immune
  globulin 824
  thrombocytopenia 339-342
Immunomodulatory therapy 435
Immunotherapy 219
Implanon implant 708*f*
Implantation 206
  abnormal 254
Implants 707
In vitro fertilization 507
Inadequate myometrial contraction 424
Incidental causes 195, 196
Index pregnancy, interval from 215
Indocin 812
Indomethacin 812, 813
Induction
  failure of 412
  nonpharmacological methods of 405
  of labor
    contraindications of 409
    risks associated with 410
Infant
  antiretroviral therapy prophylaxis 639
  feeding 639
Infection 6, 8, 62, 195, 243, 274, 394, 425
Infertility 137, 199
  preferred for 204
Inflammatory role 13
Influenza 8
  vaccine 572
Informed consent 682
Infusion
  continuous 39
  set 405*f*
Inhalation analgesics 775
Inhalational agents 38
Inhalational halogens 66
Inherited hemolytic anemia 312
Inherited thrombophilia 243, 351*t*
Initiating insulin therapy, guidelines for 276*t*
Inlet contraction, moderate/severe 89
Instrumental delivery 326

Instrumental injuries 103
Instruments 735
Insulin 276, 278, 283*t*, 287, 287*t*, 290*t*
- amount of 290
- classification of 277*fc*
- delivery device 280
- detemir 279
- glargine 279
- glulisine 279
- injection sites 281*f*
- intermediate-acting 279
- mechanism of action of 277*f*
- pharmacokinetics 279*b*
- pump 280
- regimens 279, 280
- resistance 272
- sensitivity 251
- storage of 281
- types of 278, 278*t*
- use, barriers to 282

Intensive care unit indications 559
Intermittent boluses 39
Internal anal sphincter 109
Internal pudendal artery 93
Internal rotational maneuvers 141
Interpersonal therapy 360
Interrupted sutures 109
Intestinal ileus 788
Intrahepatic cholestasis 330
Intrahepatic cholestasis 330
- of pregnancy, management of 332*t*

Intraoperative cell salvage 157
Intrapartum
- care 49*f*
- fetal heart rate 387
- fetal heart rate monitoring 387, 542
  - prevalence of 388*t*, 543*t*
  - rationale for 387, 542
- management 293, 298, 308, 442, 447
- period 316
- ultrasonography 21, 23, 28
- ultrasound 86

Intrathecal analgesia, continuous 40
Intraumbilical oxytocin 28
Intrauterine
- contraceptive devices 199
- sepsis 74
- transfusion 461

Intrauterine fetal death 413, 414, 628
- causes of 633, 633*t*
- complications of 633
- confirmed 632
- induction 635*t*
- management of 631
- suspected 631

Intrauterine growth restriction 174, 190
- types of selective 538*t*

Intravenous fluids 335
Intravenous immunoglobulin 435
Invasive mole 210, 216, 233
Invasive prenatal diagnostic procedures 221
Involution 13
Iodine demand, increased 345
Iron 8
- overload 159
- supplement 4, 803

Iron deficiency anemia 269, 313, 314
- diagnosis of 314
- prevention of 314

Ischemic heart disease 324
Isoxsuprine 820
Isthmocele 206-208
- ultrasound features of 207*f*

J

Jadelle implant 707*f*
Japanese encephalitis 575
Jaundice 330, 331
- causes of 330, 330*t*
- peculiar 330

K

Karyotype 212
Kegel's pregnancy 104
Ketamine 38
Kidney size 250
Kielland's forceps 758, 758*f*
Knee-chest position 148, 148*f*
Knots 150
Kocher's forceps, pair of 408*f*
Kocher's hemostatic forceps 753, 754*f*

L

Labetalol 790
Labor 1, 247
- abnormal 30, 30*f*
- abnormalities, types of 31
- active 13
- augmentation 14, 89
- cardinal movements of 19, 19*f*
- care guide 21, 23, 50*f*, 51, 51*t*
- course of 74
- durations of abnormal 31*t*
- fetal risk factors for abnormal 32*t*
- induction of 175, 178, 400, 402, 411, 413, 415
- management 631
  - of normal 22
  - strategies for abnormal 33*t*
- maternal risk factors for abnormal 32*t*
- mechanism of 16, 74, 82
- normal 16, 30*f*
- physiology of 10
- primary dysfunctional 30*f*
- progression, normal 16, 20, 30
- risk factors for abnormal 32
- setting for induction of 411
- stages of 20, 323
- success of induction of 411
- suite management 23
- third stage of 24
- types of abnormal 31*t*

Labor analgesia 36, 37*t*
- pharmacological agents for 38*t*

Labor and delivery 288, 326, 432, 509
- management 120, 342, 614*t*

Labor induction 14, 59, 403, 796
- and effectiveness 407
- mechanical methods of 406

Labor pain
- arises 36
- impact of untreated 37*t*
- neuroanatomy of 36

Lactation suppression 564, 567*b*
- complications of 568*t*
- indications for 564, 565*t*
- pharmacological agents for 565*t*

Lactation, physiology of 564
Lambda sign 536*f*, 537*f*
Laminaria tent 753, 753*f*
Lamotrigine 306, 309
Landon's uterine retractor 750, 750*f*
Langenbeck retractor 773, 773*f*
Laparoscopy 204
Laparotomy 204

Laqshya targets 515*t*
Late decelerations 382
Late infections 559
Late pregnancy 622*t*, 796
  complications 440
Lateral vesicouterine approach 132
Left ventricular dysfunction 428
Leopold maneuvers 18, 72, 183, 187
Lethargy 800
Levetiracetam 306
Levo bupivacaine 779
Levonorgestrel
  emergency contraceptive 711*f*
  prevalence 713
Lidocaine 779, 782
Lifestyle factors 394
Liquid chromatography, high-performance 268
Lisinopril 795
Live virus vaccines 825
Liver
  changes, normal 330
  disorders 330
  function tests 332
  transplantation 336
Local perineal infiltration 780
Lochia 167
Long cord 151, 151*f*
Long curved obstetric forceps 754, 754*f*
Long straight
  hemostatic forceps 742, 742*f*
  scissors 743, 743*f*
Long-acting insulins 279
Loop diuretics 784, 786
Lovset's maneuver 79
Low fetal fraction, causes of 489
Lower segment formation 12
Lower uterine segment 60*f*, 618
Low-lying placenta
  management of 372
  with bleeding, management of 372
Low-molecular-weight heparin 823
Lupus anticoagulant 243
Lymecycline 803

M

Macerated fetus 634*f*
Machine learning 392
Macrosomia 174, 185, 274, 445
Magnesium sulfate 583, 585*t*, 731, 792, 802, 803, 812
  dosing regimens for 584*t*
  mechanism of action of 583*f*
  monitoring on 302
  therapy 301, 302
  toxicity 732*t*, 803
Malaria 670
  diagnostic tools for 672*t*
  epidemiology of 670*t*
  fetal complications of 671*t*
  management strategies for 673*t*
  maternal complications of 671*t*
  preventive measures for 673*t*
Malignancy 348
Malpresentation 145
Manchester's operation 245
Mandatory cesarean sections 137
Maneuver, all-fours 141
Manual removal confirmation 60
Manual repositioning 66
Manual vacuum aspiration syringe 225
Manual vaginal elevation 148
Marcaine 778, 781
Marfan syndrome 11
Martius flap technique 522*f*
Massive intraperitoneal hemorrhage 425
Massive transfusion protocol 154, 157, 426
  criteria 157*t*
Maternal assessment 45
Maternal body's unique adaptations 418
Maternal care, three delays in 463*t*
Maternal cotyledons 253
Maternal death 463
Maternal early warning trigger 168, 168*t*
Maternal efforts 16
Maternal exhaustion 33
Maternal fever 40
Maternal health
  care 644
  risks 444
Maternal infection 409
Maternal management 320, 661, 666, 672
Maternal manifestations 659, 665, 671
Maternal monitoring 333
Maternal morbidity 445
Maternal mortality 74, 445
Maternal near miss
  mortality 463
  review process steps 465*t*
Maternal obesity 140
  artifact 630
Maternal outcome indices 466*t*
Maternal parameters 44
Maternal pelvis 469
Maternal pulse 547
Matrix metalloproteinases 12
Mature placenta, layers of 254*t*
MC twin pregnancies, complications of 536
McDonald's stitch 245
McRoberts maneuver 141
Mean corpuscular
  hemoglobin 269
  volume 269
Measles, mumps, and rubella 7, 573
Mechanical methods 405
Mechanical sweeping 406
Meconium, prolonged passage of 175
Meconium-stained amniotic fluid 174
Medical abortion protocol 226
Medical comorbidities 244
Medical disorders 265
Medical eligibility 713
Medical grounds 224
Medical management 202
Medical nutrition therapy 275
Medical termination of pregnancy 224, 226, 684
  act 224
  indications for 224
Medical therapy 429
Medicine, ethical principles in 681*t*
Mediolateral episiotomy 115, 115*f*, 118
Melatonin 299
Membranes
  perform artificial rupture of 408
  premature rupture of 190, 413
  preterm prelabor rupture of 161
  preterm premature rupture of 190, 453
Mendelson's syndrome 171
Meningococcal vaccine 574

Menopause 559
Menstrual changes 562
Mental depression 800
Metabolic acidosis 388
Metabolic complications 158
Metabolic demands 420
Metabolism 796
Metastases
  number of 215
  site of 215
Metastatic tumors 256
Metformin 282, 287, 287*t*
  contraindications of 285*t*
  indications of 285*t*
  prolongs gestation 299
  pros and cons of 286*t*
  role of 284*t*
Methotrexate 202
Methyldopa 788
Methyldopate 788
Methylergometrine 26
  injection 797
Metoprolol 325
Microcytic anemia, differential diagnosis of 269*t*
Microinvasive disease 678
Middle cerebral artery doppler 380*f*
Mild placental disease 476
Mild proteinuria 249
Minimally invasive techniques 104
Minocycline 803
Minor inlet contraction 89
Minute ventilation 249
Miscarriage 193
  complete 193
  management 196
  subtypes 194*t*
Misgav Ladach preference 602*f*
Misgav Ladach technique 600
  steps of 600*f*
Misoprostol 26, 27, 28, 230, 401*f*, 426, 795
  dosing 635*t*
Missed abortion 230
Missed miscarriage 193
Missed pill
  management 703
  protocols 703*t*
  threshold 703
Mitigation 647
Mitral regurgitation 325
Mitral stenosis 325
  grading of 325*t*
  management of 325
  pregnancy and management of 325
Mitral valve
  disorders 325
  prolapse 325
  replacement 326
Mobile partograms 51
Mobility 23
Modified Bishop's score 411, 412*t*
Modified early obstetric warning score 167, 167*t*
Modified Misgav Ladach technique 600, 601*f*
Molar pregnancy 195, 196, 209
  complete 234*f*
  management of 213
Molding 21
Mole
  partial 212, 213, 233
  pathogenesis of
    complete 211*f*
    partial 211*f*
Molecular basis 268
Molecular testing 269
Monitor fetal heartbeat 768
Monitors fetal heart rate 377
Monochorionic twin 473, 473*t*, 531
  delivery timing for 540*t*
  pregnancy 534
    epidemiology of 535*t*
  risk specific to 472
Monozygotic twinning 528*t*
Montevideo units 16
Mood disorder questionnaire 359
Morbidly adherent placenta 469
Mortality 589
MTHFR gene variation 3
Mucus
  extractor 740
  sucker 740*f*
Multifetal pregnancies 527, 527*t*
  diagnostic clues for 529*t*
  fetal complications of 530*t*
  management of 530
  maternal complications of 530*t*
  physiology of 527
Multi-organ failure 434
Multipara 31
  average 30*f*
Multiple gestations 185
Multiple pregnancy 78, 213
Multiple-toothed vulsellum 737, 738*f*
Muscle rigidity 783
Myocardial infarction 429
Myomectomy 59
Myometrial changes 12
Myometrial contractile mechanisms 13*t*
Myometrial contractions 13
Myometrial oxytocin receptor concentration 402
Myometrial priming 12, 12*t*
Myometrial stretching triggers 14

N

N-acetylcysteine 336
Nails, yellow staining of 175
Nasal hypoplasia 824
Nasal insulin 280
National Institute of Health and Family Welfare 514
Natural iron supplements 804
Natural micronized progesterone 230
Natural prostaglandins 798
Natural supplements 806, 807
Nausea 40, 186, 776, 781, 800, 807, 811
Needle holder 116
Neglected transverse lie
  complications of 74*t*
  management of 75
Neonatal care 308, 342
Neonatal complications 459, 342
Neonatal deaths 445
Neonatal effects 585
Neonatal management 661, 666, 672
Neonatal manifestations 659, 665, 671
Neonatal risk 119, 612
Neoplasia 209
Neuraxial analgesia techniques 39*t*
Neuraxial anesthesia 342
Neuraxial techniques 39
Neurogenic collapse 65
Neurological toxicity 40
Neuromuscular block 812
Neuroprotection 585
  magnesium sulphate for 164
Nicardipine 809
Nifedipine 792, 810

Nifedipress 792
Nitrates 430
Nitric oxide 11, 355
  deficiency 298
  donors 299
Nitroglycerin 793
Nitropress 792
Nitrous oxide 775
  with oxygen 775
Noncontraceptive benefits 703, 705
Nondelivery management 341*t*
Nonepileptic attack disorders 304
Nonhemorrhagic hypovolemic shock 426
Nonimmune fetal hydrops, causes of 492
Noninvasive attempts 60
Noninvasive prenatal screening 480, 487, 488
Noninvasive tests 471
Nonlocking suture, continuous 109
Nonpharmacological methods 41
Nonpharmacological techniques 37, 37*t*
Nonstress test 377
  physiological basis of 382
Non-surgical management 521
Normotensive shock 419
Norplant 707*f*
Novocain 780
Nuchal translucency 481
Nulli parous woman 53
Nullipara 31, 48*f*
Nulliparous 185, 186
Nutrition 446
Nutritional deficiencies 394
Nutritional interventions 3, 184

O

Oasis 108*f*
  repair 110*f*
Obesity 8, 444
  effect of 444
Obstetric
  anal sphincter injuries 98, 100*f*
  care 292, 294, 321
  factors 382
  grips 73*f*
  indications 410
  injuries 98
  ultrasound 508
Obstetric hemorrhage 128, 132, 154
  initial stabilization in 154*t*
Obstetric high dependency units
  admission, contraindications for 646*t*
  admission, indications for 646*t*
  mitigation strategies for 647*t*
Obstetric shock 418, 421-423
  strikes 417
Obstructed labor 135
  causes of 135*t*
  clinical features of 136*t*
  complications of 136*t*
  etiology 135
  management protocol for 137*t*
  prevention strategies for 138*t*
Ointment 818
Oldham's perforator 762, 762*f*
Oligohydramnios 80, 174, 374, 375, 375*t*, 623, 624, 624*f*
  by severity, classification of 624*t*
  causes of 625*t*
  management 625
    algorithm for 375
  mimicking demise, severe 630
Oliguria 297
Operative management 101
Operative vaginal delivery ventouse 53
Opioid analgesics 776
Opioid toxicity 41
  management 39
Optic atrophy 824
Oral heart failure drugs 327
Oral hypoglycemic agents 282, 283*t*
Oral route and intravenous 810
Organ system 166
Orlistat 801
Osteoarthritis 813
Overlapping repair 109
Overt cord prolapse 145
Overt diabetes, diagnosis of 274
Overt hyperthyroidism 345, 346
Overt hypothyroidism 347
Ovulation suppression 702
Ovum
  forceps 749, 749*f*
  migration 199
Oxidative metabolites 305
Oxygen 775
  carrying capacity 154
  consumption 249
  saturation 168
  therapy 154, 155
Oxytocics 170
Oxytocin 14, 26, 45, 402, 592, 592*t*, 795, 796
  administration of 403
  ampoule containing 404*f*
  infusion reference 403*t*
  receptor 12
    sensitivity 173
  side effects of 405
  titration 404*f*

P

P57 expression 212
Packed red blood cells 155
Pain 207, 229
  management 117, 308
  moderate to severe 777
  pathways 36
Palpation 72
Paperless partogram 47
Paracervical block 39
  agents 779
Parathyroid hormone 251
Parental chromosomal abnormalities 243
Parenteral medications 38
Parent-to-child transmission
  prevention 638*t*
  risk factors for 637*t*
Parous women 53
Partogram 43, 51*t*
Parturition
  fetal contributions to 14*t*
  phases of 11, 11*t*
Pathological retraction ring 74
Patient counseling 567, 598
Patient-centered strategies 609
Pelvic
  abscess 200
  adhesions 199
  assessment 79
  diameter, external 773
  examination 200
  floor exercises 104, 110
  inflammatory disease 199
  masses, bilateral 200
  pain 186
Pelvimetry 772, 772*f*
Pelvis, planes of 17*t*
Percutaneous balloon mitral valvuloplasty 326
Perforating mole, postsurgery management in 218*f*

Perimortem cesarean section 685
Perinatal morbidity 146
Perinatal mortality 146, 388
Perineal body 116
Perineal care 137
Perineal inspection 192
Perineal massage 104
Perineal muscles 109
Perineal preparation 137
Perineal skin 116
Perineal stretching 36
Perineal tear 106
  classification of 99*t*, 107*t*
  second-degree 107*f*
Perineorrhaphy 101
Perineum, incision of 114
Periodontal therapy 162
Peripartum cardiomyopathy 326, 428
  management of 429
Persistent incontinence 101
Persistent occiput posterior position, management of 83*t*
Persistent trophoblastic disease, risk of 213
Pethidine 38, 776
Pharmacotherapy 276
Phenelzine 777
Phenotype 269
Phenytoin 306, 801
  interacts 802
Physical activity recommendations 446
Physiological anemia 247, 312, 313
Physiological cardiac changes 323*t*
Physiological changes 420*f*
Physiological management 28
Physiological renal adaptations 355*t*
Pinard's fetal stethoscope 767, 767*f*
Pinard's horn 767, 767*f*
Pinard's maneuver 79
Placenta
  abnormalities of 254
  adherens 60
  development of 253, 254
  functions of 256
  manual removal of 61
  pathological examination of 256
  percreta 129
  previa 119, 254, 371, 372
  structure of 253
  synthesizes 14
Placenta accreta 59, 255
  antepartum diagnosis of 485
  index 364
  suspected 61
Placenta accreta spectrum 59, 119, 128, 206, 363, 603, 603*f*
  complications of 154, 365
  delivery timing for 131*t*
  disorders 128
  epidemiology 363
  management, complications of 132*t*
  pathophysiology 364
  prevention 366
  risk factors with 485
  risk stratification 363
Placental abnormalities 259
Placental abruption 424
Placental circulation 254, 258
  facilitating 420
Placental deiodinase 345
Placental delivery, physiology of 24
Placental development 253, 257
Placental functions 260
Placental hormones 252
Placental infarction 255
Placental insufficiency 394, 476
Placental involvement, degree of 485
Placental pathology 260
Placental role 14
Placental separation
  normal 58
  signs of 24, 69*f*
Placental shapes and sizes, abnormal 255*t*
Placental site trophoblastic tumor 210
Placental structure 258
Placental tumors 256
Plasma volume increases disproportionately 420
Platelet 155, 297
  count 339
    thresholds 342
  low 301
  transfusions 342
Pneumococcal conjugated vaccine 574
Point-of-care testing 157
Policy-level strategies 609, 610*t*
Polycystic ovarian disease 243
Polyhydramnios 374, 375, 375*t*, 624, 625, 627
  classification of 626*t*
  etiopathogenesis of 626*t*
  management algorithm for 376
Poor positive predictive value 378
Poor predictive value 392
Postabortion care 231
Postdated pregnancy 413
Posterior retrograde hysterectomy 132
Posterior reversible encephalopathy syndrome 553
Postexposure prophylaxis 667
Postgraduate insight 78
Postmaturity syndrome 174, 175
Postnatal care 68, 117
Postnatal management 308
Postnatal treatment 490
Postpartum 247, 294, 315, 326, 341, 361
  cardiomyopathy 171
  care 293, 336, 430, 447, 509, 532, 640
  collapse 166, 168
    causes of 166, 166*t*
  depression 552
  eclampsia 301, 552
  endometritis 558*t*
  follow-up 299
  glucose testing 293*t*
  period 359
  practices 361
  preeclampsia 552
  psychosis 359, 361, 362
  reversal 252
  thyroiditis 345, 348, 553
  urinary tract infection, treatment for 559*t*
Postpartum hemorrhage 14, 27, 119, 154, 169, 418, 423, 588, 796
  cause of 58, 595*t*
  kit contents 170*t*
  management 425
  prevention 592*t*
  primary 588
  risk factors for 589*t*
  secondary 588, 595
  severity, clinical signs of 593, 593*t*
  treatment of 427*f*

Postprocedural care 226
Post-repair check 109
Post-seizure care 300
Post-term pregnancy 173, 176, 180*fc*
  management of 176, 179*fc*
  prevalence 180*t*
  prevention of 176
  risk of recurrence of 174
Post-transfusion purpura 159
Potassium-sparing diuretics 785, 787
Precipitate labor 32, 33
Preconception 292, 320
  and Pre-Natal Diagnostic Techniques Act 690
  care 3
  counseling 307, 321, 446
Preconceptional care 9
  components of 3
Preeclampsia 185, 296, 339, 342
  mainstay for 344
  risk factors for 297*t*
  severe 299, 300
  superimposed 296
  symptoms of 356*t*
Preexisting diabetes 272, 292
Pregestational diabetes 381
Pregnancy 272, 413, 612, 684, 794, 797
  after cesarean delivery, complications of 122
  category 306
  complications with leiomyomas 501*t*
  failure 235*f*
  intrahepatic cholestasis of 413, 415
  normal 198*f*, 355*t*
  of unknown location 193
  prolonged 173
  risks with 119, 613
  safety of 676
  use in 361
  with one previous cesarean, management of 121, 614
  with previous cesarean delivery 119
Pregnancy-induced hypervolemia 420
Prehormone replacement therapy workup 560
Prehospital prolapse 149
Preinduction cervical assessment 409
Prematurity 78
Premix regimen 279
Prenatal diagnosis 128
Prenatal screening for aneuploidy 480
Prenatal testing 320
Preterm birth 145, 185, 821
  provider-initiated 161
Preterm delivery 190
Preterm infants 164
Preterm labor 59, 161, 190
  diagnosis of 163
  management of 164
  prevention 14
  risk factors for 161
Preterm prelabor rupture of membranes
  complications with 456*t*
  risk factors with 453*t*
Preterm prom 413
Previous cesarean
  delivery, complications after 122*t*
  section 612*t*
    after one 120, 613
    management after two 121, 614
Previous ectopic pregnancy 199
Previous tubal surgery 199, 425
Primary villus 253
Primigravida 293
  average 30*f*
Prior uterine surgery 59
Probenecid 814
Procaine 780
Procarbazine 777
Procedure-related fetal loss rate 221
Procoagulant activity 421
Prodromal symptoms 300
Progesterone 11, 230, 251, 421, 561
  role of 236
Progesterone-only pills 199, 701, 702*f*
Programmed intermittent epidural boluses 40
Prolactin 251
Prophylactic measures 137
Prophylaxis 315, 557
Propofol 784
Propylthiouracil 347
Prostacyclin 11, 798
Prostaglandin 14, 298, 400, 795, 798
  analogs 798
  E1 799
  F receptors 12
  side effects of 402
  surge 173
Prosthetic heart valves 327
Prosthetic mitral valves 325
Proteinuria 250, 296, 297
Proteoglycans 12
Protracted descent 31, 33
Protracted dilatation 31, 33
Pruritus 40, 331
Pseudoseizures 304
Psychiatric disorders 359, 360*t*
  pharmacological management of 361*t*
Psychoeducation 360
Psychological implications 445
Psychological interventions 105
Psychotherapy 360
Public health measures 668
Pudendal block 39
Puerperal infections, diagnostic investigations for 557*t*
Puerperal sepsis 550, 556
  diagnostic investigations for 551*t*
Puerperium 13, 350, 552*t*
  abnormal 550
Pulling methods 148
Pulmonary edema 297
Pulmonary embolism 432
  management of 432
Pulmonary thromboembolism 171, 350
Pulse 229
  rate 167
Pushing methods 148
Pyosalpinx 200

Q

Quintero classification 474

R

Rabies 575
Rarely bone marrow suppression 203
Reactions, acute 158
Reactive nonstress test 377*f*

Reapproximate perineal muscles 116
Recurrence risk, paternal role in 174
Recurrent abortions 444
Recurrent pregnancy loss 236, 239, 345
  causes and investigations for 237t
  investigation for 232
Recurrent seizures 584
Red cell distribution width 269
Reduce cesarean section rates 606, 607
Reduce cord compression, maneuvers to 148
Reduce tubal peristalsis 199
Regional anesthesia 39
Relaxin 11, 355
Remifentanil 38
Renal changes 250t
Renal disorders 355
  pregnancy-related 356
Renal hemodynamics 249
Renal impairment 203, 334
Renal pelvic
  anteroposterior diameter 489
  dilation 489
    causes of 489
Renal plasma flow 250
  change 355
Renal system 249
Renin–angiotensin–aldosterone system 428
Reproductive medicine 682, 682t
Reproductive system 166
Resistance syringes, novel loss of 40
Resource constraints 361
Respiratory changes 249t
Respiratory depression 40
Respiratory rate 167, 229, 249
Respiratory system 166, 167, 248
Resulting pregnancy type 528
Resuscitation cart contents 169t
Retained placenta 27, 58
  complications of 62t
  delivery timing of 58t
  fragments 61
  management protocol for 61t
  pathophysiology of 59t
  risk factors for 59t
  types 60t
  without inversion 65
Retrograde bladder filling 148
Revised maternal healthcare model 644
Rh alloimmunization 458
  fetal complications of 459t
  maternal complications of 459t
  mechanisms of 458
Rh alloimmunized pregnancy, management of 461
Rh prophylaxis 231
Rheumatic heart disease 324, 325
Rheumatoid arthritis 813
Rh-negative
  blood group, prevalence of 458
  cases 213
  patients 204, 825
  pregnancy, management of 460
  women 226
Rhoclone 824
Rising cesarean section rates, reasons for 606
Ritodrine 817
  hydrochloride 817
Road traffic accidents 98
Robotic surgery 507
Routine testing 268
Rubella 573
Rubin maneuver 141
Rupture of membranes, diagnostic tests for 454t
Rupture risk 123, 125
Ruptured chocolate cyst 200
Ruptured ectopic pregnancy 424

S

Safe cesarean section 617
Safe motherhood 512t
Salpingectomy 204
Salvage therapy 219f
Scarred uterus 119, 612, 613
Screening barriers 270
Second maneuver 18
Second trimester 225
  screening 479
Second twin, delivery of 532t
Seizure 8, 40
  disorders 6
  frequency
    causes of increased 305, 305t
  management 308
  partial 304
  primary generalized 304
Selective arterial embolization 95
Selective episiotomy 104, 117, 118
Selective intrauterine growth restriction 538
Septate 240
Septic abortion 194, 196, 200
Septic shock 170, 433, 434
  management of 434, 435
Septicemia 137
Serosal myomectomy 502
Serum 732
  bile acids 331
  creatinine 250, 355
  ferritin 269
  urea 250
Severe sepsis 170
Sevoflurane 38
Sex workers, care of 685
Sexual assault 103
Sher's classification 370
Shock 226, 417, 422
  classification of 422, 422t
  management 137
  obstructive 431, 432
  treatment 137
Short cord 150f
Shoulder dystocia 139, 140, 142
  complications of 142t
  diagnostic criteria for 140t
  management steps for 141t
  maneuvers, success rates of 142t
  mechanisms of 139t
  risk factors for 140t
Sickle cell
  anemia 312
  disease 270, 318
Simple rubber catheter 735, 735f
Simple tears 111
Simpson's forceps 773, 773f
Sims double-bladed posterior vaginal speculum 736
Single balloon device 406
Single intrauterine death 539
Single umbilical artery 149, 151
Single-agent chemotherapy 214
Singletons 535
Sinusoidal pattern 390, 545
Skin 109, 175
Slurred speech 801
Smart pumps 40
Smear, peripheral 268
Social grounds 224

Sodium
  nitroprusside 792
  oxybate 801
  reabsorption 250
  retention 790
Special obstetric care 285
Special precaution during labor 290
Speculum examination 192
Sphincter injuries 98
Sphincteroplasty 101
Spinal anesthetics 781
Spinal injection 781, 782
Spinning sensation 781
Spironolactone 785, 787
Split mix regimen 279
Sponge holding forceps 749, 749*f*
Spontaneous abortion 232
  in first trimester, management of 228
  management of 228, 229
Spontaneous breech 79
Spontaneous multiple gestation 527
Spontaneous preterm labor 161
Stabilizing induction 75
Stable angina, chronic 792
Standard skin incision 599, 599*f*
Standardized protocols ensure safety and efficacy 156
Stasis 350
Stem villi 254
Stillbirth 274
  increased risk of 445
Stomatitis 203
Straddle injuries 98
Structured intermittent auscultation 388, 543
Subchorionic hematoma 195, 232, 232*f*
Subclinical hyperthyroidism 345-347
Subcutaneous insulin infusion, continuous 279
Subsequent contacts 186
Subsequent pregnancies 219
Substance abuse 8
Suction curettage 213
Suction evacuation 233
Suitability 201
Suman services 515*t*
Supercharged blood volume 418
Superficial external pudendal artery 93
Supernumerary vessels 149
Supportive care 335
Supralevator hematomas 95
Surgical complications 119
Surgical correction 67
Surgical management 95, 204, 521
Surgical methods 226, 408
Surgical prerequisites 447
Surgical principles 101
Surgical technique 109, 599
Surgical treatment 558
Surveillance 219, 220
Suture
  continuous 117
  materials 117
Swift fluid replacement 428
Symmetric fetal growth restriction 395*t*
Symphysiotomy 141
Syncope 304
Syntometrine 26
Systemic blood pressure 355
Systemic lupus erythematosus 381
Systemic methotrexate 208
Systolic blood pressure 167, 168, 355

T

Tachycardia 389, 783
Target glucose levels 275*t*
Tear
  full-thickness 109
  partial-thickness 109
Teeth 739
Telemedicine 578, 580
  applications 578*t*
  limitations of 579*t*
Temporal lobe 304
Teratogenic effects 306*t*
Teratogenic risk 203
Terbutaline 815
  sulfate 815
Terminally ill patients, care of 685
Termination, methods of 225
Tertiary villus 253
Tetanus, diphtheria, and pertussis 7
Tetracycline, absorption of 812
Thalassemia 267, 312, 318, 319
  major 270, 321
  management of 320
  minor 320
Theca lutein cysts 212, 214
Therapeutic interventions 396*t*
Thiazide diuretics 784, 785
Third maneuver 19
Third stage
  complications of 27, 27*t*
  management of 25
    uterotonic drugs for 26*t*
Threatened abortion 213, 229
Threatened miscarriage 193
Three-swab test 519*f*
Thrombin 594
Thrombocytopenia 339
  affects 343
  causes of 339
  common causes of 340*t*
  evaluation of 340
  laboratory tests for 341*b*
  management of 341
  severe 343
  severity classification of 339*t*
Thromboelastography 157
Thromboembolic events 421
Thromboembolism 552
Thrombophilia 237, 351
Thromboprophylaxis 351, 352, 352*t*, 599
Thrombotic microangiopathics 339, 342
Thyroid 8
  disorders 5, 345
    classification of 346*t*
    prevalence of 345*t*
  dysfunction 243
  function 630
    test 240
  nodules 348
  physiology 345
Thyroid-binding globulin, increased 345
Thyroid-stimulating hormone 251
Tidal volume 249
Tinzaparin 823
Tissue 594
Titrate oxytocin 403
Tivorbex 812
Tocolysis 149, 585
  acute 163
Tocolytic 66, 372, 809
  agent 802
  drugs 822
Tonic-clonic, generalized 299
Topiramate 306

Toxicity 302, 800, 803
levels 585
management of 586
Toxoplasmosis 658
diagnostic tools for 660t
epidemiology of 658t
fetal complications of 660t
management strategies for 661t
maternal complications of 660t
Trachelectomy, role of 679
Traction 140
Tractocil 821
Tramadol 777
Tranexamic acid 26-28, 230
use of 426
Transabdominal cerclage 246
Transdermal patch 818
Transfusion 155
alternatives to 157
complications 154
protocols 156, 426
targets 155t
Transfusion-associated
circulatory overload 158
graft-versus-host disease 159
immunomodulation 159
Transfusion-related sepsis 158
Transperineal ultrasound 94, 96
Transperitoneal ovum migration 199
Transvaginal ultrasound 207, 372
Transverse lie 72
causes of 73t
diagnosis 72
etiology 72
fetal positions in 74t
management of 75, 75t
prevalence of 72
Trapped placenta 59
Trauma 594
Traumatic vaginal delivery 98
Tremors 801
Trendelenburg position 148
Triamterene 785
Triggers 129
Trophectoderm differentiation 253
Trophoblastic invasion, abnormal 297
Trophoblastic tissue 202
Trophoblastic tumors 210
True knot 150, 150f, 151
T-sign 537f
ultrasound images of 536f
Tubal ligation 716
methods of 718f
Pomeroy method of 718f
reversal of 721
techniques of 717
Tubal rupture and hemorrhage 425
Tubular function 249
Turnaround time 222
Turtle sign 140
Twin
anemia-polycythemia sequence 537
gestation 472, 472t
monitoring in 473
reversed arterial perfusion sequence 538
with coexisting mole 213
Twin-to-twin transfusion
management options of 474
syndrome 185, 474, 536
diagnosis and management of 473
Quintero staging for 536t
Twisted ovarian cyst 200
Typhoid 575
Typical gestation 226

U

Ulipristal acetate emergency contraceptive 712f
Ultrasonography 73
Ultrasound 229
findings 212
role of 480
sign 364
surveillance 535
schedule 531t
technique 482t
Ultrasound-guided
fetal blood sampling 470
intraperitoneal transfusion 471
intravascular transfusion 471
Umbilical artery Doppler 538
normal 380f
Umbilical cord 767
abnormalities 149, 151t
Umbilical cord prolapse 144
classification 145, 145t
management strategies for 148t
preventive strategies for 147t
risk factors for 145, 146t
Uncomplicated vaginal delivery 343
Uncontrolled diabetes mellitus 243
Underpowered trials 392
Unexplained factors 129
Unfractionated heparin 352, 823
Unilateral shoulder dystocia, maneuvers for 141
Universal cervical length screening 162
Universal screening 346
Untreated engorgement, complications of 564
Untreated pain 41
Ureteral dilatation 250
Ureteral smooth muscle, progesterone relaxes 249
Urinary complications 559
Urinary stasis, hydronephrosis increases risk of 249
Urinary tract infections 356
Urine
analysis 296
glucose 250
output 167
pregnancy test 200
protein excretion 355
retention of 200
Urogynecology 507
Urological injuries 132
Urological protection 131
Ursodeoxycholic acid 332
Uterine 59
abnormalities 78
anomalies, assessment of 244
atony 59
closure 602
contractility, inhibitors of 11t
contraction 13, 16, 36, 44, 45
curette 751, 751f
dressing forceps 752, 752f
effects 586
hyperstimulation 405
incision 602
extensions, managing 619
inertia 33, 74
injuries 102
massage 25
muscle physiology 13
perforation 226
quiescence 11
relaxation 66
size 212, 214

- sound 744, 744*f*
- stimulants 795
- tone assessment 28
- transformation of 11

Uterine artery
- diastolic notch in 379*f*
- embolization 208

Uterine inversion 27, 62, 64, 66, 70, 171
- classification of 64*t*
- complications of 66*t*
- differential diagnosis of 66*t*
- manual repositioning of 67*f*

Uterine rupture 74, 119, 125, 405
- risks 125*t*

Uterine scar
- integrity 122
  - factors affecting 123*t*
- types of 119, 612

Uteroplacental circulation 254
Uteroplacental insufficiency 174
Uterotonic administration 25
Uterotonic agents 26, 426
Uterus 11, 618

V

Vaccination 8, 570, 667
- principles of 570

Vaccines
- classification of 571*t*
- types of 570, 571*t*
- use of specific 573

Vacuum delivery 53
Vacuum-assisted birth 54
Vagina 109
Vaginal birth after cesarean 604
- complications of 125, 126*t*
- contraindications for 123, 124*t*

Vaginal bleeding 80, 190, 199, 207, 228
- persistent 214

Vaginal delivery 16, 99, 139, 326, 342
Vaginal discharge 186, 200
Vaginal examination 19, 53, 65, 73, 86
Vaginal injuries 102
Vaginal mucosa 116
Vaginal progesterone 162
Vaginal speculum, posterior 736*f*
Valproate 306
Valve area 325, 328
Valvular heart disease 429
Variable decelerations 382
Varicella 7, 573
Vasa previa 149, 151, 256
- management of 257*t*

Vascular abnormalities 149, 394
Vascular compromise 424
Vascular resistance 355, 421
Vasopressors 435
Vasospastic angina, management of 792
Velamentous cord insertion 256
Velamentous insertion 149, 149*f*, 151
Venous drainage 93
Venous stasis 350
Venous thromboembolism 350, 432
- risk factors for 351*t*, 552*t*

Ventilatory changes 248
Ventouse cup 760, 761*f*
Ventricular arrhythmias 783
Verapamil 811
Vertigo 801
Vesicovaginal fistula 517, 522*fc*
- classification of 518*t*
- etiology of 517*t*
- management of 524
- principles of 523
- types of 518*f*

Vibroacoustic stimulation 384, 392
Villus, secondary 253
Violence issues 685
Virchow's triad 350
Visible mass 65
Visual biofeedback 23
Visual disturbances 297
Vital signs 192
Vitamin B_{12} deficiency anemia 317
Volume depletion 424
Vomiting 186, 776, 781, 800
Vulva, anatomy of 92
Vulval injuries 101
Vulvar hematoma 92
- management strategies for 94*t*
- risk factors for 92*t*
- with ecchymosis 93*f*

W

Warfarin 352, 824
- embryopathy 824

Warning scores 172
Warren flap method 101
Water intoxication 405
Weight gain 446
Whole blood 156
Willet scalp traction forceps 766, 766*f*
Woods Corkscrew maneuver 141
Wound care 110, 117
Wrigley's forceps 757, 757*f*

X

Xylocaine 779, 782

Y

Yellow fever 575

Z

Zavanelli maneuver 141
Zhang's partogram 48